An Osteopathic Approach
to Diagnosis and Treatment

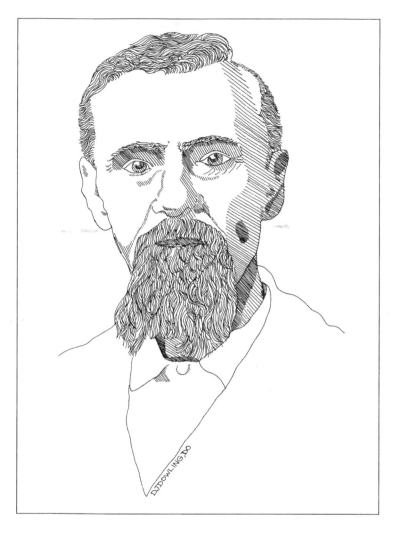

Andrew T. Still

An Osteopathic Approach to Diagnosis and Treatment

Second Edition

EDITED BY

Eileen L. DiGiovanna, DO, FAAO
Assistant Dean of Student Affairs
Professor and Chairperson
The Stanley Schiowitz, DO, FAAO Department
of Osteopathic Manipulative Medicine
New York College of Osteopathic Medicine
New York Institute of Technology
Old Westbury, New York
Fellow of the American Academy of Osteopathy

Stanley Schiowitz, DO, FAAO
Dean, Provost
Professor and Former Chairperson
The Stanley Schiowitz, DO, FAAO Department
of Osteopathic Manipulative Medicine
New York College of Osteopathic Medicine
New York Institute of Technology
Old Westbury, New York
Fellow of the American Academy of Osteopathy

ILLUSTRATED BY

Dennis Dowling, DO
Associate Professor and Associate Chairperson
The Stanley Schiowitz, DO, FAAO Department
of Osteopathic Manipulative Medicine
New York College of Osteopathic Medicine
New York Institute of Technology
Old Westbury, New York

With 23 Contributors

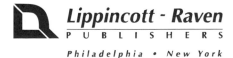

Lippincott - Raven
P U B L I S H E R S
Philadelphia • New York

We dedicate this book
To our grandchildren who were born as this book was written:
Diona Marie Amen and Justine Esta Ellis.
To osteopathic students and physicians who share our
belief that our hands are channels of healing.
To our patients who have taught us so much.

Acquisitions Editor: Richard Winters
Developmental Editor: Erin O'Connor
Senior Production Editor: Virginia Barishek
Production Service: Textbook Writers Associates, Inc.

Compositor: Maryland Composition Company
Printer/Binder: Maple Press
Cover Designer: Thomas M. Jackson
Cover Printer: Lehigh Press

Second Edition

Library of Congress Cataloging-in-Publication Data

An osteopathic approach to diagnosis and treatment / edited by Eileen
    L. DiGiovanna, Stanley Schiowitz ; illustrated by Dennis Dowling;
    with 23 contributors.—2nd ed.
        p.   cm.
    Includes bibliographical references and index.
    ISBN 0-397-51581-2
    1. Osteopathic Medicine.   I. DiGiovanna, Eileen L.
    II. Schiowitz, Stanley.
    [DNLM: 1. Osteopathic Medicine.   WB 940 084 1997]
    RZ341.0696   1997
    615.5'33—dc20
    DNLM/DLC   96-41775

Care has been taken to confirm the accuracy of the information presented and to describe generally accepted practices. However, the authors, editors, and publisher are not responsible for errors or omissions or for any consequences from application of the information in this book and make no warranty, express or implied, with respect to the contents of the publication.

The authors, editors and publisher have exerted every effort to ensure that drug selection and dosage set forth in this text are in accordance with current recommendations and practice at the time of publication. However, in view of ongoing research, changes in government regulations, and the constant flow of information relating to drug therapy and drug reactions, the reader is urged to check the package insert for each drug for any change in indications and dosage and for added warnings and precautions. This is particularly important when the recommended agent is a new or infrequently employed drug.

Some drugs and medical devices presented in this publication have Food and Drug Administration (FDA) clearance for limited use in restricted research settings. It is the responsibility of the health care provider to ascertain the FDA status of each drug or device planned for use in their clinical practice.

9   8   7   6   5   4   3   2

Contributors

MARY BANIHASHEM, DO
Instructor
The Stanley Schiowitz, DO, FAAO Department
  of Osteopathic Manipulative Medicine
New York College of Osteopathic Medicine
New York Institute of Technology
Old Westbury, New York 11568

NANCY BROUS, DO
Assistant Professor
Director of Islip Clinic
New York College of Osteopathic Medicine
New York Institute of Technology
Old Westbury, New York 11568

LISA R. CHUN, DO
Private Practice
4733 Bethesda Avenue, Suite 804
Bethesda, Maryland 20814

ALBERT R. DeRUBERTIS, DO
Private Practice
Physical Medicine and Rehabilitation
228 Oak Street
Frankford, Illinois 60423-1612

EILEEN L. DiGIOVANNA, DO, FAAO
Assistant Dean of Student Affairs
Professor and Chairperson
The Stanley Schiowitz, DO, FAAO Department
  of Osteopathic Manipulative Medicine

New York College of Osteopathic Medicine
New York Institute of Technology
Old Westbury, New York 11568

JOSEPH A. DiGIOVANNA, DO
Clinical Associate Professor, Family Medicine
New York College of Osteopathic Medicine
New York Institute of Technology
Old Westbury, New York 11568

MICHAEL J. DiGIOVANNA, DO
Clinical Assistant Professor
The Stanley Schiowitz, DO, FAAO Department
  of Osteopathic Manipulative Medicine
New York College of Osteopathic Medicine
New York Institute of Technology
Old Westbury, New York 11568

DENNIS J. DOWLING, DO
Associate Professor and Associate Chairperson
The Stanley Schiowitz, DO, FAAO Department
  of Osteopathic Manipulative Medicine
New York College of Osteopathic Medicine
New York Institute of Technology
Old Westbury, New York 11568

BARRY S. ERNER, DO
Private Practice
40 East Putnam Avenue
Cos Cob, Connecticut 06807-2606

HUGH ETTLINGER, DO
Associate Professor
The Stanley Schiowitz, DO, FAAO Department
  of Osteopathic Manipulative Medicine
Director of Residency Program in Osteopathic
  Manipulative Medicine
New York College of Osteopathic Medicine
New York Institute of Technology
Old Westbury, New York 11568

JONATHAN F. FENTON, DO
Private Practice
67 Lincoln Street
Essex Junction, Vermont 05452-3176

MARY-THERESA FERRIS, DO
Intern
St. Barnabas Hospital
3rd Avenue and 183rd Street
Bronx, New York 10457-2594

BONNIE RITT GINTIS, DO
Adjunct Assistant Professor
The Stanley Schiowitz, DO, FAAO Department
  of Osteopathic Manipulative Medicine
New York College of Osteopathic Medicine
New York Institute of Technology
Old Westbury, New York 11568

DONALD V. HANKINSON, DO
Private Practice
2 Granite Ridge
Cape Elizabeth, Maine 04107-1640

MARY E. HITCHCOCK, DO, FAAO (deceased)
Former Assistant Professor
The Stanley Schiowitz, DO, FAAO Department
  of Osteopathic Manipulative Medicine
New York College of Osteopathic Medicine
New York Institute of Technology
Old Westbury, New York 11568

DAVID J. MARTINKE, DO
Private Practice
115 Willow Breeze Road
Buffalo, New York 14223-1355

MICHAEL F. OLIVERIO
Undergraduate Fellow
The Stanley Schiowitz, DO, FAAO Department
  of Osteopathic Manipulative Medicine
New York College of Osteopathic Medicine
New York Institute of Technology
Old Westbury, New York 11568

DONALD PHYKITT, DO
Private Practice
707 Second Street
Athens, Pennsylvania 18810-1429

BARBARA POLSTEIN, DO
U.S. Public Health Service
P.O. Box 368
Kayenta, Arizona 86033-0368

PAULA D. SCARIATI, DO
Private Practice
P.O. Box 480
Syracuse, New York 13210-0480

STANLEY SCHIOWITZ, DO, FAAO
Dean, Provost
Distinguished Professor and Former Chairperson
The Stanley Schiowitz, DO, FAAO Department
  of Osteopathic Manipulative Medicine
New York College of Osteopathic Medicine
New York Institute of Technology
Old Westbury, New York 11568

CHARLES J. SMUTNEY III, DO
Osteopathic Manipulative Medicine Resident
St. Barnabas Hospital
3rd Avenue and 183rd Street
Bronx, New York 10457-2594

LILLIAN SOMNER, DO
Private Practice
Ryan's Run Apartments #1206
55 East King's Highway
Maple Shade, New Jersey 08052-2007

TONI SPINARIS, DO
Private Practice
16 Sherman Road
Bethpage, New York 11804-1424

SANDRA D. YALE, DO
Private Practice
1001 Humboldt Parkway
Buffalo, New York 14208-2221

Preface

The instruction of students in the concepts and principles of osteopathic medicine, as well as in the skills of manipulative medicine, began in a tiny frame building in Kirksville, Missouri, almost 100 years ago today. Andrew Taylor Still was the founder and professor of that school. He wrote down many of his thoughts and ideas, which were later collected into the first books of this profession.

Since that time, only a few books have been published on osteopathy, with most of the educational process relying on personal instruction and demonstration. To add to this, much of the information is scattered in obscure journals not available to everyone. Those texts which are available are generally limited to one or a few types of techniques.

Our goal here has been to prepare a text that organizes currently taught concepts and techniques into one comprehensive volume which might then serve as a reference for osteopathic medical students, as well as practicing physicians. The result is a book which presents an integrated method for both the diagnosis and treatment of somatic and visceral problems manifesting in the soma. We have also added an extensive section on practical applications to serve as a demonstration of examples of osteopathic concepts integrated into the management of some commonly encountered conditions.

The osteopathic approach to diagnosis and treatment is unique. We hope this text will make it more readily available to all osteopathic medical students.

Eileen L. DiGiovanna, DO, FAAO
Stanley Schiowitz, DO, FAAO

Acknowledgments

We wish to acknowledge the able assistance given us in preparing this book by a group of dedicated fellows of osteopathic principles and practice from our department. We also wish to express our gratitude to Anna Moon and Adele Gordon for their help in preparing and handling the manuscript and correspondence. A special thanks goes to the New York College of Osteopathic Medicine of the New York Institute of Technology for allowing us the time to complete this work. And of course, thanks to our spouses, Joseph DiGiovanna, DO, and Lillian Schiowitz for being there.

Contents

1

Introduction to Osteopathic Medicine

WHAT IS OSTEOPATHIC MEDICINE?
Eileen L. DiGiovanna

Osteopathic medicine represents one of two distinct schools of medicine in the United States. Osteopathic medical institutions issue Doctor of Osteopathy (D.O.) degrees, and allopathic medical institutions issue Medical Doctor (M.D.) degrees. The educational process is similar in both kinds of institutions. Most applicants to osteopathic medical schools have an undergraduate degree, exceeding the requirement of three years of an undergraduate education, and many have earned a master's or other postgraduate degree.

The four years in osteopathic medical school are spent in the study of basic and clinical sciences, much as in nonosteopathic medical schools, but with an added focus on osteopathic principles and concepts and intensive study of osteopathic manipulative medicine. The third and fourth years allow rotations into clinic, office, and hospital settings with introductions to inner-city, suburban, and rural types of practice.

After graduation the D.O. may complete a rotating internship for 1 year and then enter a residency to specialize in any branch of medicine. The D.O. is qualified to write prescriptions, perform surgery, deliver babies, and undertake other medical services as needed for promoting good patient health. As of April 1985, D.O.'s were certified in all specialties, including family practice.

The uniqueness of osteopathic medicine lies in the application of osteopathic concepts. Osteopathic medical practitioners follow accepted methods of physical and surgical diagnosis and treatment; they are also trained to expertly evaluate the neuromusculoskeletal system and seek to achieve normal body mechanics. Osteopathic physicians recognize the body's ability to both regulate itself and mount its own defenses against most pathologic conditions.

Osteopathic medicine thus recognizes the neuromusculoskeletal system as crucially important to the full expression of life. The viscera subserve the neuromusculoskeletal system by providing nourishment to it and removing its wastes. As George Northrup noted in *Osteopathic Medicine, An American Reformation*,

The musculoskeletal system is intimately connected with all other systems of the body through both the voluntary and the involuntary nervous systems. . . . Thus, indications are that the musculoskeletal system is a mirror of both health and disease, responding as it does to inflammation and pain from disorder in other body systems.

An Osteopathic Approach to Diagnosis and Treatment, second edition
Eileen L. DiGiovanna and Stanley Schiowitz
Lippincott–Raven Publishers, Philadelphia © 1997.

Therefore, when assessing the patient, the osteopathic physician considers the body as an integrated unit comprising multiple complex functions and interrelated structures.

Another important principle in osteopathic medicine is that structure and function are intimately interrelated. An abnormality in the structure of any body part can lead to abnormal function, whether expressed locally or distantly from the deranged structure. To correct the mechanical disorders, the osteopathic physician undertakes therapeutic manipulation. This manipulation is gentle and controlled; it may be directed toward joint motion or directed toward the muscles or fasciae. It is also used to affect circulation, lymphatic drainage, and nervous impulses.

The heart of osteopathy is the recognition of the body's ability to cure itself, with some external help, of many pathologic conditions. This tenet echoes the belief enunciated by Hippocrates more than 2,000 years ago: "Our natures are the physicians for our diseases."

Osteopathic medicine continues to grow even as it remains in a minority position in the health care system. From five schools in 1962, there are presently 17 schools with several more in the planning stages. The 1995 directory of the American Osteopathic Association numbers osteopathic physicians at 36,013. Norman Gevitz, in *The D.O.'s*, published in 1982, estimated at that time that D.O. physicians and surgeons were providing health care services for more than 20 million Americans, or in excess of 10% of the population. More importantly, most osteopathic physicians tend to go into the primary care specialties and to practice in underserved areas.

The osteopathic profession has changed even as it has grown. It has achieved recognition as a significant part of the American health care system. It is now carefully defining its special contributions to medicine and is undertaking various kinds of research to prove the effectiveness of its manipulative techniques. With these and similar steps toward full realization of the potential of osteopathic medicine, the profession is securing its position in the modern medical climate.

HISTORY OF OSTEOPATHY
Eileen L. DiGiovanna

Andrew Taylor Still, the founder of osteopathy, was born in 1828 in Lee County, Virginia, of Scottish-Irish descent. His father was a circuit-riding minister in the Methodist Church, a physician, a farmer, and a millwright.

As a young boy, Still suffered severe headaches. One day, during such a headache, he went to sit in a rope swing his father had hung for him from a tree branch. Feeling ill, he removed the board from the swing and lay on the ground with the back of his neck resting against the rope. The pain eased, and he fell asleep. When he awoke the headache was gone. He did this many times when a headache would occur. This observation contributed to later ideas, eventually leading to the development of osteopathy.

Being a hunter, as most men on the frontier were, Still would skin the animals he killed and developed a lifelong fascination with their muscles, bones, and joints. He never ceased his study of anatomy. He acquired his formal education in small schoolhouses as his father was moved ever further to the West. His informal education consisted of his incessant reading and information he learned as he followed his father on his rounds as minister-physician to the farms and small communities scattered around the countryside. Still gained his education in medicine primarily as a preceptor, although he had some formal training in Kansas City and was issued an M.D. degree by the state of Missouri.

Even as a youth, Still held strong opinions on controversial subjects. One of the first concerned slavery. He and his father were such strong abolitionists that his father was moved from Missouri, a border state supporting slavery, to an Indian reservation in Kansas. Here Andrew Taylor Still continued his fight against slavery. He also joined the Kansas militia during the Civil War and rose from captain to the rank of major. Later, as a member of the Kansas legislature, he assisted Kansas in becoming a state.

In the 1850s and 1860s, American medical practitioners were frequently poorly trained and had little understanding of the causes of disease. Treatments were unsophisticated to the point of being dangerous. Some common remedies used in those years included laxatives, purgatives, bloodletting (sometimes to the point of unconsciousness), calomel (a mercury compound), narcotics, and drugs with alcohol bases. Drug addiction, alcoholism, and mercury poisoning were among the results. Often the treatments were more dangerous than the illnesses.

Epidemics of typhoid, tuberculosis, measles, and meningitis, as well as other infectious diseases, often ran rampant across the frontier. An epidemic of meningitis took the lives of three of Still's children; orthodox medicine was unable to save them. In his autobiography, Still reflected on this episode: "In sickness, had God left man in a world of guessing? Guess what is the matter? What to give and guess the result?" Still sought answers to these perplexing questions and began to develop a systematic method of treatment that would eliminate guesswork and bring health without the disastrous results of current therapies. He worked largely with and through the musculoskeletal system and recognized the importance of the vascular system. He believed in natural immunity, that the body had its own "pharmacy" for healing itself. He developed a form of manipulation to help keep the body fit with unobstructed circulation and innervation.

Still broke with allopathy, as he called orthodox medicine, on June 22, 1874, when he "flung the banner of osteopathy to the breeze." He eventually moved back to Missouri to establish his practice in the town of Kirksville. As his fame grew, huge crowds gathered for his new treatment.

Many requests came to Still to teach his new method of healing. He first attempted to do so at Baker University in Baldwin, Kansas, an institution to which he and his brothers had contributed substantial financial support. He was not successful; osteopathy was considered quackery.

In 1892 Still purchased a small two-room building and started the American School of Osteopathy (ASO) in Kirksville, Missouri. The first class graduated in 1893 and included five women. Still quickly realized that 1 year was not enough and increased the curriculum to 2 years and then 3 years.

Dr. William Smith, a graduate of the prestigious Edinburgh University Medical School, came to Kirksville to meet the legendary osteopath and stayed on to become the first anatomy professor at the school. After he left, Jenette Bolles, a graduate of the ASO, became the anatomy professor.

Still trained his brothers, his children, his patients, and other M.D.'s in his new profession. He never wrote a technique book because he believed that his students should know anatomy exceptionally well and be able to devise their own techniques based on that knowledge.

Still died in 1917 at the age of 89, six months after a statue in his honor was unveiled in the Kirksville courthouse square, where it stands today. He left behind a struggling profession and school. Many battles lay ahead for osteopathy to be accepted into the American health care system.

By the 1960s there were six stable osteopathic schools located in Kirksville, Kansas City, Chicago, Philadelphia, Los Angeles, and Des Moines. In 1962 the profession suffered a major setback when the American Medical Association (AMA) changed its policy of fighting osteopathy and offered an alliance to D.O.'s in California, urging them to join the California Medical Association. The school at Irvine was turned into an M.D.-granting institution that offered an M.D. degree to California D.O.'s (and for a small fee to D.O.'s all over the country). The state would no longer license D.O.'s to practice in California. To the amazement of the AMA, most D.O.'s rejected this offer and began a fight to reestablish osteopathy within the state, including a licensing board, a new Osteopathic Medical Society, and a new school located in Pomona. As of 1996 there were 17 schools of osteopathic medicine. D.O.'s are licensed in all 50 states; Vermont was the first and Mississippi the last to license them.

Many people have contributed to the growth of the profession. It would be impossible to name them all, but some outstanding contributors should be noted.

J. Martin Littlejohn graduated from the American School of Osteopathy and joined the faculty there. He encouraged the teaching of physiology and other "more scientific" subjects. He and his brothers moved to Chicago, where they founded the Chicago College of Osteopathy. He later moved to London and was instrumental in founding the British School of Osteopathy, one of the best-known and respected European schools.

William Garner Sutherland was another student of Still. When the grooves in the suture of a temporal bone caught his eye, he was led to the development of cranial osteopathy and spent many years developing its theories and techniques, many of which are used today.

Harrison H. Fryette was a D.O. who studied the motion of the spine and of individual vertebrae through the use of fluoroscopy; his work produced the *Physiologic Laws of Vertebral Motion*.

Fred Mitchell, Sr., did extensive work with sacral motion and its relation to gait. He also helped develop the muscle energy technique.

Irwin Korr, Ph.D., a physiologist, spent years teaching in Kirksville, Michigan, and Texas at the osteopathic colleges. His strong commitment to osteopathy led him to do research in the field of somatic dysfunction, and he published some of the finest work in this area, including *The Physiologic Basis of Osteopathy*. He is still alive and a vocal advocate of osteopathic medicine.

Lawrence Jones was a general practitioner in Oregon, where he developed the theories and techniques of strain/counterstrain. He recently died.

Stanley Schiowitz, dean of the New York College of Osteopathic Medicine, developed the technique known as facilitated positional release, one of the newest techniques to be introduced to the profession. He is also coeditor of this textbook and has devoted his life to improving the educational system within the profession, ensuring that osteopathic principles will be included in that system.

Many others have made significant contributions of their knowledge, talents, and skills, for which we thank them all.

THE PHILOSOPHY OF OSTEOPATHIC MEDICINE
David J. Martinke
Dennis J. Dowling

The precepts discussed in this section are ideals. Those who do incorporate them into their practice will have a more realistic view of health and disease.

Osteopathic medicine is not merely a combination of traditional western medicine and osteopathic manipulations. Rather, the principles and philosophy of osteopathic medicine apply not only to manipulative treatment but also to surgery, obstetrics, emergency medicine, internal medicine, geriatrics, and many other areas of care traditionally subsumed by nonosteopathic medicine. In fact, osteopathic principles and philosophy permeate all aspects of health maintenance and disease prevention and treatment.

The *American Heritage Dictionary* defines a philosophy as an "inquiry into the nature of things based on logical reasoning rather than empirical methods." By contrast, a principle is defined as a "rule or law concerning the functioning of natural phenomena or mechanical process." Unlike philosophies, these rules or laws can be proved by experimental design or laboratory analysis. With these definitions in mind, it will be clear that the precepts outlined below are properly termed philosophies, not principles, since for the most part they are based on logical reasoning rather than on experimental design.

The first four of the following precepts were developed in 1953 by the osteopathic faculty committee at Kirksville College of Osteopathic Medicine, Kirksville, Missouri. The rest, which were added by common usage, were enumerated by Sarah Sprafka, Robert C. Ward, and David Neff, in the *Journal of AOA*, September 1981.

1. "The body is a unit."

The human body does not function as a collection of separate parts but as an integral unit. Obviously the body does consist of parts—the heart, the lungs, the musculoskeletal system, and so forth—all working to benefit the organism in totality. However, the osteopathic physician refrains from exalting any part above the whole. The kidneys, of interest to a nephrologist, or the heart, of interest to a cardiologist, are regarded by the osteopathic physician as components subserving the greater interest of the body. Uniting the body's parts is the fascia, a deep fibrous tissue investing the muscles and organs and acting as a ground substance to support and unite the whole body from head to foot. Thus the fascia is a fluid mechanism of profound functional significance. Osteopathic medicine simply understands that the person is a whole unit consisting of mind, body, and spirit.

2. "Structure and function are reciprocally interrelated."

Any body part carries out a function dictated by its structure. As an example, lung structure dictates that gases, carried by the red blood cells and dissolved in the blood, pass through the pulmonary arteries to the small capillaries in close approximation to the alveoli, where gas exchange takes place. As structure governs function, similarly, abnormal structure brings about dysfunction. In the case of abnormal lung structure, as in pulmonary fibrosis or interstitial pneumonia, the gradient between the alveolar gases and blood gases is increased, resulting in decreased gas exchange. Function also modifies structure. As an example, certain bony protrusions, such as the mastoid process, do not exist in the newborn infant. Through the use of the sternocleidomastoid muscles, upright positioning of the head is facilitated. The chronic use of these muscles brings about elongation of the bony attachments. Abnormal function also results in alteration of related structures. Constriction of blood vessels under sympathetic nervous influence brings about changes in these blood vessels as well as in other structures, such as the heart, kidneys, and eyes.

3. "The body possesses self-regulatory mechanisms."

Many examples of this precept can be considered. First, neuronal reflex mechanisms are constantly monitoring body functions. For example, the carotid sinus and baroreceptors monitor blood pressure and adjust the heart rate and cardiac contractility in response to changes in blood pressure. Second, hormonal pathways are involved in self-regulation. The releasing hormones of the hypothalamus cause the release of the stimulating hormones from the pituitary, which causes release of end-organ products (such as hormones or steroids); these products in turn provide feedback and regulate the activity of the hypothalamic-pituitary axis. These hormonal pathways are part of the complex endocrine system that is involved in the self-regulation of the body. Third, many organs such as the heart and kidneys are able to regulate blood flow. This vascular autoregulation allows the organ to maintain the appropriate blood flow in the setting of a changing vascular status. These examples represent only a few of the many ways in which the body can regulate its functions.

4. "The body has the inherent capacity to defend itself and repair itself."

The first lines of defense commonly recognized are the skin and mucous membranes. Once these are violated, elements of the cellular immune system are called on to protect the body from present and future invaders. Defense mechanisms are constantly working to protect the body as it contacts thousands of microorganisms daily.

The body's ability to repair itself is easily substantiated by observing the healing of a laceration or a fracture. Granulation tissue and the regenerative properties of certain tissues allow healing to take place. The physician may facilitate the process, but the inherent capacity of the body to repair itself brings about the actual healing. The physician's contribution is to remove obstacles to the body's performance.

5. "When normal adaptability is disrupted, or when environmental changes overcome the body's capacity for self-maintenance, disease may ensue."

Disease is caused by adverse environmental factors that overwhelm the body's defenses, or by the body's inability to adapt to a situation. The cause may be the body's inability to adapt, as in the case of an abnormal structure or abnormal function. The physician who is presented with a symptom, dysfunction, or disease—the effect—then embarks on a search for the cause. A physician who only treats a disease is merely treating an effect and may have no great impact on the cause. The osteopathic physician who helps correct the cause by restoring proper structure (at either the organ, tissue, or cellular level) facilitates proper function or adaptability. Once the cause is corrected, the body can heal itself through its inherent capacity for repair to the extent to which it is capable.

6. "Rational treatment is based on the previous principles."

Osteopathic manupulative treatment was not mentioned in these precepts of osteopathic philosophy. When Still first announced his philosophy in 1874, he did not mention manipulation, and it was about five years later that he began using manipulation as a tool for diagnosis and treatment. Manipulation is not the only aspect of osteopathic philosophy, nor is it the most important. However, with recognition of the importance of the somatic component of disease, the value of manipulation will be correspondingly better appreciated.

Even though conventional osteopathy did not incorporate the use of other interventions, such as pharmacological ones, today many contemporary osteopathic physicans do use pharmacological interventions. This is not in contrast to the principles, but rather, in further analysis, applies these principles. For example, medications such as antibiotics, through bacteriostatic properties, may maintain or reduce the absolute load of bacteria at a point where the individual's immunologic mechanisms can recover and produce adequate defense against and removal of the invaders.

In addition to the basic principles of osteopathic philosophy, there are other corollary principles that help direct and govern the osteopathic physician's approach to a patient:

1. "Movement of body fluids is essential to the maintenance of health."

The arteries and other tubular structures play a crucial role in carrying nutritive elements to their destination and carrying away waste materials to be expelled. Disturbances in the circulation will produce pathology, such as acute or chronic inflammation, atrophy, irritation, or trauma. If the vessels to these areas are compromised by intrinsic or extrinsic damage, flow will be inadequate. Such an environment could delay or even stop the healing process. For example, if the compromised artery is a coronary artery, angina or myocardial infarction might occur.

The osteopathic physician focuses on areas of structural dysfunction that influence the circulation to an area involved by a pathologic process. If such dysfunction is corrected, oxygen delivery by the arteries might increase, the venous conges-

tion be dispelled, and the healing process initiated. This process frees the body to make the repairs necessary for return of health.

2. "The nervous system plays a crucial part in controlling the body."

The nervous system is a major factor controlling blood flow. Impaired autonomic nervous control of the upper thoracic spinal cord traveling to the cervical sympathetic ganglia can produce a vast array of vascular changes in the somatic dermatomes supplied by these nerves. The somatic changes possible when such a dysfunction occurs include increased temperature locally, moisture, tenderness, and edema. These signs, recognizable on palpation, are adaptive vascular responses to an abnormal autonomic nervous supply.

Once dysfunction has been corrected, normal autonomic tone should resume, vascular response and a higher level of health should occur. Therefore, thinking osteopathically requires a knowledge of anatomy and the ability to reason from the region of pathologic manifestation to the site of autonomic control, not ignoring any of the tissues en route that may contribute to their dysfunction.

3. "There are somatic components to disease that are not only manifestations of disease but also are factors that contribute to maintenance of the diseased state."

The somatic component of the disease process may be caused by a direct bodily injury (such as a blow to the skeletal structures), or it may represent the response of viscera to pathology.

For example, in abdominal visceral pathology, such as acute appendicitis or peritonitis, one may observe spasm or guarding of the abdominal musculature. Other musculoskeletal effects may develop at a segmentally related spinal region, creating osteopathic somatic dysfunctions. These somatic components of the visceral disease are major diagnostic clues. The mechanism of this somatic response is probably the segmentally integrated viscerosomatic reflex. The nervous system is the most important system connecting and integrating the visceral and skeletal organs.

In many instances, illness is an imbalance between the neuromuscular system and the visceral systems. This must be mitigated before the body can heal itself.

What is so "osteopathic" about these precepts? Still's purpose was not to violate or rewrite basic scientific principles of his time, but rather to elucidate them and position them centrally on a system of therapeutics that emphasized the promotion of the body's ability to regulate itself toward health, given an appropriate environment and adequate nutrition. Osteopathic medicine is generally applicable to all conditions; the osteopathic physician does not address one organ system or structure at the expense of another but considers the person as an integral unit.

SOMATIC DYSFUNCTION
Eileen L. DiGiovanna

The term *somatic dysfunction* has been adopted by the osteopathic profession as a substitute for the older designation, *osteopathic lesion*. Somatic dysfunction is a condition of the musculoskeletal system that is recognized solely by the osteopathic profession and was first defined by Ira Rumney. The accepted definition in the *Glossary of Osteopathic Terminology* is as follows:

Somatic Dysfunction is an impaired or altered function of related components of the somatic (body framework) system: skeletal, arthrodial and myofascial structures, and related vascular, lymphatic, and neural elements.

It is apparent that the term can be applied to a wide variety of problems and therefore is a little too general in scope.

Not all somatic lesions are somatic dysfunctions. Fractures, sprains, degenerative processes, and inflammatory processes are not somatic dysfunctions. A useful observation has been given by Fred Mitchell, Sr.: "Implicit in the term 'somatic dysfunction' is the notion that manipulation is appropriate, effective, and sufficient treatment for it."

A somatic dysfunction is a change in the normal functioning of a joint and is diagnosed by using specific criteria. These criteria may be remembered as the T-A-R-T of diagnosis.

1. *T* denotes tissue texture changes. The soft tissues around a joint in somatic dysfunction undergo palpable changes. These changes occur in the skin, fascia, or muscle.
2. *A* denotes asymmetry. The position of the vertebrae or other bones or other structures is asymmetrical.
3. *R* denotes restriction of motion within the bound of physiologic motion. The involved joint does not have a full, free range of motion. The restriction involves one or more planes; it most frequently involves the minor motions of any given joint. This restriction is found by motion-testing the joint in all planes.
4. *T* denotes tenderness. Although not purely objective, tenderness is produced during palpation of the tissues where it should not occur if there was no somatic dysfunction.

Tissue Texture Changes
Tissue texture changes are a significant diagnostic tool. They occur in response to a variety of factors, including the following:

A. Neurologic factors
  1. Somatic manifestations
    a. Hyperresponsiveness of segmentally related functions
     i. Hypertonic muscles
     ii. Muscle spindle overactivity
    b. Sudomotor activity either increased or decreased
    c. Vasomotor activity, either constriction or dilation of vessels
  2. Reflex manifestations
    a. Tenderness to palpation
    b. Rigidity of tissues at reflex site
    c. Sudomotor activity may increase or decrease
    d. Changes in pulse rate (increase or decrease)
    e. Changes in skin temperature
B. Circulatory factors
  1. Macroscopic changes
    a. Temperature changes

b. Erythema
c. Swelling
d. Changes in pulse and cardiac rate
2. Microscopic changes
   a. Hyperemia of soft tissues
   b. Congestion and dilation
   c. Edema
   d. Minute hemorrhages
   e. Fibrosis
   f. Local ischemia
   g. Atrophy

CRITERIA FOR EVALUATION OF SOFT
TISSUES

Tissue texture changes vary somewhat between acute and chronic somatic dysfunctions. In the spinal area the changes tend to occur at the articulations of the vertebrae, over the transverse processes, and over the spinous process. The following is a chart of findings in acute and chronic somatic dysfunctions:

	Acute	*Chronic*
Temperature	Increased	Slight increase or decrease (coolness)
Texture	Boggy, more rough	Thin, smooth
Moisture	Increased	Dry
Tension	Increased, rigid, board-like	Slight increase, ropy, stringy
Tenderness	Greatest	Present, but less
Edema	Yes	No
Erythema test (red reflex)	Redness lasts	Redness fades quickly or blanching occurs

Definitions of some of these terms from the *Glossary of Osteopathic Terminology* are as follows:

Bogginess. A tissue texture abnormality characterized by a palpable sense of sponginess in the tissue, interpreted as resulting from congestion due to increased fluid content.
Ropiness. A tissue texture change characterized by a cord- or stringlike feeling.
Stringiness. A palpable tissue texture abnormality characterized by fine or stringlike myofascial structures.

Asymmetry

On palpation of a joint involved in somatic dysfunction, the bone involved will be found to lie in an asymmetric position with respect to its normal position and to the position of bones contiguous to it. For example, the spinous process of a vertebra involved by somatic dysfunction may lie to one side of the line formed by the spinous processes of other vertebrae (which should lie in the midline), or one transverse process may be more posterior than the contralateral one. There may be an approximation of one transverse process to the vertebra below while the opposite transverse process is separated from the one below it.

Restriction of Motion

A joint involved by somatic dysfunction has a restricted range of motion. It is said to meet an abnormal "barrier" to motion. In the normally functioning joint there are two barriers to motion (Fig. 1-1):

1. The physiologic barrier is that point to which the patient may actively move any given joint; it represents a functional limit within the anatomic range of motion. Passive motion is still possible (Fig. 1-2A).
2. The anatomic barrier is that point to which the joint may be passively moved beyond the physiologic barrier (Fig. 1-2B). Restriction at this point occurs because of bone, ligament, or tendons. To pass the anatomic barrier, a disruption of tissue has to occur (Fig. 1-2C).

A pathologic barrier may occur as the result of disease or trauma. An example is joint fusion due to spondylitis or osteophytes in an arthritic joint. Inflammation or joint effusion will restrict normal motion. The osteopathic restrictive barrier is one that lies within the physiologic range of motion and that prevents a joint from moving symmetrically within the physiologic range of motion (Fig. 1-3).

In somatic dysfunction, a joint is restricted, or meets a barrier, in one or more planes of motion. Motion in the opposite direction is normal or free. For example, a vertebra may move freely into flex-

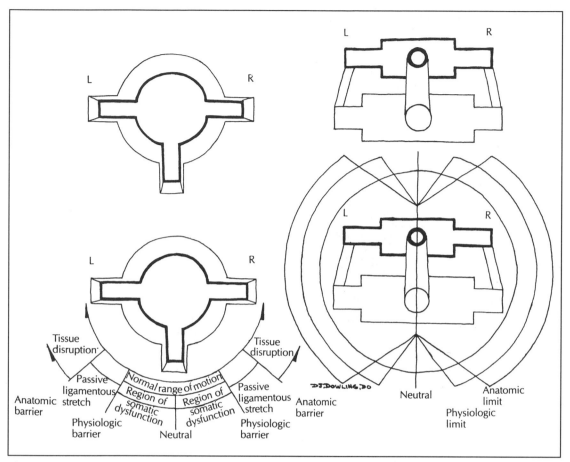

Figure 1-1. Barriers to motion.

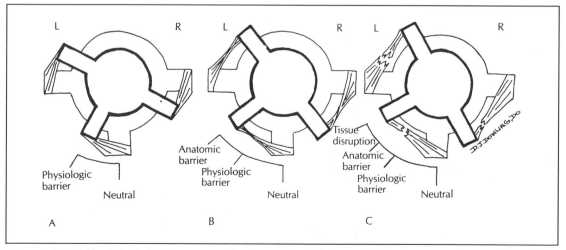

Figure 1-2. **(A)** Physiologic barrier engaged by the patient. **(B)** Anatomic barrier engaged passively, with ligaments stretched. **(C)** Anatomic barrier has been passed, causing tissue disruption.

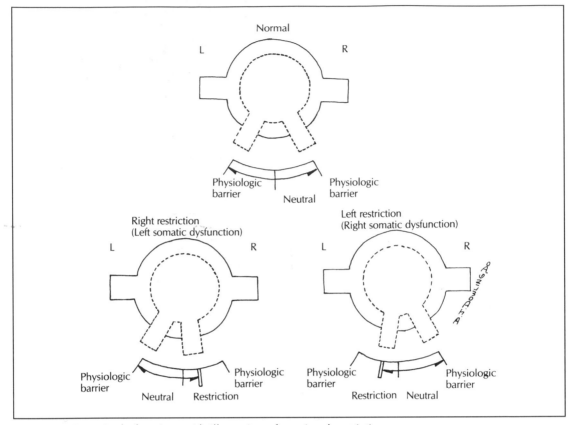

Figure 1-3. Somatic dysfunction, with illustration of rotational restrictions.

ion but not be able to move all the way to the physiologic motion barrier of extension.

It is important to understand that motion may be restricted as a result of "tethering" by a tight muscle rather than from hitting against an obstacle.

Tenderness

Tenderness is the subjective sensation of pain or soreness that is reported by the patient in response to palpation of tissues by the physician. This sensation is almost always present in tissues surrounding a somatic dysfunction with no more than normal pressure by the physician. Pressing too firmly on soft tissues will always cause pain or tenderness. Pressure that should not normally cause pain will do so in tissues around a dysfunctional joint. Recognizing that these tissues are tender should cause the physician to deal with them gently.

Diagnosing Viscerosomatic Reflex Dysfunctions

A tenet of osteopathic medicine is that visceral reflexes to the soma are an important cause of somatic dysfunction and are of major diagnostic significance. Dysfunctions caused by these reflexes may be either acute or chronic.

Acute viscerosomatic reflex dysfunctions are probably indistinguishable from any other acute somatic dysfunction. Chronic viscerosomatic dysfunctions have a few characteristics that may aid in differentiating them from somatic dysfunctions of other causes.

1. The skin tends to be more atrophic over the involved area.
2. The tissues display a firm, dry sponginess, as opposed to the bogginess of an acute dysfunction. The texture is very firm.
3. Joint motion is more restricted and seems more

fixed than the usual dysfunction. Attempts to elicit motion in the involved joint produce a sluggish, rigid movement. The end feel at the barrier tends to be more "rubbery."

4. When such a dysfunction is corrected, it will tend to return to a dysfunctional state within 24 hours.

It is important to know the location of sympathetic innervation in relation to the thoracic vertebrae so that viscerosomatic reflex dysfunctions may be used for diagnostic purposes.

Naming Somatic Dysfunctions

A standard terminology has been devised for the purpose of recording somatic dysfunctions. In the case of vertebrae, it is traditional to refer to a functional vertebral unit, consisting of two vertebrae and the intervening disc, with the upper of the vertebrae being the one with restricted motion. The somatic dysfunction is always named for its freedom of motion, that is, the directions in which the vertebra can move most easily. For example, if the C3 vertebra is restricted in the motions of extension, side-bending to the right, and rotation to the right, C3 is said to be flexed, side-bent to the left, and rotated to the left on C4. This is denoted as C3 F SlRl.

The terminology reflects the fact that the vertebra assumes the position of its freedom of motion. T7 E SrRr indicates that the seventh thoracic vertebra is extended, side-bent to the right, and rotated right on T8. In this case the seventh thoracic vertebra is restricted in the motions of flexion, side-bending to the left, and rotation to the left.

Somatic dysfunctions are classified as type I or type II dysfunctions. Type I dysfunctions follow Fryette's first principle of physiologic motion (see Chap. 4, Physiologic Motion of the Spine) and are group curves involving more than one vertebra. If rotation and side-bending are involved, the rotation is opposite to the side-bending. Although type I dysfunctions are group curves, they are distinct from idiopathic scoliosis.

Type II dysfunctions follow Fryette's second principle of physiologic motion. Rotation and side-bending are in the same direction. These are single dysfunctions and are often traumatic in origin.

Type I and type II dysfunctions refer only to somatic dysfunctions in the thoracic and lumbar vertebrae because Fryette's principles only apply

to these areas. However, in common usage somatic dysfunctions in the cervical spine may be called type II.

Somatic dysfunctions in other areas of the body, such as the extremities, are still named for their freedom of motion. For example, the radial head may move anteriorly or posteriorly. If it moves freely posteriorly and is restricted in anterior motion, it is named a "posterior radial head."

Because of some difficulty in standardization, some osteopathic physicians still use terminology indicating barriers to free motion. In this case, in the interest of clarity, the term *restriction* should be utilized.

Predisposing Factors

Certain factors that predispose to the development of a somatic dysfunction are as follows:

1. Posture
   a. Habitual
   b. Occupational
2. Gravity
3. Anomalies
   a. Abnormal size or shape of vertebra
   b. Abnormal facets
   c. Fusion or lack of fusion
      i. Lumbarization
      ii. Sacralization
4. Transitional areas (These areas are especially prone to the development of somatic dysfunction.)
   a. Occipitoatlantal (O-A)
   b. C7-T1
   c. T12-L1
   d. L5-S1
5. Muscle hyperirritability
   a. Stress
   b. Infection
   c. Reflex from another somatic or visceral area
6. Physiologic locking of a joint, "close-pack position"
7. Adaptation to stressors—spontaneously reversible
8. Compensation for other structural deficits—stable

Etiology

The exact cause of somatic dysfunction is often debated. Some feel there is a true facet locking. Most believe that muscle dysfunction is the major

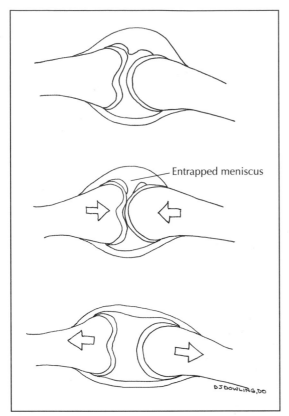

Figure 1-4. Meniscus entrapment theory. With joint motion the meniscus is trapped between the joint surfaces. Traction is required to free the meniscus.

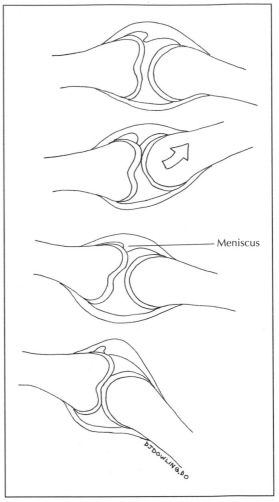

Figure 1-5. Meniscus extrapment theory. As the joint is flexed, the meniscus moves above the articular surface and occasionally is trapped there as the joint begins to extend. With further extension the meniscus bends, causing pain.

factor operating in the creation and/or maintenance of joint restrictions. Abnormal neural impulses to the muscle are probably the most significant cause of joint restriction and pain. Trauma is probably the major factor triggering an abnormal neural impulse.

Some of the theories postulated in support of the facet locking include the following:

1. Meniscoid entrapment
2. Meniscoid extrapment
3. Capsular compression

The meniscoid theory was proposed by Kos and Wolf (Bogdvk and Jull) as a mechanism of "acute locked back" and was elaborated by Bogdvk and Jull. This theory is based on the premise that there are wedge-shaped menisci in the lumbar zygapophyseal joints. It is speculated that the apex of the wedge may become trapped between the articular surfaces or, on flexion, outside the joint cavity (Figs. 1-4, 1-5).

Type I somatic dysfunctions may be due to any of the following:

1. Muscle imbalance
2. Short leg
3. Occupation
4. Trauma
5. Visceral reflexes
6. Disease or infection

OSTEOPATHIC MANIPULATION
Eileen L. DiGiovanna

Manual medicine, or manipulation, was not invented by Andrew Taylor Still. These forms of therapy were present for many centuries before his birth. Egyptian hieroglyphics show pictographs of a practitioner manipulating the body of a patient. Hippocrates writes of the use of manipulation.

In the 1800's, a popular system of treatment in Europe was "bonesetting," a secret type of manipulation passed through families and used to treat a variety of illnesses. Bonesetters jealously guarded their secrets and frequently became quite famous for their almost miraculous cures.

In many religions and among many shaman, healers, and medicine men and women, ritualistic "laying on of the hands" was common. It was believed that a healing force or some form of energy passed from the healer to the patient that would effect a cure. In more recent times Dolores Krieger, a registered nurse, has popularized "therapeutic touch" as a way of relieving many of the symptoms suffered by patients.

Still undoubtedly learned of manual medicine at some time during his early years, perhaps from European mercenaries during the Civil War, and he began to form a system of medicine using manipulation as the basis for the therapeutics of osteopathy. His success prompted him to abandon most forms of pharmacologic intervention in favor of these less harmful treatments. At one time, he advertised himself as "The Lightning Bonesetter" and as a "magnetic healer," so we know that he had knowledge of these practices.

Out of Still's system of manipulation has evolved osteopathic manipulative medicine as it is practiced in our times. New forms of treatment have come into use over time and continue to be developed by osteopathic physicians, who discover new ways to relieve patient's problems using their manual skills.

Classifications

Osteopathic techniques are classified in many different ways. They may be classified according to patient participation in the process, the position of the affected joint in relation to its movement capabilities, the goals of the treatment process, or the names of the techniques.

PATIENT PARTICIPATION
Techniques may be classified by whether or not the patient participates in them.

Passive
A technique is classified as passive if the patient takes no role in the treatment process but sits or lies passively while the practitioner performs the technique on him or her.

Active
A technique is classified as active if the patient is guided by the practitioner to assist in the treatment process. This may be done by an active, voluntary muscle contraction by the patient as directed by the physician. It may involve the use of a respiratory effort by the patient under the guidance of the physician.

MOTION CLASSIFICATION
A technique may be classified by the position used relative to the motion capabilities of the involved joint.

Direct
A technique is known as a direct technique if the starting position into which a joint is placed is "against the barrier," that is, in the direction in which the joint motion is restricted. The goal of a direct technique is to use force in such a way that motion will be created through and beyond the restrictive barrier.

Indirect
A technique is indirect when the joint is positioned into its freedom of motion, that is, away from the barrier or restriction of motion. The goal then is to allow the body's inherent neurologic or intrinsic forces to free up the restriction of motion so that the joint will regain its ability to move freely through the barrier. This may be compared to a stuck drawer that is pulled back away from the direction in which it was sticking and then

pushed freely in the direction that had previously restricted motion.

GOALS OF TREATMENT
Techniques may be classified according to the goals of the treatment or the system toward which treatment is being directed.

Musculoskeletal/Postural
The technique may be directed toward treatment of any of the components of the musculoskeletal system: bony, articular, ligamentous, muscular, or tendinous. The primary goal is to relieve pain, to improve motion, and to change abnormal conditions, primarily in the musculoskeletal system. This is probably the most common model used by manual medicine practitioners, and most techniques may be used for these purposes.

Circulatory
The main goal of the treatment may be to improve circulation or cardiovascular function. A number of techniques are designed to improve circulation. Although other effects may be accomplished, the primary one is to improve circulation—arterial, venous, or lymphatic.

Respiratory
These techniques are aimed at improving respiration. This might be done by improving motion within the musculoskeletal components of the thorax, such as the thoracic and lumbar spine, the ribs, and the sternum and clavicle; by promoting the expulsion of fluids from the respiratory tract by loosening mucus in the bronchial tree; or by assisting with lymphatic flow to help fight infections within the respiratory system.

Psychosocial
Sometimes manipulative techniques are used to reduce stress in the body or to help the patient deal with psychological problems. Patients sometimes experience an emotional release during manipulation that manifests as a period of crying or laughing, and the physician needs to be prepared to help counsel the patient through these episodes.

Bioenergetic
Osteopathic techniques may be directed toward treating the energies of the body. Some practitioners focus on the imbalances of body energies and use various techniques to improve energy balances.

TYPES OF OSTEOPATHIC TECHNIQUES
Myofascial Treatment
Myofascial techniques are directed toward the soft tissues of the body, particularly the muscles and fasciae; hence the name. They are also referred to as *soft tissue techniques*. They may be either passive or active. The active techniques are classified as direct, meaning that they treat the muscle that is having the problem, or indirect, meaning that the antagonist muscle to the problem muscle contracts. These are different from the usual definitions of the terms *direct* and *indirect* and apply only to the active myofascial techniques. In reality the active techniques are forms of muscle energy that use the Golgi tendon reflex or reciprocal inhibition of muscle.

The passive myofascial techniques usually involve a gentle stretching of the involved muscle and/or fascia to cause a relaxation or release of tension. The active use of the physiologic muscle reflexes such as reciprocal inhibition cause the muscles to relax as a result of guided patient muscle contraction.

Counterstrain
Also known as *strain/counterstrain*, this is an extremely gentle technique in which "tender points" are found in muscles, ligaments, or tendons and the involved muscle is shortened by specific positioning of the body part. The position relieves the tenderness and is held for about 90 seconds; the body part is then returned to a resting position. Since this is all done passively and the motion is always into a direction of ease of motion, the technique is "passive" and "indirect." Motion is also restored to joints that the involved muscle may have been restricting.

Muscle Energy
Muscle energy is an "active," "direct" technique. The involved joint is placed into its restriction of motion. The patient is directed to gently push in the opposite direction, the direction of freedom of motion, for about 3 to 5 seconds and then to relax the contracted muscle. After 3 to 5 seconds of relaxation, the physician moves the joint past the old barrier to the new barrier and the process is repeated. This is done a total of three times; then

the physician adds a passive stretch. This technique will restore joint motion to its physiologic limits. Other forms of muscle energy are discussed in the muscle energy section of Chapter 5.

Facilitated Positional Release

This is a passive, indirect technique that is also a positional type of technique. The area of the spine to be treated is place into a "loose-packed" position; that is, the facet joints are not engaged. A facilitating force, either compression or torsion, is added and then the joint or muscle is placed into its ease-of-motion or shortening position. This is held about 5 seconds, and then the part is returned to a resting position and the dysfunction reevaluated. These techniques may be used to treat soft tissue tension or specific joint somatic dysfunction.

Thrusting or Impulse Techniques

These techniques are "passive" and "direct." The joint is placed against the barrier or restriction, and, after careful positioning to ensure that only the involved joint will move, a gentle force is applied to the area to move the joint beyond the pathological barrier. This is the type of manipulation familiar to most people.

High-velocity, low-amplitude. High-velocity means that the force is applied very quickly, and *low-amplitude* means that the distance moved is very small. The physician directs a quick, controlled force through the joint to move it. Relaxation of the soft tissues is essential to ensure that the maneuver will be painless and the force will be the least possible.

Low-velocity, high-amplitude. In this technique, the force is applied more slowly and is slightly greater in amplitude. Again, this is a controlled and directed force.

Articulatory Technique

With this technique, the involved joint is very gently guided through its full range of motion and gently encouraged to move beyond its restrictions to motion. This is analogous to "jiggling" a stuck drawer and may also be called low-velocity, low-amplitude.

Myofascial Release Techniques

These techniques may be either "direct" or "indirect," but are always "passive" except for the occasional use of respiratory effort by the patient. The major direction of the techniques is toward the fascia, and the techniques may also be known as "fascial release techniques." The area being treated is placed either against the barrier or away from the barrier and held as the physician waits for a release of tension and restriction.

"Unwinding" techniques are fascial release techniques that follow the gradual unwinding of tense and torsioned fasciae through an extremity or through the whole body.

Osteopathy in the Cranial Field

Cranial osteopathy is directed toward improving and normalizing cranial bone motion and balancing the tension membranes of the central nervous system. This is an extremely gentle technique in which the physician monitors the cranial rhythmic impulse, an inherent motion within the cranium, and seeks to free restrictions of the cranial bones at their sutures and balance the tension membranes (falx cerebelli, falx cerebri, and tentorium). This may be done in a direct or indirect manner.

Occasionally respiratory effort by the patient is requested, but in general this is a passive technique.

Ligamentous Articular Strain

These techniques were devised by the founder of cranial osteopathy and are similar to cranial techniques except that they are applied to ligaments attached to the joints of the body. They may also be known as *balanced ligamentous tension techniques.*

Visceral

Visceral techniques are directed toward the viscera specifically. They are used to improve position, circulation, and motion of the viscera. They may be used in a variety of visceral problems, and are especially effective in treating problems of the gastrointestinal tract and pelvic organs.

Functional Techniques

Functional techniques are geared toward improving joint motion by functional positioning and mobilization. They are generally indirect and passive techniques. Low-velocity stress is applied to the restricted joint and forces are initiated that will create decreasing tissue resistance. Constant tissue monitoring is essential throughout the technique. Since the motion stress is minimal, the technique is very gentle.

Fluid Motion Techniques

These techniques are designed to move fluids in various parts of the body. Some techniques are especially for sinus drainage, and others are for moving the lymph through its thoracic channels. Some techniques are for moving lymph through peripheral areas and for removing fluid from edematous areas. There are techniques to assist the respiratory system in removing excess mucus in the airways, especially in respiratory diseases.

It behooves the student to learn as many techniques as possible. Obviously everyone will not be skilled in every technique, nor should everyone try to be. However, the more types of techniques that are mastered, the more techniques the physician will have to select from when deciding on the best management plan for the patient.

References

American Hertiage Dictionary. 1969. W. Morris, Ed. Boston: Houghton Mifflin.

Bogdvk N, Jull G. 1985. The theoretical pathology of acute locked back: A basis for manipulative therapy. Manual Medicine 1:78–82.

Booth ER. 1905. History of Osteopathy and Twentieth-Century Medical Practice. Cincinnati: Press of Jennings and Graham.

Burns L. 1907. Viscero-somatic and somato-visceral spinal reflexes. J Am Osteopath Assoc 7:51–60.

Educational Council on Osteopath Principles. 1995. Glossary. Am Osteopath Assoc Director.

Fryette HH. 1954. Principles of Osteopathic Technic. Kirksville, Missouri: Journal Printing Co. 9.

Frymann VM. 1976. The philosophy of osteopathy. Osteopath Ann 4:102–112.

Gevitz N. 1982. The D.O.'s: Osteopathic Medicine in America. Baltimore: Johns Hopkins University Press.

Greenman P. 1991. Principles of Manual Medicine. Baltimore: Williams & Wilkins.

Johnson W, Friedman H. 1995. Functional Methods. Colorado Springs: American Academy of Osteopathy.

Korr IM. 1947. The neural basis of the osteopathic lesion. J Am Osteopath Assoc 47:191–193.

———. 1967. The nature and basis of the trophic function of nerves: Outline of a research program. J Am Osteopath Assoc 66:74–78.

———. 1986. Somatic dysfunction, osteopathic manipulative treatment and the nervous system: A few facts, some theories, many questions. J Am Osteopath Assoc 86(2):109–114.

———, Appeltauer, GSL. 1970. Continued studies on axonal transport of nerve proteins to muscle. J Am Osteopath Assoc 69:76–78.

———, Chornock FW, Cole WV, Wilkinson PN. 1967. Studies in trophic mechanisms: Does changing its nerve change a muscle? J Am Osteopath Assoc 66: 79–80.

———, Wilkinson PN, Chornock FW. 1966. Studies in neurotrophic mechanisms (abstr). J Am Osteopath Assoc 65:990–991.

———, Wilkinson PN, Chronock FW. 1967. Axonal delivery of neuroplasmic components to muscle cells. J Am Osteopath Assoc 66:1057–1061.

———, Wright HM, Thomas PE. 1962. Effects of experimental myofascial insults on cutaneous patterns of sympathetic activity in man. J Neural Transm 23:22, 330–355.

Laughlin GM. 1924. The scope of osteopathy. J Osteopathy 31.

Mitchell F, Jr. 1979. Towards a definition of "somatic dysfunction." Osteopath Ann 7:12–25.

Northup GW. 1969. Orientation. In: Osteopathic Medicine. New York: McGraw-Hill.

Northup GW. 1979. Osteopathic Medicine, An American Reformation. Chicago: American Osteopathic Association.

Postgraduate Institute of Osteopathic Medicine and Surgery. 1970. The Physiological Basis of Osteopathic Medicine. New York: The Postgraduate Institute of Osteopathic Medicine and Surgery.

Rummey I. 1976. The relevance of somatic dysfunction. In: Yearbook of the American Academy of Osteopathy. Colorado Springs: American Academy of Osteopathy.

Still AT. 1908. Autobiography. Kirksville, Missouri: Andrew T. Still.

Still AT. 1899. Philosophy of Osteopathy. Kirksville, Missouri: Published by the author.

Still AT. 1920. The Philosophy and Mechanical Principles of Osteopathy. Kansas City, Missouri: Hudson-Kimberly.

Sprafka S, Ward RC, Neff D. 1981. What characterizes an osteopathic principle? Selected responses to an open question. J Am Osteopath Assoc 81:81–85.

2   Soft Tissues

THE SKIN
Eileen L. DiGiovanna

The skin is the largest organ in the body. It is in constant contact with the environment, and many of its important functions have to do with protecting the body from environmental insults or with regulating the internal milieu as the external environment changes. The skin safeguards the internal structures from chemical and mechanical irritants and seals in bodily fluids to maintain a fluid internal environment. Salt and waste products are excreted through the skin. Dilation and constriction of blood vessels in the skin and evaporation of sweat from the surface of the skin aid in regulating body temperature. Finally, the skin acts as a sensory organ, relaying information about the environment to the central nervous system.

Skin Structures

The skin consists of three layers. From exterior to interior, there are the epidermis, the dermis, and the fascia. The outer, epidermal layer is made up of dead and dying cornified cells. It has no vasculature and very few nerve endings. The middle and most important dermal layer is the least dense, consisting of about five layers of cells. It contains capillaries, small vessels, and most nerve endings. Hair and nails, specialized protective structures of the skin, are derived from dermal tissue. The deep, fascial layer of skin connects to the subcutaneous tissues. More vessels and nerve endings lie in this layer.

The circulatory elements of the skin have two functions: to conduct heat and to carry nutrition to the skin. Heat conduction, perhaps the more important of these functions, is performed by venous plexi and arteriovenous anastomoses. Nutritive components are carried by the arteries and capillaries. Other structures in the skin include two types of glands, *sudiferous*, or sweat-producing glands, and *sebaceous*, or oil-producing glands.

Innervation and Sensation

The skin is innervated by the autonomic (sympathetic) nervous system and the peripheral (sensory) nervous system. Sympathetic innervation affects the blood vessels, the muscles of the hair follicles, and the glands in the skin. Sympathetic innervation of the blood vessels in the skin contributes to vasoconstriction and vasodilation. The ends of the vasoconstrictor fibers apparently secrete norepinephrine, and it is believed vasodilation results from the secretion of acetylcholine at

An Osteopathic Approach to Diagnosis and Treatment, second edition
Eileen L. DiGiovanna and Stanley Schiowitz
Lippincott–Raven Publishers, Philadelphia © 1997.

some of the endings. Vasodilation raises the temperature of the skin, which then becomes red, in pale-complexioned persons, or darkens, in dark-complexioned persons. Vasoconstriction results in cooling of the skin and a bluish color due to the increase in deoxygenated blood. With severe or prolonged vasoconstriction the skin hue pales as blood is squeezed out of the vessels. Sympathetic stimulation also causes sweating. These effects of sympathetic stimulation contribute to osteopathic diagnosis. Increased or decreased temperature, sweating, and changes in skin texture are associated with somatic dysfunctions in the involved area.

The skin is responsive to four types of sensation—touch (pressure), heat, cold, and pain. These sensations are detected by mechanoreceptors that are expanded nerve endings in the skin. Also present are some unmyelinated, or free, nerve endings. All four sensations are elicited in skin where only free nerve endings exist; thus, the free nerve endings apparently respond to all types of stimuli. The mechanoreceptors or expanded nerve endings (Merkel's disks and Ruffini endings) and encapsulated endings (Pacini corpuscles, Meissner's corpuscles, and Krause's end bulbs) (Fig. 2-1) appear to be sensation-specific. Merkel's disks are sensitive to touch (two-point discrimination). Meissner's corpuscles are sensitive to touch, and Pacini corpuscles to deep pressure. It has been postulated that Ruffini endings are sensitive to heat and Krause's end bulbs to cold, but this is open to debate.

The Physician's Skin

Mechanoreceptors and other neural elements in the skin of the palpating physician's hand convey information about the patient. Because the dorsum of the hand is thinner-skinned than the palm, temperature is best palpated with the dorsum. Merkel's disks are most numerous in the palm and especially in the finger pads, which makes the finger pads most sensitive to touch. Thickening of the skin, as in calluses, decreases sensitivity. Because the receptors fatigue, the physician may find it necessary to rest or change fingers during palpation to ensure maximum sensitivity.

Figure 2-1. Mechanoreceptors in the skin.

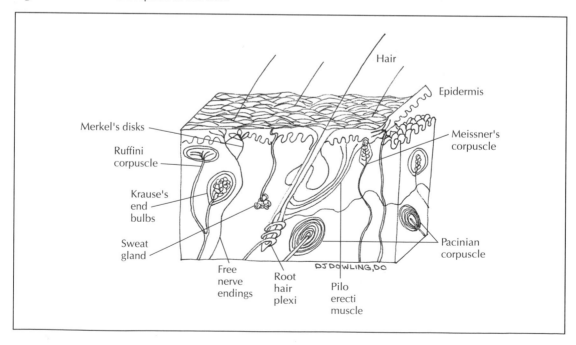

FASCIA
Nancy Brous

Anatomists define fascia as a dissectable mass of fibroelastic connective tissue. The osteopathic physician defines fascia as all the connective tissue of the body that has a supportive function, including ligaments, tendons, dural membranes, and the linings of body cavities.

Fascia is very extensive. If all other tissues and organs were removed from the body, with the fascia kept intact, one would still have a replica of human anatomy. Fascia surrounds every muscle and compartmentalizes muscle masses. It surrounds and compartmentalizes organs in the face, neck, and mediastinum. Fascia forms sheaths around nerves and vessels. It envelops the thoracic and abdominopelvic organs. It forms the pleura, pericardium, and peritoneum. Fascia connects bone to bone, muscle to bone, and forms tendinous bands and pulleys.

Fascia is continuous throughout the body. The majority of the fascial planes are arranged in a longitudinal direction. Areas of hypertonicity or muscular imbalance can impose functional restriction on the natural longitudinal glide of the body's fascial sheets. Therefore, one area of restriction can influence adjacent and distal areas.

Several functional transverse diaphragms exist in the body. Restrictions of these diaphragms can cause major alterations in the function of surrounding structures. The respiratory diaphragm permits passage of the aorta, esophagus, vena cava, azygous veins, thoracic duct, vagus, and phrenic nerves. The urogenital diaphragm supports the pelvic viscera, allows sacrococcygeal mobility, and transmits the anal canal, urethra, vagina, lymphatics, and neurovascular bundles. The cranial base and dura transmit the jugular veins and cranial nerves IX, X, and XI through the jugular foramen. Any restrictions in these major transverse diaphragms will inhibit longitudinal fascial motion above and below and thus affect function of those structures it encompasses.

The fascia has varied functions. It acts to stabilize and maintain upright posture through the lumbodorsal fascia, the iliotibial band, the gluteal fascia, and the cervical fascia. Fascia also protects and supports organs, muscles, neurovascular bundles, and lymphatic channels. It restrains and binds, enclosing muscle groups while defining their motion. This delimiting function channels muscle energy into specific action, while simultaneously preventing muscles from rupturing and tearing. Therefore, fascia coordinates the action of muscle and muscle groups for a smoother, coordinated motion.

Fascia aids the circulation of body fluids. It keeps veins open and widens them as it is tensed during muscle contraction. Fascia is inherently contractile and elastic. As it contracts along the muscle, it compresses the veins within it, increasing venous return. The elasticity of the fascia pulls the veins open after they have been squeezed by contractility, resulting in a milking action. Any contraction, tension, or imbalance in the fascia can impede or inhibit this dynamic contractile-elastic activity and result in decreased venous return and congestion.

The distribution of arterial blood to any part of the body requires adequate blood pressure and unobstructed arterial channels. The heart must be able to contract freely in the thorax without fascial or bony restrictions. Innervation to the heart must be free from mechanical irritation along its distribution. Adequate venous return is needed. Again, any restrictions in fascial sheaths housing the neurovascular bundles or even in neighboring fascial planes can decrease blood flow to an area.

The lymphatic vessels are arranged in a superficial and a deep set. Both pierce the fascia and accompany the veins. Therefore, lymphatic drainage can also be affected by restrictions in the fascial planes.

As the immediate external environment of every living cell, fascia directly or indirectly influences the metabolism of these cells. Abnormal pressure or tension will alter the diffusion of nutrients and the elimination of wastes, resulting in alterations in cell function. A cell needs proper maintenance of osmotic pressure and tissue tension of the surrounding interstitial fluid and ground substance for proper metabolism.

The most abundant cellular component of fascia is the fibroblast. The fibroblast is under control of the endocrine system. Fibroblasts are responsible for the production of collagen and ground substance, and their response to physicochemical changes is important. Under pressure, fibroblasts produce collagen organized along the same stress lines as the direction of force. Therefore, fascia can adapt to external stresses by cross-linking of collagen. This increase in strength can also decrease fascial flexibility and can cause restrictions and potential compression of vessels and nerves.

Fascia directly or indirectly influences the health of the body by being coordinated with the musculoskeletal system, by cooperating in the circulation of body fluids, and by allowing generous passageway for nerves. Derangement in the fascial planes can result in venous congestion, abnormal reflexes, and a decreased range of motion. Thus, myofascial techniques are crucial in eliminating fascial restrictions and allowing the body to return to a healthier state.

NEUROPHYSIOLOGY RELEVANT TO OSTEOPATHIC PRINCIPLES AND PRACTICE

Dennis J. Dowling
Paula D. Scariati

An understanding of neurophysiology is essential to the understanding of the mechanisms of somatic dysfunction and the logical application of osteopathic manipulation. Some basic terminology needs to be clarified:

Afferent nerve. A nerve carrying impulses toward the central nervous system (CNS).
Efferent nerve. A nerve carrying impulses from the CNS.
Ventral horn. The anterior portion of the gray matter in the spinal cord where efferent motor neurons leave the spinal cord.
Dorsal horn. The posterior portion of the gray matter of the spinal cord where afferent sensory nerves enter the spinal cord.
Contraction. Physiologic shortening of muscle length from its usual resting length.
Contracture. Abnormal, fixed shortening of muscle length.
Agonist. Muscle or muscle groups primarily responsible for performing some motion (i.e., flexion).
Antagonist. Muscle or muscle groups that oppose the motion of the agonist and produce an opposite motion (i.e., extension).

Sensory nerves carry impulses from sense organs to the spinal cord or brain. Those that enter the spinal cord do so through the dorsal horn. Those destined to terminate locally end in the gray matter of the spinal cord, where they produce local segmental responses such as excitation, facilitation, and reflex actions. They may directly affect a motor or sympathetic nerve or do so through an intermediary interneuron. These interneurons may be either excitatory or inhibitory. Those with distant terminations or other intermediaries travel to integrative areas higher in the spinal cord, the brain stem, or the cerebral cortex.

The body is artificially divided into groups of structures identified as organs, glands, ligaments, muscles, neural tissue, vessels, bone, and skin. This differentiation is anatomically correct but functionally misleading. The somatic and visceral components act synergistically to fulfill the body's needs and functions. However, this interaction is often visualized as a strictly mechanistic process in which one part of the body causes the action to be initiated, either automatically or volitionally, and the rest of the body simply carries out orders. By contrast, osteopathic medicine holds that each part of the body is in some manner responsible for and responsive to every other part.

The spinal cord is the organizer of information, which is processed from the brain to other regions. Feedback from these areas to the brain helps maintain normal function. A difficult concept to grasp is that parts of the body may communicate directly with one another without the brain's intervention. In these communications, the nervous system is less like a two-way intercom system in a large apartment house than like a fully interactive telephone system with the brain acting as the operator. A common example is the knee-jerk reflex, which occurs automatically in response to appropriate stimuli without direct intervention from the brain. Modification can be produced centrally in the brain or sometimes by other factors. Conscious attention to a hammer striking the patella tendon can blunt or eliminate the reflexive effect of knee extension. It is often necessary to use techniques of distraction such as closing one's eyes, sticking out the tongue, or performing an isometric exercise with the hands. The use of caffeine, thyroid medication, stimulants, alcohol, and the effect of stress and anxiety can all modify reflexes.

Some reflexes serve an apparent survival benefit early in life but apparently fade quickly in infancy. The Babinski reflex appears to change significantly. Initially the toes curl about a stroking stimulus and later the toes curl upwards and there is withdrawal of the foot. The Moro reflex consists of arm abduction and neck flexion in response to a sudden backwards fall. The asymmetric tonic reflex, also known as either the fencer's or bowman's reflex, results in contraction of the triceps, psoas, and hamstrings with relaxation of the biceps brachii on the side of the head and neck rotation, with the exact opposite effect on the contralateral side. There is an agonist contraction with antagonist relaxation throughout. Each of these reflexes may be considered survival mediators and apparently fade in preparation for coordinated motion. In truth, there is an inhibitory effect centrally, and these reflexes are suppressed throughout most of life. Unfortunately, they recur in response to damage of the central nervous system.

The Autonomic Nervous System

The autonomic nervous system can be thought of as an involuntary manager. It is divided into sympathetic and parasympathetic nervous systems. The autonomic nervous system controls the moment-by-moment activity of the viscera. Its components, often described as antagonistic, are more realistically understood as cooperative or complementary.

The somatic component is often discussed as a totally independent, voluntary system responsible for the musculoskeletal system. It is not customarily thought of as interacting with the autonomic nervous system. However, the somatic component has undeniable effects on the autonomic nervous system, and vice versa.

The Sympathetic Nervous System

The sympathetic chains of ganglia are bilaterally oriented in a cephalad-caudad direction at the levels of the first thoracic segment to the second or third lumbar segment. The fibers exit the cord along with the somatic motor axons as the ventral roots via the intervertebral foramina. These preganglionic fibers exit the root along the white ramus and into the ganglia. They synapse with postganglionic nerves at various levels of the chain. The postganglionic axons return to the spinal nerve via the gray ramus. For much of their course, the sympathetic nerves travel intimately with the somatic axons.

Another important anatomic feature of the sympathetic chains is their relationship to the ribs. The ganglia lie inferior to the junction between the head and neck of the ribs but posterior to the pleura. The range of influence is further extended superiorly as far as the sympathetic plexi to the head and upper extremity by the cervical ganglia and to the lower extremities by the lumbar splanchnic nerves.

The sympathetic nervous system assists the body in managing the stresses and requirements

Figure 2-2. Sympathetic chain. *B*, vertebral body; *G*, sympathetic trunk ganglion; *T*, sympathetic trunk; *D*, intervertebral disk.

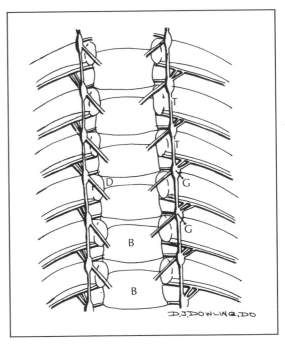

of the external environment. It is responsible for the "flight or fight" response. Reactions are constantly moderated and adjusted in response to information received by higher centers. Visceral function is fine-tuned. Circulation, metabolism, smooth muscle tone, intestinal motility, cardiac function, and pulmonary response are regulated (Fig. 2-2).

The Parasympathetic System

The parasympathetic system is also known as the craniosacral portion of the autonomic nervous system because of the sites of origin of the preganglionic fibers. The cranial portion has ganglia associated with the 3rd, 7th, 9th, and 10th cranial nerves. Spinal cord segments S2, S3, and S4 make up the sacral portion.

The parasympathetic ganglia are located close to the innervated organ. Fibers from the oculomotor, facial, and glossopharyngeal nerves supply ganglia for organs found in the head, while the remainder of the visceral organs receive their innervation from the vagus and the sacral axis. The vagus alone supplies the heart, lungs, trachea, liver, gallbladder, esophagus, stomach, pancreas, spleen, kidneys, small intestine, and the ascending and transverse colons. The nervi erigentes, constituting the pelvic nerve, send fibers to sex organs, external genitalia, and the bladder and its sphincters. There is no parasympathetic innervation of the extremities.

Despite the fact that the parasympathetic nerve fibers innervate various organs, there are regions of the body where greater than 50 percent of the fibers are actually sensory in nature. The visceral organs are under dual control of the sympathetic and parasympathetic nervous systems. The process is a synergistic rather than a competitive one, with activation usually occurring reciprocally. The primary function of the parasympathetic system is internal maintenance, including digestion

Figure 2-3. Sympathetic pathways. *D*, dorsal root; *V*, ventral root; *DRG*, dorsal root ganglion; *S*, splanchnic; *R*, recurrent meningeal; *g*, gray rami communicantes; *W*, white rami communicantes; *G*, sympathetic trunk ganglion; *T*, sympathetic trunk.

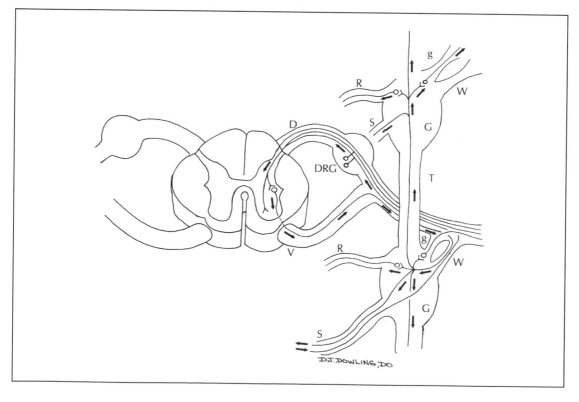

and excretion. Among other functions, the cranial axis causes constriction of the pupil and decreases in heart rate. The parasympathetic division operates most effectively during times of recovery and rest.

Skeletal Muscle System

The skeletal or somatic nervous system is under voluntary control, although some processes can be performed automatically. The typical spinal nerve is formed by a joining of the ventral and dorsal roots inside the vertebral canal. Sensory fibers have their cell bodies in the dorsal root ganglion and then synapse in the dorsal horn. The ventral root contains the motor neurons. The rami of the 31 pairs of spinal nerves split into a dorsal and ventral ramus. These in turn are subdivided into other branches. The structure is fairly consistent but is best represented by the thoracic nerves. All of the skeletal muscle nerves arise or terminate in common origins in the spinal cord and exit via the vertebral foramina. The sympathetic pathways are shown in Figure 2-3.

Neuromuscular Reflexes

Ventral motor neurons give rise primarily to two types of nerves that exit the anterior horn to innervate skeletal muscle, alpha motor neurons and gamma motor neurons. Alpha motor neurons transmit impulses via Ar nerve fibers to innervate large skeletal muscle fibers. A single alpha motor neuron excites a few to several hundred skeletal muscle fibers known as the *motor unit*. Gamma motor neurons transmit impulses via Ar nerve fibers to innervate small skeletal muscle fibers called *intrafusal fibers*. These fibers contribute to the muscle spindle apparatus (Fig. 2-4).

Two primary and separate muscular reflex systems, each with its own apparatus, function, and response, play major roles in stabilizing and modulating muscular activity. The muscle spindle re-

Figure 2-4. Muscle spindle and detail of components.

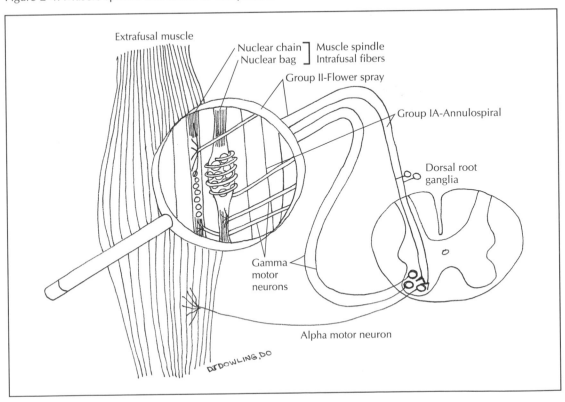

flex sends information to the nervous system about muscle length or the rate of change in muscle length. The Golgi tendon reflex sends information to the nervous system about muscle tension or the rate of change in tension.

MUSCLE SPINDLE REFLEX

Muscle spindles are intrafusal mechanoreceptors that are widely distributed between skeletal muscle fibers in the belly of the muscle. They occur in parallel with the much larger extrafusal skeletal muscle fibers, and the connective tissue around the muscle spindles is continuous with the connective tissue around the other muscle fibers. The muscle spindles mediate a response to a load placed on the muscle; this is known as the *load reflex*. Muscle spindles have a dampening function as well: they prevent some types of oscillation and jerkiness in body movement. In fact, the tremors noted especially during times of extreme anxiety or stimulants represent a failure to dampen this response smoothly. In addition to serving at a subconscious level, the muscle spindle reflex is invoked in voluntary motor activity.

Muscle spindles are composed of two types of intrafusal muscle fibers: nuclear bag fibers and nuclear chain fibers. The nuclear bag fibers have nuclei that appear to be bunched in the center of the cell, and the nuclear chain fibers have their nuclei lined up in single file in the center as in a series. There are 2 to 5 nuclear bag fibers and 6 to 10 nuclear chain fibers in a typical muscle spindle. The central portions of either type of fiber have very poor contractile ability, whereas the ends that are attached have greater contractility. The components of an intrafusal muscle spindle are diagrammed in Figure 2-4.

The sensory afferents of the muscle spindle comprise group Ia fibers (primary endings), which send branches to every intrafusal fiber in the muscle spindle, and group II fibers (secondary endings), which innervate the nuclear chain endings only. The larger primary endings (Ia) surround the center of the muscle spindle much like a coil, while the smaller secondary endings (II) terminate on either side of the primary endings in a branchlike fashion. The Ia fibers are known as *annulospiral endings*, and the type II fibers are called *flower-spray endings*. Although both respond to length changes, the nuclear bag/annulospiral complex responds primarily to rate of change and the nuclear chain/flower-spray complex reacts more to absolute length change. They both react somewhat to both conditions.

Stimulation of the muscle spindle occurs either with lengthening of the whole muscle, which stretches the midpoint and excites the receptors, or with contraction of the endpoints of the intrafusal fibers, which also stretches the midpoint and excites the fiber. Stretching the muscle spindle increases the rate of firing, whereas shortening the muscle spindle decreases the rate of firing. In the so-called neutral position, a baseline background of firing occurs (Fig. 2-5A). However, in a compacted or hypershortened position, theoretically cessation of the firing may occur. Thus, the musculoskeletal system can send a positive signal or no signal to the spinal cord to indicate the status of the muscle.

The nerve fiber from the type Ia or II group passes through the dorsal horn into the ventral region of the spinal cord. There the effect is stimulation of the alpha motor neuron. Stimulation of this fiber results in activation and contraction of the larger extrafusal muscle component. This results in shortening of the whole muscle unit. The submerged and smaller muscle spindle is then shortened, resulting in a decrease or elimination of the firing in the sensory fibers.

A simple example of the muscle spindle reflex is the patellar tendon reflex. The knee, when flexed to 90 degrees, places the quadriceps muscle into a relatively stretched position. The sudden strike of a hammer against the tendon results in a dynamic stretch of the spindle and firing of the Ia (and possibly II) fiber; the alpha motor neuron is then stimulated and in turn induces quadriceps contraction and knee extension (Fig. 2-5B).

Slow stretch of the length of the receptor portion of the muscle spindle produces the static stretch reflex. The number of impulses transmitted from both the primary and secondary endings increases in proportion to the amount of stretch, and signals are transmitted as long as the muscle is stretched. The static stretch reflex is thought to be mediated primarily by nuclear chain fibers, since these are the only fibers innervated by both primary and secondary endings. The static gamma fibers, which mainly excite the nuclear chain fibers, enhance the static reflex but contribute little to the dynamic reflex.

Motor efferents of the muscle spindle consist of static and dynamic gamma fibers, which make dif-

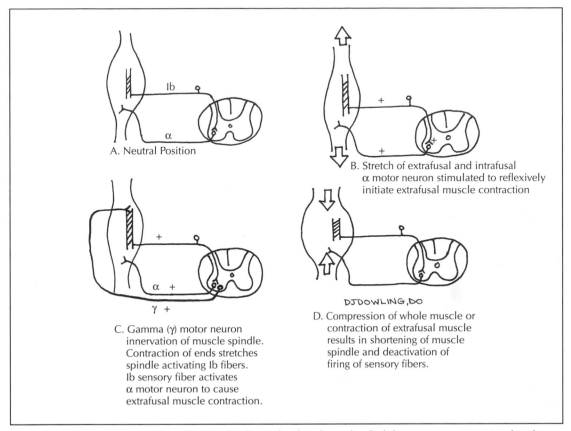

Figure 2-5. **(A)** Neutral position. **(B)** Stretch of extrafusal and intrafusal alpha motor neuron stimulated to reflexively initiate extrafusal muscle contraction. **(C)** Gamma motor neuron innervation of muscle spindle. Contraction of ends stretches spindle, activating Ib fibers. Ib sensory fiber activates alpha motor neuron to cause extrafusal muscle contraction. **(D)** Compression of whole muscle or contraction of extrafusal muscle results in shortening of muscle spindle and deactivation of firing of sensory fibers.

ferent contributions to the stretch reflex mediated by the muscle spindle. Static gamma fibers primarily innervate nuclear chain fibers, producing tonic activity in Ia afferent fibers. Dynamic gamma fibers primarily innervate nuclear bag fibers, generating phasic activity in Ia afferent fibers. Overall, the gamma motor neurons serve two functions: (1) they cause the intrafusal fibers to contract, thereby stretching the central portion of the muscle spindle and causing activity of the sensory endings (this is theorized to be the mechanism for maintaining postural tone); and (2) they cause the intrafusal fibers to contract sufficiently to stretch the muscle spindle toward threshold, thereby increasing the sensitivity of the muscle spindle apparatus (Fig. 2-5C).

The gamma motor neurons are very numerous and in some regions may actually constitute 70% of the motor neurons exiting the spinal cord. The effect of establishing or maintaining a steady state of the spindle also leaves the system vulnerable to overregulation. The resultant contraction of the end portions of the spindle results in greater susceptibility to further stretch (Fig. 2-5D). Too constant, rapid, or frequent firing or maintenance of firing past the time required results in a high gain set. Sudden stretching of muscular tissue that has not been prepared with concomitant gamma stimulation results in an even more powerful response. Inappropriate maintenance of the gamma motor neuron stimulation may result in a stretch reflex despite the fact that the muscle is actually in the neutral or a relatively shortened position.

Neuronal Circuitry of Muscle Spindle Reflexes
The monosynaptic pathway, in which sensory input fibers synapse directly with motor output fibers, governs the primary endings (Ia) that mediate the dynamic stretch reflex. The type II fibers may occasionally terminate monosynaptically, but most terminate on multiple interneurons in the gray matter of the spinal cord. Type II fibers transmit more delayed signals to the anterior motor horn.

GOLGI TENDON REFLEX

Golgi tendon organs, sometimes called tendon spindles, are encapsulated sensory mechanoreceptors located in mammalian tendons between the muscle and the tendon insertions. There is one tendon organ for every 3 to 25 muscle fibers. Tendons, because of their more fibrotic, less contractile nature, are subject to a stretching effect while there is contraction of the muscle belly. Golgi tendon organs detect the degree of skeletal muscle tension and convey this information to the CNS. The Golgi tendon organs are in series with the extrafusal fibers and are stretched whenever the muscle contracts.

Afferent neurons from the Golgi tendon mechanoreceptor are larger, myelinated neurons of the Ib group. Upon entering the gray matter of the spinal cord, the afferent Ib neuron synapses with inhibitory interneurons. It also synapses with other interneurons that ascend to higher CNS levels. The inhibitory interneurons synapse with the large alpha motor neurons located in the anterior gray horn of the spinal cord. The alpha motor neurons that are inhibited are to the same muscle in which the Ib afferents originate (Fig. 2-6). This results in reflex relaxation of the muscle.

Increased tension in a skeletal muscle distorts

Figure 2-6. Golgi tendon reflex.

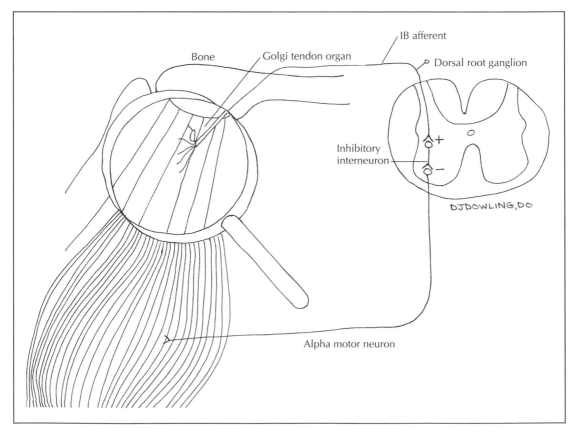

the Golgi tendon organ, producing a generator potential that initiates an action potential. The action potential travels over the Ib neurons to the spinal cord. Afferent action potentials activate the interneurons, which inhibit the alpha motor neurons back to the skeletal muscle. The increased muscle tension that initiates the reflex can result from contraction of the skeletal muscle or from marked passive stretch of the muscle.

Interneurons, as the name implies, are bipolar neurons that connect two other neurons. They are located in all areas of the spinal cord, not just the anterior horn. Interneurons are small, highly excitable, and often spontaneously active. They can fire as rapidly as 1,500 times per second.

Certain interneurons located in the anterior horn in close association with the motor neurons constitute the Renshaw inhibitory system, which causes inhibition of neurons surrounding the motor neuron carrying a given excitatory impulse. This phenomenon is known as *recurrent inhibition*. The function of the Renshaw inhibitory system is to sharpen the signal of the motor unit. It prevents the signal from diffusing into adjacent nerve fibers, which would weaken the signal.

Since the basic Golgi tendon reflex results in reflexive inhibition of the muscle, the opposite effect of the stretch reflex produced by the muscle spindle, it is sometimes called the *inverse stretch reflex*. This autogenic inhibition is more commonly known as the *lengthening reaction* or the *clasp-knife reflex*. Like a pocket knife, increased muscular tension may result in sudden relaxation. An example is the sudden extension of the elbow in the loser of an arm-wrestling contest.

Both the muscle spindle and the Golgi tendon organ reflexes serve the same basic purpose: to prevent disruption of the tissue. In the case of the muscle spindle, it is to dynamically prevent tearing or overstretching of the belly of the muscle. The Golgi apparatus protects the tendinous portion from tearing or even avulsion of the bony attachment. Both, when inappropriately set or activated, create or maintain abnormal muscle function.

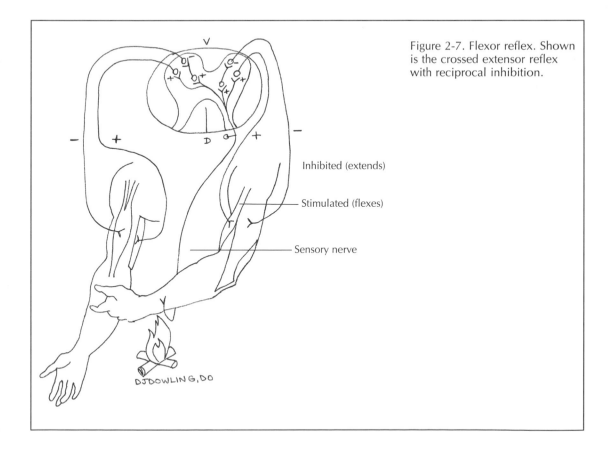

Figure 2-7. Flexor reflex. Shown is the crossed extensor reflex with reciprocal inhibition.

Inhibited (extends)

Stimulated (flexes)

Sensory nerve

DJDOWLING,DO

Flexor Reflexes

CROSSED EXTENSOR REFLEX

The crossed extensor reflex is the response elicited by stimulation of a given muscle (e.g., the biceps of the right arm, causing flexion) in the muscle of opposite function on the opposite side of the body (e.g., contraction of the triceps in the left arm, creating extension). The crossed extensor reflex is mediated via many sensory and motor interneurons in the spinal cord. Some act to inhibit the contralateral agonist and stimulate the contralateral antagonist. The reflex usually occurs in response to prolonged stimulation (200–500 msec) after a painful stimulus and continues long after the provoking stimulus has been withdrawn (Fig. 2-7). The effect is necessary for coordinated balanced activity such as walking, crawling, climbing, and running. As one arm extends, the opposite flexes.

RECIPROCAL INNERVATION

Reciprocal innervation is the stretching of a given muscle, stimulating the contraction of that muscle via the muscle spindle. The antagonist muscle is inhibited.

Segmentalization

Dermatome mapping of the cutaneous innervation is an established method of localizing a pathologic disease process to a particular segment. Although variations might exist in a given individual, the overall pattern is fairly consistent (Fig. 2-8). A different type of segmentalization is not as well known: the sympathetic system also shows segmental preference in regard to the visceral organs. According to *Gray's Anatomy*, the afferent fibers that accompany the preganglionic and postganglionic fibers of the sympathetic system occur in a segmental arrangement. Painful stimuli to the viscera are carried back to the cord via the sympathetics (Fig. 2-9). When all clues are combined, knowledge of this segmentalization can assist in the diagnosis of visceral disorder. For example, pain fibers from the heart pass to the first five thoracic spinal cord segments mainly through the middle and inferior cardiac nerves. Ischemia of the heart muscle often produces pain substernally with radiation to the chest, shoulder, neck, jaw, and abdomen.

Pain secondary to appendicitis is generally

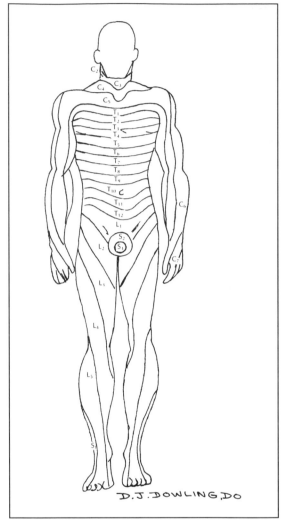

Figure 2-8. Dermatome map of cutaneous innervation.

noted to be initially in the periumbilical region. Anatomically the appendix is not within this region of the abdomen. However, the innervation for the appendix is derived from the 10th thoracic segment, as is the area around the umbilicus. This segmental relationship demonstrates the intertwining of different regions anatomically. The typical progression of pain in the right lower quadrant of the abdomen only results when an inflamed appendix makes contact with a sensitive peritoneum in that region. This represents direct mechanical and inflammatory impingement rather than a neurological pattern.

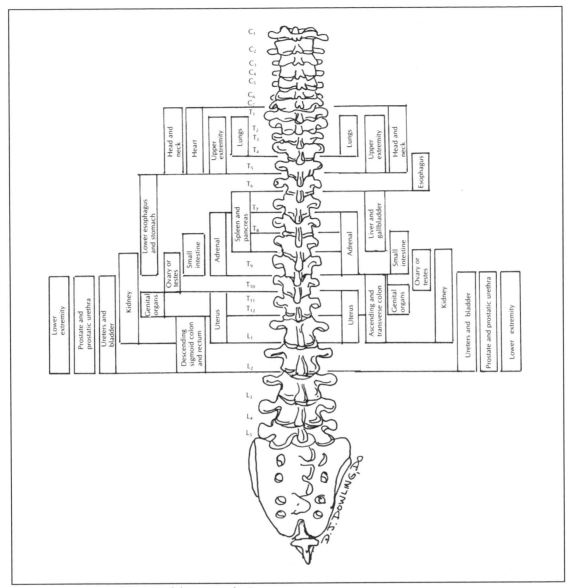

Figure 2-9. Segmentalization of the sympathetic nervous system.

Viscerosomatic Reflexes

A viscerosomatic reflex is one in which disruption, irritation, or disease of an internal organ or tissue results in reflex dysfunction of a segmentally related musculoskeletal region. In 1907, Louisa Burns, D.O., attempted, through experiments on animals, to demonstrate the physiologic processes occurring in viscerosomatic and somatovisceral reflexes. By stimulating various visceral organs, she elicited contractions of segmentally related muscles. Irritation of the visceral pericardium and the heart muscle initiated contractions in the second through sixth intercostal and spinal muscles. Stimulation of abdominal organs similarly yielded results (Korr, Wilkinson, and Chornock, 1966, 1967; Korr, Chornock, Cole, and Wilkinson, 1967; Korr and Appeltauer, 1970). The importance of these findings has yet to be determined, but it is readily apparent that disruption by compression would limit or eliminate any benefits obtained from this nutrition. With complete separation of the axon, Wallerian degeneration occurs and innervated fibers are lost. Interestingly enough, Dr. Still wrote about the "nerves of nourishment" as important in the maintenance of normal functioning. An in-depth examination of his writings indicates that there was no confusion of vascular structures with nerves in regard to this observation.

Facilitation

Facilitation indicates that an area of impairment or restriction develops a lower threshold for irritation and dysfunction when other structures are stimulated. It may be activated by reflexes of either the somatosomatic or viscerosomatic type. These low-threshold segments showed reflex hyperexcitability in response to pressure placed on the corresponding spinous processes, in response to pressure placed on the spinous processes of distant, high-threshold segments, and in response to

impulses from proprioceptors associated with positioning, from remote areas of skin, and from higher centers (Denslow et al., 1947) (Fig. 2-10). Facilitated segments are chronically hyperirritable and hyperresponsive. Muscles in the region are maintained in a hypertonic state, which constricts the available spinal motion. All of the supportive structures and their innervations may become afferent sources of facilitation. Reasonably, the neural controls would be expected to accommodate to the high level of activity, and this does occur in some cases. According to one theory, the muscle spindles, which monitor muscle length through gamma neuron control, are improperly set and therefore react inappropriately to stimuli. In comparison with messages sent from normally reactive neighboring neural tissue, messages sent from inappropriately reactive tissues are presented to the spinal cord and higher centers as confused. In other theories the spinal cord itself is considered able to adapt to the higher activity level and to channeling impulses to the affected region as if it were a "neurologic lens" (Korr, 1986).

Figure 2-10. Facilitated vertebral segment. **(A)** Facilitated segment (*shaded region*) shows increased activity. **(B)** Force or stress applied some distance away from the facilitated segment produces hyperreactivity. **(C)** Both the stressed segment and the facilitated segment exhibit hyperreactivity.

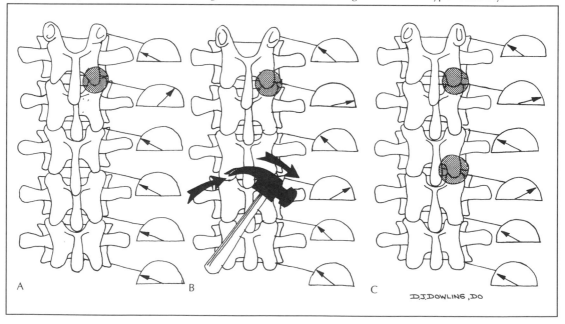

Nociception

At a local level pain can be appreciated by several sensory endings that have a high concentration, especially in the skin. Local biochemical neuropeptides such as substance P, calcitonin gene-related peptide (CGRP), histamines, and interleukins mediate inflammatory changes and also increase local neural and tissue sensitivity. The fascia and adventitia of muscular blood vessels have numerous unmyelinated group IV and small group III myelinated fibers. Pressure, stretch, prolonged contractions, thermal and chemical changes, and ischemia may excite or sensitize these fibers. There is a high concentration of nociceptive sensitive neurons in laminae I, II, IV, and X in the spinal cord. Some of these mediate local responses, and others project to the central nervous system via the spinothalamic, spinoreticular, and spinohypothalamic tracts. Higher-center involvement of the hypothalamus, the locus coeruleus, and the pituitary lead to involvement of neuro-endocrine-immune as well as cortex responses. The cyclic nature of pain–inflammation–restriction of motion–contraction–histochemical changes–dysfunction is well known. The persistence of this recurring cycle depends on many factors, not the least of which is duration of the condition.

Causes of Muscle Pain

Muscle spasms of diverse origin can cause pain. Prolonged muscle contractions irritate the splinting muscle and the associated ligaments and tendons, producing further spasm and initiating a pain cycle. The severity of the pain reflects the duration of a sustained contraction.

Ischemia, or localized anemia due to obstruction of blood at a specific site, is a well-known cause of muscle pain, occipital tension headaches, and intermittent claudication. Retention of irritating metabolites and waste products also causes muscle pain. Blood flow to the area must be increased to remove these substances. Proper delivery of oxygen, glucose, and other nutritive substances cannot occur if impedances persist.

Pain due to trauma or irritation (e.g., by an osteophyte) can be alleviated with the use of therapies that decrease muscle tension and improve local tissue circulation, affording subjective and objective relief from pain and spasm.

Failure of calcium to accumulate in the sarcoplasmic reticulum, abnormal interaction between the muscle fibril's actin and myosin, and anxiety may all cause muscle pain.

Manipulation

The goal of manipulation is to restore the whole body to a state of homeostasis. This is not some standardized posture to be rigidly applied in all cases but is individually tailored to the patient. The discovery of somatic dysfunctions describes the regions to be treated. In the case of facilitated segments, whether one imagines resetting the gamma gain or reestablishing a coherent neural communication, the end goal is to bring about normal, comfortable motion.

Somatovisceral reflexes produce unmeasured changes on the internal organs. Sympathetic stimulation may promote or maintain a disease process. Relief of this source, if performed early enough, should alleviate the symptoms and the disease process. The viscerosomatic reflex is less amenable to cure. Manipulating the affected soma should have a beneficial effect in reducing symptoms, but the overall effect on the visceral component is indeterminable at this time. If we postulate a "tape loop" that promotes the whole process, then anything that breaks the cycle is of importance.

The changes created by osteopathic manipulative treatment are mediated at a local level but have the potential to be far-reaching and interactive. Proper control of muscle function depends on local excitation in conjunction with continuous feedback from the brain about muscle status.

Practical Applications of Neurophysiology in Osteopathic Manipulative Treatment

MYOFASCIAL / MUSCLE TECHNIQUES

1. **Stretch reflex.** Quick stretch of a muscle excites the muscle spindle, causing reflex contraction. To prevent this reflex, myofascial therapy is done slowly for correction of contracted or contractured muscles. A quick stretch can be employed if the goal of therapy is to stimulate muscle tone.

2. **Moist heat** applied to muscle usually increases its **elastic** response to stretch. It also aids in increasing circulation. Dry heat is not as effective and does not penetrate as deeply as moist heat.

The application of **ice** may seem to have a para-
doxical effect, especially when one sees that
heat increases local tissue relaxation and
stretch. Cold has a multiple effect. It is an analgesic and when applied to a region may even
increase local circulation. The timing in the application of one of these modalities may effect
the response significantly. Heat in the initial inflammatory stage may actually increase localized edema. Cold may produce or increase muscle contraction. Applications of 15 or 20
minutes with equivalent latency periods may be
more effective than constant use. Some patients
even respond to alternating heat and cold.
3. Connective tissue placed under prolonged **mild
tension** shows plastic elongation.
4. **Servo-assist function of the muscle spindle reflex.** If the extrafusal fibers contract less than
the intrafusal fibers, the muscle spindles will
maintain a stretch reflex to further excite the
extrafusal fibers. This technique is used in active resistive myofascial therapy.
5. **Golgi tendon organ reflex.** When tension on the
tendon becomes extreme, the inhibitory effect
from the tendon organ can become so great that
it causes a sudden relaxation of the entire muscle. This technique is used in active resistive
myofascial therapy.
6. **Reciprocal innervation.** When a stretch reflex
excites one muscle, it simultaneously inhibits
the antagonist muscle. Reciprocal innervation
is of use in active indirect myofascial therapy,
with or without resistance.
7. **Crossed extensor reflex.** When a stretch reflex
excites one muscle, it simultaneously excites
the contralateral antagonist muscle; the motion
created crosses from one side of the spine to the
other side in an X pattern. The crossed extensor
reflex is helpful in active myofascial therapy,
usually with isokinetic resistance.

COUNTERSTRAIN AND FACILITATED
POSITIONAL RELEASE TREATMENTS

The theories of counterstrain and facilitated positional release treatments are discussed in detail in
later chapters.

Prolonged shortening of a muscle allows shortening of both the intrafusal (muscle spindle) and
extrafusal fibers. The gamma motor neurons then
increase their firing rate to maintain tone in the
muscle, resulting in hypersensitive muscle spindle fibers in the shortened muscle. If the shortened, hypersensitive muscle is now lengthened

rapidly (the muscle spindle responds to both
length and rate of change of length), a reflex over-
stimulation of the alpha motor neurons will occur
and muscle spasm will ensue. The sensory signals
also travel to the higher centers of the CNS, which
are not capable of interpreting them properly and
thus respond with excessive gamma motor stimulation, which maintains the spasm.

Reshortening the muscle allows the muscle
spindle to shorten and resume normal firing. The
CNS is now able to interpret the signals properly,
so it resets its gamma motor neurons. This takes
about 90 seconds to accomplish.

Adding a facilitating force along the axial spine
with the addition of passive positioning in muscle
shortening may compress the muscle spindle and
reduce and eliminate the firing of annulospiral
and flower-spray endings and reset the gamma
motor neuron influence in a more immediate
fashion.

MUSCLE ENERGY TECHNIQUES

Muscle energy treatment combines elements of
the Golgi tendon reflex, reciprocal innervation,
and elastic stretch. Muscle energy techniques that
use the Golgi tendon reflex are much like active
myofascial techniques in that extreme tension is
used to create an inhibitory effect that will produce a sudden relaxation.

To engage the mechanism, the physician must
resist the patient's efforts with an isometric force
after placing the muscle group or joint into its
pathologic barrier. The patient contracts for 3 to
5 seconds with sufficient minimal force to activate
the local muscles. The Golgi organ initiates reflexive relation of the muscle by inhibiting the alpha
motor neuron. After a brief period, the physician
may slowly stretch the involved muscles and engage a new barrier.

Direct muscle pull causes an elastic stretch,
such as occurs during periods of relaxation between active contractions and also at the passive
stretch administered at the end of muscle energy
treatment.

In reciprocal innervation when a stretch excites
one muscle, it simultaneously inhibits its antagonist.

HIGH-VELOCITY, LOW-AMPLITUDE
THRUST (HVLA)

Although it is not necessarily thought of as a soft
tissue technique, HVLA may result in regional
changes in the musculature. Usually the surrounding soft tissues should be relaxed before the

technique is used. The effect of the quick thrust of low amplitude, as long as it does not initiate a stretch reflex, may be to reduce local proprioceptive and nociceptive impulses from the joint. The sudden restoration of normal movement may help interrupt the cycle of pain–inflammation–restriction of motion–contraction–histochemical changes–dysfunction. The full mechanism is not well understood.

FASCIAL RELEASE (MYOFASCIAL RELEASE)
Fascia is a tissue that intimately covers all tissue, and the tension that results from spasm cannot separate the combination of fascia and muscle. As a substance that acts like a sheath and a colloid, fascia begins to show histochemical changes after trauma or prolonged stress. Resolution of somatic dysfunction must involve reversing such tensions.

INHIBITION/STIMULATION
The theories concerning the process of inhibition are not well documented. One of the oldest techniques of manipulation, its application is very similar, and perhaps no different from, accupressure. The physician grasps or pushes a location, usually with one or two fingers; some practitioners use elbows and large surface areas such as the forearm or palm of the hand. The pressure engaged is firm and constant. After a period of time, the tissue appears to soften and the patient may describe that pain or sensitivity has diminished. When this technique is applied to the thoracic or other spinal regions related to visceral innervation, the objective is to reduce stimulation, sympathetic or parasympathetic, to an organ or system. Some theories stress that the effect is simply muscular and may be due to localized ischemia. Others state that painful stimuli or muscular contraction reduces because of accommodation. Accommodation occurs many times during the day. A person who wears eyeglasses becomes unaware of the stimuli of the frame resting on the bridge of the nose. We become less aware of our clothing as we proceed through the day. However, a collar or waistband that intermittently irritates may be more noticeable than one, however tight, that is constantly irritating.

Stimulation, also used for thousands of years, may be directed toward the muscle or the underlying structures. A flaccid muscle may be stimulated to activity by pressuring or kneading. This may activate some of the stretch receptors, such as the muscle spindle apparatus, and the body of the muscle contracts. When used to address visceral concerns, the effect may be stimulation of the parasympathetic or sympathetic underlying components. Stimulation in the suboccipital region or along the sacrum may initiate the former, whereas activity in the thoracolumbar spine may involve the latter.

With either of these techniques, the physician may intend to accomplish a certain goal, but it is the patient's response that is important. Changes in health may not occur so much because of a simple "knob turning" approach. As physicians using manipulative medicine, we facilitate the individual's own ability to reset his or her condition back to the more normal, functional state.

PALPATION
Eileen L. DiGiovanna

Palpation is a particularly important means of uncovering information. Palpation can disclose subtle changes in the texture of the soft tissues of the body—the skin, fascia, muscles, ligaments, and tendons. Tissue changes that occur in response to the effects of sympathetic innervation may be manifested by an increase or decrease in skin temperature or moisture. Edema of the underlying soft tissues may produce a palpable bogginess. Changes in the quality of joint motion may be felt before they produce visible symptoms. Deeper palpation is used to search for masses, outline organ size and consistency, test muscle tone, and feel the impulse of the heart.

During palpation, the physician concentrates on the sensations received through the fingers and hands. The distribution and depth of receptor organs determine which part of the hand is most useful in specific tests. Since the heat receptors lie deep, the ulnar or dorsal aspect of the hand, where the skin is thinner than on the palms, should be used to test for temperature changes.

Touch receptors such as Merkel's disks and Meissner's corpuscles are most numerous in the pads of the fingers, making these the most sensitive areas.

Observation is an important aid to palpation. The area being examined should be inspected for color changes (pallor) or erythema (redness). Increased erythema may indicate infection or inflammation and commonly occurs with acute somatic dysfunction. Pallor may occur with chronic somatic dysfunction. The physician should also look for signs of trauma, such as scars, bruises, lacerations, abrasions, and swelling. Blemishes or masses on the skin's surface should be noted.

Palpation

The following is an organized approach to the development of palpatory skills.

Temperature Changes
1. Palpate lightly. Pressure or friction causes vasodilation, creating temperature changes.
2. See which area of the hand is most sensitive to temperature: the back or side of the hand, the fingertips, the wrist. (Thinner-skinned areas are most sensitive.)
3. Palpate various areas of the back to discriminate temperature differences. The thoracic area is usually warmer because of the underlying heart and great vessels. Compare the skin temperature in several individuals.

Evaluation of Skin Drag
1. Slide fingertips lightly across the surface of the skin to see if any drag can be felt on the fingertips.
2. Increased drag may be due to a fine film of moisture.
3. A decrease in drag may be due to excessive moisture, oily skin, or abnormally atrophic skin.

Evaluation of Skin Texture
1. Palpate for roughness or smoothness. Compare individual skin differences.
2. Feel for sebaceous activity (oiliness).
3. Try palpating through cloth to get the feel of its effect on sensations.

Palpation of Fluid in Tissues
1. Excess fluid in tissues is called *edema*. Edema results in a spongy or boggy feel to the tissues.

Edema of significant proportions may accumulate over the sacrum or anterior aspect of the lower legs and ankles. It is also found in hives or welts.

Turgor (Elastic Rebound of the Skin)
1. Pick up the skin, then release it.
2. Observe how it returns to its former tautness. If the skin returns to its original state immediately, it has normal turgor. If the skin remains tented, it has poor turgor.

Evaluation of Erythema (Red Reflex)
1. Rub the skin with the fingers in a firm stroke. Observe for blanching (whiteness) or erythema (redness). Note the length of time required for the skin color to return to normal.

   Note: Are both sides equally red? Does the redness fade equally? Does one side remain red longer than the other? Areas of acute somatic dysfunction tend to remain red longer.

Lack of turgor is found in dehydration, aging, and certain metabolic diseases.

Tenderness
1. Tenderness is a subjective rather than an objective finding. Palpation of certain areas may cause the sensation of pain to the patient. This is known as tenderness. Because it is subjective, this finding is not as reliable as the objective findings of the physician.

LAYER-BY-LAYER PALPATION
During palpation, it is helpful to mentally visualize the depth of the palpation. A gradually increasing pressure of the fingertips gives the sensations and textures of structures deeper and deeper in the body.

Subcutaneous Tissues
Beneath the surface of the skin lie the subcutaneous tissues, consisting of various connective tissues, fascia, and fat. These tissues normally have a slightly spongy feel. Edema fluid may collect here and produce a "doughy" feel.

In these tissues lie some of the superficial blood vessels. Palpate veins over the back of the hand or in the antecubital fossa. Occlusion with a tourniquet makes the veins more prominent. Note the springy feel. Palpate the radial and carotid arteries. Note that they are much firmer than unoccluded veins. Palpate the back for any abnormal tensions in the subcutaneous tissues. This may indicate contracture or fibrous changes of the fascia.

Muscle
Muscle tissue consists of bundles of fibers arranged in parallel fashion.

1. Press more deeply into the tissues until you contact the firmer muscle tissues.
2. Select several large muscles (trapezius, biceps, sternocleidomastoid, deltoid) and follow the directions of their fibers to the muscle attachments.
3. Palpate the paraspinal muscles, feeling for the following:
   a. **Tone:** The normal feel of a resting muscle (if palpation is too rough it may change the tone):
      i. *Hypertonic*—an increase in normal tone
      ii. *Hypotonic*—a decrease in normal tone
      iii. *Atonic*—no tone; a limp, flaccid muscle
   b. **Contraction:** Normal tension built up in muscle as it shortens
   c. **Contracture:** Abnormal fixing of a muscle in a shortened position with fibrous changes in the tissue
   d. **Spasm:** Abnormal contraction maintained beyond physiologic need
   e. **Bogginess:** Increased fluid in a hypertonic muscle; feels like a wet sponge
   f. **Ropiness:** Cordlike or ropelike feel to a muscle that has been chronically contracted
   g. **Stringiness:** A finer version of ropiness—the muscle feels as if it were made of tense strings

Tendons
Tendons are fibroelastic strands of connective tissue attaching muscle to bone.

1. Palpate the Achilles tendon at the heel and the biceps tendon at the elbow.

Ligaments
Ligaments are tough fibrous bands that connect bone to bone. Since they lie very deep, they are difficult to palpate. Some are not accessible to palpation.

1. The lateral collateral ligament of the knee may be palpated by asking the patient to cross his or her legs so that one ankle lies on the knee of the other leg. The knee should be flexed and the thigh externally rotated. The ligament may be palpated crossing the joint space laterally and slightly posteriorly.

References

Barry G. 1984. Lecture, Physiology. Old Westbury, NY: New York College of Osteopathic Medicine.

Becker FR. 1975. The meaning of fascia and continuity. Osteopath Ann 3:8–32.

Bullock J, Boyle J III, Wang MB, Ajello RR. 1984. The National Medical Series for Independent Study: Physiology. New York: John Wiley.

Cathie AG. 1966. Manual of Osteopathic Principles and Practice—Second year, article C-17. Philadelphia: Philadelphia College of Osteopathy.

Denslow JS, Korr IM, Krems AD. 1949. Quantitative studies of chronic facilitation in human motoneuron pools. Am J Physiol 150:229–238.

Ettlinger H. 1987. Myofascial Release. Osteopathic Principles and Practice. Old Westbury, NY: NYCOM.

Ganong WF. 1981. Review of Medical Physiology. Palo Alto, Calif: Lange Medical Publications.

Guyton AC. 1986. Textbook of Medical Physiology, 7th ed. Philadelphia: W.B. Saunders.

Hollinshead HW. 1974. Textbook of Anatomy, 3rd ed. Hagerstown, Md: Harper & Row.

Kandel E, Schwartz JH. 1985. Principles of Neural Science. New York: Science Publishing.

Korr IM, 1986. Somatic dysfunction, osteopathic manipulative treatment and the nervous system: A few facts, some theories, many questions. J Am Osteopath Assoc 86(2):109–114.

————, Appeltauer, GSL. 1970. Continued studies on axonal transport of nerve proteins to muscle. J am Osteopath Assoc 69:76–78.

————, Chornock FW, Cole WV, Wilkinson PN. 1967. Studies in trophic mechanisms: Does changing its nerve change a muscle? J Am Osteopath Assoc 66:79–80.

————, Wilkinson PN, Chornock FW. 1966. Studies in neurotrophic mechanisms (abstr). J Am (Osteopath Assoc 65:990–991.

————, Wilkinson PN, Chornock FW. 1967. Axonal delivery of neuroplasmic components to muscle cells. J Am Osteopath Assoc 66:1057–1061.

Langley LL, Telford IR, Christensen JB. 1980. Dynamic Anatomy and Physiology. New York: McGraw-Hill.

Moritan T, Moramatsu S, Neuo M. 1987. Activity of the motor unit during concentric and eccentric contractions. Am J Physiol 66:338–350.

Nicholas AS. 1978. Palpation in osteopathic medicine. Osteopath Ann 67:36–42.

Patterson MM, Howell JN, eds. 1992. The Central Connection: Somatovisceral/Viscerosomatic Interaction: 1989 International Symposium. Athens, Ohio: University Classics, Ltd.

Sauer GC. 1980. Manual of Skin Diseases, 4th ed. Philadelphia: J.B. Lippincott.

Schiowitz S, DiGiovanna E, Ausman P. 1981. An Osteopathic Approach to Diagnosis and Treatment Westbury, NY:NYCOM.

Smith PE, Copenhaver WM, eds. 1984. Bailey's Textbook of Histology. Baltimore: Williams & Wilkins.

Taber W. 1970. Taber's Cyclopedic Medical Dictionary, 2nd ed. Philadelphia: F.A. Davis.

Upledger JE, Vredeboogd JD. 1983. Craniosacral Therapy, chap. 5. Seattle: Eastland Press.

Willard FH, Patterson MM, eds. 1994. Nociception and the Neuroendocrine-Immune Connection: 1992 International Symposium. Athens, Ohio: University Classics, Ltd.

Williams PL, Warwick R, eds. 1980. Gray's Anatomy, 36th ed. Philadelphia: W.B. Saunders.

3

Static Symmetry

STATIC SYMMETRY
Stanley Schiowitz

Any observation of a patient that can be used to differentiate normal from abnormal function is an asset in determining a differential diagnosis. Changes in skin color, gait, or regional motion restrictions are used daily to this end. This chapter describes ideal and variant postures of an immobile, upright patient as seen in the sagittal, anterior, and posterior planes. The technique of examination and common causes of abnormal findings are described in the next section.

Sagittal Plane Symmetry
In an ideal erect posture, a plumb line dropped from the ceiling along the body's midline would pass through the following points:

1. Slightly posterior to the apex of the coronal suture
2. Through the external auditory meatus
3. Through the bodies of most of the cervical vertebrae
4. Through the shoulder joint
5. Through the bodies of the lumbar vertebrae
6. Slightly posterior to the axis of the hip joint
7. Slightly anterior to the axis of the knee joint
8. Slightly anterior to the lateral malleolus

Any deviation from these relationships is considered a normal variant or an abnormal postural relationship.

PHYSIOLOGIC CURVES IN THE SAGITTAL PLANE
The adult has four normal sagittal curves, as follows:

1. In the cervical region, C1 to C7, convex forward, normal lordosis
2. In the thoracic region, T1 to T12, concave forward, normal kyphosis
3. In the lumbar region, L1 to L5, convex forward, normal lordosis
4. In the sacral region, the fused sacrum, concave forward

These curves are physiologic and biomechanical, and were created by the body's functional development. At birth, the cervical, thoracic, and lumbar vertebrae form one continuous kyphotic (concave forward) curve. As the cervical extensor muscles develop, allowing the head to stay raised, the normal cervical (convex forward) lordosis develops. As the child begins to stand and walk, the back muscles strengthen and normal lumbar lor-

An Osteopathic Approach to Diagnosis and Treatment, second edition
Eileen L. DiGiovanna and Stanley Schiowitz
Lippincott–Raven Publishers, Philadelphia © 1997.

dosis (convex forward) is achieved. This process begins at about age 3 years and is fully developed by the 10th year. The thoracic spine retains its kyphotic posture, but the angle of the curve is usually decreased.

TRANSITIONAL ARTICULATIONS

The normal sagittal spinal curve changes from anterior convexity to anterior concavity and back at specific articulations: C7 on T1, T12 on L1, and L5 on the sacral base. These articulations have special osteologic constructions that assist in maintaining balance and reduce local mechanical stress. A transition in the curve at any other articulation causes local strain and dysfunction.

The sagittal spinal curves are interrelated in function. An increase in lumbar lordosis will result in increased thoracic kyphosis and increased cervical lordosis. In addition, the curves promote spinal flexibility and strength, allowing the spine to withstand stress. The spine has elastic properties under force, aiding the supporting function of the ligaments and muscles. A straight spine would transmit vector forces through the vertebral bodies, contributing to fracture.

SACRAL BASE RELATIONSHIP

The normal angle between the lumbar spine and the sacral base is 25 to 35 degrees (in the sagittal plane). A greater or lesser angle will affect the lumbar curve and cause compensatory changes in the curves higher in the spine.

Flexion of the sacrum in the sagittal plane increases lumbar lordosis (anterior convexity). This will be accompanied by a similar increase in thoracic kyphosis and cervical lordosis. Extension of the sacrum reduces the lumbar anterior convexity, decreasing lumbar lordosis and providing a similar flattening of the thoracic and cervical curves.

COMMON VARIATIONS IN SAGITTAL POSTURES

1. **Kypholordotic posture** (Fig. 3-1A)
   Head forward
   Cervical spine lordotic
   Thoracic spine kyphotic
   Scapulae abducted
   Lumbar spine lordotic
   Anterior pelvic tilt
   Hip joints slightly flexed
   Knee joints extended

   Plantar flexion of ankle joints in relation to angle of legs
   Anterior bulging of abdomen
2. **Swayback posture** (Fig. 3-1B)
   Head forward
   Cervical spine lordotic, thoracic spine kyphotic
   Decreased lordosis of lumbar spine
   Posterior tilt of pelvis
   Hip and knee joints hyperextended
3. **Flat back posture** (Fig. 3-1C)
   Head forward
   Cervical spine has slightly increased lordosis
   Thoracic spine slightly kyphotic in upper portion, then flattens in lower segments
   Lumbar lordosis flattened
   Hips and knees extended
4. **Military-bearing posture** (Fig. 3-1D)
   Created by drilling in "chest out, stomach in" position
   Head tilted slightly posteriorly
   Cervical curve and thoracic curve normal
   Chest elevated, creating anterior cervical and posterior thoracic deviation from plumb line
   Increased lordosis of lumbar curve
   Anterior pelvic tilt
   Knees extended
   Ankles plantar flexed
5. **Anterior postural deviation** (Fig. 3-1E)
   Entire body leans forward, deviating anteriorly from the plumb line
   Patient's weight supported by metatarsals
6. **Posterior postural deviation** (Fig. 3-1F)
   Entire body leans backward, deviating posteriorly from plumb line
   Balance maintained by anterior thrust of pelvis and hips
   Marked lordosis from midthoracic spine down
7. **Rotary posture** (Fig. 3-1G)
   Body rotated to right or left
   Entire body may be involved, with rotation beginning from ankles and proceeding up
   Lateral alignment appears completely different when viewed from right and left sides; in scoliotic posture, rotation primarily of thorax, in direction of scoliotic convexity
8. **Lumbar lordosis**
   Number of variations, described by increase in lumbar curve and height of curve
   Simple lordosis: lordotic curve increased but contained within the lumbar region
   High lordosis: lumbar lordotic curve passes into thoracic region, including half to two thirds of thoracic spine in anterior convexity; apex

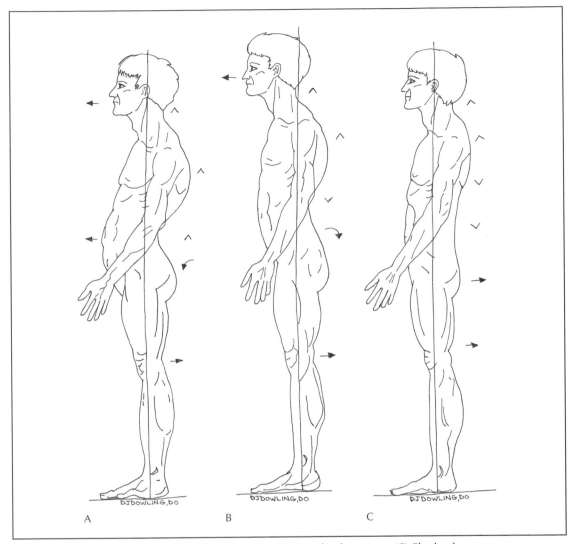

Figure 3-1. **(A)** Kypholordotic posture. **(B)** Swayback posture. **(C)** Flat back posture.

of curve moves upward toward first lumbar vertebra

These described variations of posture are commonly created by changes in pelvic, hip, and knee angles, or by multiple combinations of muscle hypo- and hypertonicities.

LOCALIZED THORACIC FLATTENING

The examiner may find a localized area of thoracic spine, encompassing no more than three contiguous vertebrae, that exhibits severe flattening of the usual kyphotic pattern. This relationship can occur at an area of change of direction of a scoliotic curve, such as a right convexity becoming a left convexity. If rotation in both directions is severe, the spinous processes of the vertebrae involved will be rotated off the midline. Failure of these processes to point directly posteriorly causes the flattened appearance.

Localized thoracic flattening may also be due to chronic somatic dysfunction in two contiguous

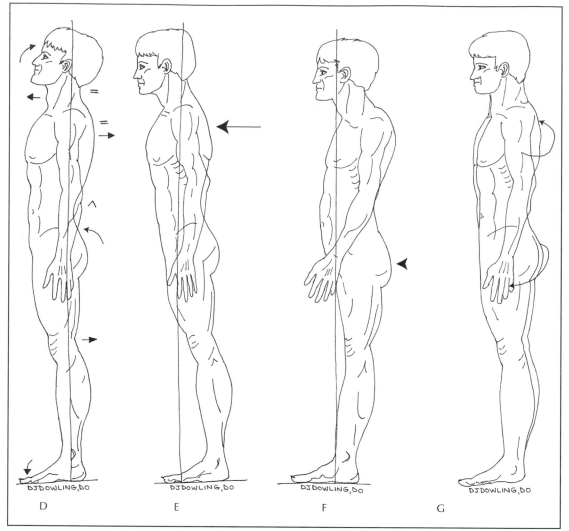

Figure 3-1. *(continued)* **(D)** Military-bearing posture. **(E)** Anterior postural deviation. **(F)** Posterior postural deviation. **(G)** Rotary posture.

vertebrae. The examiner should look for a segmentally related visceral-somatic reflex pattern as the underlying cause. Chronic visceral pathology can cause this condition.

Posterior Plane Symmetry

In a completely symmetric posture (Fig. 3-2), a plumb line dropped from the ceiling to the floor would pass through the following points:

1. The inion
2. The midline of the vertebrae

3. The midline of the sacrum
4. The midline of the coccyx
5. A point midway between both medial malleoli

In addition, all the points of reference described for sequential observation in the next section (Technique of Static Symmetry Examination) should be level and symmetric.

SCOLIOSIS

Muscles and ligaments balance the spine bilaterally. A second group of muscles maintains the position and alignment of the scapular girdle with

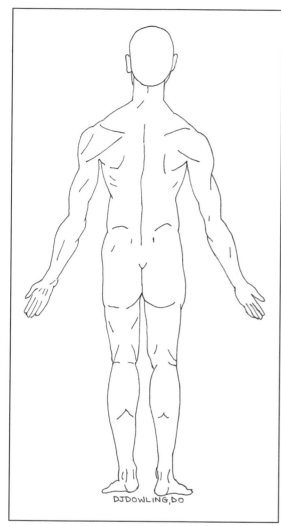

Figure 3-2. Posterior view of the body. An ideal plumb line alignment is shown.

respect to the spine. A difference in function between muscles and ligaments on the two sides of the spine will pull the spine out of alignment. The spine is not rigid but is made up of multiple movable vertebral links. In response to asymmetric pull, one or more vertebrae will move from the position of symmetry. This vertebral motion can occur in three planes—the sagittal plane (flexion-extension), horizontal plane (rotation), or frontal plane (side-bending)—and always represents a combination of multiple planar motions.

Scoliosis is defined as an appreciable deviation of a group of vertebrae from the normal straight vertical line of the spine, as viewed in the posterior plane. Scoliosis can be structural (organic) or functional. A structural curve is fixed: when the patient side bends into the convexity of the curve, it does not straighten out. A functional scoliotic pattern will correct with side-bending. If an acute muscle contracture is causing a scoliotic appearance, placing the patient in the prone position will straighten the curve. A functional scoliotic curve that remains uncorrected for a number of years can give rise to musculoskeletal changes and become a fixed structural curve.

Harrison Fryette in *Principles of Osteopathic Technique* discussed specific coupled motion patterns. Of relevance here, when the spine is at rest, normal lateral flexion in one direction will cause the vertebral body to rotate in the opposite direction. (This rule applies only to the thoracic and lumbar regions.) If a group of vertebrae side-bends toward the right, the vertebral bodies will rotate to the left. If this vertebral position is fixed, the patient would have a scoliotic curve. The scoliosis is said to have a *left convexity*. The spinous processes are deviated to the right of the midline and the left transverse processes are rotated posteriorly. If the thoracic region is involved, the rib cage will rotate and side-bend with the vertebrae. The ribs will be more posterior and separated on the left side. The scapular girdle may follow the rib cage in its displacement.

Muscle imbalance, representing unilateral hypo- or hypertonicity, will create scoliotic patterns. The examiner must be aware of the line of force of the muscles involved, and of the complexity of multiple muscle actions at one region. The assignment of cause or effect to postural changes requires a thorough understanding of functional anatomy.

What happens to the spine when the sacral base is not level? In the frontal plane, sacral base unleveling will cause a lumbar scoliotic pattern convex in the direction of the inferior sacral side, if the spine is flexible. The convexity may continue up through the thoracic region to create one thoracolumbar C-shaped scoliotic curve (Fig. 3-3). The body tries to compensate for the imbalance created by the C curve by creating a secondary, compensatory curve above the first lumbar curve. The side of convexity of the second curve is opposite that of the primary curve, producing an S-shaped curve (Fig. 3-4). Additional compensatory scoliotic curves can develop higher in the spine, into

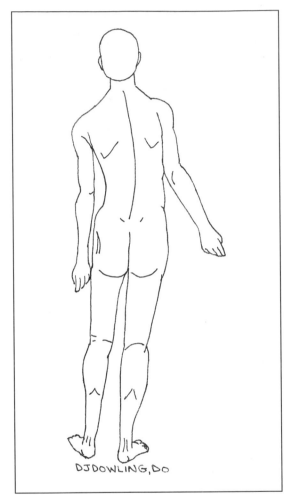

Figure 3-3. C-shaped curve due to sacral base unleveling, posterior view.

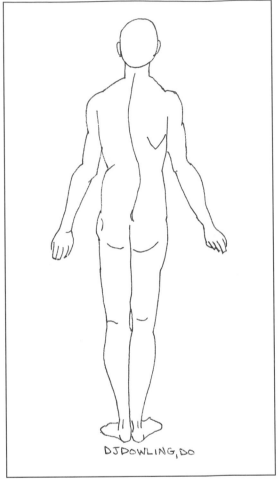

Figure 3-4. S-shaped curve compensating for thoracolumbar scoliosis, posterior view.

the cervical region, with alternating convexities. Because the body always attempts to maintain the eyes on a level plane, the last compensatory maneuver may be side-bending of the head. The body waist crease lines usually follow the pattern of the largest scoliotic asymmetry. The waist crease would have the most acute angle at the site and side of the greatest lateral flexion concave curve.

FACTORS THAT COMMONLY INFLUENCE OR CAUSE SCOLIOSIS (see Chap. 27)
1. Structural or organic scoliosis—all causes
2. Bone deformities caused by congenital etiology, trauma, or disease
3. Muscle tone changes due to hypo- or hypertonicity, hypertrophy, or atrophy
4. Postural changes created by habits or occupation
5. Unilateral structural changes: Short leg or unilateral flat foot or pronation. Tibial torsion, knee deformity, or hip deformity. Sacral torsion or pelvic torsion
6. Somatic dysfunctions
7. Compensatory and noncompensatory fascial patterns (see Chap. 24)

Common Variations of Frontal Postures
1. **Right-handedness**
   a. Upper thoracic scoliosis, concave to right
   b. Right shoulder lower than left
   c. Right buttock deviated away from midline

2. **Left-handedness**
   a. Upper thoracic scoliosis, concave to left
   b. Left shoulder lower than right
   c. Left buttock deviated away from midline
3. **S-type compensated structural scoliosis**
   a. The lumbar and thoracic scoliotic convexities are in opposite directions
   b. The rib cage will rotate posteriorly with the thoracic convexity
   c. The shoulders may be level
   d. The iliac crest heights may be level
   e. The buttocks are not deviated away from the midline
4. **C-type compensated structural scoliosis**
   a. Thoracic and lumbar scoliotic convexity form one continuous curve in same direction
   b. Rib cage rotated posteriorly with thoracic convexity
   c. Buttocks not deviated away from midline
   d. Iliac crest heights may be level
5. **Lateral pelvic tilt functional curve, cephalad on right, C-type**
   a. Thoracic and lumbar curves continuous and convex to left
   b. Scapula lower on right
   c. Rib cage rotated posteriorly on left

d. Waist crease has more acute angle on right
e. Neck laterally tilted to left

6. **Lateral pelvic tilt functional curve, cephalad on right, S-type**
   a. If compensated, should act as described in item 3, except that iliac crest height is higher on right
7. **Unilateral erector spinal muscle hypertonicity**
   a. Side-bending of spine in direction of hypertonic muscle
   b. Scoliotic convexity in opposite direction
   c. Elevated iliac crest on side of hypertonicity
   d. Placing patient prone should change above findings
8. **Unilateral upper trapezius muscle hypertonicity**
   a. Head tilted toward side of hypertonic muscle
   b. Shoulder girdle elevated on affected side
   c. Scapula on hypertonic muscle side-rotated upward and slightly adducted

The patterns of asymmetry described in this chapter are not all-inclusive. The body exhibits various biomechanical responses to all factors that influence the musculoskeletal system.

TECHNIQUE OF STATIC SYMMETRY EXAMINATION
Stanley Schiowitz

A postural examination begins with the patient and physician in a fixed, reproducible position, so that observations may be correlated with observations made on future examinations. The patient stands on a level surface, without shoes. All extremities should be in full extension. The feet are placed 6 to 8 inches apart with the heels in the same frontal plane and the toes abducted about 15 degrees. The physician stands facing the aspect of the patient to be evaluated (front, back, or side) and at a sufficient distance to permit a complete body view. In the course of the examination the physician will step closer to observe local areas of interest. The examiner's eyes should be at the level of the part being viewed, which may entail crouching or kneeling during evaluation of lower body portions. Light palpation may be used to confirm anatomic landmarks or observations. Areas of observation are highlighted in Figure 3-5.

Posterior View
For posterior inspection, a good method is to observe the patient in the following sequence:

DISTANT EVALUATION, POSTERIOR VIEW
1. General observation of gross body symmetry and asymmetry
2. Achilles tendon
3. Medial malleoli
4. Popliteal lines
5. Gluteal creases
6. Greater trochanters
7. Posterior superior iliac spines
8. Heights of iliac crests
9. Thoracolumbar spines for deviations from midline symmetry, or flattening
10. Waist creases
11. Level of inferior angles of scapula, abduction-adduction

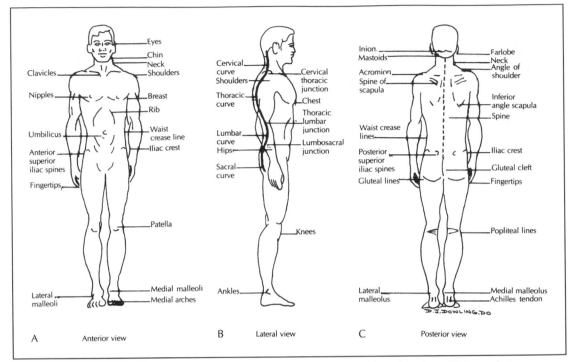

Figure 3-5. Points of interest on the static symmetry examination. (**A**) Anterior view. (**B**) Lateral view. (**C**) Posterior view.

12. Rib cage rotation or scapular rotation
13. Level of shoulders
14. Level of fingertips
15. Deviation of cervical spine and skull from midline
16. Level of earlobes

Note the following factors:

1. Head
2. Earlobes
3. Neck
4. Shoulders
5. Shoulder girdles
6. Spine
7. Rib cage
8. Waist crease lines
9. Iliac crests
10. Gluteal creases
11. Fingertips
12. Popliteal creases
13. Achilles tendons
14. Heels

After gaining an overall impression, the examiner steps within arm's length of the patient and adds palpation to confirm visual observation. The sequence of observations is repeated.

CLOSE EVALUATION WITH PALPATION, POSTERIOR VIEW

1. Is the head straight? Palpate the inion. Is it in the midline?
2. With one finger on the inion, place a finger of the other hand at the gluteal cleft. Are they in a line directly above each other?
3. Touch the earlobes; measure their heights. Touch the tips of the mastoid bones. Are they level?
4. Are the neck and head tilted?
5. Put one finger of each hand on the right and left trapezius muscles where the neck meets the trunk. Are they level?
6. Slide those fingers laterally to the top of each acromium process. Are they level?
7. Place one finger at the inferior angle of each

scapula, about the level of the seventh thoracic vertebra. Are they level?

8. Move both fingers up the vertebral borders of the scapulae to their spinous processes. Are they level?

9. Place a palm flat on the posterior surface of each scapula, with your fingers resting on the superior scapular border. Are the scapulae rotated? Are they level?

10. Have the patient bend forward. Slide your palms over the angles of the ribs. Is there an exaggerated rib hump indicating scoliotic convexity?

11. Place one finger on the spinous process of the first thoracic vertebra. Slide it down the spine, one vertebra at a time, to the sacrum. Are the spinous processes symmetric with respect to each other in all three planes?
    a. *Frontal plane*—feel for deviation from the midline.
    b. *Sagittal plane*—feel for depression or prominence.
    c. *Horizontal plane*—feel the space between the tips of the spinous processes. Are they equal?
    d. Do areas of the spine seem flat?

12. Follow the waist crease lines. Are the angles equal? Does the more acute angle coincide with the concavity of a spinal scoliosis?

13. Measure the posterior superior iliac spines bilaterally. Place your thumb or index finger at each dimple in the lower back. Identify the most prominent (posterior) bony point. Bend down by flexing your knees, so that your eyes are at finger level. Note the following:
    a. Are they at the same height?
    b. Are they of the same depth?

14. Move these fingers up the iliac crest until they are resting on the uppermost portion of the ilium bilaterally. Are the crest heights level?

15. Place a finger of each hand at the gluteal lines. Move your eyes to that level. Are the lines level?

16. Bend down further and measure the heights of the popliteal lines. Are they level?

17. Measure the distance from the fingertips to the floor.

18. Trace each Achilles tendon to its insertion. Are they bowed or straight?

Anterior View

The sequence for anterior observation is as follows:

DISTANT EVALUATION, POSTERIOR VIEW
1. General observation of gross body symmetry and asymmetry
2. Medial longitudinal arches
3. Medial malleoli
4. Patellas
5. Greater trochanters
6. Anterior superior iliac spines
7. Heights of iliac crests
8. Waist creases
9. Rib cage angle
10. Rib cage rotation
11. Nipple levels—males or children only
12. Level of shoulders
13. Level of fingertips
14. Deviation of cervical spine and skull from midline
15. Level of earlobes
16. Level of eyes

Note the following factors:

1. Head
2. Eyes
3. Neck
4. Chin
5. Shoulders
6. Clavicles
7. Chest wall
8. Rib angle
9. Nipples
10. Umbilicus
11. Iliac crests
12. Patellas
13. Fingertips
14. Medial malleoli
15. Medial arches

After completing the general evaluation, the examiner moves forward and adds palpation to confirm visual observations.

CLOSE EVALUATION WITH PALPATION, ANTERIOR VIEW
1. Is the head straight? Palpate the earlobes.
2. Are eyes level?

3. Is the chin deviated from midline?
4. Palpate and measure the shoulder heights at the top of the acromium processes. Are they level?
5. Palpate and measure the clavicle heights. Are they level?
6. Note chest wall symmetry and rotation. If asymmetric, does it match the posterior view findings?
7. Note nipple heights (men and children only).
8. Measure the rib cage angle and the angle of the arm at the elbow.
9. Is the umbilicus at the midline? Are there scars on the abdomen?
10. Palpate the waist crease lines and note their length and angle.
11. Palpate the anterior superior iliac spines and note their heights and anterior posterior orientation (examiner's eyes at that level).
12. Follow the iliac crests to their greatest heights and measure them (examiner's eyes at that level). Are they equal?
13. Palpate the superior aspect of both patellae and measure their heights (examiner's eyes at that level). Are they level? Do they point anteriorly, medially, or laterally?
14. Measure the heights of the tips of the fingers from the floor. Are they equal? Are the hands internally rotated?
15. Measure the heights of the lowest aspect of each medial malleolus from the floor. Are they equal?
16. Measure the height of each medial arch. Are they equal?

Sagittal Plane View

DISTANT EVALUATION, SAGITTAL VIEW
1. Head
2. Cervical curve
3. Cervical-thoracic junction
4. Thoracic curve
5. Thoracolumbar junction
6. Lumbar curve
7. Lumbosacral junction
8. Sacral curve
9. Shoulders
10. Hips
11. Knees
12. Ankles
13. Anterior silhouette, chest to abdomen

With these observations in mind, the examiner moves forward and adds palpation to confirm visual observations, reproducing the sequence of evaluation.

CLOSE EVALUATION WITH PALPATION, SAGITTAL PLANE VIEW
1. Is the head displaced anteriorly?
2. Is the anteroposterior cervical curve exaggerated or flattened?
3. Is the transition from the cervical lordosis to thoracic kyphosis a smooth minimal curve?
4. Is the upper thoracic posterior convexity increased?
5. Is the thoracic posterior convexity a smooth curve? Is its kyphosis exaggerated? Do segments seem flattened?
6. Is the thoracolumbar junction at the articulation of the 12th thoracic and first lumbar vertebrae? Is the transitional curve smooth?
7. Is the lumbar anteroposterior curve smooth? Is it exaggerated or flattened?
8. Is the lumbosacral junction a smooth transitional curve? Does the lumbosacral angle appear normal?
9. Is there marked posterior angulation of the sacrum?
10. Look directly at the nearest shoulder. Is it forward, depressed, rotated? Can you see the other shoulder without moving your head?
11. Repeat the same examination with the scapulae and rib cage. Are they rotated?
12. Is the body rotated?
13. Bend down and look at the hips. Are they rotated? Are they fully extended?
14. Look at the knees. Are they rotated? Are they fully extended? Are they hyperextended?
15. Look at the ankles. Are they rotated?
16. Look at the anterior silhouette. What is the shape and position of the chest? What is the shape and position of the abdomen? What is the relationship of the chest to the abdomen, in position and size?
17. Does the body seem displaced from the midline anteriorly or posteriorly?

FACTORS THAT COMMONLY INFLUENCE THE SAGITTAL CURVES
Osseous-Muscular Factors
1. Bone deformities, of which the most common result from:

a. Congenital deformities of the vertebrae

b. Trauma creating fracture or dislocation

c. Diseases such as tumors, infections, and osteopenia

2. Ventral or dorsal muscle tone changes, commonly caused by:

a. Muscle disuse or atrophy secondary to neurologic disease, immobilization, or age

b. Obesity or pregnancy, creating abdominal muscle stretch

c. Contracture of muscles due to burns, overdevelopment, injuries, or viscerosomatic reflexes

Structural-Mechanical Factors

1. Change in location of transitional areas of the sagittal curves, commonly caused by:

a. Congenital vertebral formation

b. Sacral base imbalance in the sagittal or frontal plane

c. Localized regional scoliotic patterns

d. Organic kyphoscoliosis

e. Wearing high heels

f. Habit or occupation

2. Endomorphic characteristics (usually increase the lordotic curve)

3. Hereditary characteristics (increase lordotic curve)

4. Foot defects such as pronation or calcaneal valgus (increase lumbar lordosis)

5. Genu valgus or varus (influences lumbar curve)

6. Hip joint changes such as femoral ante/retroversion or femoral valgus/varus (influence lumbar curve)

7. Localized somatic dysfunctions (flattened thoracic kyphosis)

General Considerations

In all close examinations, the examiner should use palpation whenever it can help confirm visual observations. The eyes should be at the level of the body part observed during close examinations. Looking up or down can distort the findings. The examiner may bend down by flexing the knees or sit in a suitable chair.

The first observations should be from a distance. The examiner first develops a sense of body symmetry, then uses closer observation and palpation to confirm or rule out initial impressions.

References

Basmajian JV. 1978. Muscles Alive. 4th ed. Baltimore: Williams & Wilkins.

Calliet R. 1975. Scoliosis. Philadelphia: F.A. Davis.

Fryette HH. 1954. Principles of Osteopathic Technique. Colorado Springs: Academy of Applied Osteopathy.

Heilig D. 1978. Some basic considerations of spinal curves. Osteopath Ann 311:318.

Kapandji IA. 1974. Physiology of the Joints, 2nd ed, vol 3. Edinburgh: Churchill Livingstone.

Kendall FP, McCreary EK. 1983. Muscles: Testing and Function, 3rd ed. Baltimore: Williams & Wilkins.

MacConaill MA, Basmajian JV. 1969. Muscles and Movements, 2nd ed. Huntington. NY: Robert E. Krieger.

Northup GW. 1972. Osteopathic lesions. J Am Osteopath Assoc 71:854–864.

Schiowitz S. 1980. Static symmetry and asymmetry. Osteopath Ann 8:9.

4

Spinal Motion

PHYSIOLOGIC MOTION OF THE SPINE
Dennis J. Dowling

In 1918, Harrison Fryette presented a paper on physiologic movements of the vertebral column at the American Osteopathic Association convention. What is now regarded by the osteopathic profession as important diagnostic theory was, by Fryette's account, not enthusiastically received. Much of his work was based on an earlier book by Robert Lovett, *Spinal Curvatures and Round Shoulders.* Before reading this work, Fryette experimented with radiographs and a spine mounted in soft rubber. He analyzed the movement of the vertebral column and developed several principles, now frequently referred to as Fryette's laws. They are not so much laws as guidelines for discriminating different types of dysfunction, determining diagnoses, and delineating treatment.

Physiology of Spinal Motion
In analyzing vertebral motion, it is useful to know the phylogeny involved. Humans were originally quadripeds with the spine in a basically horizontal state. In this position, all weight-bearing was carried by the articular facets (Fig. 4-1). The facets are hard, compact, and sturdy trabecular bone, as opposed to the more cancellous bone of the vertebral bodies.

In the vertical orientation, the articular bodies and intervertebral disks are subject to stresses that gradually compress the disks and further define the shape of the body. Humans are subject to stress fractures, herniations, and bulging disks, conditions virtually unknown in four-footed species. Gravity causes a further approximation of the superior and inferior facets while increasing the overall contribution of the vertebral body joints to spinal movement (Fig. 4-2).

Fryette credited Lovett with conceptualizing the backbone as consisting of two columns (Fig. 4-3). The anterior column is defined by the vertebral bodies and intervertebral disks. As this column is bent, the disks and bodies attempt to accommodate the distortion by moving away from the concave side (Figs. 4-4 through 4-6). The posterior or dorsal column is constituted by the facets, their capsules, and the ligaments. This column behaves as a flexible ruler with its edges oriented laterally. To induce side-bending in this column, Lovett theorized, the region bent must also rotate away from the concave side and toward the convex side. Forward and backward bending can occur without

An Osteopathic Approach to Diagnosis and Treatment, second edition
Eileen L. DiGiovanna and Stanley Schiowitz
Lippincott–Raven Publishers, Philadelphia © 1997.

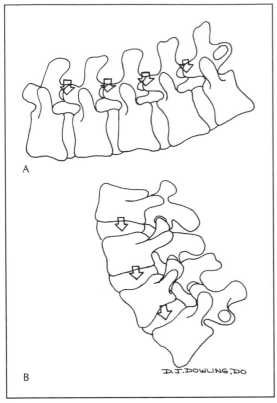

A

B

D.J.DOWLING,DO

Figure 4-1. Weight-bearing in an animal with a horizontal spine (**A**) and in an animal (human) with a vertical spine (**B**).

a secondary rotary movement unless some restriction is present. Together the two columns act synergistically to produce total vertebral motion.

Forward and backward bending in a normal vertebral column occurs with the facets gapping in the first instance and approximating in the second instance (Fig. 4-7). In the nondysfunctional thoracic and lumbar spine, the actions of side-bending and rotation are coupled and occur in opposite directions because of the flexible ruler action of the facets and their attachment.

An exception to coupled motion occurs in the cervical region and is caused by the extreme lordosis, planar relationship, and convergence of the facets. The mechanics in this region dictate that side-bending and rotation are coupled and occur in the same direction (Figs. 4-8 and 4-9).

In the lumbar and thoracic spine, when one vertebra locks on another and a combination of extension–rotation–side-bending or flexion–side-bending–rotation occurs, then the rotation and side-bending are in the same direction. In this situation, as the vertebra moves in any one plane, simultaneous movement is created along the other two component planes.

These observations are summed up in the three principles known as Fryette's principles I, II, and III.

PRINCIPLE I
When any part of the lumbar or thoracic spine is in neutral position, side-bending of a vertebra will be opposite to the side of rotation of that vertebra.

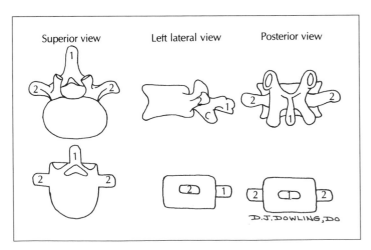

Superior view   Left lateral view   Posterior view

D.J.DOWLING,DO

Figure 4-2. Orientation of the vertebrae (**1**) spinous process; (**2**) transverse process.

Figure 4-3. Lovett-Fryette conception of the backbone as consisting of two columns, the vertebral bodies and intervertebral disks (**A**) and the facets, capsules, and ligaments (**B**), which unite to form the spinal column (**C**).

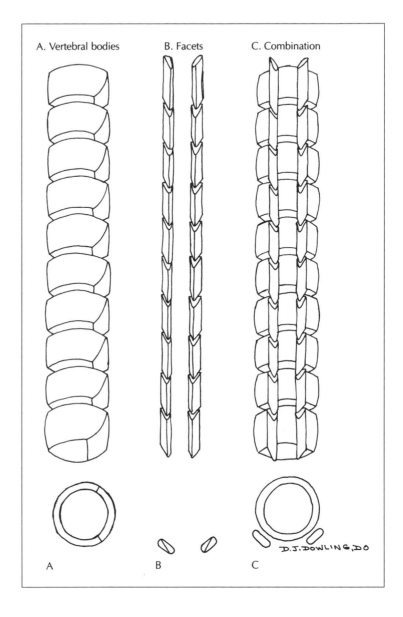

Although this description applies chiefly to the lumbar and thoracic spine in neutral (normal resting) position, it also applies to moderate truncal flexion and extension. The facets must not be in a locked position, nor should there be single-sided tautness of ligaments. Therefore, on clinical examination of the vertebral column, the expected findings should be side-bending and rotation in opposite directions (i.e., when side-bent to the right, the vertebral body will rotate counterclockwise to the left; Fig. 4-10).

Fryette's first principle is of use in analyzing dysfunctions that are most often initiated or maintained by muscle. Ideally the vertebral joints are free from restriction initiated by muscles. The vertebral column acts as a bow, with the muscles acting as a cord that induces a curve when single-sided contraction occurs (Fig. 4-11). The spinal segments compensate for this side-bending by rotating in the opposite direction (Fig. 4-12), and the posterior facets or transverse processes are palpable on the convex side of the lateral curve. A curve

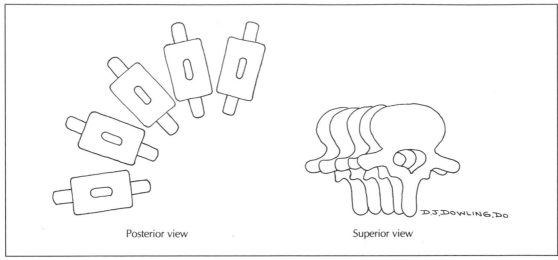

Figure 4-4. Pure (nonphysiologic) vertebral side-bending without the influence of the facet joints.

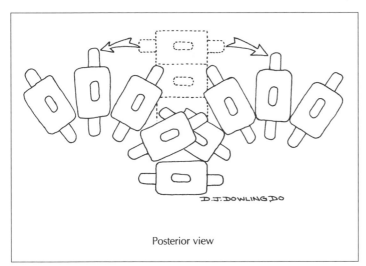

Figure 4-5. Pure (nonphysiologic) vertebral side-bending, without the influence of the facet joints, to each side.

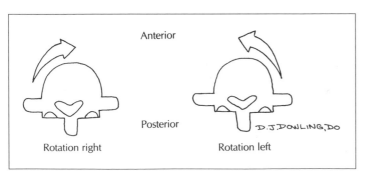

Figure 4-6. Orientation of rotation.

Figure 4-7. Flexion (forward bending) and extension (backward bending) of the spinal column, producing, respectively, gapping and approximation of the articular facets.

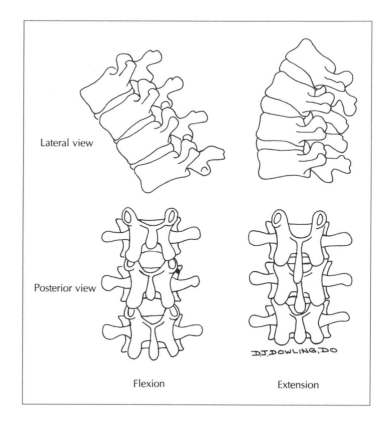

Lateral view

Posterior view

Flexion   Extension

Figure 4-8. Pure (physiologic) cervical vertebral side-bending. Side-bending in the cervical vertebrae occurs in the same direction as rotation.

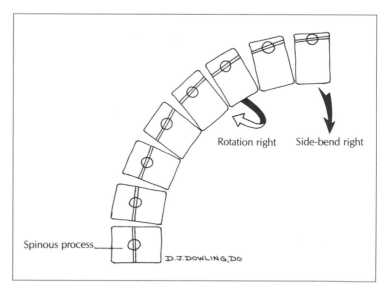

Rotation right   Side-bend right

Spinous process

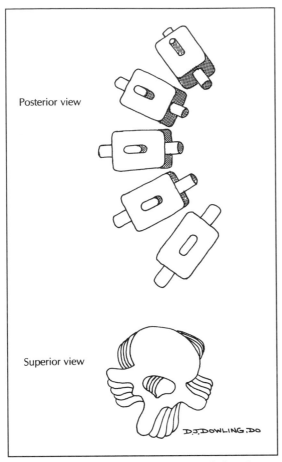

Posterior view

Superior view

D.J.DOWLING.DO

Figure 4-9. Normal cervical motion. Side-bending and rotation occur in the same direction.

of this sort may also represent a response to dysfunction occurring higher or lower in the spinal column (e.g., an unlevel sacral base), in which case it is generally more gradual in onset.

The shorthand notation for the lateral group curve is T3–8N Sr Rl. The 3 denotes the third thoracic segment at the top of the curve and the 8 denotes the eighth thoracic segment at the bottom of the curve. The S indicates the direction of side-bending freedom, in this case to the right, with coupled rotation (R) to the opposite side (left) in the thoracic spine.

PRINCIPLE II
When any part of the spine is in a position of hyperextension or hyperflexion, the side-bending of a vertebra will be to the same side as the rotation of that vertebra.

A type II dysfunction (Fig. 4-13) is primarily a single-segment lesion. The movement has become pathologic and the segment is locked. Muscular involvement may occur but is second in importance to the restriction of the vertebral segment. Any attempt to move the segment along a single plane, whether sagittal, coronal, or horizontal (flexion-extension, side-bending, and rotation, respectively), will produce motion in all planes, thereby initiating a helical movement (Fig. 4-14). The locked segment, rather than alleviating the compression by rotating away when side-bent or by side-bending away when rotated, compensates by side-bending and rotating to the same side.

This phenomenon can be observed when the region of the spine is side-bent with the locked region on the concave side of the curve and the whole spine is flexed or extended. With flexion and extension, the locked segment becomes more noticeable as it is moved in its direction of restriction (Fig. 4-15).

Palpation of single-segment somatic dysfunctions is important for localizing the area of involvement, but the sine qua non for diagnosis is the observation that it follows type II mechanics.

Pain, tenderness, and restricted motion are frequently noted at the site. The onset can be quite abrupt, with the patient aware of the time, duration, and direction of the precipitating event. Such situations may be brought about by unexpected or severe disruption, which may be initiated by sudden movement. Frequently the patient is at the extreme in one plane of the range of motion, then attempts to move in another plane(s) (e.g., the patient is fully flexed, then twists or turns to the side) (Table 4-1).

The single-segment aspect of type II dysfunction does not exclude the occurrence of a series of somatic dysfunctions that all behave in the prescribed manner. In fact, type II dysfunctions are often observed at the beginning, apex, and end of a type I group curve.

Fryette's observations on hyperflexion and hyperextension developed from his study of the movements of cadaver spines, which exhibit the biomechanics of a type II dysfunction when placed at extremes of motion. However, cadaver spines are significantly relaxed and not subject to the stresses of living spines.

Figure 4-10. Type I mechanics: the thoracic and lumbar vertebrae, when side-bent in one direction, will rotate in the opposite direction.

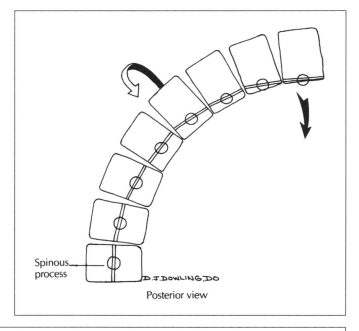

Spinous process

D.J.DOWLING,DO

Posterior view

Figure 4-11. Bowing effect produced by contracted paravertebral muscles.

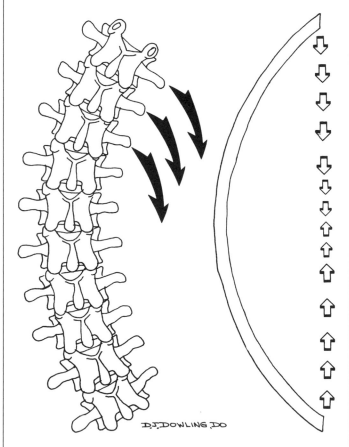

D.J.DOWLING,DO

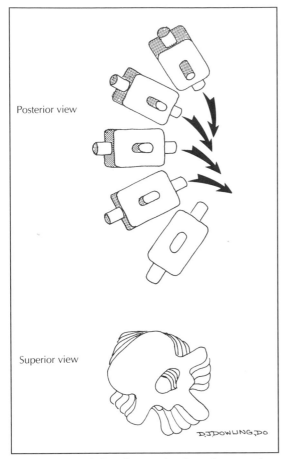

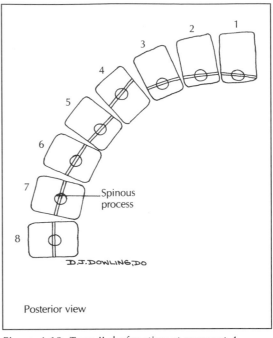

Figure 4-13. Type II dysfunction at segment 4.

Figure 4-12. Side-bending under the influence of the facets: side-bending and rotation occur in opposite directions (Fryette's first principle).

The notation used to describe a type II somatic dysfunction indicates both the single-segment nature and the status of its freedom of movement. L3 E Sl Rl denotes a locking of L3 on L4 in which the top segment moves more easily into side-bending and rotation to the left and extension.

Table 4-1. Summary of Dysfunctions

	Type I Dynamics	Type II Dynamics
Number of segments	Multiple	Single
Rotation/side-bending	Opposite side	Same side
Position of spine	Neutral	Flexion or extension
Clinical appearance	Lateral curve	Flattening or exaggeration of anteroposterior curve
Onset	Usually gradual	Usually abrupt
Site of pain	Either on concave side, because of contracted muscle, or on convex side, because of stretched muscles	Usually over posterior facet

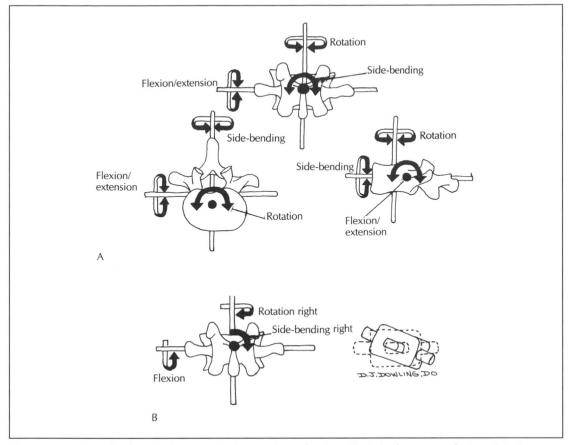

Figure 4-14. **(A)** Helical axes of movement in type II mechanics. **(B)** A single-segment lesion, F Sr Rr.

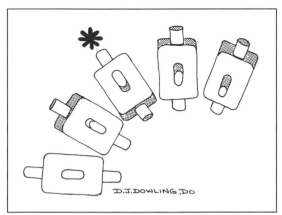

Figure 4-15. Type II dysfunction. Segment marked by asterisk is side-bent and rotated in the same direction, whereas nondysfunctional segments side-bend and rotate in opposite directions.

PRINCIPLE III

Initiating motion of a vertebral segment in any plane of motion will modify the movement of that segment in other planes of motion.

The third principle of coupled action alerts the clinician to spinal limitations. In type I dynamics, an example is the side-bent scoliotic curve. Normal coupled motion includes rotation to the opposite side. An attempt to induce further side-bending is easier when bending is continued in the direction already established. Rotation is similarly modified. Movement in a direction opposite to the established direction is limited. The same observations apply to type II dynamics: movement produced in a direction opposite to the freedom of motion is restricted.

BIOMECHANICS OF JOINT MOTION
Stanley Schiowitz

All bones that have freedom of movement will move on other bones at their respective joints. Several factors influence these motions. Knowledge of why, when, and how joint motion is induced is essential for the understanding of functional anatomy and for the diagnosis and treatment of osteopathic somatic dysfunctions.

General Principles
None of the articulatory surfaces of the body are truly flat. They are ovoid or sellar (saddle-shaped) (Fig. 4-16). The joints that have evolved are an attempt at a mating of these forms: sella to sella, and ovoid convex to ovoid concave. The articulations thus formed are not truly congruent, permitting greater freedom of joint movement and geometrically created coupled and accessory motions.

Figure 4-16. Bony shapes. At this articulation an ovoid shape sits in a sellar shape. Convex and concave surfaces are shown.

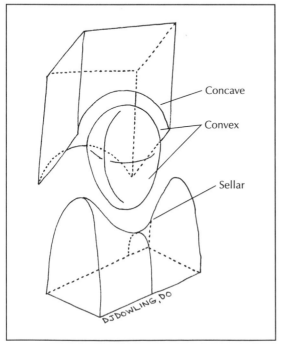

Individual joint motions can be described in terms of spin, roll, and slide. *Spin* is defined as one bone rotating on its mechanical axis, in place, on another bone. *Roll* is defined as movement resulting from an increase or decrease in angle between the two articulating bones. *Slide* (glide) is a translatory motion of one bone sliding over the surface of another bone (Fig. 4-17).

The curved articular surfaces, moving one upon another, develop complex patterns of motions. The coupled motions created by convex-concave mating articulations follow specific patterns. When a concave surface moves on a convex surface, the roll and slide motions are in the same direction. However, when a convex surface moves on a concave surface, the roll and slide motions are in opposite directions.

Femoral extension on the tibia follows these patterns of motion. As the stance leg extends in gait, the femur rolls anteriorly with posterior slide on a fixed tibia (Fig. 4-18). However, the swing leg on extending creates tibial roll and slide anteriorly (in the same direction) on the distal femur (Fig. 4-19). Full femoral extension can be described as an anterior femoral roll with a posterior slide, accompanied at full extension by a medial femoral spin upon the tibia.

The fully extended knee undergoes another prescribed motion in its final stage of extension. This is a conjunct rotation created by the geometry of the articulating surfaces (see Chap. 20, The Knee Joint).

Motion is affected by ligamentous relationships. A "close-packed" joint position is one in which the ligaments have twisted, bringing the bones together into maximum congruence. The bones cannot be separated without first loosening the ligaments. Joint motion is lost, and forces are more easily transmitted through this joint into the next one. Tangential force will more likely cause fracture than sprain.

In weight-bearing joints, the close-packed position replaces muscle activity for maintenance of support. In the spine, motion is transmitted through the bodies of close-packed vertebrae into the first movable zygapophyseal articulation. So-

Figure 4-17. **(A)** Spin, **(B)** roll, **(C)** slide.

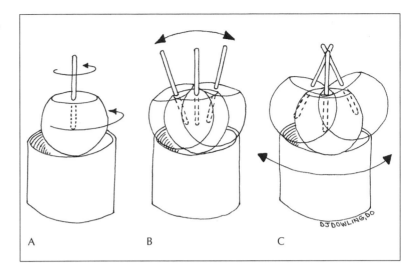

Figure 4-18. Femoral extension on fixed tibia. Roll and slide occur in opposite directions.

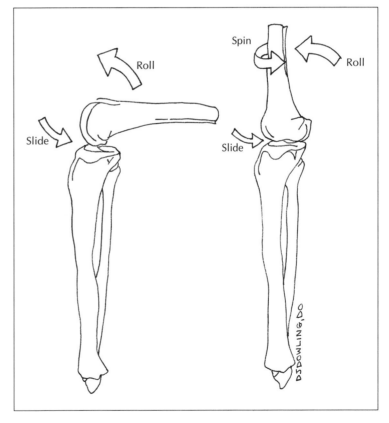

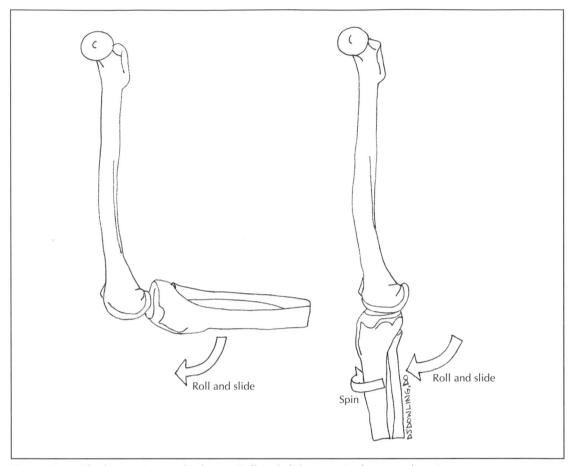

Figure 4-19. Tibial extension on the femur. Roll and slide occur in the same direction.

matic dysfunction can result. The principle of transmittal of motion through close-packed joints is used therapeutically in high-velocity, low-amplitude thrusting techniques.

Articular stability is a combined function of the shape of the joint, its ligamentous and muscular attachments, the strength of its capsule, and the balance of joint pressure to atmospheric pressure. Variation in any of these factors may contribute to somatic dysfunctions.

It is usual to describe motion as occurring in cardinal planes about fixed axes. Shoulder abduction would be described as motion in a frontal plane about an anteroposterior axis. However, we know that the head of the humerus, a convex surface, moves on the concave glenoid fossa with an upward roll and downward slide. Since this is a coupled, continuous motion, it cannot be about a fixed axis. This type of motion is said to be about an *instantaneous axis of rotation*. This axis defines multiple motions, rotary and translatory, that occur simultaneously in the same plane. The abduction motion would require continuous determinations of its instantaneous axis as it moved. This would give a true pathway of the joint motion. This motion is still only in one plane.

In full extension the femur rolls, slides, and spins. The motion is multiplanar and involves more than one axis; it is said to occur on a *helical axis*. The helical axis completely defines a three-dimensional motion between two rigid bodies. Active functional motions, appendicular as well as vertebral, are usually motions about helical axes.

The addition of force to joint motions may bring into play accessory motions. Accessory motions cannot be performed voluntarily; they can only be activated against resistance or by an outside force. An example is long-axis traction on the phalangeal articulations. The restriction of small accessory motions is a major factor in the creation of somatic dysfunctions, especially in the articulations of appendages.

Biomechanics of the Upper Extremities
SHOULDER GIRDLE

Five joints are primarily involved in shoulder girdle function. Three, the glenohumeral, acromioclavicular, and sternoclavicular, are true joints. The suprahumeral and scapulothoracic joints are pseudojoints (Fig. 4-20). These joints may be divided into two functional groups. Joints in the first group, the glenohumeral and suprahumeral joints, act in unison to produce the early motion of shoulder abduction. Joints in the second group, the scapulothoracic, sternoclavicular, and acromioclavicular joints, act in unison to produce the mid to late motions of shoulder abduction.

The movements of the humerus on the glenoid fossa include the following:

1. Flexion and extension in the sagittal plane.
2. Abduction and adduction in the frontal plane.

True adduction is absent because of the presence of the trunk. Relative adduction is the return of the humerus toward midline from the position of abduction. Flexion adduction is humeral movement across the front of the body. Extension adduction is humeral movement across the back of the body.

3. Axial rotation: internal and external rotation of the humeral head.
4. Horizontal plane rotation: flexion plus adduction anteriorly or extension plus adduction posteriorly.
5. Circumduction: the conical motion of the distal end of the humerus as the shoulder moves through all planes.

Abduction-adduction and axial and horizontal rotations are coupled in that angular motions are accompanied by translatory slides. The caudal slide of the humeral head with abduction confers increased freedom of motion on the supraspinatous tendon beneath the coracoacromial ligament.

In addition to the slide motions, the joint exhibits the accessory motion of long-axis extension.

The movements of the individual joints are as follows:

Figure 4-20. Shoulder girdle, anterior view.

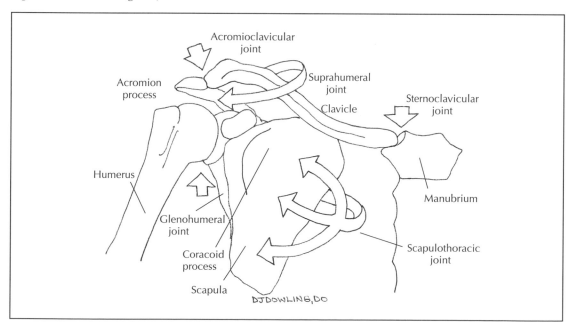

1. The glenohumeral joint has three degrees of cardinal motion: flexion and extension, abduction and adduction, and internal and external rotation.
2. The suprahumeral joint acts in concert with the glenohumeral joint.
3. The scapulothoracic joint movements are related to scapular motions. The motions are medial and lateral movements of the scapula on the thorax (abduction-adduction), elevation and depression of the scapula, and upward and downward rotation of the scapula (tilt), all relative to the glenoid fossa.
4. The sternoclavicular joint moves cephalad and caudad in the frontal plane, moves ventrad and dorsad in the horizontal plane, and rotates on its mechanical axis (Fig. 4-21). All cephalad-caudad and ventrad-dorsad movements are accompanied by translatory slides.
5. The primary motion of the acromioclavicular joint is axial rotation.

The combined axial rotation of the sternoclavicular joint (30 degrees) and the acromioclavicular joint (30 degrees) allows the normal 60 degrees of rotation of the scapula on full abduction of the shoulder.

Total abduction of the shoulder joint can be divided into three phases. During the **first phase** (0 to 90 degrees), the supraspinatus and deltoid muscles are involved. At the beginning of the movement the supraspinatus is very efficient in abduction and in maintaining joint stability, while the deltoid is very inefficient and tends to produce superior dislocation. As abduction progresses, the deltoid's efficiency increases while that of the supraspinatus decreases. These actions are a direct result of the changes in position of the muscles' origins and insertions that accompany the motion.

In the **second phase** (90 to 150 degrees), upward rotation of the scapula causes the glenoid fossa to face upward. This is accomplished by concomitant rotations of the sternoclavicular and acromioclavicular joints. In the **third phase** (150 to 180 degrees) the spinal column is displaced laterally by the action of the contralateral spinal muscles. Bilateral abduction would require an exaggeration of the lumbar lordosis, since the spinal column would be otherwise synergistically balanced. These combined motions are known as the *scapulohumeral rhythm*.

Total flexion of the shoulder joint can also be divided into three phases. In the **first phase** (0 to 60 degrees), the muscles used are the anterior fibers of the deltoid, the coracobrachialis, and the clavicular fibers of the pectoralis major. Motion is limited by the tension of the coracohumeral ligament and by the resistance offered by the teres minor, teres major, and infraspinatus muscles.

In the **second phase** (60 to 120 degrees) the function is similar to the second phase of abduction in that scapular rotation is added and the glenoid fossa is facing upward and anteriorly. In the **third phase** (120 to 180 degrees), both unilateral and bilateral flexion require the same motion of the spinal column as for complete abduction.

In diagnosing somatic dysfunctions involving shoulder girdle motion, the clinician must be aware that dysfunctions limiting motion reflect involvement of multiple joints, muscles, tendons, ligaments, the synovium, and the joint capsules. Functional anatomic knowledge and diagnostic ability should include knowledge of the following:

1. The functioning of accessory and coupled motions
2. The origins and insertions of the shoulder muscles
3. The influence of these muscles on the entire spinal column

Figure 4-21. Sternoclavicular joint motion.

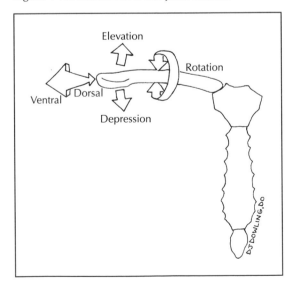

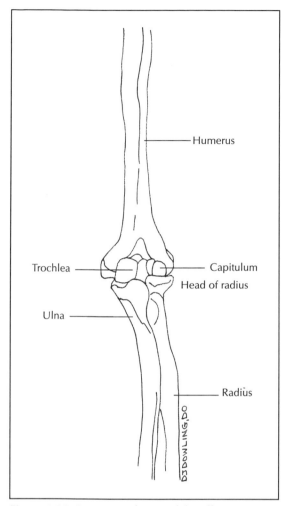

Figure 4-22. Bony articulation of the elbow joint.

4. The relationship of the thorax and rib cage to all scapular motion
5. How the first rib, at its sternal attachment, is directly influenced by clavicular motion

The entire shoulder girdle, thorax, rib cage, and vertebral column must be evaluated for a comprehensive diagnosis of somatic involvement in shoulder girdle dysfunction. The plan for therapy should be similarly comprehensive.

ELBOW JOINT

The distal end of the humerus articulates with the ulna and radius, forming two articulations: the **humeroulnar,** between the trochlea of the hu-

merus and the trochlear notch of the ulna, and the **humeroradial,** between the capitulum of the humerus and the head of the radius (Fig. 4-22).

The elbow joint has the composite motions of elbow flexion, with forearm supination, and elbow extension, with forearm pronation. Therefore, the superior radioulnar joint and its motions complicate, and are part of, elbow joint motion.

Humeroulnar articulation. The trochlea of the humerus consists of a central groove with a convex wing on each side. The central groove lies in an oblique sagittal plane. The obliquity creates the carrying angle of the arm. The trochlear notch of the ulna has a corresponding shape.

The major motion of the articulation is flexion-extension. However, extremes of supination and pronation create a rocking motion and the accessory motions of adduction with supination and abduction with pronation. Restrictions of these accessory motions influence normal flexion-extension and must be sought and normalized in elbow joint treatment.

Humeroradial articulation. This consists of the concave head of the radius articulating with the convex-shaped capitulum of the humerus. Motion of this articulation must accompany humeroulnar flexion-extension. This angular motion is accompanied by ventral and dorsal translatory slide of the radius on the humerus: dorsal radial slide with extension, ventral radial slide with flexion (Fig. 4-23). Extension stress is the major cause of posterior radial head somatic dysfunction.

The proximal radioulnar articulation consists of the cylindric rim of the head of the radius articulating with the radial notch of the ulna. The annular ligament encompasses the head of the radius and is attached to the anterior and posterior margins of the radial notch. In conjunction with the distal radioulnar articulation, its main motions are supination and pronation. The axis of these motions is represented by a line drawn through the center of the head of the radius, with the distal end of the radius swinging around and in front of the ulna. The proximal end of the ulna moves backward and laterally during pronation and forward and medially with supination (Fig. 4-24). This means that the axis of rotation of the head of the radius does not remain constant. The accessory motions therefore consist of the previously mentioned dorsal-ventral radial slide on the capitulum, similar motion on the radial notch, and dorsal and ventral ulnar slide on the radius. All of

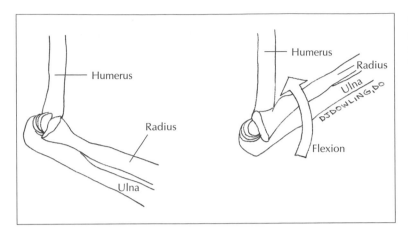

Figure 4-23. Translatory slide of the radius on the capitulum. Roll and slide occur in the same direction.

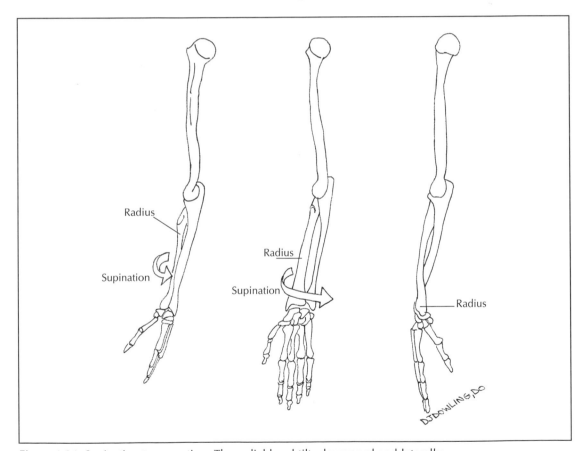

Figure 4-24. Supination to pronation. The radial head tilts downward and laterally.

Figure 4-25. Bony articulation of the wrist.

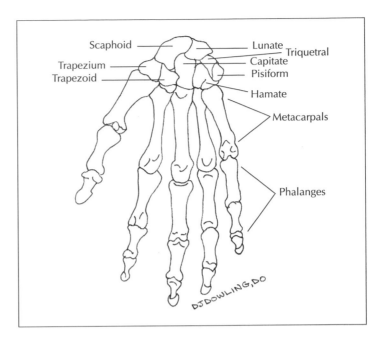

these motions may contribute to somatic dysfunctions.

The motions of supination and pronation are also greatly influenced by the function of the interosseous membrane and the distal radial ulnar articulation.

WRIST JOINT

The wrist joint consists of 15 bones, each with multiple articulations. A good example is the capitate bone, which articulates with the second, third, and fourth metacarpals and with the lunate, scaphoid, trapezoid, and hamate bones (Fig. 4-25). The wrist acts as a functional unit, exhibiting flexion, extension, adduction (ulnar deviation), abduction (radial deviation), and circumduction.

The articular complex of the wrist can be divided into three functional units:

1. The radiocarpal joint, consisting of the distal end of the radius articulating with the scaphoid and lunate
2. The midcarpal joint, consisting of the combined articulations between the proximal and distal rows of the carpal bones (Fig. 4-26)
3. The ulnomeniscotriquetral pseudojoint, consisting of the distal end of the ulna, the triquetrium, and the meniscus between the two

The movements that occur at the radiocarpal and midcarpal joints can be considered together because these joints act as a combined mechanism. Flexion involves the combined motion of both units, with midcarpal motion somewhat greater than radiocarpal motion. The roles are reversed in extension: radiocarpal motion is greater (Fig. 4-27). In adduction, most of the motion occurs at the radiocarpal and the ulnomeniscotri-

Figure 4-26. Midcarpal joint of the wrist.

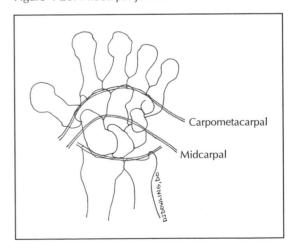

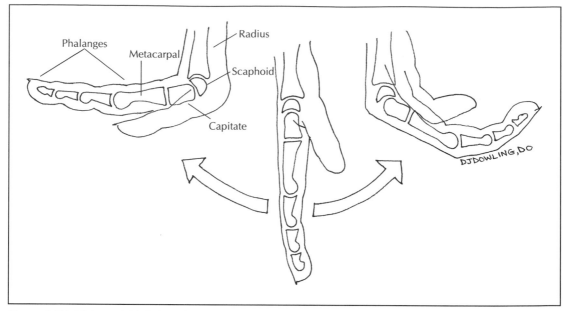

Figure 4-27. Major wrist joint motion.

quetral joints. Abduction involves primarily the midcarpal joint. There is a complex torsion movement of the carpal bones about their long axes during abduction and adduction. Circumduction of the hand is not axial rotation, but a series of movements: flexion followed by adduction, extension, and abduction, or the same movements in reverse order.

Accessory movements are greatest at the radioscaphoid and radiolunate articulations. These movements are ventral-dorsal slide, axial rotation, slight side-to-side slide, and long-axis traction. Similar accessory motions can be found at all carpal articulations, but in greatly diminished degree.

The close-packed position of the wrist is full extension. Falling on the wrist in this position will readily cause fracture. In a relaxed, loosely packed position, the joints are relatively mobile. For the performance of any task involving wrist action, the articulations must enter into a combination of interdependent locked positions, creating a solid structure that can bear the strain of torsional motion. In turning a doorknob, for example, the wrist joint changes from a sack of loose bones into a solid functional unit for the transmission of force.

An infinite number of partially close-packed positions of the wrist articulation can be created by muscle contraction and tightening of the ligaments. The close-packed articulation transmits force to the end of its total unit. Acting as a lever, it produces maximum force impact at one end or at one articulation. Somatic dysfunctions may easily develop in this manner, without sustaining direct trauma. The dysfunctions usually are loss of accessory motions.

HAND
With the exception of the thumb, the movements of the carpometacarpal articulations consist of flexion-extension and abduction-adduction. The accessory motions are dorsal-ventral slide, axial rotation, and long-axis traction. The thumb is a sellar articulation, permitting the motions of flexion-extension, abduction-adduction, rotation, and circumduction. The accessory motions are axial rotation and long-axis traction.

The intermetacarpal joints are limited to slight gliding of one on another. The accessory motion is axial rotation. The metacarpophalangeal articulations have the following movements: flexion-extension, adduction-abduction, limited rotation, and circumduction. The accessory motions are axial rotation, dorsal-ventral slide, and long-axis traction.

The interphalangeal joints are limited to flexion-extension motions. Flexion is usually accompanied by a conjunct rotation to assist in thumb-finger approximation. The accessory motions are dorsal-ventral slide, abduction-adduction, axial rotation, and long-axis traction.

The early motion dysfunctions caused by arthritic involvement of the hands are manifested in loss of accessory motions.

Biomechanics of the Lower Extremities

HIP JOINT

The anatomic relationships of the hip joint are similar to those of the glenohumeral joint. It is a ball-and-socket articulation, allowing 3 degrees of motion plus circumduction (Fig. 4-28). The entire weight of the body is transmitted through the hip joints, which therefore must have a greater degree of stability than the shoulder joints. Increased stability is afforded by a deeper acetabulum, the acetabular labrum, and the strong supportive hip ligaments. The acetabulum is in the innominate bone and relates to spinal, sacral, and ilial movements.

During normal gait, the stance leg starts in hip flexion. At midstance, hip extension begins until a close-packed position is achieved. The vector force transmitted from the ground passes into the innominate bone and causes rotation of the ilium.

Disturbances of gait will create iliosacral joint dysfunctions.

Movements of the hip joint include flexion-extension, abduction-adduction, internal and external rotation, and circumduction. The range of flexion depends on the action of the knee joint. Hip flexion is always greater with the knee flexed (Fig. 4-29). Greater hip flexion can be achieved passively than actively. Both hips can undergo full passive flexion when both knees are approximated to the chest. This is accompanied by a posterior pelvic tilt and lumbar flattening. The range of flexion motion is 90 degrees with the knee extended, 120 degrees with the knee flexed, and more than 120 degrees in passive flexion.

Hip extension is greater when the knee is in extension (Fig. 4-30). Passive extension is greater than active extension. Active hip extension is 10 degrees with the knee flexed and 20 degrees with the knee extended; passive extension can reach 30 degrees.

The gluteus maximus muscle is the major extensor muscle of the hip. Its ability to create extension depends on the planar relationships of its origin and insertion. According to the rule of muscle detorsion, all muscles attempt to align their origins and insertions into the same plane when contracting. Therefore, as the pelvis is tilted anteriorly, the

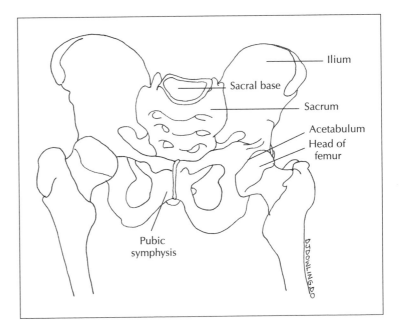

Figure 4-28. Bony anatomy of the hip joint.

Ilium

Sacral base

Sacrum

Acetabulum

Head of femur

Pubic symphysis

DJDOWLING DO

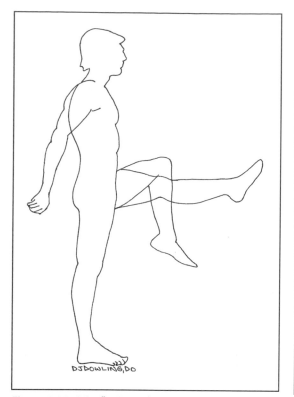

Figure 4-29. Hip flexion. Shown are ranges of motion with the knee in different positions.

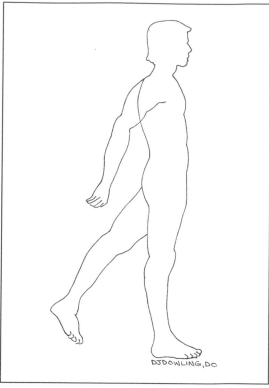

Figure 4-30. Hip extension.

origin of the gluteus maximus changes its planar relationship, allowing for femoral extension in an attempt to align the origin and insertion of the muscle into one plane. Maximum extension (anterior dance splits) creates marked anterior pelvic tilt accompanied by lumbar lordosis. The abduction of one joint is accompanied by pelvic tilt to the weight-bearing side and bilaterally equal abduction of the legs in relation to the pelvis. Maximum abduction creates a 90-degree angle between the two legs (45 degrees for each limb in abduction).

True adduction is not possible because of the midline interference of the other limb. Relative adduction is the return from abduction. As in shoulder motion, there can be adduction-flexion and adduction-extension motions. A complex motion of adduction of one hip accompanied by abduction of the other hip is achieved by a pelvic tilt in the frontal plane to the abduction side, with accompanying increased lumbar convexity.

Internal and external hip rotation can be easily measured with the patient prone and the knee flexed to 90 degrees. From the true vertical position, moving the foot laterally causes internal rotation (30 to 40 degrees). Moving the foot medially causes external rotation (60 degrees). The same test can be performed with the patient sitting on a table with the feet dangling. The position of greatest hip instability is in sitting with the legs crossed (abduction, flexion, and external rotation).

The accessory hip motions consist of slide with abduction-adduction and internal-external rotation and long-axis traction.

Of major importance in function and dysfunction, many large hip joint muscles involve the function of both the hip and the knee. Muscle contraction always involves an attempt at motion of both joints. Limiting the motion to one joint requires stabilization of the other joint by other muscles.

Pure extension of the hip joint would require the synergistic actions of the gluteus maximus, gluteus medius and minimus, the hamstrings, the rectus femoris, and the adductor magnus muscles. The gluteus maximus and hamstrings, along with the iliopsoas and erector spinae, are major factors in maintaining the stability of the pelvis and the lumbar lordosis.

The somatic dysfunctions related to hip joint dysfunction may involve the lower spine, sacrum, ilium, ischium, acetabulofemoral joint, femoral shaft, and the knee joint.

KNEE JOINT

The knee joint is the largest appendicular articulation. In function it resembles a hinge joint. However, it is a compound articulation within one joint cavity. It consists of two condylar joints between the corresponding condyles of the femur and tibia, with convex-concave relationships, and an additional sella-shaped joint between the patella and the femur.

The knee joint is one of the few joints of the body that have menisci. Menisci contribute to stability, weight-bearing, and mobility of the joint.

The patella's articulation allows it to slide up and down on the femur and act as a pulley for its musculotendinous attachments. The joint has an intricate ligamentous network to create stability while still permitting joint mobility.

The major movements of the knee joint are flexion and extension. These motions are a classic example of coupled roll and slide. The passive range of motion is 0 degrees at extension and 135 degrees at flexion.

With the foot on the ground, the final 30 degrees of femoral extension is accompanied by a conjunct medial femoral rotation (Fig. 4-31). This conjunct rotation results from the geometry of the articulating surfaces and the action of the ligaments. In full extension, the knee is in close-packed position, which confers greater stability and strength on the joint. As in all close-packed joints, trauma can more easily cause fracture. However, the more common ligamentous tears occur in mid- or loose-packed positions. With the foot off the ground, extension is associated with conjunct lateral rotation of the tibia.

The voluntary movements of axial internal and external rotation also occur in the knee. These motions are best observed with the knee in a flexed position. Passive internal and external rotation are each about 10 degrees.

The accessory motions of the femorotibial joint consist of passive internal and external rotation, conjunct rotation, dorsal and ventral tibial slide, abduction, adduction, and long-axis traction.

Besides the possibility of multiple soft tissue dysfunctions, the major somatic dysfunctions of joint motion affect abduction and adduction, or dorsal and ventral slide.

The patella, with the knee semiflexed, can be passively moved in the dorsal-ventral, cephalad, caudad, and side-to-side directions.

Figure 4-31. Tibial-femoral extension accompanied by conjunct rotation of the tibia.

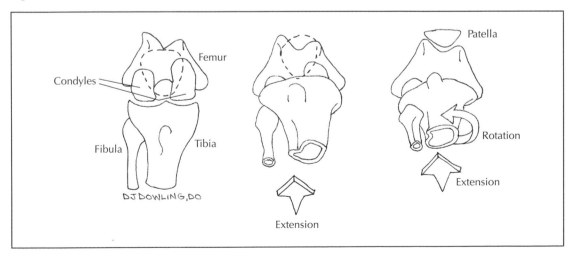

TIBIOFIBULAR JOINTS

The superior tibiofibular joint is a plane oval artic-ulation. The tibial facet lies on the posterolateral aspect of the rim of the lateral tibial condyle. It faces obliquely posteriorly, inferiorly, and lat-erally.

The inferior tibiofibular joint is a syndesmosis. The tibial facet is a rough concave notch into which the convex fibular facet fits. This fibular facet con-tinues below as the fibulotalar articulation.

Dorsiflexion and plantar flexion of the ankle au-tomatically create motion in both tibiofibular joints. Dorsiflexion causes the lateral malleolus to move laterally, to move vertically in a cephalad direction, and to rotate medially. This causes the superior tibiofibular joint to move in an upward posterior direction while rotating medially. The reverse occurs in plantar flexion.

The most common somatic dysfunction found in this area is a posterior fibula at the superior tibiofibular joint. This may be secondary to ankle dysfunction and marked dorsiflexion. To resolve the superior tibiofibular dysfunction, it is impor-tant to evaluate the ankle joint and treat any dys-functions found in that region.

FOOT AND ANKLE

The foot and ankle joints constitute a complex unit of 28 bones that must be strong enough to bear the body's weight yet elastic enough to allow adapta-tion to terrain, walking, jumping, or the stress of additional weight (Fig. 4-32).

The patient must be examined both in the static position and while walking, with the shoes on and off. Static examination is conducted with and without weight-bearing to determine changes in arch as well as bony relationships.

Pediatric examination of the feet prior to weight-bearing is very important. The early diag-nosis of congenital deformities may allow a non-operative therapy while increasing the quality of the results obtained.

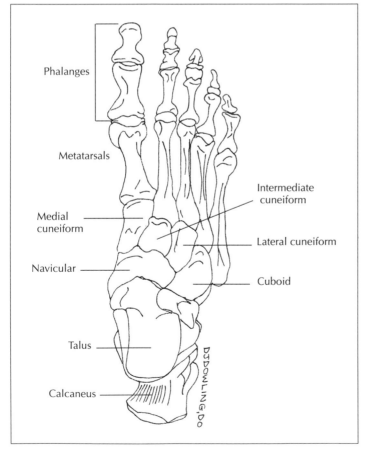

Figure 4-32. Bony anatomy of the foot.

Phalanges

Metatarsals

Intermediate cuneiform

Medial cuneiform

Lateral cuneiform

Navicular

Cuboid

Talus

Calcaneus

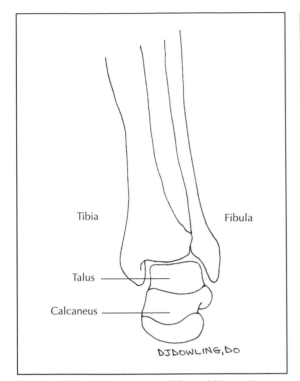

Figure 4-33. Bony anatomy of the ankle mortice articulation.

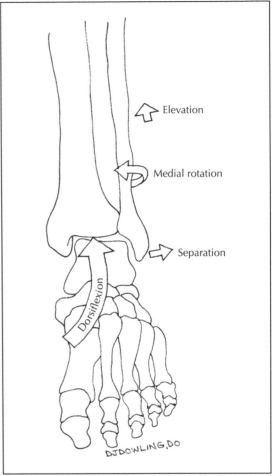

Figure 4-34. Dorsiflexion of the ankle with the accompanying motions.

The distal end of the tibia, along with the lateral malleolus, forms a concave surface into which is fitted the body of the talus. This is the ankle mortice articulation (Fig. 4-33). This hinge joint permits the major motions of dorsiflexion and plantar flexion of the foot on a transverse axis. The tibial malleolus extends about one third of the way down the medial surface of the body of the talus and is anterior to the lateral malleolus. The fibular malleolus extends down the entire lateral aspect of the talus.

The body of the talus is wedge-shaped, with its anterior portion larger. Dorsiflexion creates a close-packed position with medial rotation and elevation and separation of the fibula in relation to the tibia (Fig. 4-34).

The active motions of this articulation are dorsiflexion and plantar flexion. With the articulation in the loose-packed position, accessory motions of the side-to-side slide, internal and external rotation, abduction and adduction, and long-axis traction motion are permitted. Somatic dysfunction involving joint motion restriction usually occurs in abduction or adduction, as evidenced by the large number of inversion and eversion ankle sprains encountered.

The posterior portion of the foot consists of the talocalcaneal, talonavicular, and calcaneocuboid articulations. The calcaneus can move into abduction (valgus) or adduction (varus) in relation to the talus (Fig. 4-35). The other motions are best described as combined talocalcaneal-navicularcuboid efforts. Inversion in relation to a stable talus can be described as a medial rotation of the calcaneus and navicular bone, increasing the height of the medial arch, accompanied by the cuboid rotating downward on the calcaneus (Fig. 4-36). Motion of the anterior tarsus and plantar flexion will increase this movement. Eversion is the reverse of the above.

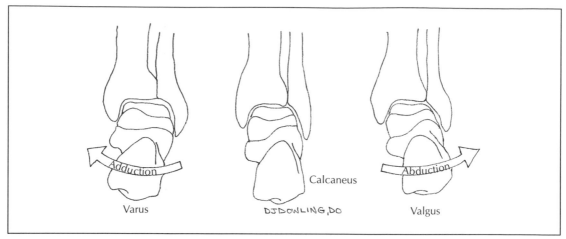

Figure 4-35. Calcaneal motion on the talus as viewed from the rear.

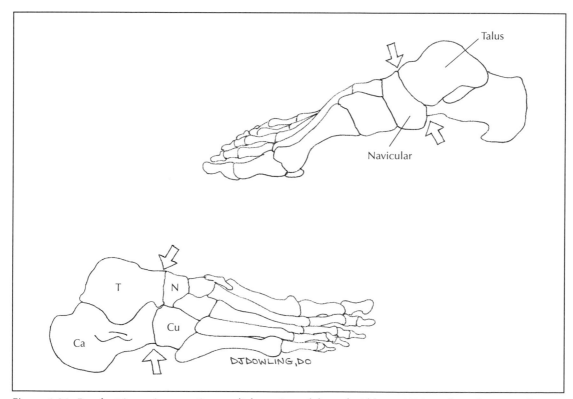

Figure 4-36. Forefoot inversion creating medial rotation of the cuboid bone (*Cu*) on the calcaneus (*Ca*) and the navicular bone (*N*) on the talus (*T*).

With weight-bearing, the distal tarsus and metatarsals become involved, creating the combined motions of pronation and suppination. *Pronation* of the foot consists of a combination of calcaneal abduction (valgus), eversion, foot abduction, and dorsiflexion. The opposite motions, calcaneal abduction (varus), inversion, foot adduction, and plantar flexion produce suppination.

The accessory motions of these articulations are slide and conjunct rotations.

Somatic dysfunction restricting joint motion will affect the motions of slide and conjunct rotation. An example is the conjunct rotation of the cuboid on the calcaneus with eversion and inversion of the foot.

The movements of the cuneiforms, cuboid, and navicular bones, in relation to each other, are primarily gliding and conjunct rotations. Accessory motions of increased glide and rotation can be created, especially if accompanied by long-axis traction.

The primary motions of the tarsometatarsal joints are flexion and extension. The axis of flexion and extension of the fourth and fifth metatarsals is oblique. This raises and lowers the transverse metatarsal arch with flexion and extension movements of these metatarsals. The intermetatarsal joint movement is primarily that of slide. Accessory motions of the tarsometatarsal and intermetatarsal joints consist in exaggeration of all sliding motions, especially when accompanied by long-axis traction. The metatarsophalangeal articulations allow active motions of extension-flexion and adduction-abduction. Accessory motions are sliding, axial rotation, and long-axis traction.

The active interphalangeal motions are flexion and extension. The accessory motions are abduction and adduction, axial rotation, and long-axis extension.

Biomechanical and functional relationships of the foot. To perform its weight-bearing and elastic mobile activities, the longitudinal arch is constructed in two different anatomical forms. The *lateral longitudinal arch* is a firm osseous structure consisting of the calcaneus, cuboid, and the fourth and fifth metatarsals. It resembles the classical architectural definition of an arch, having a keystone (the cuboid) with a flank stone (calcaneus and metatarsal) on each side. It is low, of limited mobility, and built to transmit weight and thrust to and from the ground (Fig. 4-37).

The *medial arch* is higher, without firm osseous support, and can be increased or reduced to meet the needs of motion or terrain. MacConaill describes the subtalar area as functioning as a twisted plate. It is flattened transversely along the line of the metatarsal heads and vertically at the calcaneus. It can be elongated or untwisted in pronation, dropping the medial "arch," or, with suppination, become more twisted, raising the medial arch (Fig. 4-38).

The medial arch is controlled by the rotation of the calcaneus on a longitudinal axis (calcaneal valgus-varus). Extreme adduction of the standing feet (crossing one foot over the other) causes posterior clockwise rotation of the calcaneus (varus) and a high medial arch. Extreme abduction of the standing foot with dorsiflexion of the ankle causes counterclockwise rotation of the calcaneus (valgus) with a dropping of the medial arch.

Therefore, the structure and motions of this area of the foot can be said to twist and untwist the foot in various positions.

If on examination the foot arch changes in con-

Figure 4-37. Lateral longitudinal arch of the foot.

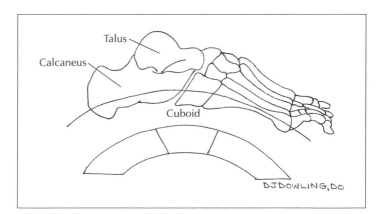

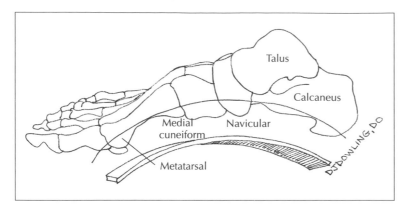

Figure 4-38. Medial longitudinal arch of the foot and its associated torsion.

formity with these principles, the feet are not structurally flat. Calcaneal valgus can have far-reaching structural and mechanical effects. It can reduce the medial arch, exaggerating foot pronation and increasing toe abduction and the tendency for eversion. This is very evident when observing gait. Calcaneal valgus also increases genu valgus, anterior pelvic tilt, and lumbar lordosis. The evaluation and treatment of foot imbalance is an integral part of the osteopathic examination.

Biomechanics of Intervertebral Joint Motion

The general rules of motion discussed with regard to appendicular articulations pertain as well to spinal synovial articulations. The vertebral articulations, however, have a tripod arrangement, which further complicates their motions. This tripod consists of an anterior synarthrosis, the vertebral bodies with intervertebral disks, and a pair of matched posterior synovial articulations. These three articulations are involved simultaneously in every vertebral motion.

A functional unit of the vertebral column is composed of two segments: an anterior segment that consists of two neighboring vertebral bodies separated by an intervertebral disk, and a posterior segment consisting of the two neural arches, their pedicles, laminae, superior and inferior articulations, transverse processes, and a spinous process (Fig. 4-39).

The main functions of the anterior segment are supportive, weight-bearing, shock-absorbing, and, in combination with the posterior segment, protection of the spinal cord. The posterior segment

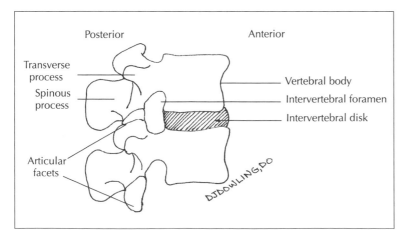

Figure 4-39. Functional unit of the vertebral column.

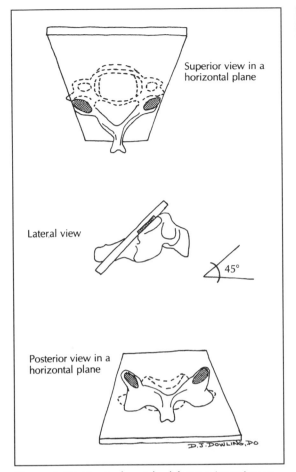

Figure 4-40. Cervical vertebral facet orientation at the level of C4.

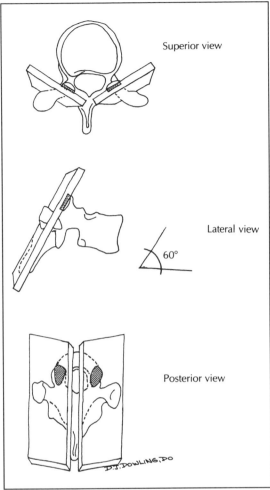

Figure 4-41. Thoracic vertebral facet orientation at the level of T6.

primarily effects directional guidance of joint motion. In the upright position it is almost non-weight-bearing.

Common factors that influence segmental motion include the design and spatial relationships of the individual facets; the vertebral ligamentous and muscular attachments and their function; the size and health of the intervertebral disks; the osteology of the vertebra; and the age, sex, and health of the patient. In addition, preload, gravity, and tone, and the amount and direction of applied load and stress must be taken into account.

DESIGN AND SPATIAL RELATIONSHIPS OF FACETS

The facets of the typical cervical vertebrae, C3 through C7, are flat and oval. Their average spatial orientation is a 45-degree angle between the horizontal and frontal planes. The superior facets face backward and upward (Fig. 4-40). They therefore have great freedom of motion in all planes. Because of the 45-degree spatial planar relationship, the coupled motions of rotation and lateral flexion always occur in the same direction.

The thoracic articular facets are flat, with the superior facets facing backward, upward, and laterally. The spatial orientation is a 60-degree angle from the horizontal to the frontal plane, and a 20-degree rotation from the frontal to the sagittal plane in a medial direction (Fig. 4-41). Without the rib attachments, the coupled motions of lateral flexion and rotation would be excellent. Flexion

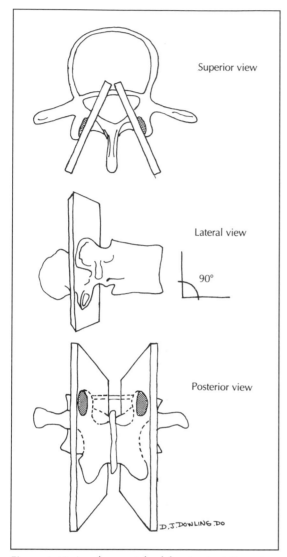

Superior view

Lateral view

90°

Posterior view

D.J. DOWLING DO

Figure 4-42. Lumbar vertebral facet orientation at the level of L3.

is greatly reduced by the 60-degree angle toward the frontal plane. Combined lateral flexion with rotation can be in the same or opposite directions.

The lumbar facets have curved surfaces. The superior facets are concave and face backward and medially. The inferior facets mirror them by being convex, facing forward and laterally. The rules of concave-convex relationship are evident with joint motion. Lateral flexion is a coupled roll-and-slide motion. This creates a slight rotary move-

ment. As in the thoracic region, lateral flexion and rotation can be in the same or opposite directions.

The average lumbar facet spatial orientation is a 45-degree angle from the frontal to the sagittal plane, turning in the lateral direction (Fig. 4-42). The greatest motion is found in flexion-extension; some lateral flexion is present with slight rotation. The described typical motion patterns may vary segmentally if other factors intervene.

The motion found at transitional intervertebral segmental levels is unpredictable. The additional stress created by changes in curve directions, and the osseous shape variations, create a climate for the development of somatic dysfunctions.

The anterior and posterior longitudinal ligaments limit extension and flexion, respectively. Posteriorly they are joined by the interspinous and supraspinous ligaments and the ligamentum flavum. Collectively they create a firm connection, linking all the vertebrae together. This supports and limits excessive motion. Dysfunction can develop when degenerative disks allow a loosening of the supportive ligaments, and posterior or anterior spondylolisthesis occurs.

The muscular attachments are commonly described as bilaterally symmetric. Unfortunately this is not the case. Everyone has asymmetric development. This causes unstable hypo- or hypertonic muscular development. Even simple spinal motions would become imbalanced, but for the synergistic or stabilizing assistance of other groups of muscles. All motions are susceptible to dysfunction because of these factors. The greater the imbalance, the greater is the tendency for the development of somatic dysfunction.

When evaluating muscle function or using muscle contractive force therapeutically, the clinician must be cognizant of the differences in strength and action between the superficial, powerful muscles and the deep, weaker muscles. The deep muscles, because of their vertebral attachments, create localized intervertebral balancing movements. The clinician uses the localized but lesser strength of the deep muscles in muscle energy therapy.

INTERVERTEBRAL DISKS
The intervertebral disks influence joint motion in a number of ways. The annulus consists of layers of fibroelastic fibers that are attached to the superior and inferior vertebral endplates. These fibers

intertwine in oblique patterns that permit rolling, rotation, and translation of one vertebra on another. The relative size of the disk with reference to its attached veretebrae is proportional to the motion allowed.

Disk degeneration, with a reduction in height, creates an imbalance of the articular facet relationship. The possible ligamentous effect was discussed earlier.

Osteology

The various shapes and structures of the vertebrae may also affect their motions. The cervical vertebral bodies are sella-shaped, which encourages freedom of motion. The joints of Lushka modify the translatory lateral motion of the cervical vertebral bodies. The shingle effect created by the thoracic spinous processes can restrict extension. A similar restriction can occur in the lumbar region if the spinous processes are elongated. The rib cage restricts lateral flexion and unilateral joint rotation.

The fifth lumbar vertebra is subject to a greater number of congenital abnormalities than any other bone. These abnormalities affect motion and create the tendency for dysfunction. A very common abnormality of this region, usually not reported radiologically, entails a change in the fifth lumbar vertebra-sacral base articular facet relations. It is common to find atypical bilateral horizontal articulations or one horizontal and one vertical facet articulation in this region. This creates an imbalance that develops into low back dysfunction.

Preload and Gravity

Normally, the effects of preload (gravity, weight, and muscle tone) are greater at the fifth lumbar vertebra than at the fifth cervical vertebra in the upright subject. However, the cervical muscles of a patient who has been living with constant stress may be chronically contracted, with a marked increase in tone. The disks would be subjected to a constant increased preload. Slight force can create great dysfunctions. The effect of scoliosis at any level creates an imbalance in muscle tone, with increased preload on one side of the disk. One-sided muscular overdevelopment, a common occurrence over time in most humans, can produce dysfunction in this manner.

Normal gravitational force directly affects the functional spinal unit. A gravitational force that is not directed toward the center of gravity of an object creates a secondary rotary force vector. None of the functional spinal units are completely horizontal to the earth. There are normal or abnormal lateral physiologic spinal curvatures, and multiple compensatory scoliotic patterns. Thus, spinal muscles are in a constant state of hypertonicity, trying to maintain an upright stature against gravity's rotary force. All of these factors affect articular motion and function.

Vertebral Motion at the Functional Spinal Unit

Coupled motions are normally present in a functional spinal unit. **Flexion** is the rotary motion of anterior vertebral approximation coupled with ventral translatory slide. **Extension** is the rotary motion of anterior vertebral separation coupled with dorsal translatory slide.

Rotation right is the turning of the anterior aspect of the body of the vertebra toward the right, coupled with a diminution of intervertebral disk height, described as vertical translatory compression (Fig. 4-43).

Rotation left is the turning of the anterior aspect of the body of the vertebra toward the left, coupled with the previously described vertical translatory compression. As the vertebra turns back toward the midline, either from right or left rotation, the intervertebral disk returns to its usual height.

Lateral flexion right or left is a rotary motion that causes the side of upper vertebral body to approximate the one below it, right or left, accompanied by a contralateral translatory slide (Fig. 4-44).

Each of these described coupled motions occurs in a single plane and on an instantaneous axis of rotation. If two of these coupled motions occur simultaneously, i.e., lateral flexion accompanying rotation, then multiple planes are involved, and the combined motions occur on a helical axis of rotation.

When the somatic dysfunction diagnosis is T4 ESr Rr, the motion of the fourth thoracic vertebra on the fifth thoracic vertebra is greater in the directions of extension, right lateral flexion, and right rotation. These three coupled motions occur in three planes simultaneously on a helical axis of rotation (Fig. 4-45). The barriers to freedom of the described motion would all be in the opposite directions, but on the same helical axis of rotation.

Many osteopathic diagnostic and therapeutic approaches can be explained by combining the

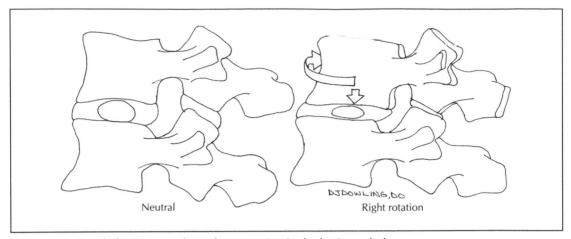

Figure 4-43. Coupled rotation and translatory motion in the horizontal plane.

laws of physiologic motion, vertebral biomechanics, and the kinetic principle of the effect of resistance to linear motion. The effect of resistance to linear motion can be described as follows: If an object in linear motion encounters an obstacle or resistance, it will turn about its point of contact with the interfering factor.

Example: On palpation, the transverse process of the fourth thoracic vertebra is more prominent posteriorly on the right. Is it part of a somatic dysfunction complex involving three planes and six motions on a helical axis? The vertebra is placed into a position of flexion. The right transverse process becomes more prominent posteriorly. It is assumed that this has happened because there is a barrier present to the motion of flexion, and the vertebra is responding according to the rule of the effect of resistance on linear motion. That is, on

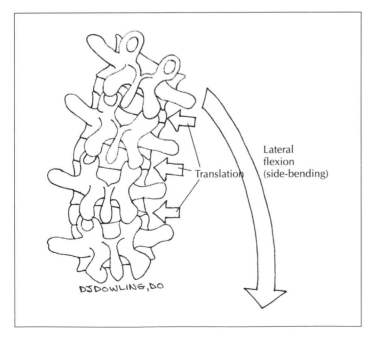

Figure 4-44. Coupled rotator and contralateral translator motions in the frontal plane that occur during lateral flexion.

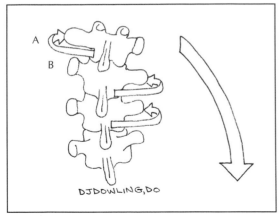

DJDOWLING, DO

Figure 4-45. **(A)** Type II: side-bending and rotation in same direction. **(B)** Type I: side-bending and rotation in opposite directions.

meeting this flexion barrier, the vertebra turns away from and around it in the direction of allowable freedom of motion, or right rotation.

Two parts of the diagnosis are now available. Freedom of motion in extension (flexion barrier), and right rotation. According to the laws of physiologic motion, if flexion or extension is involved in the motion diagnosis, then lateral flexion is in the same direction as the motion of rotation. Therefore, the diagnosis is T4 ESr Rr, moving on a helical axis.

To treat this dysfunction, the vertebra is placed in a position duplicating its helical axis. This allows it to move into or away from the barriers of motion. A force is then applied along this same helical axis of rotation in the direction desired, depending on whether direct or indirect treatment procedures are used.

MOTION TESTING
Donald E. Phykitt

The diagnosis of somatic dysfunctions of the axial skeleton includes assessment of symmetry of spinal motion. This assessment occurs on a number of levels, ranging from evaluation of movement of a complete section of the spine (regional motion testing) to evaluation of movement of a single spinal functional unit (rotoscoliosis testing, intersegmental motion testing). This section describes the goals, theories, and interpretation of these techniques. The techniques themselves are described in later chapters.

Regional Motion Testing
The goal of regional motion testing is to assess the overall motion of a section (cervical, thoracic, lumbar) of the axial skeleton. Gross motion of the spine is modified by numerous conditions, including osseous deformities (e.g., structural scoliosis), ligamentous imbalances, muscle spasm (acute or chronic), articular disease (e.g., degenerative joint disease), somatic dysfunction, and pain, usually due to one or more of the preceding conditions. These conditions limit both the degree and the quality of motion. Limitations can occur in one (or more) of three planes. Limitation of flex-

ion-extension occurs in the sagittal plane, limitation of rotation occurs in the horizontal plane, and limitation of lateral flexion occurs in the frontal plane.

Regional motion testing is used as a screening procedure to:

1. Determine a region to be more closely evaluated.
2. Provide a measurement with which a patient's progress can be assessed.
3. Identify regions that could benefit from general techniques such as myofascial treatment.

The evaluation of regional motion entails evaluation of the degree of motion, the symmetry of motion (e.g., right rotation vs. left rotation), and the *quality* of motion (restrictions may be due to one or more of the conditions listed in the section on the biomechanics of joint motion in this chapter).

Assessment of Group Curves (Type I Somatic Dysfunctions)
The goal of assessment of group curves is to identify groups of adjacent vertebrae (usually three or

more) that are dysfunctional in such a way that they obey Fryette's first law of vertebral motion.

Lateral group curves can occur in any region of the axial skeleton. They are most often caused by (1) asymmetric muscle contraction or contracture producing a "bowstring" effect on the spine, (2) structural asymmetries elsewhere in the body (e.g., short leg), for which they are compensating (functional or physiologic scoliosis), and (3) structural scoliosis secondary to known or idiopathic etiologies.

As a result of the prevailing conditions, the vertebrae in a group curve exhibit type I motion (side-bending and rotation occur to opposite sides). The techniques involved in diagnosing group curves address both the side-bending and rotational components of the dysfunction. These techniques are as follows:

1. **Observation of the standing patients.** Lateral deviation of a group of vertebrae from the midline can be observed when the patient is examined from behind. The rational component can be observed as posterior prominence of the paravertebral musculature, scalpula, or ribs on one side of the body. This prominence is usually located on the side opposite to the direction of side-bending (on the same side as the convexity of the curve). This is a result of side-bending and rotation occurring in opposite directions. The prominence is more obvious if the patient is asked to bend forward.

2. **Rotoscoliosis testing.** This technique evaluates the rotational component of group curves when the spine is in the neutral position. Vertebrae involved in a group curve display rotation opposite to their direction of side-bending. This is detected by palpating the transverse processes, which should be more prominent on the side of the direction of rotation of the involved vertebrae. Flexion or extension of the individual vertebra should not alter this rotation factor. From Fryette's first law of vertebral motion it can be inferred that the group is laterally flexed to the opposite side. It should be noted that the biomechanics of the cervical region are such that rotoscoliosis testing cannot be used to evaluate group curves. Static symmetry examination of landmarks of the skull and evaluation of range of motion are the best means of diagnosing group curves in this region.

3. **Interpretation.** A group curve in the thoracic or lumbar spine in which the vertebrae are side-bent left and rotated right would display the following features: a lateral curve with its convexity facing right; more prominent musculature, ribs, or scapula on the right; and posterior transverse processes on the right when palpated in neutral position.

Individual Vertebral Motion Testing

ROTOSCOLIOSIS TESTING

The goal of rotoscoliosis testing is to detect somatic dysfunctions of single vertebral functional units, by comparing the rotational position of vertebrae when they are in flexion to that when they are in extension. Somatic dysfunctions usually involve restrictions in three planes: the sagittal plane (restriction noted on flexion-extension), the horizontal plane (noted on rotation), and the frontal plane (noted on lateral flexion). These restrictions affect static position as well as motion. A vertebra's position is always away from its restriction (i.e., toward its freedom of motion) in all three planes.

A principle of physics states that when a moving object encounters a barrier, it will change direction to follow the path of least resistance. Similarly, when a vertebra encounters a barrier in one plane, it tends to move further in the direction of its freedom of motion in the other two planes. A three-dimensional example is a box that is pushed along the floor. If the front of the box (the vertebra) hits a pole (barrier), it has encountered restriction in motion. If the portion of the box that contacts the pole is away from the midline (as is usually the case in a somatic dysfunction), pushing the box further (moving it into its barrier) causes the box to rotate around the pole. In contrast, pulling the box back away from the pole allows straight sliding (no rotation).

Rotoscoliosis testing is based on the assumption that placing a vertebra into its flexion-extension barrier results in rotation of the vertebra in the direction of its freedom of motion. For example, in T4 ERr Sr, T4 is extended on T5. The barriers to motion are flexion, left side-bending, and rotation. Placing T4 into flexion would further accentuate the restrictive forces (the box hits the pole). In an attempt to follow the path of least resistance, T4 would rotate and flex laterally to the right.

By palpating the transverse process or articular

pillars, the clinician can detect the rotational position of a vertebra. Noting whether rotation to a certain side is greatest in flexion or extension allows discrimination of the freedom of motion in the sagittal plane (i.e., the position opposite to that in which the greatest rotation was noted). The freedom of motion in the frontal plane (side-bending) is deduced from Fryette's second law of vertebral motion, according to which rotation and lateral flexion occur in the same direction when either flexion or extension barriers are present.

Of aid in rotoscoliosis testing are the following observations:

1. The position (flexion-extension) in which rotation is the greatest is the barrier of motion.
2. The side on which the transverse process is more posterior denotes the direction of rotational freedom of motion.
3. Since, in single somatic dysfunctions, rotation and side-bending occur in the same direction, the side-bending component is named for the same direction as the rotational component. For example, the left transverse process of T3 is most prominent when it is placed in flexion. The dysfunction is designated as T3 E Rl Sl.

DIRECT INTERSEGMENTAL MOTION TESTING

The goal of direct intersegmental motion testing is to dynamically diagnose somatic dysfunction of single vertebral functional units by directly assessing the symmetry of motion in all three planes.

The clinician localizes motion in a single vertebral level, then induces motion in all three planes. Symmetry of motion may be noted in flexion versus extension, rotation right versus rotation left, and right lateral flexion versus left lateral flexion. The somatic dysfunction is named for the directions of freedom of motion. This method can be used in the cervical, thoracic, and lumbar regions. The somatic dysfunction is named for the directions of freedom of motion, using the accepted nomenclature, e.g., T3 E Rr Sr.

INDIRECT INTERSEGMENTAL MOTION TESTING WITH TRANSLATORY MOTION

The goal of this form of testing is to dynamically detect somatic dysfunctions of single vertebral functional units (usually in the cervical region) by indirectly assessing asymmetry of lateral flexion.

The method incorporates the principle that lateral flexion of a vertebra to one side is accompanied by translation of that vertebra to the opposite side in the frontal plane (see the first section on palpation in this chapter). Interpretation indicates that asymmetric lateral flexion will be accompanied by asymmetric translation to the opposite side. Furthermore, asymmetry of translation (and therefore of lateral flexion) is most noticeable when the vertebra is placed into its barrier in the sagittal plane (flexion or extension). This latter point can be explained by the fact that placing a vertebra into its barrier of motion in one plane of motion enhances the restrictive forces to motion in the other two planes. Finally, as previously mentioned, side-bending and rotation occur to the same side. Therefore, by determining in which direction asymmetry of translatory motion in present, by determining if the asymmetry of translation is greatest in flexion or extension, and by applying knowledge of cervical vertebral biomechanics, the clinician can diagnose a somatic dysfunction in the cervical region in all three planes. As a nomenclatural example, C3 translates easier from right to left when placed in flexion, so the dysfunction is named C3 E Sr Rr.

References

Basmajian JV. 1978. Muscles Alive, 4th ed. Baltimore: Williams & Wilkins.

Cailliet R. 1968. Foot and Ankle Pain. Philadelphia: F.A. Davis.

———. 1981. Neck and Arm Pain. Philadelphia: F.A. Davis.

Ealton WJ. 1970. Textbook of Osteopathic Diagnosis and Technique Procedures, 2nd ed. Colorado Springs, Colo: American Academy of Osteopathy.

Fryette HH. 1918. Physiologic movements of the spine. J Am Osteopath Assoc 18:1. Reprinted in 1950 Yearbook of Selected Osteopathic Topics, pp 91–92. Ann Arbor, Mich: Academy of Applied Osteopathy.

———. 1954. Principles of Osteopathic Technique. Kirksville, Mo: American Academy of Osteopathy.

Fujiwara M, Basmajian JV. 1975. Electromyographic study of two joint muscles. Am J Phys Med 54: 234–242.

Hoag JM, Kosok M, Moser JR. 1960. Kinematic analysis and classification of vertebral motion. J Am Osteopath Assoc 54:894,982.

Hoover HV, Nelson CR. 1950. Basic physiologic movements of the spine. In: 1950 Yearbook of Selected Osteopathic Topics, p. 63. Ann Arbor, Mich: Academy of Applied Osteopathy.

Jones L. 1955. The Postural Complex. Springfield, Ill: Charles C. Thomas.

Kapandji IA. 1974. The Physiology of the Joints, 2nd ed, vols 1, 2, 3. Edinburgh: Churchill Livingstone.

Kraus H. 1970. Clinical Treatment of Back and Neck Pain. New York: McGraw-Hill.

MacConaill MA. 1949. The movements of bones and joints. J Bone Joint Surg [Am] (31B)1:100–104.

———, Basmajian JV. 1977. Muscles and Movements. Huntington, New York: Robert E. Krieger Publishing.

Mitchell FL Jr, Moran PS, Pruzzo MT. 1979. An Evaluation and Treatment Manual of Osteopathic Muscle Energy Procedures. Valley Park, Mo: self-published.

Moore KL. 1980. Clinically Oriented Anatomy. Baltimore: Williams & Wilkins.

Project on Osteopathic Principles Education. 1982. Glossary of Osteopathic Terminology. Chicago: Educational Council on Osteopathic Principles.

Rasch PJ, Burke RK. 1978. Kinesiology and Applied Anatomy, 6th ed. Philadelphia: Lea & Febiger.

Schiowitz S, DiGiovanna EL, Ausman PJ, eds. 1983. An Osteopathic Approach to Diagnosis and Treatment. Old Westbury, NY: New York College of Osteopathic Medicine.

Warwick R, Williams P. 1973. Gray's Anatomy, 35th British ed. Philadelphia: W.B. Saunders.

Wells KF, Luttgens K. 1976. Kinesiology, 6th ed. Philadelphia: W.B. Saunders.

White AA, Panjabi MM. 1978. Clinical Biomechanics of the Spine. Philadelphia: J.B. Lippincott.

5

Principles of Osteopathic Manipulative Techniques

MYOFASCIAL TECHNIQUES

Toni Spinaris
Eileen L. DiGiovanna

Myofascial techniques are a group of specific maneuvers that, in general, achieve the same goals. They can be used as the primary modality of treatment or in combination with other methods.

The term *myofascial* comes from the root words *myo*, meaning "muscle," and *fascia*, which is self-explanatory. Myofascial techniques are among the soft tissue techniques. Muscle and fascia are most commonly thought of as the tissues treated by these techniques, but all of the fibroelastic connective tissues, as well as skin, tendons, ligaments, cartilage, blood, and lymph, may be affected.

The musculoskeletal system comprises a large percentage of the human body, and myofascial techniques can and do have significant effects on the body. Dysfunction of musculoskeletal and neuromuscular components can be as disabling as infectious organ diseases or metabolic disorders. Myofascial techniques aid in achieving the primary goal of the human body—homeostasis, or the restoration and preservation of optimal bodily function. The effects of myofascial techniques on homeostasis include, but are not limited to, the following:

1. Relaxation of contracted muscles, which de-

creases the oxygen demand of the muscle, decreases pain, and allows normalized range of motion across a joint
2. Increased circulation to an area of ischemia, therefore supplying blood carrying oxygen and nutrients to the tissues and removing harmful metabolic waste products
3. Increased venous and lymphatic drainage, thereby decreasing local swelling and edema
4. A stimulatory affect of the stretch reflex in hypotonic muscles

The schematic diagram in Figure 5-1 explains the tissue changes that lead to impaired mobility and the function, pain, and soft tissue changes seen and felt in the human body at various stages. The initiating insult or trauma may be subtle or quite dramatic. Cailliet defines *trauma* as "a wound or injury with implication of a force applied externally or internally causing a tissue reaction. Pain is the resultant which has varying degrees of intensity and effective interpretation with numerous avenues of transmission."

The initiating trauma may be anything that causes soft tissue irritation. The irritation is interpreted as pain. The body's usual reaction to pain

An Osteopathic Approach to Diagnosis and Treatment, second edition
Eileen L. DiGiovanna and Stanley Schiowitz
Lippincott–Raven Publishers, Philadelphia © 1997.

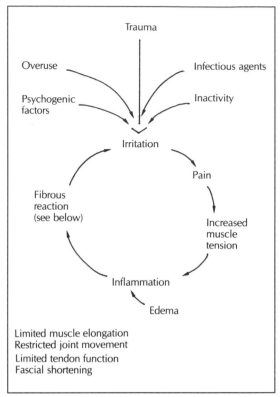

Figure 5-1. Cycle of soft tissue changes/pain/soft tissue changes following traumatic insult.

is an increase in muscle tension. A vicious cycle ensues: a positive feedback mechanism informed by pain leads to increased muscle tension, which leads to increased pain, and so on. The increase in muscle tension plays an important role in tissue ischemia. The cycle continues, with tissue ischemia hindering provision of nutrients to the tissue and permitting buildup of waste products in the tissues. These waste products act as noxious stimuli, causing further irritation of the tissues, pain, and inflammation.

To this point the process can be thought of as acute. If the process continues, it may become chronic. The next step is fibrous tissue reaction. If this occurs, it is believed to be permanent, which makes the soft tissue damage less reversible. An effect of the fibrous reaction is limited muscle elongation or stretch, which allows muscle shortening to develop, which in turn may limit movement across a joint. Other effects are limitation in tendon function and fascial shortening. All lead

to a decrease in the functional ability of the body part and person.

Myofascial techniques are useful in breaking the pain-muscle tension-pain cycle. Increasing the circulation to and drainage from the tissues may aid in diminishing the inflammatory response.

Some of the physiologic principles applied in myofascial techniques include the following:

1. **Extensibility of the connective tissues.** Connective tissue placed under prolonged mild tension shows plastic elongation.
2. **Stretch reflex.** The stretch of a muscle excites the muscle spindle, resulting in reflex contraction of that muscle. This is to be avoided when applying passive myofascial techniques to contracted or contractured muscles. It can be avoided by applying slow, even force and releasing that force slowly and evenly. However, the stretch reflex is to be used during active myofascial techniques for the purpose of stimulating muscle tone in hypotonic muscles.
3. **Heat.** Heat applied to a muscle usually results in an increase in elastic response of the muscle to stretch.
4. **Muscle spindle reflex.** This is used in active resistive myofascial techniques. If the extrafusal fibers contract less than the intrafusal fibers, the muscle spindle will maintain a stretch reflex, further exciting the extrafusal fibers.
5. **Golgi tendon organ reflex.** This is used in active myofascial techniques. When the tension on the tendon becomes extreme, the inhibitory effect from the Golgi tendon organ can cause sudden relaxation of the entire muscle.
6. **Reciprocal inhibition.** This is used in active myofascial techniques with or without resistance. When a stretch reflex stimulates one muscle, it simultaneously inhibits the antagonist muscle; e.g., if the stretch reflex excites the biceps, reciprocal inhibition inhibits the triceps.
7. **Crossed extensor reflex.** This is used in active myofascial techniques with resistance. When a stretch reflex excites one muscle, it simultaneously excites the contralateral antagonist muscle. Motion is created that crosses from one side of the spine to the other in an X pattern; e.g., the stretch reflex excites the right biceps, and the crossed extensor reflex excites the left triceps.

Passive and Active Techniques

Passive techniques are used by the physician with the patient relaxed. Passive techniques entail application of a manual traction force in one of four directions:

1. Linear pull at either end of the muscle
2. Linear pull at both ends of the muscle at the same time
3. Pushing the muscle in a direction perpendicular to the long axis of the muscle fibers, thus creating stretch
4. Pulling the muscle in a direction perpendicular to the long axis of the muscle fibers, thus creating stretch

In **active** techniques the patient assists the physician by actively contracting certain muscles under the guidance of the physician. There are two forms of active myofascial techniques. **Active direct** techniques are those in which the patient is asked to contract the involved muscle. These techniques use the Golgi tendon organ reflex to relax the involved muscle(s). In these techniques the physician applies isometric resistance to the contraction. (*Isometric resistance:* The physician applies resistance to the patient's contraction such that little shortening of the muscle is permitted but a great increase in muscle tension results.)

Active indirect techniques are those in which the patient is asked to contract the muscles antagonistic to those being treated. This method uses the reciprocal inhibition reflex to relax the muscles being treated. In these techniques the physician applies isokinetic resistance to the patient's contraction. (*Isokinetic resistance:* The physician applies a resistive force such that the muscle contraction increases very little with the gradual decrease in muscle length; i.e., the joint is allowed to move and the resistance is gradually increased.)

General Considerations

There are a few general rules to follow when applying myofascial techniques.

1. The patient should be in a position of comfort and be relaxed.

2. The physician should be in a position of comfort and be at ease.
3. The physician should minimize energy expenditure and use body weight whenever possible instead of upper arm strength.
4. The force must be of low intensity, is slowly applied and maintained for 3 to 4 seconds, and is slowly released.
5. The force applied must not create pain.
6. Always push or pull muscle away from bone, since it is painful to push into bone.
7. Push or pull muscle in a direction perpendicular to the long axis of the muscle fibers.
8. Avoid rubbing or irritating the patient's skin by the friction of your fingers or hands.
9. Use leverage whenever possible.
10. When treating muscles with myofascial techniques, the physician's fingertips and the thenar and hypothenar eminences are used to apply pressure.
11. When a transverse force (push or pull) is applied across a muscle body, a counterforce may also be applied to maintain the patient's position.
12. Muscle stretch may also be achieved by applying traction in a lengthwise direction of the muscle fibers at the insertion or attachment of the muscle, thus lengthening the distance between the two.
13. Compression may be used in areas of multiple muscle layers in order to reach the deeper tissues.

Inhibitory Techniques

In muscle tissue, areas of tension and tenderness may develop as a result of trauma, inflammation, or stress. These areas exhibit palpable changes and are tender to pressure.

Firm pressure may inhibit nerve impulses that maintain the muscle tension. This may be done by pinching a muscle, such as the trapezius, between two fingers, or pressing firmly into the tense area with the thumb, or on occasion in large muscles with the elbow. The pressure should be maintained for 60 to 90 seconds. The tissue will be felt to soften and the tenderness will gradually diminish.

MUSCLE ENERGY TECHNIQUES
Dennis J. Dowling

As a technique, muscle energy was first formulated by Fred Mitchell, Sr., D.O., FAAO, in cooperation with Neil Pruzzo, Peter Moran, and Fred Mitchell, Jr., D.O., FAAO. A collection of descriptive techniques was published in *An Evaluation and Treatment Manual of Osteopathic Muscle Energy Procedures* in 1979. Their work may have been based on that of another osteopathic physician, T. J. Ruddy, D.O., who used pulse-timed procedures in and around the head and neck. Many osteopathic practitioners had used similar techniques over the decades, but this was the first coordinated, unifying work. Since then another work, *Outline of Muscle Energy Techniques* by Kenneth Graham, D.O., has become available.

A basic tenet of the muscle energy modality is that muscles cause and/or maintain somatic dysfunctions. For type II somatic dysfunctions, the small spurt-and-shunt muscles such as the rotator brevis or the intertransversii may become or remain in a state of hypertonicity. This allows some regional motion but restricts single intervertebral motion. A type II somatic dysfunction may also be theorized to occur because of locking of the involved facets. In this case, the position of the vertebrae may cause stress on the small muscles that respond by contracting. After treatment with techniques such as high-velocity, low-amplitude techniques, the joint may be more mobile but the tonicity of these small muscles may not be reduced. The continued, inappropriate contraction may return the vertebral or other joint to its dysfunctional position. This pattern may account for the need to treat patients several times a week if articulatory techniques are the sole ones employed. Thus, by using muscle energy techniques, one can improve or resolve the dysfunction. These techniques can also be utilized prior to or in combination with other techniques such as high-velocity, low-amplitude thrust.

It is postulated that muscle energy, when used directly on involved restrictions, uses the Golgi tendon reflex. The physician localizes the muscles surrounding and acting across a joint by placing the joint into its barrier or restriction in all involved planes. The patient is instructed to move that portion of his or her body toward the diagnosed relative freedoms of the joint. The physician resists by using an isometric counterforce. This is held for 3 to 5 seconds. After complete relaxation, the joint is further moved into the barriers and the whole procedure is repeated three to five times. A passive repositioning must occur after the last sequence to adequately restore more normal motion. After the technique is completed, the region is retested. The Golgi tendon reflex is activated by the resisted contraction and the muscles relax by neurophysiological reflex. Another theory is that a temporary muscle fatigue takes place and that simple contraction-relaxation allows for further stretching without reflex contraction of the inappropriately contracted muscles.

Diagnosis requires that testing be localized to the target joint. Restriction of motion is the primary criterion, but asymmetry, soft tissue tension changes, and tenderness may be used to further localize and corroborate the diagnosis. There are specific muscle energy techniques for each region of the body. However, a few basic principles apply to all areas. Once one knows the joint, the origins, insertions, and actions of the muscles, the findings of the relative freedoms, and the restrictions of motion, a treatment can be formulated.

Dr. Graham summarized some of the principles in his book. The following is a paraphrase of his eight essential steps.

1. Accurate structural *diagnosis* must be made. Each location can be defined by its somatic dysfunction diagnosis. An example would be C4 ESr Rr or C4 ES Rr, which informs us that flexion, side-bending, and rotation right are the barriers to be engaged.
2. Engage the restrictive *barrier* in all three planes. Spinal motion would involve restriction in flexion-extension, side-bending, and rotation. Appendicular restrictions frequently involve flexion-extension, supination-pronation (internal-external rotation), and abduction-adduction. The barrier engagement should not cause distress to the patient. Even though the final effect is greater motion at a joint, the physician must

be aware of the soft tissue muscular barrier. Some physicians describe this as "feather edge" barrier placement.

3. Unyielding *counterforce* (operator force = patient force) in the form of isometric resistance is necessary to activate the Golgi tendon reflex. Inaccuracy could lead to counterproductive force.

4. Appropriate patient *muscle effort:*
   a. Correct amount of force, which is light to moderate in effort (ounces to pounds)
   b. Correct direction of effort (away from the restrictive barrier)
   c. Correct duration of effort (3–5 seconds)

5. *Complete relaxation* after the muscle effort (both operator and patient relax their forces simultaneously).

6. *Repositioning* to the new restrictive barrier in all three planes; the physician motion-monitors with palpation. In most cases, this will involve maintaining monitoring with one hand throughout the whole treatment. Reengagement in most cases will involve small motions in each direction.

7. Steps 3 through 6 are *repeated* three to five times.

8. The region is *retested* (structural diagnosis is repeated).

Dr. Graham also notes some of the most common errors made by physicians when they are first learning and practicing muscle energy techniques:

1. The physician does not accurately monitor with palpation of the involved joint.

2. The patient uses a muscle contraction that is too forceful. This may prevent the treatment from being localized because other muscles and joints are recruited. The larger muscles may overlie the smaller muscles' effort and reduce the effectiveness. Conversely, too little effort may not activate the target muscles enough.

3. The muscle contraction is too short in duration. In this case the Golgi tendon organ would not be activated. If one supposes a simple contract-relax mechanism, there may not be enough fatigue to allow stretch.

4. The patient is not allowed to totally relax before repositioning into new restrictive barriers. This may lead to inefficient localization, or the new barriers may not be engaged at all.

5. The examiner forgets to retest. Any improve-ment may not be noted. Further treatment may or may not be necessary.

The muscle energy techniques are very effective and well tolerated in many conditions and by a wide age range of patients. Spasm, either primary or secondary, that is reduced will almost always be accompanied by some reduction of pain.

Muscle energy techniques may also be used over wider regions, especially for type I group curve spinal dysfunctions. In this case, the barriers of side-bending and rotation are applied and the region does not move from neutral in the sagittal plane (there is no flexion or extension component). The same principles as stated previously are employed. Whether used segmentally or regionally, these forms of muscle energy are direct, in that barriers are engaged, and active, in that the patient performs some activity.

Other forms of muscle energy can likewise be employed. Active indirect techniques of muscle energy employ a crossed extensive reflex. Contraction of antagonist muscles results in reflex relaxation of the target agonist muscles. Typically, the target muscles are large regional muscles. Initially, the region is placed into its relative freedoms and the target muscles are shortened. The patient is directed to push toward the barriers. The physician provides an isokinetic counterforce that allows movement toward the barrier. In other words, the patient pushes against resistance but slowly moves in the prescribed directions. After pushing as far as possible without discomfort, the patient is instructed to relax. The physician then gently pushes a few degrees into the barriers. The region is again repositioned into the relative freedoms and the procedure is repeated at least twice, with each successive time involving more effort on the part of the patient and coordinated resistance on the part of the physician. Crossed extensor or reciprocal inhibition results in reflex activation of inhibitory interneurons, which limit or prevent motorneurons from activating muscle.

Isolytic procedures involve lengthening involved muscles while the patient actively contracts them. In theory, adhesions and fibrotic changes could be broken and the muscle permitted to perform in a more physiologic manner.

Isotonic contractions can be of an eccentric or concentric fashion and generally involve large regional muscle groups. This type of muscle energy is directed toward the development of muscle strength, stamina, enlargement, and/or definition. Many of the well-known exercise apparatuses use this principle. Concentric activity occurs when a force is overcome by the patient by the continued constant tone of the muscle. In the case of eccentric isotonic contraction, the muscle is stretched while maintaining relatively the same tone. During forward bending from the waist, the muscles of the back activate to help maintain fluidity of motion and balance while gravity and the flexor muscle promote the motion. Machinery-assisted exercise is more efficiently used when the patient exerts a smooth range of motion while maintaining tension in both agonist and antagonist groups.

COUNTERSTRAIN
Eileen L. DiGiovanna

The counterstrain technique was developed by Lawrence Jones, an osteopathic practitioner in Oregon. He spent many years perfecting the technique before introducing it to the profession.

In *Strain and Counterstrain,* Jones offers two definitions of the technique:

1. "Relieving spinal or other joint pain by passively putting the joint into its position of greatest comfort."
2. "Relieving pain by reduction and arrest of the continuing inappropriate proprioceptor activity. This is accomplished by markedly shortening the muscle that contains the malfunctioning muscle spindle by applying mild strain to its antagonists."

The theory of counterstrain is based on the belief that somatic dysfunction has a neuromuscular basis (Fig. 5-2). With trauma or muscle effort against a sudden change in resistance, or with muscle strain incurred by resisting the effects of gravity (e.g., bending over) for a period of time, one muscle at a joint is strained and its antagonist is hypershortened. When the shortened muscle is suddenly stretched, the annulospiral receptors of the muscle spindles in that muscle are stimulated, causing a reflex contraction of the already shortened muscle. The proprioceptors in the short muscle now fire impulses as if the shortened muscle were being stretched. Since this inappropriate proprioceptor response can be maintained indefinitely, a somatic dysfunction has been created. The joint is restricted, within its physiologic range of motion, from achieving full range of motion by this shortened muscle. It is therefore an active process rather than a static injury, such as is usually associated with strain (Fig. 5-3).

In counterstrain, the diagnosis is made by finding reflex "tender points." Each involved joint has its own specific tender points, either anterior or posterior. The point may lie in the shortened muscle or in a more distant area to which it has been referred reflexly. It is about the size of a dime and can be palpated as tissue change—a tense, slightly fibrotic area. It is tender to an amount of pressure that would not normally cause pain. The tender points may very well be related to trigger points (Travell points) and acupuncture points; there are similarities in distribution.

The treatment technique is positional. According to Jones, positioning the joint in the position that shortens the involved muscle will relieve the pain and dysfunction. In treatment, therefore, the joint is positioned in such a manner that pressure on the tender point no longer elicits tenderness. The physician should be able to palpate a softening of the tissues.

The technique is passive in that the patient is requested to allow the muscle being treated to relax completely. It is indirect because the joint is positioned into its ease of motion (away from the barrier).

To position the joint, the physician makes a gross adjustment toward the position of comfort and then fine-tunes. For example, the joint may require flexion to reduce the degree of pain, and then a little rotation or side-bending to remove the remaining tenderness. Jones refers to the final position as the "mobile point." The position is held for 90 seconds, the amount of time usually

Figure 5-2. Muscular activity. Bar gauge represents extent of muscle fiber stretch; circular gauge indicates impulses from muscle stretch receptors. (**A**) Arm flexed. (**B**) Arm hyperflexed. (**C**) Arm extended. (**D**) Arm hyperextended.

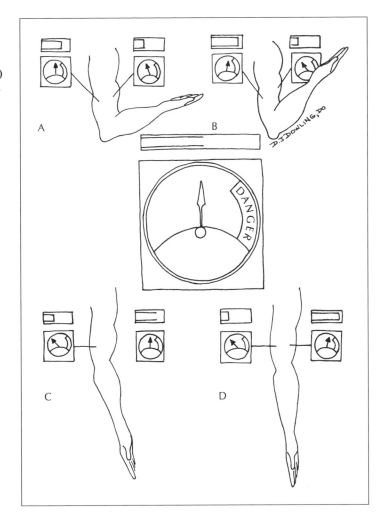

required for the proprioceptive firing to decrease in frequency and amplitude.

The next step is important. The joint is returned slowly to its neutral position. The slow motion prevents reinitiation of the inappropriate proprioceptive firing. The point should be monitored at all times because it is possible to palpate the changes occurring in the muscle, and therefore perhaps less than 90 seconds may be needed for treatment.

The patient is cautioned that some muscle sore-ness may result, but since this is not a somatic dysfunction, the muscle will return to normal quickly.

Counterstrain treatment is an extremely effective and nontraumatic treatment. It is especially good for elderly or hospitalized patients, and any others for whom gentleness is desirable. Patients who have experienced an acute strain respond well. Certain positions may be uncomfortable or undesirable for some patients, so the physician must use judgment when selecting the treatments.

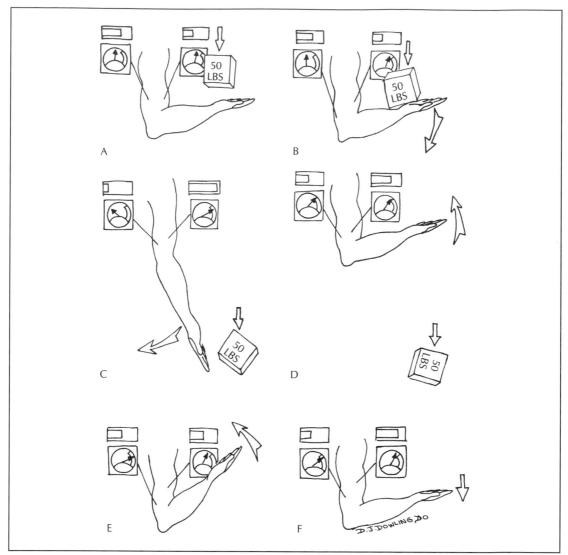

Figure 5-3. Etiology of tender point. **(A)** Both flexors and extensors are in easy normal position. **(B)** Force is suddenly exerted counter to the flexors, forcing the arm into extension. **(C)** Fibers and stretch receptors indicate that a danger point has been reached. Extensor fibers are hypershortened. **(D)** Arm is relatively flexed, exciting the muscle stretch receptors. **(E)** Rapid rate of flexion overstimulates extensor stretch receptors. **(F)** Arm is in same position as in **A**, but stretch receptors continue to respond as if muscle were being rapidly stretched.

FACILITATED POSITIONAL RELEASE
Stanley Schiowitz

Facilitated positional release uses a modification of indirect myofascial release techniques, enhanced by placing the region in the neutral position and adding compression or torsion. The advantage of this technique is its ease of application and speed of response. In addition, if the desired results do not occur immediately, it may be repeated or other methods of treatment can be added.

This treatment is directed toward the normalization of hypertonic muscles, both superficial and deep. It is this author's belief that most of the vertebral joint motion restrictions diagnosed as somatic dysfunctions are caused and/or maintained by hypertonicity of the small, deep, intervertebral muscles. These hypertonic muscles respond well to facilitated positional release, thus immediately restoring normal joint function.

A possible explanation for the effectiveness of this treatment relates to the action of the muscle spindle gamma loop when the gain is suddenly decreased. According to Carew, with a sudden decrease in load, the spindles in the muscle become unloaded and the Ia fiber discharges from these spindles cease and no longer excite motor neurons controlling the extrafusal muscle fiber. The muscle then begins to relax until it lengthens. This physiologic change may well account for the immediate effect felt when facilitating force is used in these techniques.

General Procedure

The physician modifies the patient's sagittal posture in the region to be treated, adding a facilitating force and placing the dysfunction into its freedoms of motion.

In general, hypertonic muscle tissue found along the posterior aspect of the spine is shortened with backward bending and side-bending to the same side. If tissue hypertonicity is found anteriorly, forward bending is usually required. Some muscles have a contralateral side-bending function or a rotary component; these muscles must be placed in their individual shortened positions. Careful localization of the component motions of facilitation, forward and backward bending, sidebending, and rotation to the area of the hypertonicity will produce more accurate results.

Specific Techniques

TECHNIQUE FOR MODIFYING SUPERFICIAL AREAS OF MUSCLE HYPERTONICITY

1. The patient assumes a relaxed position.
2. The physician flattens the anteroposterior spinal curve of the area to be treated.
3. The physician places the muscle into its ease of motion (i.e., shortened).
4. The physician applies a facilitating force (compression, torsion, or a combination of these forces). Steps 3 and 4 may be applied in reverse order.
5. The position is held for 3 to 4 seconds.
6. The physician releases the position and reevaluates the dysfunction.

TECHNIQUE FOR TREATING INTERVERTEBRAL MOTION RESTRICTIONS, SECONDARY TO HYPERTONICITY OF DEEP INTERVERTEBRAL MUSCLES

The procedures are the same as for treating superficial muscle hypertonicity, except for step 3: the physician places the vertebra into its planes of freedom of motion. For example, a somatic dysfunction diagnosed as C5 F Sr Rr is treated by placing the fifth cervical vertebra into a position of flexion, right lateral flexion, and right rotation with respect to the sixth cervical vertebra. Springing, which exaggerates the freedoms of motion, may be added to completely release articular dysfunctions.

THRUSTING TECHNIQUES
Eileen L. DiGiovanna

Most thrusting techniques are direct techniques, in that the dysfunctional unit is placed into at least one of its barriers to motion and the physician thrusts through that barrier. The techniques are considered passive because the physician provides the treating force and the patient remains passive.

High-Velocity, Low-Amplitude Techniques

The best known of all manipulative techniques are the high-velocity, low-amplitude techniques. In these techniques, the physician positions the patient in such a way that the restricted joint is placed into its barriers to motion. The physician then quickly applies a small amount of force to the joint in such a way as to move it through the barriers. Improved joint motion should result.

To achieve the best results with as little pain as possible, the surrounding tissues should be relaxed before the thrusting force is applied. Myofascial (soft tissue) techniques or other nonthrusting techniques may be used for this purpose. When the muscles and soft tissues are relaxed, less force is needed to move the joint and the treatment will be less painful.

High-velocity, low-amplitude techniques may have been the first type of manual medicine ever devised. They are the therapeutic maneuvers most commonly used by chiropractors and many osteopathic physicians, as well as other practitioners of manual medicine.

Low-Velocity, High-Amplitude Techniques

In some thrusting techniques a greater force is applied slowly with the goal of moving the joint through the barrier. Care must be taken to avoid joint or soft tissue damage. These techniques, when applied skillfully, are quite useful, but the force must be carefully controlled. Again, relaxation of the soft tissues before force is applied makes the procedure safer and less painful.

Springing Techniques

Springing techniques are similar to high-velocity, low-amplitude techniques except that a full force is not applied. The joint is positioned as before, then gently sprung several times against its barriers. This maneuver gently nudges the joint motion through its barrier. The springing force is much less than that applied in high-velocity, low-amplitude techniques.

With repeated springing thrusts against the barrier, the joint may be moved as effectively as with high-velocity, low-amplitude thrusting but with less danger of trauma. Springing techniques are useful in more painful joints, older persons, and children, and whenever a stronger force is contraindicated.

General Principles of Thrusting Techniques

1. Prepare the joint to be treated by relaxing the soft tissues so that the joint may be moved more easily with less resistance from the soft tissues.
2. Place the joint into its barriers of motion. If only one barrier is to be engaged, it is essential that all other joint motions be "locked" out.
3. Once a joint has been placed into its barriers of motion, this position must be held firmly by the physician and the "locking" thus created not lost as the force is applied.
4. The force must be controlled by the physician. Maximum force should never be applied in the hope that the joint will move. Only force sufficient to create the motion desired should be used. Force should never replace skill.
5. Treatment must be localized and applied to the specific restricted joint. A "shotgun" approach to an entire area of the spine is inappropriate and harmful.

Pops and Cracks

Particularly with high-velocity, low-amplitude techniques, a popping or cracking sound may be heard, similar to the sound made by cracking the knuckles. Some observers believe the sound is due to the breaking of a vacuum in the joint, others that it is caused by release of a nitrogen bubble. Whatever its cause, eliciting this noise is not essential to the correction of a dysfunction. Feeling the joint move is more important than hearing it pop.

Many patients feel the treatment is successful only if they hear this sound. Others are frightened by it, fearing bones may be breaking. The patient must be assured that the sound is harmless, as well as unnecessary.

EXERCISE THERAPY
Stanley Schiowitz
Albert R. DeRubertis

The average physician, before prescribing a specific drug, will have arrived at a working diagnosis and a therapeutic plan. The physician is expected to know the appropriate drug dosage, its side effects, its compatibilities with other drugs, and its effects on other clinical entities that the patient might have.

These minimal requirements of physician capability hold equally true in the prescription of exercise as a therapeutic modality. All physicians encounter patients who are voluntarily pursuing some form of exercise or for whom an exercise program should be prescribed. This chapter addresses the primary care physician's use and prescription of exercise therapy for musculoskeletal dysfunctions.

Biomechanics of Muscle Function

Muscle tissue has the properties of extensibility, elasticity, and contractility. *Extensibility* is the ability of muscle fiber to lengthen, usually to an additional 50% of its resting size. As one bends forward to touch the toes, the back muscles lengthen to accommodate the stretch.

Elasticity is the ability of muscle fiber to return to its original length. When one straightens up after touching the toes, the back muscles return to their former length.

Contractility is the ability of muscle fiber to shorten its length up to 50%. Only muscles have this capability, and it is the muscle property that is usually acknowledged.

In the example of forward bending, inability to touch the toes has no relationship to the contractile property of the abdominal muscles. Loss of extensibility of the hamstrings might be the culprit. Therefore, exercises would be directed toward increasing the extensibility of the hamstrings, and not toward strengthening the abdominals.

In daily usage, "tight, shortened, hypertonic" muscles need restoration of extensibility. "Flaccid, stretched, atonic" muscles have lost their elasticity, and "weak, hypotonic" muscles require increased contractility. The type of exercise, massage, and myofascial therapy prescribed is different for each of these dysfunctions.

MOMENT OF FORCE

Muscle power is used to move one part of the skeletal system around another part, with their articulation acting as a fulcrum. This creates a torque or *moment of force*. The torque around any point equals the product of the amount of force and its perpendicular distance from the direction of force to the axis of rotation (*moment arm*). If one were to hold a 5-pound weight in the palm, with the elbow flexed at a 90-degree angle, and if the distance from the elbow joint to the weight were 1 foot, then 5 foot-pounds of flexor muscle effort would be needed to maintain this position. If the elbow were flexed at a 45-degree angle, the force, the 5-pound weight, would stay the same but the moment arm would be reduced. Less than 5 foot-pounds of flexor muscle effort would be needed to maintain this position.

LEVER ACTION

The use of the joint as a fulcrum brings into play Newton's laws of levers.

1. A first-class lever has the fulcrum placed between the point of effort and resistance.

2. A second-class lever has the resistance placed between the fulcrum and the point of effort.
3. A third-class lever has the point of effort between the fulcrum and resistance.

Of the three levers, the second-class lever is most efficient with regard to minimizing effort needed to move a resistance. A wheelbarrow is an example of such a lever. Most of our long muscles act as third-class levers. The biceps muscle's flexion effort in moving the forearm is an example of such a lever action. The triceps' action causing forearm extension is an example of a first-class lever. First-class lever action usually requires less effort for motion than third-class lever action.

An interesting demonstration of lever action is afforded by the brachialis muscle in flexion. Simple forearm flexion represents a third-class lever action; however, with a weight in the palm, lowering the forearm from a position of flexion to one of extension reverses the designations, in that gravity becomes the effort or moving force, while the insertion of the brachialis becomes the resistant force. This creates a second-class lever action.

SPURT-AND-SHUNT ACTION
MacConaill and Basmajian defines the spurt and shunt action of muscles as follows. When a muscle contracts it creates two vector forces with regard to the articulation. One is a swing (rotation) force around its axis (spurt action). The second is transarticular motion into the joint in relation to its axis (shunt action). Both of these motions are present simultaneously, but in different proportions in all muscles. A large spurt-to-shunt ratio permits greater rotary motion with diminished joint stability. The reverse is true with an increased shunt-to-spurt ratio.

The biceps flexion motion of the forearm is primarily a spurt action at the elbow, but contraction of the long head of the biceps is a stabilizing, shunt action at the glenohumeral articulation.

A third motion is created by muscle contraction—spin motion. The amount of spin will depend on the difference in the planes of the origin and insertion of the muscle. Spin motion plays a part in the second law of myokinematics, described below.

LAWS OF MYOKINEMATICS
The first law of myokinematics (MacConaill and Basmajian, 1977), the law of approximation, states

that "when a muscle contracts it tends to bring its attachments (origin and insertion) closer together." In most activities the effect of this law is modified by using other muscle activity or resistant force to stabilize either the insertion or origin end of the muscle. This creates motion at one end of the muscle only.

The second law, the law of detorsion, states that "when a muscle contracts it tends to bring its line of origin and its line of insertion into one and the same plane." A simple example is sternocleidomastoid action. Unilateral contraction creates ipsilateral side-bending, extension, and contralateral rotation of the head.

A less commonly recognized application of this principle is in hip extension. Pure gluteus maximus contraction tightens the hip joint and raises the femur somewhat toward the ilium in the frontal plane. To achieve hip extension, the pelvis rotates anteriorly in the sagittal plane. This rotation changes the planar relationships of the origin and insertion of the muscle. The law of detorsion is activated, and the insertion will try to match the plane of muscle origin. The more the pelvis is rotated, the greater will be the hip extension.

Gravity
Gravitational force is the attraction of each mass-particle in the universe for every other mass-particle. Gravitational force has three unique characteristics:

1. It is applied constantly.
2. It is applied in one direction only.
3. It acts on each mass-particle of the body.

This force is constantly exerted on all parts of the musculoskeletal system. Its effects, however, can be modified by body position. In the upright, anatomic position, gravity assists in stabilizing the hip, knee, and ankle joints. At the same time it creates instability of the glenohumeral articulation. In the supine position, gravitational force on all these joints is markedly different. The physician must be aware of the action of gravity when using exercise therapy. Bending the head forward in the upright position does not exercise the cervical flexor muscles. Gravity is the primary force involved. Extensor muscles are brought into play if control of the speed of forward bending is desired. In the supine position, forward bending or bringing the chin to the chest would necessitate use of the neck flexors.

An important aspect of all exercises is the patient's position and its relationship to gravitational force.

Muscle Contraction Definitions

1. **Concentric contraction.** The muscle shortens, using the property of contractility to perform the task.
2. **Eccentric contraction.** The muscle lengthens, using extensibility to perform the task.
3. **Static contraction.** The muscle is in partial or complete contraction without changing its length. There is no rotary joint motion.

Note: In the previous example of forward bending of the head:

1. In the upright position, the eccentric contraction (lengthening) of the extensor muscles controls the speed of forward bending. These muscles are exercised.
2. In the supine position, the concentric (shortening) contraction of the flexor muscles lifts the head off the floor. These muscles are exercised.
3. In the prone position, the patient may try to bend forward, but the floor will prevent the motion. This will create static contraction of the neck flexors, which are exercised.

Classification of Exercise

1. **Isotonic.** A dynamic exercise with a constant load. The resistance is the product of the load and the resistance arm (moment arm), and therefore is not constant.
2. **Isokinetic.** A dynamic exercise in which the speed of motion is controlled by varying the resistance.
3. **Isometric.** A static exercise in which the muscle contracts with little or no shortening (static contraction).

Note: The previous example of elbow flexion by contraction of the biceps with a weight held in the palm can be described as follows:

1. As flexion proceeds from a position of 90 degrees, the moment arm lessens; therefore, the resistance lessens. If the contraction force of the biceps is maintained constant, then the speed of flexion will correspondingly increase. This is an example of isotonic exercise.
2. If, as the moment arm lessens, the weight in the palm correspondingly is increased, then the resistance continually increases with flexion. The speed of flexion will remain constant. This is an example of isokinetic exercise, which can only be performed by using machines designed for this purpose.
3. If the weight in the palm were too heavy to be moved, then, as the biceps contracted, flexion would not be created, the muscle would not change its length, and the moment arm and resistance would be constant. This is an example of isometric exercise.

Isokinetic exercise increases the work a muscle can do more rapidly than either isometric or isotonic exercise. It is more efficient. *Isometric* exercise should be used when motion of the joint is contraindicated or creates pain. For skill training, the best form of exercise is isotonic repetition of the motions needed in performing those skills.

Indications for Exercise Therapy

1. To develop a sense of good postural alignment
2. To relax or lengthen contracted or shortened musculature
3. To achieve flexibility of joint motion within its normal range of motion
4. To increase muscle strength as needed to attain and maintain proper function.

Other chapters of this book describe methods for determining if these indications exist: static symmetry scan, regional motion testing, joint motion testing, palpation, and intersegmental motion testing. The only dysfunction testing not yet described is that used for muscle strength.

Testing for Muscle Function (Strength-Contractility)

The general procedure for strength testing is to direct the patient to concentrically contract the muscle to be tested, and then quantitatively measure the results and classify the findings.

1. Procedure for strength testing
   a. Place the segment in a completely relaxed position with minimal influence of gravity.
   b. Position the segment of the body involved so that the motion being tested can occur.
   c. Have the patient contract the involved muscle in an attempt to achieve concentric contraction and joint motion.
   d. Evaluate results.
2. Classification
   a. No contraction at all—paralysis—grade 0.
   b. Contraction felt by examiner's fingers, but no motion—grade 1.
   c. Contraction with motion achievable only on elimination of gravity—poor—grade 2.
   d. Contraction with motion against gravity—fair—grade 3.
   e. Contraction with motion against resistive force—good—grade 4.

Inactivity and Hypokinetic Disease

Kraus and associates reported on studies performed to measure strength and flexibility of the trunk and leg muscles in children. Whereas only 8.7% of European children failed this test, 57.9% of American children failed. The poor American showing may be explained by the high degree of mechanization available.

In addition to mechanization, civilization has inhibited the "fight or flight" response. Urbanized man lives in an almost constant alert reaction phase. This imbalance in our lives—excessive unresolved stimulation—combined with insufficient exercise keeps us living in a potentially pathogenic environment.

The terms *tension neck, tension headache*, and *tension back pain* are common to the primary care physician. These syndromes are difficult to diagnose and even more difficult to treat. A multifactorial approach, incorporating behavior modification with relaxation and lengthening exercises, is advisable. Prevention by means of universal relaxation and lengthening exercises and stress modification techniques should begin in childhood and continue throughout life.

Kraus-Weber Test (Modified)

The modified Kraus-Weber test is a scanning procedure for evaluating groups of muscles acting together to perform specific body motions. Tests 1

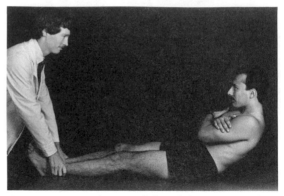

Figure 5-4. Test of upper abdominal–psoas muscle strength.

through 5 primarily evaluate muscle strength. As the primary agonist muscles are contracted, the antagonist muscles are stretched. Contracture of these antagonist muscles might lead to a false interpretation of agonist muscle weakness. Tests 6 and 7 primarily test for muscle shortening (loss of extensibility).

Physicians treating musculoskeletal dysfunctions should use some form of screening to assist in prescribing effective exercise therapy. Numerous other tests are available, in addition to the one described here.

Test 1 tests upper abdominal-psoas muscle strength (Fig. 5-4):

1. **Patient position:** Supine, with hands folded across chest, and legs fully extended.
2. **Physician position:** At foot of table holding patient's feet down.
3. Patient is instructed to curl head and body up, off the table. If the back is elevated 30 degrees or more off the table, the upper abdominal muscles are functioning adequately. If the back is elevated more than 60 degrees to the fully upright position, psoas muscle strength is being used and tested.

Test 2 tests abdominal muscle strength without psoas involvement (Fig. 5-5):

1. **Patient position:** Supine, with hands folded across chest, hips and knees flexed, with feet flat on table.
2. **Physician position:** Holding patient's feet down flat on table.

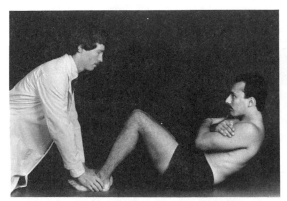

Figure 5-5. Test of upper abdominal muscle strength without psoas involvement.

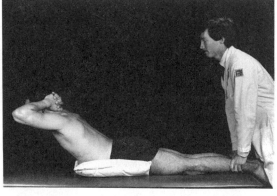

Figure 5-7. Test of upper back muscle strength.

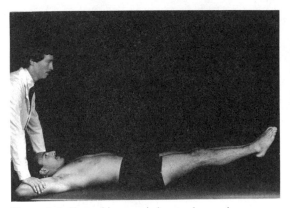

Figure 5-6. Test of lower abdominal muscle strength.

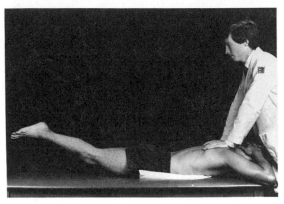

Figure 5-8. Test of lower back muscle strength.

3. Patient is instructed as before to curl the body up to a seated position.
4. Measure degree of compliance.

Test 3 tests lower abdominal muscle strength (Fig. 5-6):

1. **Patient position:** Supine with hands behind neck and both legs extended.
2. **Physician position:** At head of the table, holding patient's shoulders to the table.
3. Patient is instructed to lift both feet off the table, with legs extended, to a height of 10 inches, and to hold this position for 10 seconds.
4. Measure degree of compliance.

Test 4 tests upper back muscle strength (Fig. 5-7):

1. **Patient position:** Prone, with pillow under abdomen, legs fully extended, hands clasped behind back.
2. **Physician position:** At foot of table, holding patient's hips and legs down to table.
3. Patient is instructed to raise his chest and abdomen off the table, and hold this position for 10 seconds.
4. Measure degree of compliance.

Test 5 tests lower back muscle strength (Fig. 5-8):

1. **Patient position:** Prone, with pillow under abdomen, legs fully extended, hands clasped behind neck.
2. **Physician position:** At head of table holding patient's shoulders down.

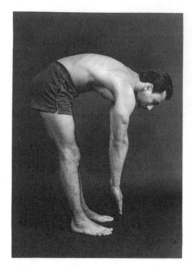

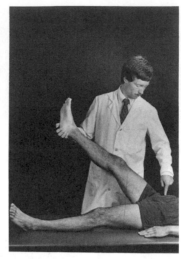

Figure 5-9. Test of hamstring extensibility.

Figure 5-10. Test of hamstring extensibility.

3. Patient is instructed to raise both legs off the table, without bending the knees, and to hold this position for 10 seconds.
4. Measure degree of compliance.

Test 6 tests hamstring extensibility (Fig. 5-9):

1. **Patient position:** Upright, completely erect, feet together, hands at sides.
2. Patient is told to bend forward, trying to touch the floor, without bending the knees.
3. Physician measures the distance of the fingertips from the floor to determine degree of compliance.

Test 7 tests hamstring extensibility (Fig. 5-10):

1. **Patient position:** Supine, both legs fully extended.
2. **Physician position:** At side of hamstrings to be tested.
3. Physician places one hand under the patient's heel. The physician's other hand is at the ipsilateral anterior superior iliac spine.
4. Physician passively raises the fully extended leg off the table until rotary motion is felt at the anterior superior iliac spine.
5. Measure the degree of hip flexion. Less than 60 degrees of flexion is considered loss of hamstring extensibility.
6. Flexion of 80 to 90 degrees indicates good extensibility of the gluteus maximus muscle. More

than 90 degrees of flexion indicates good extensibility of the erector spinae muscle.
   Note: The interpretation of this test can be invalidated by the presence of radiculitis or hip joint restriction.

Planning an Exercise Program—General Principles

1. Do not perform if exercise causes pain.
2. Evaluate the gravitational force and patient's position.
3. Evaluate the effect of exercising two joint muscles on both joints.
4. Start with relaxing (postural) exercises, then add mild corrective exercise, gradually increase to strenuous corrective exercises, specifically planned and to patient's tolerance.
5. Do not stop exercising abruptly. Return to mild exercises and relaxing exercises, gradually tapering off.
6. Instruct patient to relax between individual exercises.
7. Change position of patient and vary the exercises.
8. Multiple repetitions of identical movements should be avoided. Perform only two or three of the same exercise in one session.
9. All exercises are performed slowly and smoothly.
10. Avoid patient fatigue.
11. Perform regimen regularly.

General Precautions

These precautions should be taken into account when writing exercise prescriptions.

1. Protect one body segment from strain while exercising another part.
2. Be aware of the needs, expectations, and limitations of the older patient.
3. Be aware of the needs, expectations, and limitations of debilitated patients.
4. Patients may have illness that may be worsened with active exercises.
5. Always prescribe specific therapy for specific purposes.
6. Avoid overdose of exercise therapy.
7. Do not cause pain by movement.
8. Prescribe supportive medications as indicated.
9. Prescribe follow-up treatments.
10. Prescribe home therapy and exercise as you would prescribe drug therapy.

Relaxing Exercises

There are many variations and styles of relaxing exercises. The one described here uses static muscle contraction.

Patient position: Supine, legs extended and arms at sides. Instruct patient as follows:

1. Bring your ankles and toes into full dorsiflexion; now try to push the foot and toes into further dorsiflexion. Hold for a count of 4, relax.
2. Contract your calf muscles statically, hold for a count of 4, relax.
3. Contract your buttocks statically, hold for a count of 4, relax.
4. Bend your hips and knees and place your feet on the floor. Push your low back to the floor as firmly as possible, hold for a count of 4, relax.
5. Raise your back off the floor so that you are supported by your feet, upper spine, and shoulders. Push down on your upper spine and shoulders. Hold for a count of 4, relax.
6. Contract your hands, making a firm fist. Hold for a count of 4, relax.
7. Contract your forearm muscles statically. Hold for a count of 4, relax.
8. Contract your biceps muscles statically. Hold for a count of 4, relax.
9. Shrug your shoulders up toward your ears, as far as possible. Hold for a count of 4, relax.
10. Bring your shoulders forward, trying to meet in the midline. Hold for a count of 4, relax.
11. Tuck your chin in, then push your neck firmly backward toward the floor. Hold for a count of 4, relax.

Writing an Exercise Prescription

The exercise prescription must do the following:

1. Be specific for musculoskeletal dysfunctions
2. Take into account the patient's physical and mental condition
3. Take into account the patient's muscle function:
   a. Ability to shorten—*contractility*
   b. Ability to lengthen—*extensibility*
   c. Ability to return to normal size—*elasticity*

Below is an example of an exercise prescription.

Patient's name: _____

Date: _____

Goals: _____

_____

Procedures to follow:

1. Patient position: perform the following relaxing exercises:

   a. _____   time _____

   b. _____   time _____

   c. _____   time _____

   d. _____   time _____

2. Rest; change position; perform the following mild exercises (specific for goals):

   a. _____   time _____

   b. _____   time _____

   c. _____   time _____

3. Rest; change position; perform the following more difficult exercises, without pain (specific for goals):

a. _____ time _____

b. _____ time _____

c. _____ time _____

4. Rest, repeat item 2.

5. Rest, repeat item 1.

You have completed this set of exercises. It should have taken _____ minutes to complete them.

Repeat this set of exercises _____ times daily.

You are to continue these exercises until your next appointment at this office

on _____ (date).

Warning: *Do not perform any of the prescribed exercises if they create pain. Call my office for advice before continuing with this program.*

References

Ashmore EF. 1981. Osteopathic Mechanics. London: Tamor Pierston.

Bove AA, Lowenthal DT. 1983. Exercise Medicine. New York: Academic Press.

Cailliet R. 1977. Soft Tissue Pain and Disability. Philadelphia: F.A. Davis.

Carew TJ. 1985. The control of reflex action. In Kandel ER, Schwartz JH, eds., Principles of Neural Science, 2nd ed. New York: Elsevier, p. 464.

Daniels L, Worthingham C. 1972. Muscle Testing, 3rd ed. Philadelphia: W.B. Saunders.

——— Worthingham C. 1977. Therapeutic Exercise, 2nd ed. Philadelphia: W.B. Saunders.

De Lateur B, Lehmann J, Stonebridge J. 1972. Isotonic versus isometric exercise. Arch Phys Med Rehabil 53:212–217.

Gowitzke BA, Milner M. 1980. Understanding the Scientific Basis of Human Movement. Baltimore: Williams & Wilkins.

Graham K. 1985. Outline of Muscle Energy Techniques. Tulsa, OK: Oklahoma College of Osteopathic Medicine.

Greenman PE. 1987. Models and mechanisms of osteopathic manipulative medicine. Osteopath Med News IV:11–14,20.

Guyton AC. 1986. Textbook of Medical Physiology. Philadelphia: W.B. Saunders.

Hoag JM, Cole WV, Bradford SG. 1969. Osteopathic Medicine. New York: McGraw-Hill.

Hutton RS, Nelson DL. 1986. Stretch sensitivity of Golgi tendon organs in fatigued gastrocnemius muscle. Med Sci Sports Med 18(1):69–74.

Jones LH. 1981. Strain and Counterstrain. Colorado Springs: American Academy of Osteopathy.

Kendall FP, McCreary EB. 1983. Muscles: Testing and Function. 3rd ed. Baltimore: Williams & Wilkins.

Kraus H. Clinical Treatment of Back and Neck Pain. New York: McGraw-Hill Book Co.

———, Hirschland RP. 1954. Minimum muscular fitness tests in school children. Res Q 25(2):178–188.

———, Prudden B, Hirschorn K. 1956. Role of inactivity in production of disease: A hypokinetic disease. J Am Geriatr Soc 4(5).

MacConaill MA, Basmajian JV. 1977. Muscles and Movement. Huntington, New York: Robert E. Krieger.

Mitchell FL Jr, Moran PS, Pruzzo NA. 1979. An Evaluation and Treatment Manual of Osteopathic Muscle Energy Procedures. Valley Park, Mo: Mitchell, Moran, and Pruzzo Assoc.

Moffroid M, Whipple R, Hofkosh J, et al. 1969. A study of isokinetic exercise. Phys Med Ther 49:735–746.

Rasch PJ, Burke RK. 1978. Kinesiology and Applied Anatomy, 6th ed. Philadelphia: Lea & Febiger.

Schiowitz S. 1990. Facilitated positional release. J Am Osteopath Assoc 901:145–155.

Spulman JM, Hauffer EK. 1986. Morphological observations of motor units connected in series to Golgi tendon organs. J Neurophysiol 55(1):147–162.

Stauffer EK, et al. 1986. Responses of Golgi tendon organs to concurrently active motor units. Brain Res 375:157–162.

Stiles EG. 1984. Manipulation: A tool for your practice? Patient Care 18:137–189.

Thistle HG, Hislop HJ, Moffroid M. 1967. Isokinetic contraction: A new concept of resistive exercise. Arch Phys Med Rehabil 48:279–282.

Wells KF, Luttgens K. 1976. Kinesiology, 6th ed. Philadelphia: W.B. Saunders.

6

Evaluation of the Cervical Spine

FUNCTIONAL ANATOMY AND BIOMECHANICS
Jonathan Fenton

The cervical spine is made up of the seven cervical vertebrae. Functionally it is divided into two areas: the articulations between the occiput, atlas, and axis, and the articulations between the third through seventh cervical vertebrae.

Occipitoatlantal Joint
The occipitoatlantal articulation consists of the superior articular facets of the atlas and the two occipital condyles. The superior facets of the atlas face backward, upward, and medially and are concave in both anteroposterior and transverse diameters. The surfaces of the occipital condyles match the facets of the atlas, and the joint is best thought of as a sphere (the occiput) gliding on the articular surfaces of the atlas (Fig. 6-1). The freely movable occiput is limited by its muscular and ligamentous attachments, which make flexion-extension the primary motion, producing a small-amplitude nodding of the head. Flexion of the occiput on the atlas is accompanied by a posterior translatory slide of the occiput; extension is accompanied by an anterior translatory slide.

Side-bending and rotation of the occipitoatlantal joint always occur in opposite directions, in part because of the position of the lateral atlanto-occipital ligament. When the occiput rotates left on the atlas, the lateral atlanto-occipital ligament causes the occiput to slide (translate) to the left and therefore side-bend to the right (Fig. 6-2). Somatic dysfunctions of the occipitoatlantal joint most often involve the minor motions of side-bending and rotation.

Atlantoaxial Joint
The atlantoaxial articulation is specially adapted for (nearly) pure rotation. In addition to the inferior articular facets of the atlas and the superior articular facets of the axis, movement other than rotation is limited by the anteriorly located odontoid process (dens) of the axis. The odontoid process is held close to the anterior arch of the atlas by the transverse ligament of the atlas, which allows only a slight amount of flexion of the atlas on the axis.

There is no true lateral flexion at the atlantoaxial joint, only a wobble created by the articulation of the superior axial and inferior atlantal articular facets. Unlike most facets, these four facets are all convex in shape (Fig. 6-3). During rotation of the

An Osteopathic Approach to Diagnosis and Treatment, second edition
Eileen L. DiGiovanna and Stanley Schiowitz
Lippincott–Raven Publishers, Philadelphia © 1997.

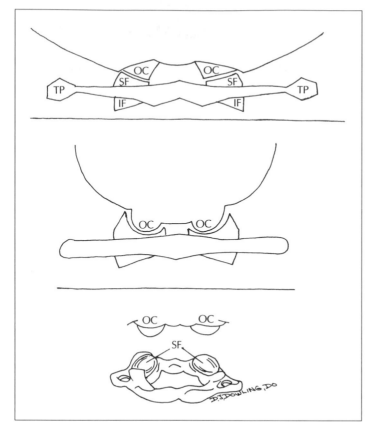

Figure 6-1. Bony anatomy of the occipitoatlantal joint, posterosuperior view. *OC*, occipital condyle; *SF*, superior facet; *IF*, inferior facet; *TP*, transverse process.

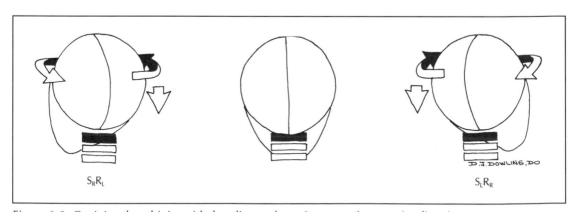

Figure 6-2. Occipitoatlantal joint: side-bending and rotation occur in opposite directions.

Figure 6-3. Atlantoaxial articulation. *AT*, anterior tubercle; *PT*, posterior tubercle; *TF*, transverse foramen; *SP*, spinous process; *IFa*, inferior facet of atlas; *IFax*, inferior facet of axis; *SFa*, superior facet of atlas; *SFax*, superior facet of axis.

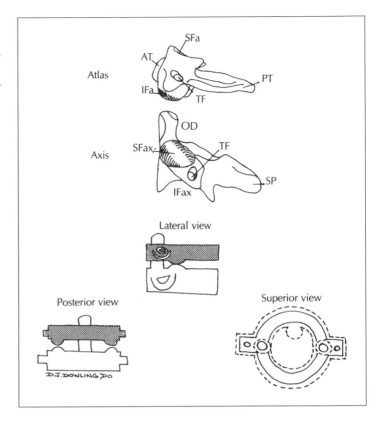

atlas on the axis to the right, the left articular facet of the atlas in effect slides uphill on the left articular facet of the axis, while on the right the atlas slides downhill on the axis. This wobble motion is not true lateral flexion.

Somatic dysfunction at the atlantoaxial joint occurs in rotation.

The complex of the occipitoatlantal plus the atlantoaxial joints is known as the *suboccipital articulation*. Its range of motion makes it function as a universal (swivel) joint. Many consider the suboccipital articulation the final compensator of the spine, by which the body adjusts to any dysfunctions occurring below. Compensatory adjustment is needed to keep the eyes level in two planes, to promote binocular vision.

The articulation between the second (C2) and third (C3) cervical vertebrae sustains tremendous stress because of its position between the final compensator above and the rest of the spine below. Therefore, it is a common location for chronic somatic dysfunction.

Third to Seventh Cervical Vertebrae (C3–C7)

This portion of the cervical spine allows for a great deal of motion, with special adaptation to meet the demands of mobility and stability placed upon it. The cervical intervertebral disks are the relatively thickest of the spinal disks; the ratio of disk height to vertebral body height in this section of the spinal column is 2:5. The disks are wedge-shaped and thicker anteriorly than posteriorly (Fig. 6-4). In conjunction with the anteroposterior convexity of the vertebral endplates, the wedge shape maintains the flexible cervical lordosis.

The facet joints in this area are located posterolaterally. Two articulating facets, one superior and one inferior, form the palpable articular pillars. The superior articular facets face backward and upward. The plane of the facet joints lies midway between the horizontal and frontal planes in normal lordosis (Fig. 6-5). This orientation causes rotation and side-bending to be coupled motions, always occurring in the same direction. When the

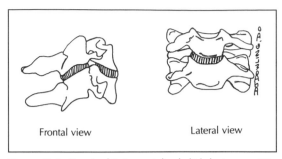

Figure 6-4. Cervical intervertebral disk between C3 and C4.

The cervical vertebrae C3 to C7 move least in flexion-extension. In flexion the inferior articular facets of the upper vertebrae must slide up the superior articular facets of the lower vertebrae, up a 45-degree incline. The normal lordotic curve in this area places the cervical spine in partial extension; the cervical spine has no neutral position.

To assist in maintaining some measure of stability in the face of the large amounts of motion possible in the midcervical spine, a specialized set of synovial joints has developed as an adaptation for upright posture in humans. These joints, known as the unciform joints or the joints of Luschka, are located on the lateral edges of the cervical vertebral bodies (Fig. 6-6). The lateral lips of two adjacent vertebrae articulate and are contained within

cervical spine is placed in a more backward bending position, the facets are more oriented in the frontal plane, where side-bending is the primary motion. When the neck is brought into a forward bending position, the plane of the facets becomes more horizontal, and rotation is the major motion.

Figure 6-6. Location of the joints of Luschka (unciform joints), anterior view.

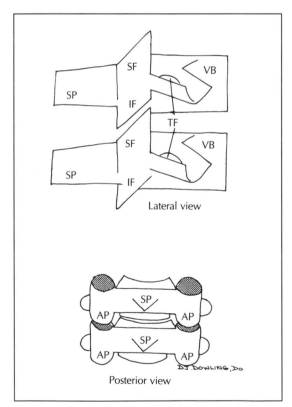

Figure 6-5. Orientation of articular facets of C3 and C4 vertebrae. *SP*, spinous process; *SF*, superior facet; *IF*, inferior facet; *VB*, vertebral body; *AP*, articular pillar; *TF*, transverse foramina.

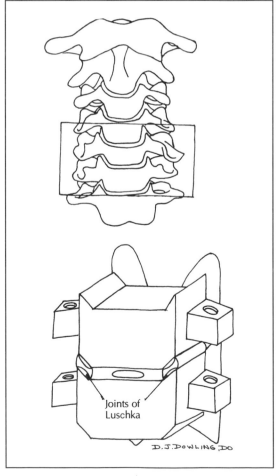

Joints of Luschka

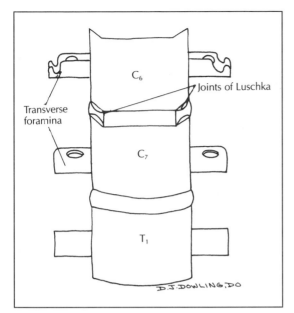

Figure 6-7. Seventh cervical vertebra. Note anatomic similarity superiorly to sixth cervical vertebra and inferiorly to first thoracic vertebra.

a small synovial capsule. These joints develop at age 8 to 10 years.

The unciform joints (joints of Luschka) act as guide rails for the motions of flexion-extension. They also limit the lateral translatory motion (side slip) that occurs simultaneously with the coupled motions of side-bending and rotation. When one vertebra side-bends and rotates on another, that vertebra will translate laterally in the opposite direction. In the cervical spine this lateral translatory motion would be excessive to the point of subluxation were it not for the unciform joints.

Somatic dysfunctions in the C3 to C7 joints occur in the coupled rotary motions of side-bending and rotation, and in lateral translation. Dysfunctions of translatory motion that accompany rotary dysfunctions create a complicated dysfunction, side slip.

Seventh Cervical–First Thoracic Joint (C7-T1)

The anatomy of the seventh cervical vertebra is transitional, resembling cervical vertebral anatomy superiorly and thoracic vertebral anatomy inferiorly (Fig. 6-7). At the cervicothoracic (C7-T1) junction, cervical lordosis normally ends and thoracic kyphosis begins. As a result, the forces placed on this area are quite complex, and of a different nature from forces sustained higher or lower in the spine. Somatic dysfunction of the cervicothoracic junction is quite common and difficult to treat.

MOTION TESTING
Sandra D. Yale

Gross Motion Testing
FORWARD BENDING
1. **Patient position:** seated.
2. **Physician position:** standing at side of patient.
3. **Technique:**
   a. Place one hand on the occiput and the other hand on the cervicothoracic junction (Fig. 6-8).
   b. Gently push the patient's head forward until you feel motion at the cervicothoracic junction (between C7 and T1).
   c. Note the angle of displacement from the upright position. This is usually 80 to 90 degrees, or until the patient's chin touches the manubrium.

BACKWARD BENDING
1. **Patient position:** seated.
2. **Physician position:** standing at side of patient.
3. **Technique:**
   a. Place one hand on the patient's forehead and the other hand on the cervicothoracic junction (Fig. 6-9).
   b. Gently push the patient's head backward until you feel motion at the cervicothoracic junction.
   c. Note the angle of displacement from the upright position. This is usually 80 to 90 degrees, or until the patient looks directly at the ceiling.

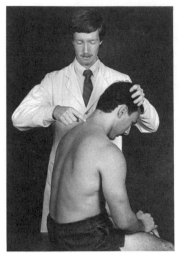

Figure 6-8. Gross motion testing of the cervical spine, forward bending.

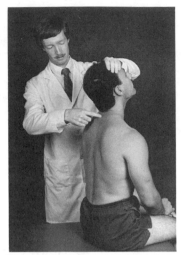

Figure 6-9. Gross motion testing of the cervical spine, backward bending.

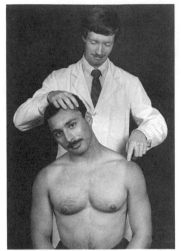

Figure 6-10. Gross motion testing of the cervical spine, lateral flexion.

SIDE BENDING
1. **Patient position:** seated.
2. **Patient position:** standing behind patient.
3. **Technique:**
   a. To flex the patient's spine laterally to the right, place one hand on the left parietal. Use the other hand to monitor left shoulder elevation (Fig. 6-10).
   b. Apply gentle pressure with the hand to bend the patient's neck to the right.
   c. Reverse hands for left side-bending. Repeat step b to the left.
   d. Note the angle of displacement from the midline. This is usually 40 to 45 degrees in either direction.

ROTATION
1. **Patient position:** seated.
2. **Physician position:** standing behind patient.
3. **Technique:**
   a. To evaluate right rotation, place your right hand on the patient's left frontal area and use the left hand to monitor shoulder rotation or motion at C7-T1.
   b. With your left hand, gently turn the patient's head to the right until you feel motion at the cervicothoracic junction (Fig. 6-11).
   c. Note the displacement from the midline. This is usually 80 to 90 degrees, or until the patient's chin is over his shoulder.

d. Reverse hands to evaluate left rotation. Repeat steps b and c.

Intersegmental Motion Testing
OCCIPITOATLANTAL JOINT
1. **Patient position:** supine.
2. **Physician position:** seated comfortably at the head of the table with forearms resting on the table.
3. **Technique:**
   a. Tissue texture changes and asymmetry
      i. Slide fingers downward and laterally from inion to sulcus, between occiput and atlas (Fig. 6-12).
      ii. Note changes in tissue texture.
      iii. Slide fingers slightly laterally toward mastoid processes and note the depth of the sulcus.
   b. Motion testing technique
      i. Keep the palpating fingers in the occipitoatlantal sulcus.
      ii. Have the patient slowly flex his head, occiput on atlas only.
      iii. Note the symmetry of flexion bilaterally. Increased sulcal depth on one side may indicate a side-bending dysfunction on the other side.
      iv. Keep your fingers in the occipitoatlantal sulcus.

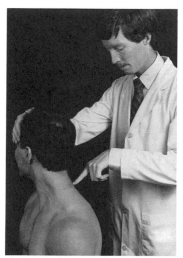

Figure 6-11. Gross motion testing of the cervical spine, rotation.

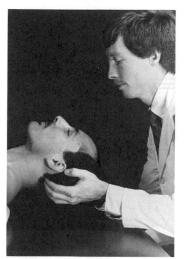

Figure 6-12. Intersegmental motion testing of the occipitoatlantal joint.

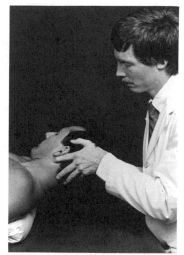

Figure 6-13. Intersegmental motion testing of the atlantoaxial joint.

v. Have the patient slowly extend his head over your fingers.

vi. Note the symmetry of extension bilaterally. Unilaterally increased sulcal depth indicates a side-bending dysfunction on the other side.

ATLANTOAXIAL JOINT

1. **Patient position:** supine.
2. **Physician position:** seated at head of table with forearms resting on table.
3. **Technique:**
   a. Tissue texture changes
      i. Slide fingers laterally along the occipitoatlantal sulcus until they are resting behind and near the tips of the mastoid processes bilaterally, and behind the transverse processes of the atlas (Fig. 6-13). Note tissue texture changes and changes in symmetry.
      ii. Move fingers anteriorly between the mastoid processes and the mandible to palpate the tips of the transverse processes of the atlas. Note any changes in symmetry. One tip more prominent posteriorly may be an indication of a rotation dysfunction in that direction.
   b. Motion testing technique
      i. Place your fingers behind the transverse processes of the atlas.

ii. Have the patient flex the occiput on the atlas (flex head) and maintain this locked position.

iii. Rotate the patient's head bilaterally until motion is felt at each transverse process.

iv. Note the degree of freedom of rotation. A decrease in rotation indicates restriction on that side and freedom in other direction.

C2 THROUGH C7

1. **Patient position:** supine with head and neck relaxed.
2. **Physician position:** seated at the head of the table with forearms resting on the table.
3. **Technique:**
   a. Tissue texture changes
      i. Palpate the spinous processes and ligaments in the midline and slightly caudad to the occipitoatlantal sulcus.
      ii. Move your fingers slightly laterally and palpate the cervical paravertebral muscles.
      iii. Palpate the articular pillars in the following manner. Slide your fingers slightly more laterally until they are in the groove between cervical paravertebral muscle masses. Then gently press your fingers medially until you palpate the bones beneath the muscles. C2 on C3 should be

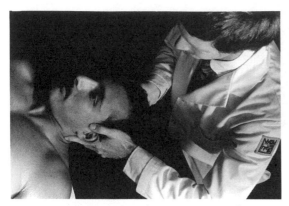

Figure 6-14. Intersegmental motion testing of C2 through C7, side-bending.

approximately 1 cm below the occipitoatlantal sulcus. To test your position, have the patient laterally flex slightly to one side. You should be able to feel the sliding motion with your palpating fingers.

   iv. Slide your fingers caudad bilaterally and palpate each pair of articular pillars. Note changes in tissue texture and in bony symmetry. When one articular pillar is more prominent posteriorly, it may indicate a rotation toward that side.

  b. Motion testing technique—side-bending (Fig. 6-14)

    i. Keep the palpating fingers on the articular pillars.

    ii. Introduce side-bending until you feel motion at your fingertips.

    iii. Note the displacement of the patient's head from the midline.

    iv. Greater motion to one side than the other indicates a side-bending restriction on the side of the decreased motion.

    v. Feel the fluidity of motion at your fingertips.

  c. Flexion-extension (Fig. 6-15)

    i. With your fingertips on the articular pillars, flex the patient's neck until you feel motion at the articular pillars.

    ii. Return the patient's head to neutral position. Introduce extension up to your palpating fingers at the articular pillars. Use your palpating fingers as fulcrums.

    iii. Feel the fluidity and amount of motion.

    iv. Note any asymmetry of motion. Decreased motion in extension indicates a flexion dysfunction. Decreased motion in flexion indicates an extension dysfunction.

Rotoscoliosis Motion Testing

When a cervical vertebra side-bends, it also rotates to the same side. A type II somatic dysfunction will exhibit restrictions in side-bending and rotation in the same direction, as well as in flexion or extension.

C2 THROUGH C7

1. **Patient position:** supine.
2. **Physician position:** seated at head of table.
3. **Technique:**

  a. Place your palpating fingers on the articular pillars bilaterally. Note the bony symmetry of articular pillars. If one side is more posterior than the other, the vertebra may be rotated to that side.

  b. Flex the patient's head to the palpating fingers (see Fig. 6-15)

    i. If the posteriorly rotated vertebra becomes more posterior, the vertebra has restricted motion in flexion. This also confirms freedom of rotation.

    ii. The posteriorly rotated vertebra will stay the same or improve in extension. This is considered an *extension dysfunction.*

  c. Extend the patient's head to the palpating fingers.

    i. If the posteriorly rotated vertebra becomes more posterior, the vertebra has restricted motion in extension.

    ii. The posteriorly rotated vertebra will stay the same or improve in flexion. This is considered a *flexion dysfunction.*

    Example: The C4 articular pillar is posterior on the left. The posterior articular pillar becomes more posterior in flexion and less posterior in extension. The somatic dysfunction is designated C4 E Rl Sl. This is a type II somatic dysfunction.

ATLANTOAXIAL MOTION TESTING

The atlantoaxial joint never leaves the neutral position, because extension is limited by bony apposition and flexion is limited by the odontoid

Figure 6-15. Intersegmental motion testing of C2 through C7, flexion-extension.

Figure 6-16. Rotoscoliosis motion testing of the atlantoaxial joint.

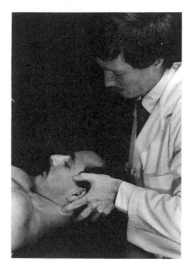 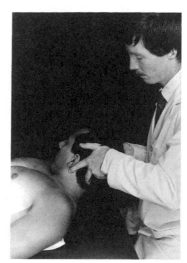

ligament. Therefore, the major motion of the atlantoxial joint is rotation.

1. **Patient position:** supine.
2. **Physician position:** seated at head of table.
3. **Technique:**
   a. Cradle the patient's occiput in your hands.
   b. Fully flex the patient's neck, locking all the cervical vertebrae in flexion. This maneuver prevents motion of the vertebrae below the atlantoaxial joint.
   c. Maintain flexion and rotate the head from one side to the other until the physiologic barriers to motion are reached (Fig. 6-16).
      i. Note the symmetry of motion to each side.
      ii. If the motion on one side is greater than on the other, there is restriction on the side of limited motion.

   Example: If rotation is greater to the right, the somatic dysfunction would be designated AA Rr (atlantoaxial rotation right).

Translatory Motion Testing

Rotoscoliosis motion testing evaluates the rotation of the vertebra. Translatory motion testing evaluates side-bending motion. Side-to-side translatory motion is coupled with individual vertebral side-bending toward the opposite direction. Translatory motion of C4 toward the right is coupled with side-bending of C4 to the left. For most cervical vertebrae, side-bending and rotation are coupled and occur in the same direction.

C2 THROUGH C7
1. **Patient position:** supine.
2. **Physician position:** seated at head of table.
3. **Technique:**
   a. Place palpating fingers on the articular pillars of the affected vertebra bilaterally.
   b. Push the pillar in a left-to-right direction, using the palpating fingers alternately. This translatory motion creates side-bending to the left. Then push right to left, creating side-bending to the right. Note any asymmetry of motion. If there is better translation to the left, the vertebra side-bends better to the right side.
   c. Flex the neck to the area of palpation and apply a translatory force toward one side and then toward the other side (Fig. 6-17).
      i. Note any asymmetry of motion.
      ii. Compare the motion with the translatory motion that occurs in the neutral position.
      iii. If translatory motion is increased to one side in flexion, the restriction is exaggerated in flexion; therefore, flexion is restricted. This is designated an *extension dysfunction.*
   d. Extend the neck to the area of the palpating fingers and apply the same type of translatory force.

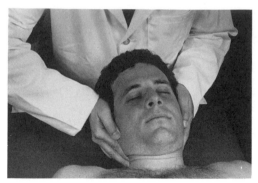

Figure 6-17. Translatory motion testing of C2 through C7.

i. Note any asymmetry of motion.
ii. Compare this motion with the translatory motion that occurs in the neutral position.
iii. If translatory motion is decreased to one side in extension, the restriction is exaggerated in extension; therefore, extension is restricted. This is designated a *flexion dysfunction*

OCCIPITOATLANTAL JOINT
1. **Patient position:** supine.
2. **Physician position:** seated at head of patient.
3. **Technique:**
   a. Flex the patient's neck slightly to the monitoring fingers in the sulcus.
   b. Stabilize the top of the head against your waist.
   c. Cup the occiput in your hands.
   d. Move the head on the neck by translating the occiput to the left. Translation to the left is coupled with side-bending to the right (Fig. 6-18).
   e. This is coupled with rotation to the left. Note any asymmetry of motion.
   f. Extend the neck slightly.
   g. Repeat steps b through d.
      Interpretation: Since rotation is opposite to side-bending at the occipitoatlantal joint, there are four possible designations for the

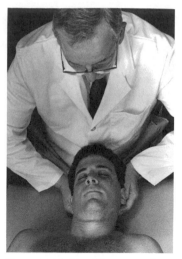

Figure 6-18. Translatory motion testing of the occipitoatlantal joint.

somatic dysfunction: OA F Sr Rl, OA F Sl Rr, OA E Sr Rl, OA E Sl Rr.

Example: If there is normal translation to the left in flexion and decreased translation to the left in extension, the somatic dysfunction is designated OA F Sl Rr (occiput restricted in right side-bending while in the extended position; its free motions are flexion, side-bending to the right, and rotation to the left).

References
Fryette H. 1954. Principles of Osteopathic Technique. Colorado Springs: Academy of Applied Osteopathy.

Kapandji IA. 1974. The Physiology of the Joints. Vol 3. The Trunk and the Vertebral Column. Edinburgh: Churchill Livingstone.

Schiowitz S, DiGiovanna E. 1981. An Osteopathic Approach to Diagnosis and Treatment. Old Westbury, NY: New York College of Osteopathic Medicine.

Warwick RW. 1973. Gray's Anatomy, 35th British ed. Philadelphia: W.B. Saunders.

White A, Panjabi MM. 1978. Biomechanics of the Spine. Philadelphia: J.B. Lippincott.

7

Treatment of the Cervical Spine

MYOFASCIAL TECHNIQUES
Toni Spinaris
Eileen L. DiGiovanna

This section describes passive, indirect active, and direct active myofascial techniques used to treat somatic dysfunction as well as muscle or fascial tension in the cervical region. These techniques may entail a passive linear or perpendicular stretch of the neck muscles or an active use of neuromuscular methods to create relaxation of the suboccipital and paravertebral muscles.

Passive Techniques

Passive techniques are performed by the physician on a relaxed patient. The purpose of the passive techniques described below is to place a stretch on the posterior extensor muscles of the cervical region.

LINEAR STRETCH ON THE MUSCLES
OF THE OCCIPITOATLANTAL REGION
1. **Patient position:** supine.
2. **Physician position:** standing at the head of the table.
3. **Technique:**
   a. The physician cups her palms to support the patient's occiput.

   b. The physician's fingers are placed in the occipital sulcus bilaterally.
   c. For best results, the patient's neck should be straight or bent slightly forward.
   d. The physician's arms should be in near or full extension, so that they can be used as long levers. This position allows the physician to use her weight as the force of traction, by rocking backward on her feet rather than relying on upper body strength (Fig. 7-1).
   e. The traction is slowly and uniformly applied, maintained for a few seconds, and slowly released.
   f. The technique may be repeated without repositioning of the physician's fingers or feet.
4. Hints for performing technique:
   a. The physician's feet should be placed far enough from the table so that she may rock back and thus apply traction without changing her stance.
   b. The physician should avoid creating friction by sliding her fingers over the patient's skin.
   c. See that the patient is comfortable and relaxed.

An Osteopathic Approach to Diagnosis and Treatment, second edition
Eileen L. DiGiovanna and Stanley Schiowitz
Lippincott-Raven Publishers, Philadelphia © 1997.

111

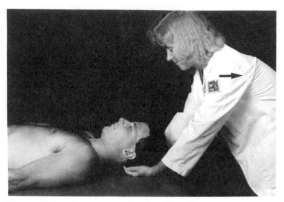

Figure 7-1. Linear stretch with the physician standing.

Seated Technique: In the seated technique, linear traction is applied to the posterior extensor neck muscles with the physician seated at the head of the table (Fig. 7-2). The technique is similar; however, the lever action is shorter, involving only the forearms. Therefore, the physician should keep her elbows close to her body while applying traction. The physician may still use body weight as the applied force, but with less efficiency because both the arms and body levers are shorter. Linear traction is applied by the physician slowly rocking back on her buttocks. As in the original technique, traction is slowly and uniformly applied, maintained for a few seconds, and released. The manuever may be repeated without repositioning.

Suboccipital Technique. A similar technique can be used in the suboccipital region. In this technique, the physician's fingers stretch the tissues of the occipital sulcus laterally while linear traction is applied.

1. **Patient position:** supine.
2. **Physician position:** seated at the head of the table.
3. **Technique:**
   a. The physician places her index and middle fingers in the occipital sulcus bilaterally but medially so that the middle fingers meet at the midline.
   b. The occiput is cupped in the physician's palms.
   c. The patient's neck is maintained in a straight or slightly forward bent position.

d. The physician applies linear traction slowly by rocking back on her buttocks.
e. Maintaining linear traction, the physician rolls her finger laterally away from the midline. With the longitudinal axis of the forearm as the rotational axis, the fingers remain in the occipital sulcus but gradually roll out laterally.
f. The physician's wrist, forearm, hand, and fingers are maintained in straight alignment and work as a single unit.
g. The technique may be repeated as needed.

LINEAR TRACTION APPLIED
TO THE LOWER NECK
1. **Patient position:** supine.
2. **Physician position:** standing or sitting at the head of the table.
3. **Technique:**
   a. The physician places her fingers on the patient's posterior neck muscles bilaterally at any cervical level.
   b. The physician applies a linear traction force to the musculature, slowly and uniformly, by rocking back on her feet or buttocks.
   c. The patient's neck is held straight or slightly forward bent as the traction is applied.
   d. Slowly release by rocking forward.
   e. Some perpendicular stretch may be added by pushing the fingers ventrally while maintaining the traction.

LINEAR STRETCH OF POSTERIOR EXTENSOR
NECK MUSCLES
1. **Patient position:** supine.
2. **Physician position:** standing or sitting at the head of the table.
3. **Technique:**
   a. The physician cradles the occiput in one hand and cups the patient's chin with the other hand (Fig. 7-3).
   b. The physician applies a linear traction force along the longitudinal axis of the cervical spine with the hand holding the occiput. The hand cupping the chin is primarily used to stabilize the neck and hold it slightly bent forward. The main force of traction is applied to the occiput.
   c. This may be repeated as necessary.

PERPENDICULAR STRETCH
OF THE MUSCLE FIBERS
1. **Patient position:** supine.

Figure 7-2. Linear stretch with the physician seated.

Figure 7-3. Linear stretch of posterior extensor neck muscles, cupping the chin.

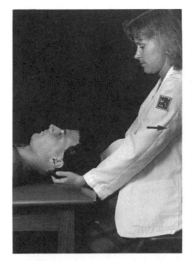

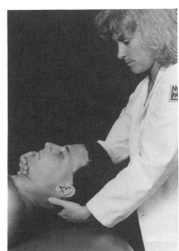

Figure 7-4. Unilateral perpendicular stretch.

Figure 7-5. Crossed arms technique.

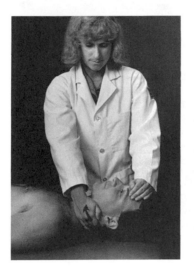

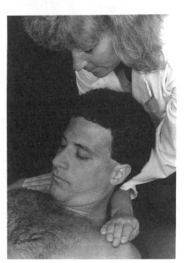

2. **Physician position:** standing at the patient's side opposite the side to be treated.
3. **Technique:**
   a. The physician places one hand on the patient's forehead to act as a stabilizing counterforce to the treating hand.
   b. The physician places her other hand across the patient's body and grasps the posterior cervical muscles of the opposite side (Fig. 7-4).
   c. A gentle stretch is applied to the muscle body by pulling it away from the spinous processes and ventrally.
   d. The stretch is maintained for a few seconds,

then slowly released. The maneuver may be repeated as needed. The hand stretching the muscle may move up and down the cervical spine.
   e. Additional stretch may be achieved by rotating the patient's head away while pulling on the muscle.

BILATERAL LINEAR STRETCH APPLIED
TO BOTH ENDS OF THE MUSCLE
1. **Patient position:** supine.
2. **Physician position:** standing at the head of the table.

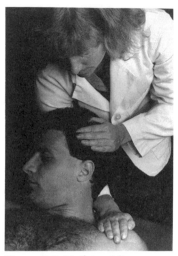

Figure 7-6. Unilateral linear stretch.

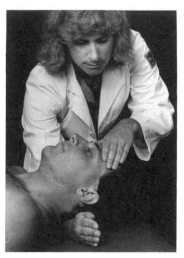

Figure 7-7. Linear stretch of suboccipital muscles.

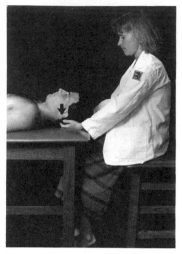

Figure 7-8. Active direct myofascial technique applied to suboccipital muscle region.

3. **Technique:**
   a. The physician crosses her forearms under the patient's occiput and neck so that the patient's head is fully supported on the physician's forearms and the physician's hands are pressing down on the patient's contralateral shoulders (Fig. 7-5).
   b. The physician gently and slowly lifts her arm, creating a lever-fulcrum effect that puts linear traction on both ends of the muscles.
      Note: The patient's neck should be bent forward to a comfortable position of maximum stretch. Careful control of the force must be used.
   c. This position is held for a few seconds and slowly brought back to neutral.
   d. When repeating the technique, the physician should bend the neck forward a bit more than the previous time. Each repetition of the technique should increase the range of motion.
4. **Modification—active direct technique:**
   a. While the physician is fully supporting the head at the maximal stretch, she may ask the patient to push back against her arms.
   b. The physician resists this motion with an isometric counterforce.
   c. The patient is allowed to push for 3 seconds, then told to relax.

d. The physician allows the patient 3 to 6 seconds of relaxation, then bends the neck forward to the new point of maximal stretch.

UNILATERAL LINEAR STRETCH APPLIED TO BOTH ENDS OF THE MUSCLE
1. **Patient position:** supine.
2. **Physician position:** standing at the head of the table.
3. **Technique:**
   a. The physician places one forearm under the patient's head with the hand on the patient's contralateral shoulder, on the side of the neck to be treated. The patient's head should be fully supported.
   b. The physician places her other hand on the side of the patient's head.
   c. The physician slowly and gently lifts the head up, forward-bending the neck (Fig. 7-6). The head is rotated away to give a stretch on the muscles opposite the rotation.

SUBOCCIPITAL MUSCLE TREATMENT
1. **Patient position:** supine.
2. **Physician position:** standing or seated at the side of the table facing the patient.
3. **Technique:**
   a. The physician places one forearm under the

patient's neck in the suboccipital sulcus so that the patient's neck rests on the forearm.

b. The other hand is placed on the patient's forehead and gentle pressure is applied downward toward the table. This stretches the muscles in the area of the occipital sulcus (Fig. 7-7).

Active Direct Techniques

Active direct techniques use the Golgi tendon reflex to cause relaxation. These techniques are described for the suboccipital muscle region and for unilateral occipital and paravertebral muscles.

SUBOCCIPITAL MUSCLE REGION
1. **Patient position:** supine.
2. **Physician position:** seated at the head of the table with her forearms resting on the table, palms facing up.
3. **Technique:**
   a. The physician places her fingertips in the patient's occipital sulcus, allowing the occiput to rest in her palms.
   b. The patient gently pushes his head into the physician's palms, with the physician's fingertips being used as a fulcrum, avoiding neck extension.
   c. As the patient pushes into her palms, the physician resists this motion with an isometric counterforce (Fig. 7-8).

      The muscles involved in this technique include the bilateral suboccipital muscles, the rectus capitis posterior major, rectus capitis posterior minor, obliquus capitis inferior, and obliquus capitis superior.
4. **Modification:**
   a. The same technique can be applied to the lower extensor muscles of the cervical region. The physician places her fingers more caudally.
   b. The patient may push his head into the physician's palms with slightly greater force the lower down the neck one is treating, since the muscles enlarge.

UNILATERAL SUBOCCIPITAL MUSCLE
TREATMENT
1. **Patient position:** supine.
2. **Physician position:** seated at the head of the

table with forearms resting on the table, palms up.
3. **Technique:**
   a. The physician places her fingertips in the occipital sulcus on the side to be treated.
   b. The physician's other hand guides the patient's head into side-bending over the fulcrum of her fingers.
   c. The patient tries to side-bend his head farther into the freedom of motion (toward the dysfunctional side).
   d. The physician resists this motion by applying an isometric counterforce with her palm.
   e. The physician should be able to feel the involved muscle contracting.
4. **Modification:** The physician may instruct the patient to push his head gently backward toward the table. This motion is similarly resisted with an isometric counterforce.

UNILATERAL SINGLE PARAVERTEBRAL
MUSCLE TREATMENT—SIDE-BENDING
AND ROTATION
1. **Patient position:** supine.
2. **Physician position:** seated at head of table.
3. **Technique:**
   a. The physician places her index or middle finger on the involved muscle. This is the monitoring finger.
   b. With her other hand, the physician grasps the patient's head under the occiput and bends it backward, side-bends, and rotates it ipsilaterally until motion of the involved muscle is felt by the monitoring finger.
   c. The patient attempts to push his head into further backward bending and ipsilateral side-bending and rotation.
   d. The physician resists this motion with an isometric counterforce for no more than 2 seconds. Relax and repeat the process.

Active Indirect Techniques

Active indirect techniques use reciprocal inhibition or the crossed extensor reflex. They are described for the paravertebral muscles.

1. **Patient position:** supine with his head off the end of the table.
2. **Physician position:** seated at the head of the table, fully supporting the patient's head.

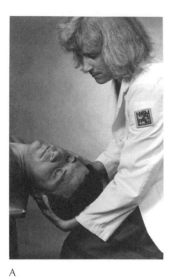 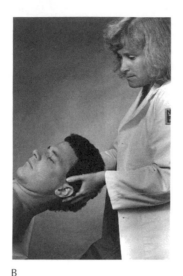 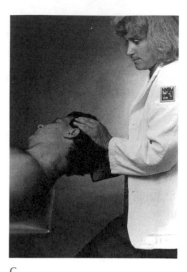

A   B   C

Figure 7-9. Active indirect stretch of the paravertebral muscles. **(A)** Starting position. **(B)** Midway through the maneuver, with the patient attempting to reverse the motions applied by the physician. **(C)** A passive stretch ends the technique.

3. **Technique:**

   a. The physician places the palm of one hand on the patient's ipsilateral parieto-occiput so that the patient's head is fully supported.

   b. The palm of the other hand is placed on the other side of the head. No pressure is placed on the patient's ear.

   c. The physician places the patient's head in a position of backward bending, side-bending, and rotation toward the side of the hand on the occiput (Fig. 7-9A).

   d. The patient tries to reverse the motions that the physician has just engaged by bringing

his neck into flexion and touching his chin to the opposite shoulder (Fig. 7-9B).

   e. The physician applies isokinetic resistance to this motion with her hand on the temporo-parietal region.

   f. The patient will stop this motion because of a restricting muscle or pain.

   g. The physician then gently applies a passive stretch of the patient's neck, manually increasing the desired muscle stretch (Fig. 7-9C).

   h. The patient relaxes. The physician returns to the starting position and repeats the maneuver.

MUSCLE ENERGY TECHNIQUES
Nancy Brous

This section describes muscle energy techniques used to treat dysfunctions of the occipitoatlantal joint, rotational dysfunctions of the atlantoaxial joint, and single dysfunctions of a typical cervical vertebral joint. Unless the dysfunction is severe, the techniques are repeated two or three times, with the motion barrier engaged at each repetition.

Occipitoatlantal Dysfunction
DYSFUNCTION IN FLEXION
Example: OA F Sr Rl
1. **Patient position:** supine.
2. **Physician position:** seated at the head of the table.
3. **Hand position:** The physician's monitoring

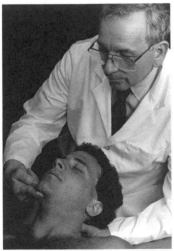

Figure 7-10. Muscle energy technique for a dysfunction in flexion of the occipitoatlantal joint.

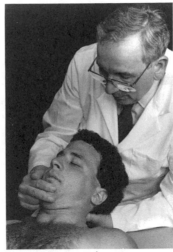

Figure 7-11. Muscle energy technique for dysfunction in extension of the occipitoatlantal joint.

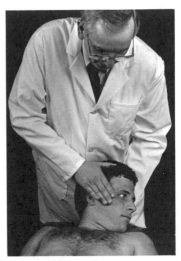

Figure 7-12. Muscle energy technique for atlantoaxial rotation restriction.

hand cradles the patient's occiput. Two fingers of the monitoring hand are in the patient's occipital sulci (medial and inferior to mastoid). The physician's other hand is placed on the inferior aspect of the patient's chin.

4. **Technique:**
   a. The physician extends the patient's head back over his monitoring hand until motion is felt at the occipitoatlantal joint (Fig. 7-10).
   b. With the monitoring hand, the physician side-bends the occiput left and rotates it right until motion is felt at the occipitoatlantal joint.
   c. The patient is instructed to push his chin down against the isometric resistance of the physician (into the freedom of motion) for about 3 seconds. *Ounces* of force are used to achieve the desired results.
   d. The patient relaxes for 3 seconds.
   e. The physician repeats steps a through d twice more, reengaging the motion barrier each time.
   f. The patient's head is returned to neutral and the lesion is reassessed for change.

DYSFUNCTION IN EXTENSION
Example: OA E Sr Rl
1. **Patient position:** supine.
2. **Physician position:** seated at the head of the table.

3. **Hand position:** The physician's monitoring hand cradles the patient's occiput. Two fingers of the monitoring hand are in the patient's occipital sulci. The physician's other hand is placed on the superior aspect of the patient's chin.

4. **Technique:**
   a. The physician bends the patient's head forward until he feels motion at the monitoring hand (Fig. 7-11).
   b. With his monitoring hand, the physician side-bends the patient's neck left and rotates it right until motion is felt at the occipitoatlantal joint.
   c. The patient is instructed to push his chin up against the isometric resistance of the physician for about 3 seconds. *Ounces* of force are used to achieve the desired result.
   d. The patient relaxes for 3 seconds.
   e. The physician repeats steps a through d twice more, reengaging the motion barrier each time.
   f. The patient's head is returned to neutral and the lesion is reassessed for change.

Atlantoaxial Dysfunction
Example: AA Rr
1. **Patient position:** supine.
2. **Physician position:** seated at head of table.

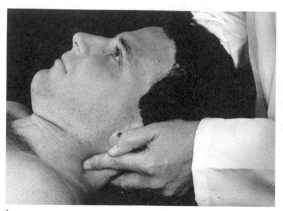

A

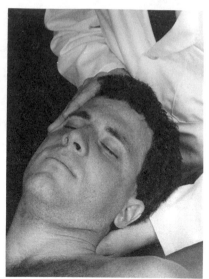

B

Figure 7-13. Muscle energy technique for dysfunction in extension of a typical cervical vertebra. **(A)** Note position of monitoring finger. **(B)** Rotation is introduced into barrier to motion of a typical cervical vertebra.

3. **Technique:**
   a. Since the motion at the atlantoaxial joint involves primarily rotation, the physician need address only the motion barrier of rotation.
   b. The physician supports the back of the patient's head with his palms.
   c. The physician bends the patient's neck and head fully forward until locking occurs below the A-A joint.
   d. Keeping the patient's neck bent forward, the physician rotates the head toward the side of the restricted rotation and engages the motion barrier (left).
   e. The physician then places the palm of his hand opposite the side of the restriction, on the patient's cheek and temple (Fig. 7-12).
   f. The patient turns his head with a pure rotary force against the isometric resistance provided by the physician's hand on the patient's cheek.
   g. After 3 seconds the patient relaxes and the physician simultaneously stops applying the counterforce.
   h. Once the patient has completely relaxed, the physician increases the rotation into the restriction, engaging a new motion barrier.
   i. Steps f through h are repeated two or three times. Symmetry of motion at the atlantoaxial joint is rechecked.
   j. The patient's head is returned to neutral position and the lesion is reassessed for change.

Typical Cervical Vertebral Dysfunctions (C2–C7)

Example: C4 E Sr Rr

1. **Patient position:** supine.
2. **Physician position:** seated at the head of table.
3. **Technique:**
   a. The physician places the fingertip of the index finger of the monitoring hand against the posterior facet at the level of the involved segment (left side) (Fig. 7-13A).
   b. The physician introduces flexion to treat an extension dysfunction, or extension to treat a flexion dysfunction. The motion is monitored and localized at the particular level being treated. The first motion barrier has now been engaged.
   c. Side-bending is introduced by placing a medial translatory force on the side of the restricted segment, resulting in side-bending into the barrier (left).
   d. Rotation is introduced by rotating the patient's head and into the restriction (left) until motion is felt at the monitored segment (Fig. 7-13B).
   e. The physician then asks the patient to move into the freedom of motion by having the patient bring his ear to his shoulder, causing a side-bending away from the barrier. (The physician could also ask the patient to rotate

his head toward the freedom). These actions are performed against isometric resistance provided by the physician's hand against the patient's cheek.

f. The patient relaxes and the physician simultaneously stops applying the counterforce.

g. Once the patient is completely relaxed, the physician engages the new motion barriers, increasing the side-bending, rotation, and flexion or extension further into the restriction.

h. Steps e through g are repeated two or three times.

i. The patient's head is returned to neutral and the lesion is reassessed for change.

COUNTERSTRAIN TECHNIQUES

Eileen L. DiGiovanna
Lillian Somner

The treatment of tender points by the Jones counterstrain method requires that the patient be completely relaxed. The goal is to shorten the involved muscle, hold it in this shortened position for 90 seconds, and then return the patient to a neutral position.

Anterior Tender Points

The anterior tender points are diagrammed in Figure 7-14. In general they are located on the antero-

Figure 7-14. Cervical anterior tender points.

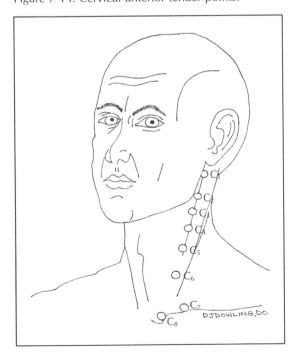

lateral tip of the articular pillars of the cervical vertebrae. C1 has two anterior points located on the posterior edge of the ascending ramus of the mandible and just below the angle of the jaw on the inferior surface of the mandible. The tender point for C7 is located on the superior surface at the medial end of the clavicle, and the point for C8 is located on the medial tip of the clavicle in the sternal notch.

1. **Patient position:** supine.
2. **Physician position:** seated at the head of the table.
3. **Technique:**
   a. C1: Rotate the head away from the tender point (Fig. 7-15).
   b. C2 and C3: Slight flexion, rotation, and side-bending away from the tender point.
   c. C4: Create extension to the vertebra, then side-bend and rotate away from the tender point (Fig. 7-16). May require flexion.

Figure 7-15. Treatment of tender point on the right side of C1. The head is rotated and bent laterally away from the tender point.

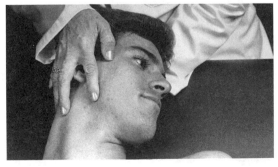

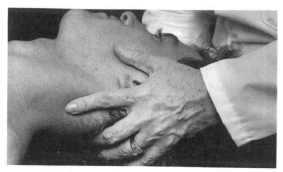

Figure 7-16. Treatment of tender point on the left side of C4. Side-bending and rotation are induced in the direction away from the tender point.

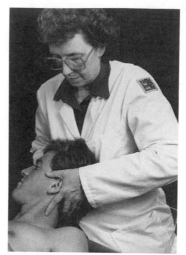

Figure 7-18. Treatment of anterior tender point on the left side of C7.

d. C5 and C6: Create flexion with side-bending and rotation away from the tender point (Fig. 7-17).
e. C7: Create moderate flexion to the C7 level, slightly rotate away, and side-bend toward the tender point (Fig. 7-18).
f. C8: Create marked flexion, marked side-bending, and rotation away from the tender point.

It is important to remember that although SARA (side-bend away, rotate away) is used to treat most anterior cervical tender points, adjustment may need to be made for individual patients who re-

quire some variation, particularly of the side-bending component.

Posterior Tender Points
The posterior cervical tender points are shown in Figure 7-19. They are generally located on the in-

Figure 7-19. Posterior cervical tender point locations.

Figure 7-17. Treatment of anterior tender point on the left side of C6.

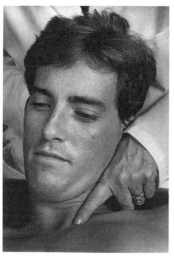

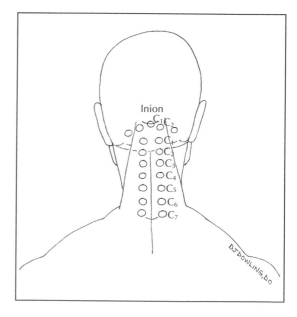

terspinous ligaments between the spinous processes or on the articular pillars more laterally. C1 has tender points on the inion and in the muscle masses laterally on the nuchal line.

1. **Patient position:** supine.
2. **Physician position:** seated at the head of the table.
3. **Technique:** While carefully monitoring with one finger on the tender point, the physician positions the neck, as noted below, until the point is no longer tender. This position is held for 90 seconds.
   a. C1: Treated in flexion for midline tender point or rotation away and side-bending toward the tender point for the more lateral points.

b. Interspinous tender points: Create extension of the neck to the segment to be treated.
c. **Articular pillar points:**
   i. C2, C4 to C7: Create extension with rotation away and side-bending toward the tender point.
   ii. C3: Create flexion with rotation away and side-bending toward the tender point. Occasionally C3 will require extension.

It is important to remember that any given point may vary from patient to patient and may require some adjustment of the side-bending, rotation, or flexion-extension component. It is more imperative to achieve a position of comfort than to follow a written description.

FACILITATED POSITIONAL RELEASE
Stanley Schiowitz

Cervical Region Techniques

All techniques for treating cervical region dysfunctions are begun with a slight flattening of the region to be treated.

SUPERFICIAL MUSCLE HYPERTONICITY, POSTERIOR RIGHT SIDE, IN REGION OF C4 VERTEBRA

1. **Patient position:** supine.
2. **Physician position:** seated at the head of the table.
3. **Technique:**
   a. The patient moves up the table until his head and neck are off the table and supported by the physician. (The head may be supported by a pillow on the physician's lap.)
   b. With the thumb, palm, and middle finger of the left hand, the physician cradles the patient's neck. His middle finger is on the tissue to be treated. The rest of the hand helps support the patient's neck.
   c. The patient's head is firmly supported in the palm of the physician's right hand, which will be used in the ensuing maneuvers.
   d. The physician gently bends the head and neck forward to flatten the cervical lordosis.
   e. From this starting position the physician gently applies axial compression on the pa-

tient's occiput, with the vector of force directed through the patient's head toward his feet (Fig. 7-20). Less than 1 pound of force is sufficient—just enough to be felt at the physician's left index finger.
   f. Maintaining axial compression, the physician bends the patient's neck backward, then side-bends it up to the physician's left index finger (Fig. 7-21). This maneuver causes shortening and relaxation of the muscle being treated.
   g. This position is held for 3 seconds, then released and the area of interspinous dysfunction reevaluated.

SOMATIC DYSFUNCTION (C4 E Sr Rr)

1. **Patient position:** supine, as described in above technique.
2. **Physician position:** seated at the head of the table, with hands placed as described in above technique.
3. **Technique:**
   a. The physician places his finger at the articular facet of C4 on C5.
   b. After flattening the curve and adding a compressive force, the physician moves the patient's neck into extension and rotation to the right.

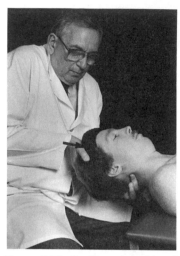

Figure 7-20. Facilitated positional release for treatment of muscle hypertonicity of the cervical region: application of axial compression.

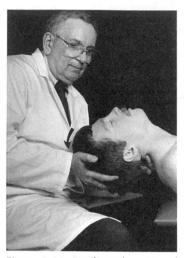

Figure 7-21. Facilitated positional release for treatment of muscle hypertonicity the cervical region, with backward bending and right side-bending added.

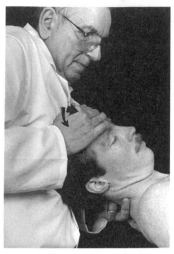

Figure 7-22. Facilitated positional release treatment for C4 flexion dysfunction (C4 F Sr Rr).

c. The physician then adds right lateral flexion of C4 on C5.

d. Immediate release of the articulation should be felt.

e. The position is held for 3 seconds, returned to the original position, and reassessed.

SOMATIC DYSFUNCTION (C4 F Sr Rr)

1. **Patient position:** supine as described in first technique.
2. **Physician position:** seated at the head of the table, with hands placed as in above techniques.
3. **Technique:**
   a. The physician gently bends the patient's neck forward to flatten the sagittal curve.
   b. From this starting position, the physician applies compression.
   c. Maintaining compression, the physician gently increases the forward bending until flexion of C4 on C5 is felt by the monitoring finger. (With compression maintained, the degree of forward bending of the neck needed to achieve the necessary vertebral flexion is greatly reduced.)
   d. The physician adds right rotation and lateral flexion, up to the monitoring finger (Fig. 7-22).
   e. After feeling an articular release, the physician holds the position for 3 seconds, then releases it and reevaluates the dysfunction.

HIGH-VELOCITY, LOW-AMPLITUDE THRUSTING TECHNIQUES

Barry Erner
Eileen L. DiGiovanna

The principles of thrusting techniques were discussed in Chapter 5. This section describes the application of high-velocity, low-amplitude thrusting techniques to correct somatic dysfunctions of the cervical spine. The vertebra may be placed into one or all of its barriers to motion. Frequently with this technique only one plane of motion is addressed. When this motion restriction is corrected, the other planes of restriction respond as well. After placing the vertebra into its barrier, the physician applies a rapid, gentle force through a very short distance to pass through the barrier.

Occipitoatlantal Joint Dysfunction

1. **Patient position:** supine.
2. **Physician position:** standing at the head of the table toward the side of the freedom of rotation.
3. **Technique:**
   a. The physician grasps the patient's head with his nonthrusting hand and flexes the neck slightly.
   b. The metacarpophalangeal joint of the thrusting hand is placed on the occiput just above the sulcus.
   c. The occiput is allowed to extend just over that finger in a backward nod.
   d. The occiput is rotated and side-bent into its barriers, taking up the slack in the soft tissues.
   e. A thrust is given as a coupled side-bending and rotational force directed toward the eye (Fig. 7-23).

Atlantoaxial Joint Dysfunction

1. **Patient position:** supine.
2. **Physician position:** standing at the head of the table toward the side of the somatic dysfunction.
3. **Technique:**
   a. The physician cups the lateral aspect of the patient's chin in his nonthrusting hand.

   b. The physician rotates the head into the motion barrier, keeping the head in the midline.
   c. The thrusting joint is positioned behind the posteriorly rotated articular pillar.
   d. The physician exerts a rapid rotary thrust through the rotational barrier (Fig. 7-24).

C3 to C7 Somatic Dysfunction

1. **Patient position:** supine.
2. **Physician position:** standing at the head of the table.
3. **Technique:**
   a. The physician flexes the neck to the level of the vertebra being treated.
   b. The physician places his second metacarpophalangeal joint behind the posteriorly rotated articular pillar.
   c. The upper neck is allowed to extend over the thrusting finger just at the level of the vertebra being treated.
   d. The neck is simultaneously rotated toward the barrier and side-bent at the thrusting finger up away from the table. All the slack is taken out of the soft tissues.
   e. The physician exerts a rapid, short rotary thrust (Fig. 7-25).

   Note: It is important to keep the head in the midline at all times when performing this technique. The technique may be modified

Figure 7-23. High-velocity, low-amplitude thrusting technique for somatic dysfunction of the occipitoatlantal joint.

Figure 7-24. High-velocity, low-amplitude thrusting technique for somatic dysfunction of the atlantoaxial joint.

Figure 7-25. High-velocity, low-amplitude thrusting technique for somatic dysfunctions of the cervical spine, C3 to C7.

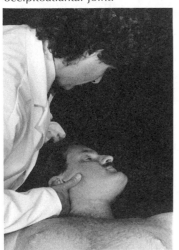
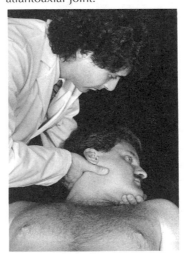
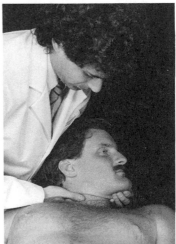

to engage all three barriers to motion prior to performing the thrust.

The direction of thrust varies with the level of vertebra being treated. For the upper cervical region the thrust is toward the eye, the middle cervicals are thrust straight across the neck, and the thrust through the lower cervicals is directed down toward the chest.

Cervical Somatic Dysfunction, Alternative Technique

1. **Patient position:** supine.
2. **Physician position:** standing at the head of the table.
3. **Technique:**
   a. The physician places the lateral aspect of the second metacarpophalangeal joint of the thrusting hand on the articular pillar opposite the posteriorly rotated one.
   b. The other hand is placed along the opposite side of the patient's head.
   c. Engage the barriers of extension-flexion, rotation, and side-bending.
   d. The physician exerts a rapid side-bending thrust through the involved vertebra (Fig. 7-26).

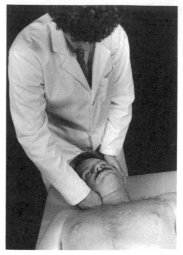

Figure 7-26. An alternative high-velocity, low-amplitude technique for the treatment of somatic dysfunctions of the cervical spine.

EXERCISE THERAPY
Stanley Schiowitz
Albert R. DeRubertis

The exercises described can be used to increase regional cervical motion (muscle stretch, extensibility), to increase regional strength (muscle contractility), or to restore structural symmetry. Many cervical muscle functions and structural changes involve the thoracic region. It is suggested that the physician review the section in Chapter 9, Exercise therapy for the thoracic spine, when writing an exercise prescription.

Regional Stretch
FORWARDING BENDING
1. **Patient position:** seated or standing, with the back erect.
2. **Instructions:**
   a. Drop your head forward; let its weight (gravity) pull it down.

   b. Add anterior (flexor) muscle contraction to bring your chin to your chest.
   c. Place both hands behind your head and passively pull your head down, chin to chest (Fig. 7-27). Do not create pain.
   d. Hold this position for 5 to 15 seconds. Relax, rest, and repeat.

BACKWARD BENDING
1. **Patient position:** seated or standing, with the back erect.
2. **Instructions:**
   a. Drop your head backward; let its weight pull it back.
   b. Add posterior (extensor) muscle contraction to increase the backward bending.
   c. Place both hands on your forehead and pas-

Figure 7-27. Exercise therapy for the cervical spine: forward bending.

Figure 7-28. Exercise therapy for cervical stretch: backward bending.

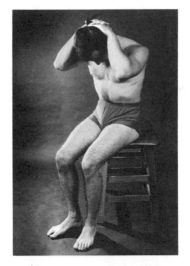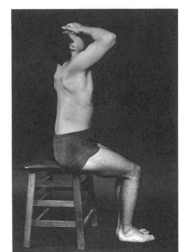

Figure 7-29. Exercise therapy for cervical stretch: side-bending.

Figure 7-30. Exercise therapy for cervical stretch: rotation.

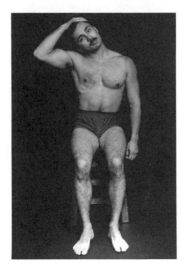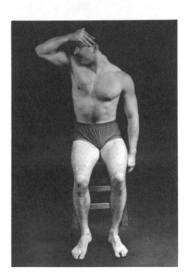

sively push your head back (Fig. 7-28). Do not create pain.
   d. Hold this position for 5 to 15 seconds. Relax, rest, and repeat.

SIDE-BENDING
1. **Patient position:** seated or standing, with the back erect.
2. **Instructions:**
   a. Without moving your shoulders, drop your head to the right; let its weight pull your right ear toward the right shoulder.
   b. Add right-sided muscle contraction to increase the side-bending.
   c. Place your right hand over your head, palm

on the left side of your head, and passively pull your head down to the right (Fig. 7-29). Try not to introduce rotation motion. Do not create pain.
   d. Hold this position for 5 to 15 seconds. Relax, rest and repeat. For left side-bending, reverse the instructions.

ROTATION
1. **Patient position:** seated or standing, with the back erect.
2. **Instructions:**
   a. Without moving your shoulders, turn your head to the right as far as you can, using right rotation muscle contraction.

b. Place your right hand in front of your forehead with the palm on the left side of your
head. Passively pull your head to the right as
far as possible (Fig. 7-30). Do not create pain.
   Note: In steps a and b, keep the chin in one
horizontal plane. Avoid adding lateral bending motion.
c. Hold this position for 5 to 15 seconds. Relax,
rest, and repeat. For left rotation, reverse directions.

Regional Strength

The exercises for promoting cervical strength use
static contraction. Exercises are described for
flexor muscles, extensor muscles, side-bending
muscles, and rotator muscles.

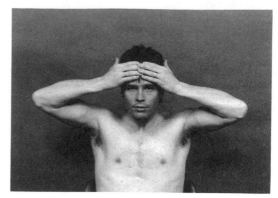

Figure 7-31. Cervical strengthening exercise: flexor muscles.

FLEXOR MUSCLES
1. **Patient position:** seated or standing, with the
back erect.
2. **Instructions:**
   a. Place both your palms on your forehead.
   b. Push your head forward against your palms.
   Resist the forward push so as to prevent all
   head motion (Fig. 7-31).
   c. Hold for 4 seconds, then relax.
   d. Repeat the exercise, gradually increasing the
   strength of the contracting force and hand resistance. Do not create pain. Do not hold a
   static contraction beyond 5 seconds.

EXTENSOR MUSCLES
1. **Patient position:** seated or standing, with the
back erect.
2. **Instructions:**
   a. Place both hands behind your head.
   b. Push your head backward against your resisting hands (Fig. 7-32). Prevent all head motion.
   c. Hold for 4 seconds, then relax.
   d. Repeat the exercise, gradually increasing the
   strength of the contracting force and hand resistance. Do not create pain. Do not hold a
   static contraction for more than 5 seconds.

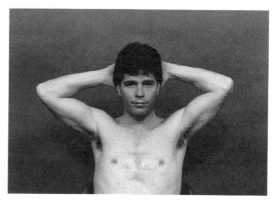

Figure 7-32. Cervical strengthening exercise: extensor muscles.

SIDE-BENDING MUSCLES
1. **Patient position:** seated or standing, with the
back erect.
2. **Instructions:**
   a. Place your right hand on the right side of your
   head, above the ear.

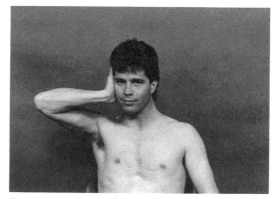

Figure 7-33. Cervical strengthening exercise: side-bending muscles.

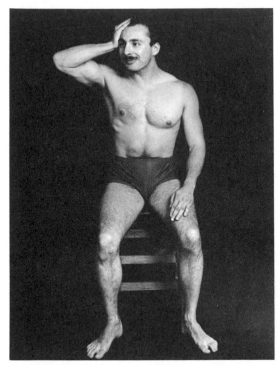

Figure 7-34. Cervical strengthening exercise: rotator muscles.

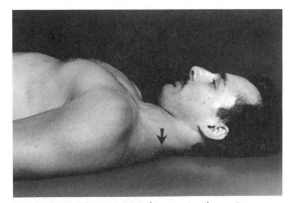

Figure 7-35. First exercise for cervicothoracic asymmetry.

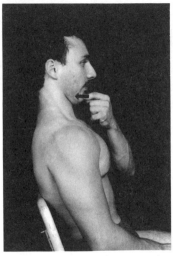

Figure 7-36. Second exercise for cervicothoracic asymmetry.

b. Push your head to the right against your resisting right hand (Fig. 7-33). Prevent all head motion.

c. Hold for 4 seconds, then relax.

d. Repeat the exercise, gradually increasing the strength of the contracting force and hand resistance. For left side-bending, reverse directions. Do not create pain. Do not hold a static contraction for more than 5 seconds.

ROTATOR MUSCLES

1. **Patient position:** seated or standing, with the back erect.

2. **Instructions:**

a. Place your right hand on the right side of your forehead.

b. Turn your head to the right against your resisting right hand (Fig. 7-34). Prevent all head motion.

c. Hold for 4 seconds, then relax.

d. Repeat the exercise, gradually increasing the strength of the contracting force and hand resistance. For left rotation, reverse directions. Do not create pain. Do not hold a static contraction for more than 5 seconds.

Cervicothoracic Asymmetry

Exercises for cervicothoracic asymmetry are designed to reduce excessive cervical lordosis and upper thoracic kyphosis (dowager's hump). Three exercises are described.

Exercise 1

1. **Patient position:** supine on solid flat surface.

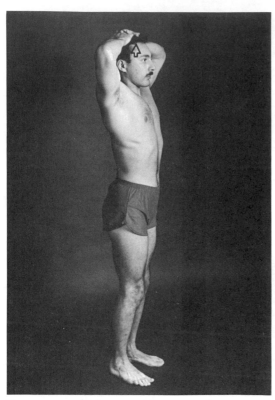

Figure 7-37. Third exercise for cervicothoracic asymmetry.

2. **Instructions:**
   a. Tuck in your chin.
   b. Try to push your neck down, flattening your neck against the surface (Fig. 7-35).
   c. Hold for 4 seconds, relax, and repeat.

Exercise 2

1. **Patient position:** seated in a chair with back pressed firmly against the back of the chair. A pillow may be used to maintain a low back lordotic curve if necessary.
2. **Instructions:**
   a. Tuck in your chin.
   b. With one hand, push your chin toward the back of your neck, trying to flatten the neck. Your chin must be kept in one horizontal plane (Fig. 7-36).
   c. Hold for 4 seconds, relax, and repeat.

Exercise 3

1. **Patient position:** standing.
2. **Instructions:**
   a. Stand straight with your back and neck stretched as tall as possible.
   b. Tuck in your chin.
   c. Place both hands on top of your head.
   d. Push your head up toward your hands, lengthening your neck. Keep your chin in one horizontal plane (Fig. 7-37).
   e. Hold for 4 seconds, relax, and repeat.
     Note: Do not increase your lumbar lordosis. Once this procedure has been mastered, keep your hands down and practice standing and walking with your chin and neck in this position, as often as possible.

8

Evaluation of the Thoracic Spine

FUNCTIONAL ANATOMY AND BIOMECHANICS

Jonathan F. Fenton
Donald E. Phykitt

The thoracic spine is a relatively immobile area, compared with the cervical or lumbar spine. The immobility has two anatomic causes. First, considerable stability is provided by the intimate connection of the thoracic spine to the thoracic cage, the ribs and sternum, via the costovertebral articulations. Second, the ratio of intervertebral disk height to vertebral body height is small (1:5), which greatly reduces intersegmental motion. By contrast, the disk height–vertebral body height ratios in the cervical and lumbar regions are 2:5 (permitting greatest motion) and 1:3, respectively.

The thoracic spine normally displays a gentle kyphosis, a C-shaped curve, convex posteriorly. This is mainly due to the wedge shape of the vertebral bodies, which are slightly higher at the posterior edge than at the anterior edge. The degree of kyphosis can vary with age and postural habits as well as with pathologic conditions, such as osteoporosis.

Although the thoracic spine has characteristic features that distinguish it from the cervical and lumbar spinal regions, it is mainly a transitional zone between the cervical and lumbar regions, as evidenced by the steady increase in height of the vertebral bodies from T1 to T12. Moreover, the inferior articular facets of T12 correspond to those in the lumbar area to allow proper articulation with L1. The different forms of articulation play a considerable role in the amplitude of various physiologic motions in the thoracic spine.

Osteology

VERTEBRAL BODY

The transverse diameter of the thoracic vertebral body is approximately equal to its anteroposterior diameter. The vertebral body is slightly higher at the posterior edge than at the anterior edge, contributing to normal kyphosis in the area. The anterior and lateral edges of the body are hollow.

The posterolateral corners of the superior and inferior vertebral plateaus bear the costal articular facets. These facets are oval, set into the body at an oblique angle, and lined by cartilage. They articulate with the heads of the ribs. Of the thoracic vertebrae, only T12 has costal articular facets only at the superior plateau.

ARTICULAR FACETS

The superior articular facets face backward, upward, and laterally. They are rotated approxi-

An Osteopathic Approach to Diagnosis and Treatment, second edition
Eileen L. DiGiovanna and Stanley Schiowitz
Lippincott–Raven Publishers, Philadelphia © 1997.

mately 60 degrees from the horizontal plane and 20 degrees from the frontal plane. In the transverse dimension they are convex.

The inferior articular facets face forward, downward, and medially. In the transverse dimension they are concave. The inferior articular facets of T12 resemble those of a lumbar vertebra in that they face laterally and anteriorly and are convex transversely.

TRANSVERSE AND SPINOUS PROCESSES

The transverse processes of the thoracic vertebrae face laterally and slightly posteriorly; they are easily palpated. They bear costal articular facets at the anterior aspects of their bulbous tips, the point of articulation with the costal tubercles of the corresponding ribs.

THE SPINOUS PROCESS

The spinous process faces posteriorly and inferiorly, the degree of inferior angulation varying with the area of the thoracic spine. The "rule of 3's" is used to locate a vertebra's spinous process in relation to its transverse process.

RULE OF 3'S

1. The upper three thoracic vertebrae (T1, T2, T3) have spinous processes that project directly posteriorly; therefore, the tip of the spinous process is in the same plane as the transverse processes of that vertebra.
2. The next three vertebrae (T4, T5, T6) have spinous processes that project slightly downward; therefore, the tip of the spinous process lies in a plane halfway between that vertebra's transverse processes and the transverse processes of the vertebra below it.
3. The next three vertebrae (T7, T8, T9) have spinous processes that project moderately downward; therefore, the tip of the spinous process is in a plane with the transverse processes of the vertebra below it.
4. The last three thoracic vertebrae (T10, T11, T12) have spinous processes that project from a position similar to T9 and rapidly regress until the orientation of the spinous process of T12 is like that of T1. That is, the spinous process of T10 is near the plane of the transverse processes of the vertebra below it, the spinous process of T11 is halfway between its own transverse processes

and the transverse processes of the vertebra below it, and the spinous process of T12 projects directly posteriorly in the plane of its own transverse processes.

Rib Articulations

COSTOVERTEBRAL ARTICULATION

The articular facets on the vertebral bodies are really demifacets (i.e., partial facets). The entire facet consists in the demifacet on the superior aspect of one vertebra and the demifacet on the inferior aspect of the vertebra above it.

The heads of the second through 12th ribs articulate with the bodies of the corresponding vertebrae and the one above, as well as with the corresponding intervertebral disk. However, the first rib articulates only with the superior aspect of T1. The costovertebral articulation is a synovial joint, with a joint capsule that is strengthened by the radiate ligament (see below, Costovertebral Ligaments).

COSTOTRANSVERSE ARTICULATIONS

The costotransverse articulation is a joint representing the articulation of the tubercle of a rib with the transverse process of the corresponding vertebra. The joint is surrounded by a weak capsule that is greatly strengthened by the costotransverse ligaments.

ANTERIOR ARTICULATIONS

The anterior end of the rib is joined to its costal cartilage by the costochondral joint. The costal cartilage articulates anteriorly in a number of ways.

1. The first rib is joined to the manubrium by a cartilaginous joint.
2. The cartilage of the second rib articulates with demifacets on both the manubrium and the body of the sternum by way of synovial joints.
3. The cartilages of the third through seventh ribs create small synovial joints with the body of the sternum.
4. The 8th through 10th costal cartilages do not join the sternum but are continuous with the costal cartilage immediately above.
5. The 11th and 12th costal cartilages are free. These ribs are known as the floating ribs.

Ligamentous Attachments

Seven ligaments connect adjacent vertebrae in the thoracic spine.

1. The anterior longitudinal ligament is attached to the anterior surface of all vertebral bodies.
2. The posterior longitudinal ligament runs down the posterior surface of all vertebral bodies.
3. Intertransverse ligaments pass between the transverse processes in the thoracic spine.
4. Capsular ligaments are attached just beyond the margins of the adjacent articular processes.
5. Ligamenta flava (arcuate, flaval, or yellow ligaments) extend from the anteroinferior border of the laminae above to the posterosuperior borders of the laminae below.
6. Interspinous ligaments connect adjacent spinous processes; they extend from the root to the apex of each spinous process.
7. The supraspinous ligament originates in the ligamentum nuchae and continues along the tips of the spinous processes.

COSTOVERTEBRAL LIGAMENTS

There are two kinds of costovertebral ligaments, interosseous ligaments and radiate ligaments, the latter consisting of three bands. Interosseous ligaments are attached to the head of the rib between the two articular demifacets and to the corresponding intervertebral disk. In the radiate ligaments, the superior band of tissue runs from the head of the rib to the vertebral body above. The inferior band runs from the head of the rib to the corresponding vertebral body, and the intermediate band runs from the head of the rib to the corresponding intervertebral disk.

COSTOTRANSVERSE LIGAMENTS

There are three kinds of costotransverse ligaments, determined by anatomic location with respect to the ribs and vertebrae—interosseous, posterior, and superior. The interosseous costotransverse ligament runs from the transverse process to the posterior surface of the neck of the corresponding rib. The posterior costotransverse ligament runs from the tip of the transverse process to the lateral border of the corresponding costal tubercle. The superior costotransverse ligament runs from the inferior border of the transverse process to the superior border of the neck of the underlying rib.

Thoracic Spinal Motion

INTERVERTEBRAL MOTION, EXCLUDING RIBS

Extension (least motion). In extension, the vertebrae approximate posteriorly. The inferior articular process of the superior vertebra glides posteriorly and inferiorly on the inferior vertebra. Motion is limited by approximation of the articular processes and spinous processes. These structures are sharply inclined posteriorly and inferiorly, and in normal anatomic relation are almost touching. The anterior longitudinal ligament is stretched, and the posterior longitudinal ligament, the ligamenta flava, and the interspinous ligaments are relaxed.

Flexion (second least motion). During flexion, the interspace between vertebrae increases posteriorly. The inferior articular process of the superior vertebra glides anteriorly and superiorly. Motion in the flexed spine is limited by the tension developed in the interspinous ligaments, the ligamenta flava, and the posterior longitudinal ligament.

Lateral flexion (second greatest motion). In lateral flexion, the articular surfaces on each side of a vertebra glide in opposite directions: on the contralateral side they glide upward, as in flexion; on the ipsilateral side they glide downward, as in extension. Lateral flexion to one side is accompanied by axial rotation to the opposite side, for three reasons: (1) One articular surface glides anteriorly while the other glides posteriorly. (2) Compression developed in the intervertebral disk, the anterior aspect of the unit, causes the vertebral body to move in the direction opposite to that of sidebending. (3) Lateral flexion tends to stretch the contralateral ligaments, located at the posterior aspect of the unit, which causes these ligaments to move toward the midline posteriorly to minimize their lengths.

Motion in the laterally flexed thoracic spine is limited by the impact of the articular processes on the ipsilateral side and by the tension developed in the contralateral ligamenta flava and intertransverse ligaments.

Rotation (greatest motion). In rotation, the orientation of the thoracic articular facets allows them to glide relative to each other with an axis of rotation near the center of the vertebral body. Thus, one vertebra can rotate around an axis, producing a simple twisting of the thoracic intervertebral disk. In contrast, the facets of the lumbar vertebrae are aligned such that the axis of rotation is at the spinous process. For rotation to occur one vertebral body must glide laterally with respect to its adjacent vertebrae. This results in shearing forces at the intervertebral disk. The articulation at T12-L1 is identical to the articulations found in the lumbar spine, so that the degree of rotation is greatly reduced. For the thoracic spine, motion in rotation is limited by multiple ligamentous tensions.

STABILITY AFFORDED
BY THE COSTAL CAGE

There are two mechanisms by which the ribs tend to increase the stability (and decrease the motion) of the thoracic spine. The first mechanism involves the articulation of the head of the ribs with the body and transverse processes of the vertebrae. The second mechanism increases the spine's moment of inertia via an increase in the transverse and anteroposterior dimensions of the spine structure. This results in increased resistance to motion in all directions.

Although no studies have compared the motion of the thoracic spine with and without intact costovertebral joints, White and Panjabi et al. have determined that the costovertebral joint plays a critical role in stabilizing the thoracic spine during flexion and extension.

The rib cage as a whole greatly enhances the stiffness of the spine, despite the flexibility of the individual components of the rib cage—the ribs, sternum, and their joints. Using a mathematical model of the thoracic and lumbar spine and the rib cage, Andriacchi et al. performed computer simulations to determine the effect of the rib cage on the stiffness of the normal spine during flexion, extension, side-bending, and axial rotation. They also studied the effect of removing one or two ribs or the entire sternum from an intact thorax. The stiffness properties of the spine were found to be greatly enhanced by the presence of an intact rib cage for all four motions, especially extension. The percentage increase in the stiffness of the spine with an intact rib cage, as compared with the spine and ligaments alone, was 27% for flexion, 132% for extension, 45% for lateral bending, and 31% for axial rotation. Removal of the sternum virtually nullified the stiffening effect of the costal cage. Removal of one or two ribs had minimal effect.

Thus, the intact thoracic cage, rather than individual elements or articulations, is a major factor contributing to the increased stability of the thoracic spine.

OVERALL MOTION OF THE THORACIC SPINE

The thoracic spine is a transitional region between the relatively more mobile cervical and lumbar regions. It is designed for rigidity and support of vital structures. The extent of each of the four physiologic motions varies throughout the region because of variable effects of the costal cage and changes in vertebral osteology from a cervical-like osteology to a lumbar-like osteology.

Flexion and extension. Flexion and extension are the least of the motions of the thoracic spine and occur to the smallest extent in the upper thoracic spine, gradually increasing in amplitude in the lower thoracic spine. This transition is largely due to the stiffening effect of the costal cage in the upper thoracic spine, which is most evident during extension. The first seven ribs are attached directly to the sternum, promoting greatest stability. The next three ribs are only indirectly attached via costal cartilage. The last two ribs are not attached at all anteriorly and therefore resemble the cylinder with a strip cut out, providing considerably less stability than the ribs higher in the costal cage.

The motions of flexion and extension in the thoracic spine are further limited by costovertebral articulations. This stabilization is lost at T11-T12 and T12-L1, as the 12th rib articulates only with the body of T12, thus losing the support found when a rib articulates with two adjacent vertebrae.

Lateral bending. Lateral bending is the second greatest motion in the thoracic spine. The amplitude of motion remains fairly constant throughout the region but is restricted by articular impingement, by ligamentous attachments (including costovertebral and costotransverse ligaments), and by the resistance afforded by the intact costal cage.

Rotation. Rotation is the greatest motion in the larger part of the thoracic spine (T1–T10). The amplitude of rotation is markedly decreased in the lower part of the region. The articular orientation of the thoracic vertebrae allows them to rotate about a point in the center of the vertebral body. The articular orientation of the lower thoracic vertebrae, however, is similar to that of the lumbar vertebrae and permits rotation only about a point near the spinous process. This rotation is greatly resisted by shearing forces in the intervertebral disk. The extent of rotation is further diminished by the resistance afforded by the intact costal cage.

MOTION TESTING
Donald E. Phykitt

Gross Motion Testing
SIDE-BENDING, T1–T12
1. **Patient position:** seated.
2. **Physician position:** standing behind patient.
3. **Technique:**
   a. The physician places his hands on the patient's shoulders with the web of the thumb and first finger over the acromion. The thumb rests posteriorly, pointing to T12, and the fingers rest anteriorly.
   b. To evaluate *right* side-bending:
      i. The physician exerts *downward* pressure accompanied by *left* translatory force on the *right* shoulder (Fig. 8-1A). The resulting force is trasmitted downward through the body of T12.
      ii. Note the ease and degree of side-bending (normal = approximately 20 degrees) and the smoothness of the right lateral curve created in the thoracic spine.

c. To evaluate *left* side-bending:
   i. The physician exerts *downward* pressure accompanied by a *right* translatory force on the *left* shoulder. The resulting force will be directed downward through the body of T12.
   ii. Note the ease and degree of side-bending (normal = approximately 20 degrees) and the smoothness of the left lateral curve created in the thoracic spine.
d. Compare the degree of side-bending in each direction.
e. Note the presence and location of any pain experienced by the patient during these maneuvers.

SIDE-BENDING, T1–T8
1. **Patient position:** seated.
2. **Physician position:** standing behind the patient.

Figure 8-1. Localization of force induced on thoracic side-bending. **(A)** T1 through T12. **(B)** T1 through T8. **(C)** T1 through T4.

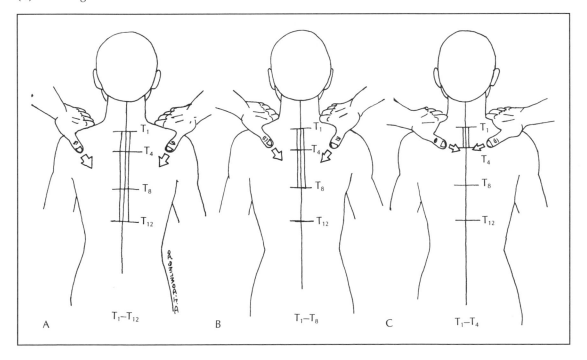

3. **Technique:**
   a. The technique is similar to that described for side-bending of T1–T12, with the following modifications. The physician's hands are placed with the web of the thumb and first finger halfway between the base of the patient's neck and the acromion process. The thumbs point toward T8. Greater force is required to induce side-bending in the T1–T8 region. The resulting force exerted by the physician is directed downward and through the body of T8 (Fig. 8-1B).
   b. Compare the degree of side-bending (left versus right), and note any difference (normal = approximately 10 degrees).
   c. Observe the smoothness of the lateral curve created.

SIDE-BENDING, T1–T4
1. **Patient position:** sitting.
2. **Physician position:** standing behind patient.
3. **Technique:**
   a. The technique is similar to that described for testing side-bending of T1–T12 and T1–T4, with the following modifications. The physician's hands are placed with the web of the thumb and first finger as close as possible to the patient's shoulders at the base of the neck. The thumbs point toward T4. Greater force is required to induce side-bending than in the previous two tests. The force induced by the physician is directed downward and through the body of T4 (Fig. 8-1C).
   b. Compare the degree of side-bending (right versus left) and note any differences (normal = approximately 5 degrees).
   c. *Note:* Asymmetry in side-bending (right versus left) can be caused by single dysfunctions, group curves, or myofascial tension in the area being examined.

Discrepancies in findings between areas of the thoracic spine (T1–T12, T1–T8, or T1–T4) may indicate an area of dysfunction and should prompt the physician to examine this area more closely with the techniques of rotoscoliosis testing and intersegmental motion testing, described below.

ROTATION IN THE THORACIC SPINE
1. **Patient position:** seated, straddling the table, with his back near the end of the table.

2. **Physician position:** standing behind patient.
3. **Technique:**
   a. The physician places a hand on each of the patient's acromion processes.
   b. Rotation is induced by the physician drawing one shoulder toward himself while simultaneously pushing away the opposite shoulder (Fig. 8-2).
      i. *Right rotation:* The physician draws the right shoulder toward himself while pushing away the left shoulder.
      ii. *Left rotation:* The physician draws the left shoulder toward himself while pushing away the right shoulder.
   c. *Note:*
      i. The degree of rotation in each direction. This is best measured by noting the deviation of the shoulder line from the frontal plane. Normal rotation is approximately 40 degrees in each direction.
      ii. The symmetry of right rotation versus left rotation.
      iii. The presence and location of pain during this maneuver.

FORWARD BENDING/BACKWARD BENDING
It is quite difficult to separate the motions of forward and backward bending in the thoracic spine from the same motions in the lumbar spine. Therefore, these motions are considered for the combined thoracolumbar region, and the technique is described in Chapter 10.

Rotoscoliosis Testing

Rotoscoliosis testing and intersegmental motion testing are two diagnostic modalities for evaluating somatic dysfunction at a vertebral level. They can be used alone or in conjunction with each other, according to physician preference.

Rotoscoliosis testing evaluates the rotational position of the vertebrae with respect to the position of the transverse processes. This position is evaluated with the spine in neutral position, in flexion, and in extension.

Vertebrae involved in a group curve will exhibit the greatest positional rotation in neutral position. From Fryette's first law, side-bending and rotation should occur in opposite directions. Single somatic dysfunctions exhibit the greatest

Figure 8-2. Positions for thoracic left rotation.

Figure 8-3. Rotoscoliosis testing for type II dysfunction in the upper thorax.

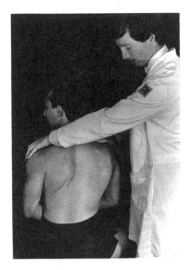 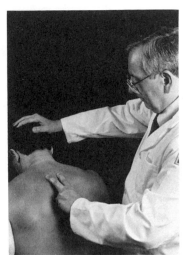

positional rotation in either flexion or extension. From Fryette's second law, side-bending and rotation should occur in the same direction. Furthermore, in single somatic dysfunctions the freedom of motion (the direction for which the dysfunction is named) in flexion or extension will be opposite to the position in which the rotation is exaggerated.

The positions described in the following sections are the positions in which the patient is examined. Examples of examination findings and the corresponding diagnoses are given at the end of the chapter.

THE DOMINANT EYE

The dominant eye is the eye through which most information about the outside world is conveyed. A dominant eye develops in every person shortly after birth and does not change for the duration of life. It has no relationship to handedness.

Technique for Determining Dominant Eye
1. Make a circle by apposing your thumb and index finger.
2. Fully extend the arm in front of you.
3. With both eyes open, locate an object at least 10 feet away so that it is enclosed in the circle formed by your two fingers.
4. Maintaining this position, close each eye alternately, so that you are looking through the circle with each eye alternately.

5. The dominant eye is the one that "sees" the object as within the circle. The nondominant eye "sees" the object as outside the circle.

ROTOSCOLIOSIS TESTING
FOR TYPE II DYSFUNCTIONS, T1–T3
1. **Patient position:** seated.
2. **Physician position:** standing behind the patient.
3. **Technique:**
   a. The physician uses his thumbs to palpate the tips of the transverse processes, located one-half inch lateral to and at the same level of the corresponding spinous process (Fig. 8-3).
   b. Evaluate for the presence of pain, increased myofascial tension, and one transverse process (right or left) more posterior than the other. The latter can be detected either by palpating a more posterior transverse process or by sensing a decreased tissue depth on the side of the posterior transverse process.
   c. At each level, have the patient begin with the neck fully flexed. Instruct the patient to slowly bring his head back into neutral position and then into full extension.
   d. Observe the changes under your palpating fingers. *Note* the position (flexion, extension) in which the maximum positional rotation occurs, and the direction of positional rotation (side of the posterior transverse process).
   e. Repeat these steps for T2 and T3.

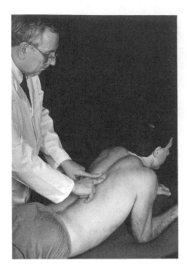

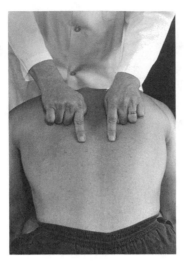

Figure 8-4. Rotoscoliosis testing for type II dysfunction in extension in midthoracic region, patient prone.

Figure 8-5. Rotoscoliosis testing for type II dysfunction in flexion in midthoracic region, patient seated.

ROTOSCOLIOSIS TESTING
FOR TYPE II DYSFUNCTIONS, T4–T12

Rotoscoliosis testing in the region of T4–T12 is identical to testing in the upper thoracic region, with the exception of differences in patient position for the different physiologic motions.

Extension

1. **Patient position:** prone, resting on his elbows. The upper thoracic musculature should be relaxed to allow full extension and to facilitate palpation (Fig. 8-4).
2. **Physician position:** seated or standing at the side of the patient, facing the patient's head. The physician's dominant eye is closest to the patient.
3. **Technique:** described under Flexion, which follows.

Flexion

1. **Patient position:** seated, with the feet supported on the floor or a stool. The hands are locked behind the neck and the patient is instructed to bend forward as far as he can (Fig. 8-5).
2. **Physician position:** standing in front of or behind patient.
3. **Technique:** (for all lower thoracic rotoscoliosis diagnoses):
   a. The physician uses the thumbs or index fingers to palpate the tips of the transverse processes, located one-half to one inch lateral to the spinous processes. (The caudad-cephalad relationship between a vertebra's spinous process and its transverse processes is governed by the rule of 3's, described earlier in this chapter.)
   b. Evaluate:
      i. Pain on palpation.
      ii. Increased myofascial tension.
      iii. Posterior transverse process. Increased musculature in this region makes direct palpation of transverse processes difficult. Posterior rotation will most likely be detected from a decreased tissue depth.
   c. The physician positions himself so that he can visualize the midline of the patient's back parallel to the spine. *Note* the relative heights of the palpating fingers. Are they even? Is one finger more posterior?
   d. Begin by examining the entire lower thoracic region in neutral position and noting findings. Then instruct the patient to move up into extension, and note findings in this position. Finally, instruct the patient to move into flexion, and note findings in this position.
   e. After evaluating the lower thoracic region in all three positions, note in which position positional rotation was greatest at each vertebral level. It may be necessary to reevaluate one or more levels to determine the position in which the transverse process was most posterior.

ROTOSCOLIOSIS TESTING
FOR TYPE I DYSFUNCTIONS
Evaluation of the thoracic spine for the detection of type I dysfunctions entails three different kinds of examinations:

1. Static symmetry scan (see Chap. 3). Observation from behind the patient may reveal side-bending of a group of vertebrae, asymmetry in the *height* of paired landmarks (e.g., shoulders), or asymmetry in the *prominence* of paired landmarks (e.g., scapulae).
2. Regional motion testing. The physician observes for asymmetric side-bending. Restricted motion to the side of the convexity is common.
3. Rotoscoliosis testing. The diagnosis of type I dysfunctions is based on detecting three or more adjacent vertebrae whose positional rotation is greatest in neutral. Testing is done separately for the upper and lower thoracic regions.

Upper thoracic region (T1–T3)
1. **Patient position:** seated.
2. **Physician position:** standing behind patient.
3. **Technique:**
   a. The patient is instructed to sit up straight, thus placing the vertebrae in neutral position.
   b. Using the thumbs, the physician palpates the transverse processes of T1 bilaterally.
   c. The physician determines which transverse process is more posterior.
   d. Repeat these steps at T2 and T3.

Lower thoracic region (T4–T12)
1. **Patient position:** prone, head resting on chin and facing forward, arms either at the side or hanging down from table (Fig. 8-6).
2. **Physician position:** standing at the side of the patient, facing the patient's head. The physician's dominant eye is closest to the patient.
3. **Technique:** Repeat test as described for rotoscoliosis testing for type II dysfunctions, T4–T12.

*Alternative Methods of
Rotoscoliosis Testing, T4–T12*
The methods described here are alternatives to conventional rotoscoliosis testing. Their advantages include ease and speed of diagnosis. The patient remains in a single position in all three methods. Furthermore, the physician can more readily compare findings in neutral, flexion, and extension. These techniques require greater palpatory skill, and should be used only by an experienced physician.

Alternate technique 1
1. **Patient position:** seated on a stool with the feet resting firmly on the ground, shoulder width apart.
2. **Physician position:** standing behind the patient.
3. **Technique:**
   a. The physician's thumbs are used to palpate the tips of the transverse processes bilaterally (Fig. 8-7).

Figure 8-6. Rotoscoliosis testing for type I dysfunction, lower thorax, neutral position.

Figure 8-7. Rotoscoliosis testing, T4–T12, hand position.

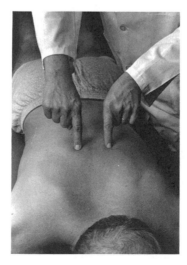

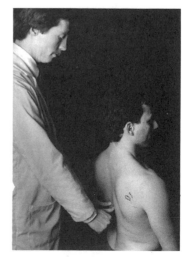

b. At each vertebral level, evaluation begins with the patient in neutral position (sitting straight up). *Note* pain, tissue changes, and vertebral rotation, as in conventional rotoscoliosis testing of T4–T12.

c. With the physician's thumbs at the same vertebral level, the patient is asked to bend over as far as possible. *Note* changes in vertebral positional rotation.

d. With the physician's thumbs at the same level, the patient is asked to sit up and position himself in extension.

  i. To evaluate T4–T8, ask the patient to thrust his chest out as far as possible.

  ii. To evaluate T9–T12, ask the patient to thrust his abdomen out as far as possible.

  iii. Note changes in vertebral positional rotation.

e. Note in which position (neutral, flexion, or extension) vertebral positional rotation is greatest.

f. Repeat these steps for all levels, T4 through T12.

Alternate technique 2

1. **Patient position:** prone, head resting on chin, arms at sides.

2. **Physician position:** standing at the patient's side, with the dominant eye closest to the patient.

3. **Technique:**

  a. The physician's thumbs or index fingers are used to palpate the tips of the transverse processes bilaterally.

  b. At each level, the physician begins by palpating the vertebra in the neutral position by pressing straight down on the transverse processes.

    i. Note tissue tension and vertebral positional rotation, as described for the conventional method.

    ii. Visualize the relative heights of thumbs, as described for the conventional method.

  c. With the thumbs at the same level, the physician evaluates the vertebrae in flexion.

    i. Roll the thumbs superiorly and press down on the superior aspect of the transverse processes, thus placing the vertebrae into flexion (Fig. 8-8).

    ii. Evaluate as above.

  d. With the thumbs at the same level, the physician evaluates the vertebrae in extension.

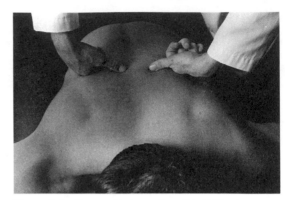

Figure 8-8. Rotoscoliosis testing, T4–T12, alternate technique 2, flexion testing.

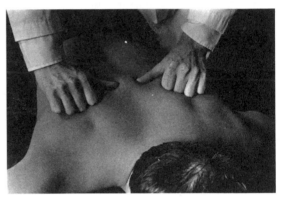

Figure 8-9. Rotoscoliosis testing, T4–T12, alternate technique 2, extension testing.

  i. Roll the thumbs inferiorly and press down on the inferior aspect of the transverse processes, thus placing the vertebrae into extension (Fig. 8-9).

    ii. Evaluate as above.

  e. Determine in which position (neutral, flexion, extension) the greatest positional rotation is found.

  f. Repeat these steps at all levels, T4 through T12.

Alternate technique 3

1. **Patient position:** prone, head resting on chin, arms at sides.

2. **Physician position:** standing at the patient's side.

3. **Technique:**
   a. The physician places his hand on the patient's back with his fingers perpendicular to the patient's spine. One finger is placed in the interspinous space above and one finger in the interspinous space below the vertebra being evaluated.
   b. **Note:**
      i. Symmetry of interspinous spaces above and below vertebra in question.
      ii. Lateral deviation of spinous process of vertebra in question.
      iii. Anteroposterior deviation of spinous process of vertebra in question.
   c. **Interpretation:**
      i. Flexion (freedom of motion) dysfunction:
         a. Superior interspinous space narrower.
         b. Inferior interspinous space wider.
         c. Spinous process more prominent.
      ii. Extension dysfunction:
         a. Superior interspinous space wider.
         b. Inferior interspinous space narrower.
         c. Spinous process less prominent.
      iii. Neutral dysfunction (group curve):
         a. Superior and inferior interspinous spaces equal.
      iv. Rotation:
         a. Spinous process deviated to the side opposite that of vertebral rotation.
      v. **Example:** The spinous process of T6 is more prominent and rotated to the left; the space between the spinous processes of T5 and T6 is narrower than the space between the spinous processes of T6 and T7. The diagnosis is T6 flexion, rotation, and side-bending to the right.
   d. Repeat these steps at each level, T4 through T12.

EXAMPLES OF ROTOSCOLIOSIS FINDINGS AND CORRESPONDING DIAGNOSES

Example 1. Transverse process of T8 is posterior on the right and most prominent in flexion. Diagnosis: T8 E Rr Sr.

Example 2. Transverse processes of T4–T10 are posterior on the right and most prominent in neutral position. Diagnosis: T4–10 N Rr Sl.

Example 3. The same finding as in example 2, except that the transverse process of T7 is posterior on the left and most prominent in extension. Diagnosis: group curve (T4–T10 N Rr Sl) with a single somatic dysfunction (T7 F Rl Sl) at the apex. *Note:* Single somatic dysfunctions can occur within a group curve. They are most common at the apex (center) and the ends of a curve.

Intersegmental Motion Testing
TISSUE TEXTURE CHANGES
AND SYMMETRY

1. **Patient position:** seated comfortably, with the hands on the thighs and the cervical spine in neutral position.
2. **Physician position:** standing behind the patient.
3. **Technique:**
   a. The physician slides one finger along the spinous processes from T1 to T12. *Note:*
      i. Deviation from midline.
      ii. Any change in the size of the space between spinous processes.
      iii. Displacement of the spinous processes in the sagittal plane.
      iv. Point tenderness along the spinous processes.
   b. Place the pads of the second and third fingers on each side of the spinous process of T1, over the transverse processes. Slide them down from T1 to T12. *Note:*
      i. Tissue texture changes (firmness, bogginess).
      ii. Posterior prominence of transverse processes.
      iii. Change in size of space between transverse processes.
      iv. Deviation of spinous process from the midline.
      v. Point tenderness.
         Interpretation: For a detailed interpretation of deviations found on static evaluation of the spinous processes, see preceding, Alternate technique 3.

INTERSEGMENTAL MOTION TESTING, T1–T4

1. **Patient position:** seated comfortably, with the hands on the thighs and the cervical spine in neutral position.
2. **Physician position:** behind and to one side of the patient. The hand farthest from the patient (the motion-inducing hand) is placed on top of the patient's head. The position of the other hand (the palpating hand) varies with the mo-

tion being tested and is described below for the individual cases.

3. **Technique:**

   a. In evaluating **flexion-extension,** the physician's palpating hand is placed so that the fingers are oriented horizontally and pointing away from the physician. The pad of the third finger lies in the interspinous space of the level being tested (i.e., for testing T1, it lies in the interspinous space between T1 and T2). The pads of the second and fourth digits lie in the interspinous spaces one level above and one level below, respectively. The patient's head is passively bent forward and backward until motion is palpated at the level in question, but not at the level below (Fig. 8-10). *Note* symmetry of flexion versus extension at the vertebral level.

   Interpretation: The dysfunction is named for the direction (flexion or extension) where greater motion is detected.

   b. To evaluate **rotation,** the physician places one or two fingers on either side of the spinous process, over the transverse processes of the vertebrae being tested. The patient's head is bent forward or backward (the direction in which least motion was detected on flexion-extension testing) down to the level in question. The patient's head is then rotated to the left until full motion is palpated at the transverse process in question (Fig. 8-11). This process is repeated to the right. *Note* symmetry of rotation right versus rotation left.

Interpretation: The dysfunction is named for the direction of greater rotation.

   c. To evaluate side-bending, the physician places one or two fingers on both sides of the spinous process, between the transverse processes of the level being tested and the level below. The patient's head is bent forward or backward (in the direction of least motion) down to the level being tested, then is bent laterally to both sides (Fig. 8-12). Side-bending is detected as separation or approximation of the transverse processes under the palpating fingers. *Note* symmetry of right side-bending versus left side-bending.

   Interpretation: The dysfunction is named for the direction of greater side-bending.

Note that side-bending on intersegmental motion testing is greatly restricted by the ribs and may be difficult to evaluate. In normal spines or in group curves, side-bending is in the direction opposite the direction of rotation. In type II single-segment somatic dysfunctions, side-bending occurs in the same direction as rotation. The diagnosis of a side-bending limitation relies primarily on the finding of asymmetric motion in flexion-extension and in rotation.

INTERSEGMENTAL MOTION
TESTING, T5–T12

The methods of diagnosing intersegmental dysfunction in the lower thoracic spine are quite similar to the techniques used in the upper thoracic

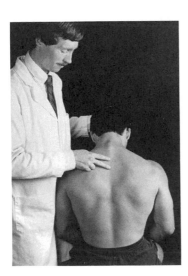 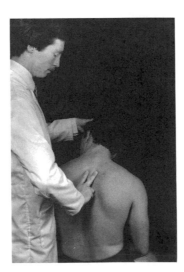

Figure 8-10. Intersegmental motion testing, flexion-extension, T1–T4.

Figure 8-11. Intersegmental motion testing, rotation, T1–T4.

Figure 8-12. Intersegmental motion testing, lateral flexion, T1–T4.

Figure 8-13. Intersegmental motion testing, rotation, T5–T12.

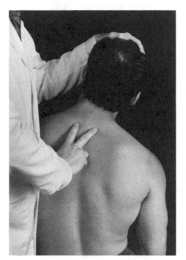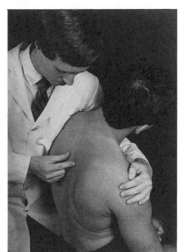

spine. The patient position is the same except that the patient must sit up straight. The positions of the palpating hand are the same. However, the physician is positioned differently with respect to the patient, and different techniques are used to induce motion in the lower thoracic spine. Only these differences are described.

1. **Patient position:** as for intersegmental motion testing of the upper thoracic spine.
2. **Physician position:** behind and to one side of patient. The hand closer to the patient serves as the palpating hand. The other arm is positioned so that the axilla rests on the patient's near shoulder. The arm reaches across the patient's sternum and the hand grasps the patient's far shoulder.
3. **Technique:**
   a. **Flexion** is induced by applying a downward and slightly anterior force to both of the patient's shoulders.
   b. **Extension** is induced by applying a caudal and slightly posterior force to both of the patient's shoulders.
   c. **Rotation** is induced by rotating the shoulders in the desired direction (Fig. 8-13).

d. Side-bending is induced by exerting a caudal force to one shoulder (the side ipsilateral to the desired side-bending), accompanied by a translatory force to the opposite side.

Palpation and interpretation are identical to those described for intersegmental motion testing of the upper thoracic spine.

References

Andriacchi TP, Schultz AB, Belytscko TB, Galante JO. 1974. A model for studies of mechanical interaction between the human spine and rib cage. J Biomech 7: 497.

Fryette H. 1954. Principles of Osteopathic Technique. Colorado Springs: Academy of Applied Osteopathy.

Kapandji IA. 1974. The Physiology of the Joints. Vol 3. The Trunk and the Vertebral Column. Edinburgh: Churchill Livingstone.

Schiowitz S, DiGiovanna E. 1981. An Osteopathic Approach to Diagnosis and Treatment. Old Westbury, NY: New York College of Osteopathic Medicine.

Warwick R, Williams P. 1973. Gray's Anatomy, 35th British ed. Philadelphia: W.B. Saunders.

White A, Panjabi MM. 1978. Biomechanics of the Spine. Philadelphia: J.B. Lippincott.

9

Treatment of the Thoracic Spine

MYOFASCIAL TECHNIQUES
Toni Spinaris

The principles of myofascial treatment were discussed in Chapter 5. Several of the techniques described in this section are good general techniques for relaxing and stretching the muscles of the thoracic and shoulder girdle.

Passive Techniques
PERPENDICULAR STRETCH
Perpendicular stretch techniques can be used to treat any muscles of the thoracolumbar region that run parallel to the spinous processes, including the erector spinae and its subdivisions.

1. **Patient position:** prone, with the head turned to the side of most comfort.
2. **Physician position:** standing at the side of the table and opposite the side being treated.
3. **Technique:**
   a. The physician places the thumb and thenar eminence of one hand at the medial edge of the muscle to be treated and lateral to the spinous processes. The thumb is parallel to the spinous processes (Fig. 9-1).
   b. He then places the thenar eminence of the other hand over the thumb of the first hand (Fig. 9-2).

c. The physician applies a slow, gentle pressure downward (toward the table) and laterally. The pressure is held for 3 seconds and gently released.
   Note: The direction of the force is lateral and parallel to the table. Do not press down into the muscle belly when using this technique.
   d. The physician may shift his hands up or down the spine to treat different areas of the thoracolumbar region.
   e. The technique may be repeated.

Treatment of Muscles Running Along Suprascapular Area from Cervical Region to Shoulder (e.g., Superior Trapezius)
1. **Patient position:** prone, with the head turned toward the physician.
2. **Physician position:** standing at the side of the table and opposite the side of the patient being treated, near shoulder level.
3. **Technique:**
   a. The physician places the thumb and thenar eminence of one hand perpendicular and slightly caudad to the fibers being treated.
   b. The other hand may reinforce the first or may be placed beside it to extend the area of treatment.

An Osteopathic Approach to Diagnosis and Treatment, second edition
Eileen L. DiGiovanna and Stanley Schiowitz
Lippincott–Raven Publishers, Philadelphia © 1997.

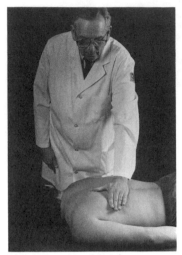

Figure 9-1. Myofascial perpendicular stretch technique: thumb position.

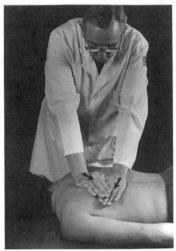

Figure 9-2. Myofascial perpendicular stretch technique: both hands in place.

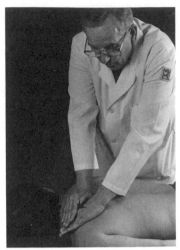

Figure 9-3. Myofascial perpendicular stretch of trapezius muscle.

c. The physician applies a slow gentle force downward and perpendicular to the muscle fibers (Fig. 9-3). This force is maintained for 3 seconds and gently released.

   Note: Always push the muscle perpendicular to the fibers.

d. The technique may be repeated.

Treatment of Superior Border of Trapezius

1. **Patient position:** prone, with the head turned to the side of most comfort.
2. **Physician position:** standing at the side of the table and opposite the side being treated, near shoulder level.
3. **Technique:**
   a. The physician places his caudal (with respect to the patient) hand over the patient's shoulder (the side to be treated).
   b. The fingers of the other hand are wrapped around the superior border of the trapezius.
   c. The physician applies gentle traction on the trapezius while applying a downward counterpressure on the shoulder. The direction of traction should be upward and perpendicular to the muscle fibers (Fig. 9-4).
   d. The traction is held for 3 seconds and gently released.
   e. The physician may slide his cephalad hand closer to the patient's neck or shoulder in order to treat other parts of the muscle.

Modification: The same technique can be performed with the patient supine (Fig. 9-5).

TREATMENT OF SUBSCAPULAR MUSCLES (E.G., SERRATUS ANTERIOR)

1. **Patient position:** prone, with the head turned away from physician.
2. **Physician position:** standing at the side to be treated, slightly cephalad to the scapula.
3. **Technique:**
   a. The patient places his hand (on the side to be treated) behind his back until the scapula abducts away from the rib cage.
   b. The physician wraps his fingers around the medial border of the scapula (Fig. 9-6).
   c. A gentle upward and lateral traction is applied, pulling the scapula away from the rib cage. This force is maintained for 3 seconds and gently released.
   d. The technique may be repeated.

PARALLEL STRETCH

1. **Patient position:** prone, with the head turned to the side of most comfort.
2. **Physician position:** standing at the side of the table and opposite the side of the patient being treated.
3. **Technique:**
   a. The physician's forearms are crossed and heels of his hands are placed on the body

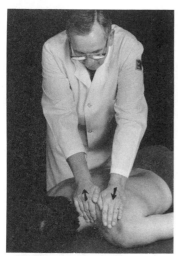

Figure 9-4. Myofascial stretch of trapezius muscle, patient prone.

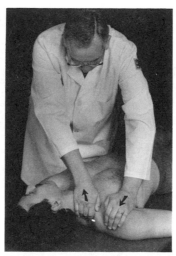

Figure 9-5. Myofascial stretch of trapezius muscle, patient supine.

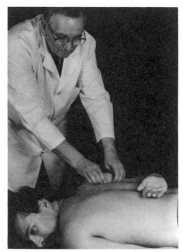

Figure 9-6. Subscapular muscle myofascial stretch.

of the muscle with the fingers of each hand parallel to each other. One hand is directed cephalad, the other is directed caudad (Fig. 9-7).

b. A gentle downward pressure is applied as the hands are separated.

Note: To avoid excessive stretching of the skin, the hands are placed approximately one inch apart, then moved together to create slack in the skin. This will bring the hands to the position shown in Figure 9-7.

PERPENDICULAR TRACTION
Upper Thoracic Region
1. **Patient position:** lying on his side, the side to be treated facing up. The hips and knees are flexed 90 degrees.
2. **Physician position:** standing at the side of the table and facing the patient.
3. **Technique:**
   a. The physician places her hands around the patient's scapula, allowing the patient's arm to hang over hers.
   b. The physician gently grasps the muscle to be treated (erector spinae, trapezius), separating it from the spine.
   c. The physician rocks her body backward while simultaneously applying a lateral and anterior (with respect to the patient) traction on the muscle (Fig. 9-8). The traction is held for 3 seconds and released.

Note: The physician's hands should not slide over the patient's skin, since this will cause friction and irritation. To avoid fatigue, the physician should use leverage and rock her body rather than apply the traction force with her arms.

d. The physician can move her hands (and body) caudad and cephalad to treat other muscle groups.

Thoracolumbar Area
1. **Patient position:** lying on his side, the side to be treated facing up. The knees and hips are flexed 90 degrees.
2. **Physician position:** standing at the side of the table, facing the patient. Her thighs rest against patient's knees.
3. **Technique:**
   a. The physician wraps the fingers of both hands around the paravertebral muscles to be treated.
      i. The fingers are directed perpendicular to the muscle fibers being treated.
      ii. The tips of the fingers are between the spinous processes and the muscle being treated.
   b. The physician rocks her body backward while simultaneously applying a gentle lateral and anterior traction to the muscle (Fig. 9-9).

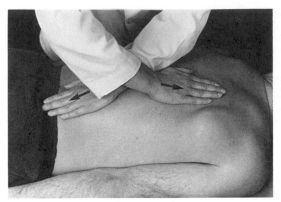

Figure 9-7. Parallel stretch of muscle.

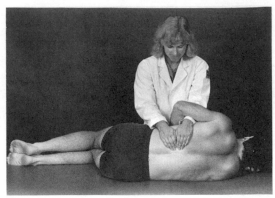

Figure 9-8. Perpendicular traction applied to muscle.

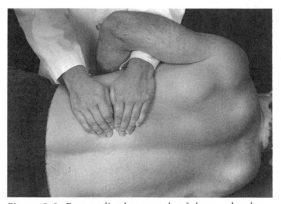

Figure 9-9. Perpendicular stretch of thoracolumbar paravertebral muscles, patient in lateral recumbent position.

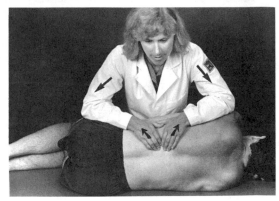

Figure 9-10. Thoracolumbar bidirectional stretch.

    i. The physician exerts a counterforce with her thighs against the patient's knees.
  c. The traction is held for 3 seconds and gently released.
  d. The physician can move her hands caudad or cephalad to treat other parts of the paravertebral musculature.

Modification of Thoracolumbar Technique
1. **Patient position:** same as above.
2. **Physician position:** same as above, except the physician need not place her thighs against the patient's knees.
3. **Technique:**
  a. The physician grasps the muscle to be treated, as above.
  b. The physician braces her cephalic (with re-

spect to the patient) elbow against the patient's axilla and the other elbow against the patient's hip. The elbows should not dig into the patient's body.
  c. The physician applies a gentle traction to the muscle while simultaneously pressing downward and cephalad on the axilla and downward and caudad on the hip (Fig. 9-10). This induces both a parallel stretch and perpendicular traction on the muscle.

Medial Scapular Area (Levator Scapulae, Rhomboids, Superior Trapezius)
1. **Patient position:** lying on his side, the side to be treated facing up.
2. **Physician position:** standing at the side of the table, facing the patient.

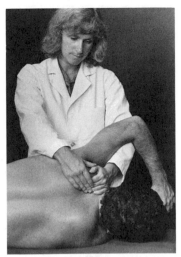

Figure 9-11. Medial scapular stretch, patient in lateral recumbent position.

3. **Technique:**
   a. The physician grasps the medial scapular muscles with her cephalic (with respect to the patient) hand and places the patient's arm over hers, toward the patient's head.
   b. The physician's other hand is placed over the inferior portion of the scapula and is used to stabilize the patient.
   c. Gentle traction is applied in a direction perpendicular to the muscle fibers (Fig. 9-11).
   d. The traction is held for 3 seconds and gently released.

Subscapular Area
1. **Patient position:** lying on his side, the side to be treated facing up.
2. **Physician position:** standing at the side of the table, facing the patient.
3. **Technique:**
   a. The physician places her cephalic (with respect to the patient) hand over the patient's suprascapular area and grasps the upper medial border of the scapula with her fingers.
   b. With her other hand, the physician reaches under the patient's arm and grasps the inferior angle and border of the scapula (Fig. 9-12).
   c. The physician applies gentle traction laterally and caudally (relative to the patient), lifting the scapula into abduction and away from the rib cage.

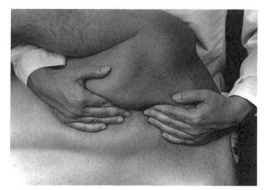

Figure 9-12. Subscapular stretch.

   i. The physician may also try to insert her fingers under the scapula and pull the scapula away from the rib cage (as previously described and illustrated in Fig. 9-6).
   ii. This technique must be done gently so as not to cause the patient discomfort.
   d. The traction is held for 3 seconds and gently released.

Active Direct Techniques: I

In the active direct techniques described below, the patient pushes his hand toward the floor. The first two techniques can be used to treat the paravertebral muscles, the rhomboids, the levator scapulae, and the trapezius muscle.

1. **Patient position:** lying on his side, the side to be treated facing up.
2. **Physician position:** standing at the side of the table, facing the patient.
3. **Technique:**
   a. With her caudal hand, the physician palpates (monitors) the muscles to be treated.
   b. The other hand grasps the patient's upper arm at the elbow such that the arm is fully supported. The patient's arm is flexed at the elbow and the fingers point toward the floor.
   c. Once the area to be treated has been localized (see below), the physician instructs the patient to push his fingers toward the floor (Fig. 9-13).
   d. The physician provides an isometric resistive counterforce to the patient's arm with her cephalic hand.
   e. To localize the muscle fibers to be treated, she monitors the muscles with her caudal

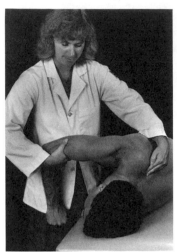

Figure 9-13. Active direct myofascial technique for thoracolumbar muscles. The patient pushes his fingers toward the floor while the physician applies an isometric counterforce.

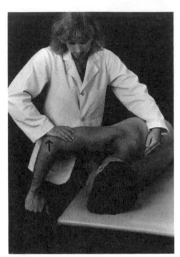

Figure 9-14. Active direct myofascial technique. The patient pushes his elbow toward the ceiling.

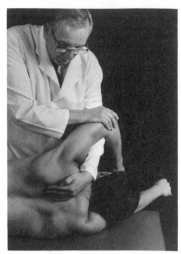

Figure 9-15. Active direct myofascial technique with patient's arm supported.

hand during the isometric contraction. The localization is controlled by the position (caudad or cephalad) of the patient's arm during isometric contraction.

   i. The further cephalad the physician positions the patient's elbow during contraction, the further cephalad are the fibers that will contract (i.e., be treated).

   ii. The further caudad the physician positions the elbow, the further caudad are the fibers being treated.

   iii. The caudal hand monitors for muscle contraction localized to the fibers being treated.

  f. The isometric contraction is held for 3 seconds, then the patient is instructed to relax.

  g. This technique can be repeated at the same location, or the elbow can be repositioned to treat a different area.

Active Direct Techniques: II

In the technique described below, the patient pushes his elbow toward the ceiling while the physician applies an isometric counterforce.

1. **Patient position:** same as for previous technique.

2. **Physician position:** same as for previous technique.

3. **Technique:**

  a. The physician's caudal hand monitors the muscle being treated, as in the previous technique.

  b. The patient's arm is positioned as in the previous technique (elbow flexed, fingers pointing toward the floor). The physician grasps the dorsal aspect of the patient's elbow, the part closest to the ceiling (Figs. 9-14, 9-15).

  c. The physician instructs the patient to push his elbow to the ceiling while she provides an isometric resistive force with her cephalic (with respect to the patient) hand.

  d. With this technique the area being treated is in a direct line with the long axis of the patient's upper arm (Fig. 9-16).

   i. If the patient's elbow is placed more cephalad, the fibers being treated are located more caudad.

   ii. If the elbow is placed more caudad, the fibers being treated are located more cephalad.

  e. The isometric force is maintained for 3 seconds; then the patient is instructed to relax.

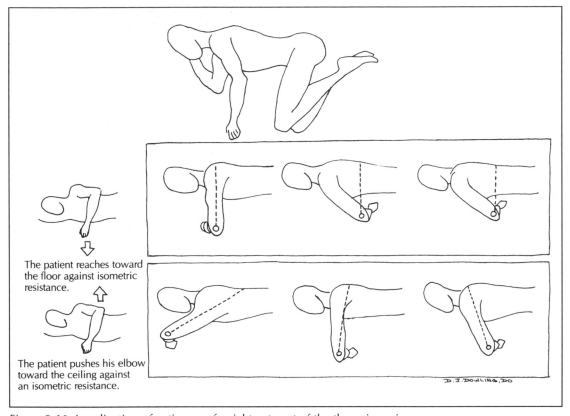

The patient reaches toward the floor against isometric resistance.

The patient pushes his elbow toward the ceiling against an isometric resistance.

D. J. DOWLING, DO

Figure 9-16. Localization of active myofascial treatment of the thoracic region.

f. The technique can be repeated at the same location, or the elbow can be repositioned to treat another area.

Active Direct Techniques: III. Scapula

This technique is good as an initial treatment to facilitate general relaxation of the entire scapular area.

1. **Patient position:** lying on his side, the side to be treated facing up.
2. **Physician position:** standing at side of table, facing the patient.
3. **Technique:**
   a. The physician grasps the superior border of the scapula with her cephalic (with respect to the patient) hand and the inferior angle with her other hand. The patient's arm rests on her caudal arm.
   b. The physician gently presses her sternum against the patient's shoulder.
   c. Using the weight of her upper torso against the patient's shoulder, the physician gently pushes the scapula medially and either superiorly or inferiorly (whichever motion is more free). The scapula is held in this position.
   d. The patient pushes his shoulder straight up against physician's chest while she applies an isometric resistive force.
   e. The contraction is maintained for 3 seconds; then the patient relaxes.
   f. The physician moves the scapula further medially and either superiorly or inferiorly.
   g. The technique is repeated three times.

Active Indirect Technique

The active indirect technique described below is a generalized technique for all the muscles in the upper and middle thoracic region.

1. **Patient position:** supine.

2. **Physician position:** standing at the side of the table near the patient's head, on the side opposite that being treated.
3. **Technique:**
   a. The patient grasps the wrist on the side being treated with his other hand. He is then instructed to rotate his upper torso away from the physician while keeping his lower body flat on the table.
   b. The physician reaches across the table and holds the patient's opposite wrist.
   c. The patient pulls the arm he is holding (the one opposite the physician) across his body toward the physician, thus rotating his torso toward the physician.
   d. The physician provides an isokinetic counterforce to this motion (Fig. 9-17).
   e. The patient's active motion will end when his upper torso is fully rotated to the side of the physician.
   f. The patient is instructed to relax.
   g. The physician applies a passive stretch to increase the rotation while stabilizing the lower body at the opposite anterosuperior iliac spine.

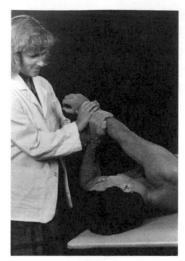

Figure 9-17. Active indirect myofascial technique for thoracic spine. The physician provides a resistive counterforce to the patient's rotation of the torso, adding a passive stretch at the end.

   h. The technique is repeated three times, with the physician providing increasingly greater counterforce each time.

MUSCLE ENERGY TECHNIQUES
Lillian Somner
Eileen L. DiGiovanna

This section describes muscle energy techniques for somatic dysfunctions, types I and II, of the thoracic spine. All of the techniques begin with the patient sitting erect and his feet adequately supported on the floor.

Type I Group Curve
1. **Patient position:** seated, feet on the floor, weight equally distributed on the buttocks.
2. **Physician position:** standing behind the patient and slightly to the side of the convexity.
3. **Technique:**
   a. The physician monitors at the apex of the curve being treated.
   b. The physician induces side-bending toward the convexity and rotation away from the convexity by applying a caudal and anterior force to the ipsilateral shoulder. Motion is induced down to the monitoring finger at the apex of the curve (Fig. 9-18).
   c. If the patient becomes unbalanced by the above movement, a translatory force should be applied toward the concavity. *Note* that the spine is kept in neutral position (i.e., no flexion or extension).
   d. The patient then side-bends toward the concavity (the freedom of motion) while the physician maintains a resistance on the shoulder closest to him (i.e., the side of the convexity).

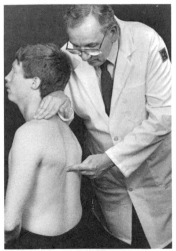

Figure 9-18. Muscle energy treatment for a type I group curve, convex right.

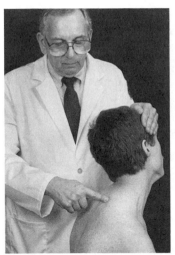

Figure 9-19. Muscle energy treatment for an upper thoracic type II somatic dysfunction.

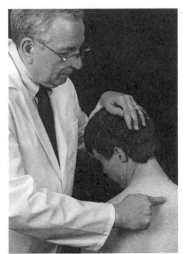

Figure 9-20. Muscle energy treatment for an upper thoracic type II somatic dysfunction. The barriers to flexion have been engaged, with left rotation and side-bending of the patient's head.

e. The force is held for 2 or 3 seconds; then the patient relaxes.
f. After 2 seconds of rest, the new motion barriers to side-bending and rotation are engaged.
g. The procedure is repeated twice more.

Type II Single-Segment Somatic Dysfunction

UPPER THORACIC REGION (T1–T4)
1. **Patient position:** seated, with feet on the floor.
2. **Physician position:** standing behind the patient and to the side of the motion barriers.
3. **Technique:**
   a. One hand monitors the involved vertebra to detect motion.
   b. The other hand holds the patient's head, or the arm is wrapped around it turban-style to control its motion and to provide a resistance to the patient's motion.
   c. The patient's neck is either flexed or extended to its motion barrier, while the physician monitors at the vertebra being treated.

The patient's head is then side-bent and rotated into the barriers to motion (Fig. 9-19).
   d. The patient is instructed to side-bend or rotate his head toward the freedom of motion against the physician's resistive force (Fig. 9-20).
   e. This is held 3 to 4 seconds; then the patient relaxes.
   f. New motion barriers are engaged.
   g. The process is repeated twice more.
   h. A passive stretch is given.

MIDDLE AND LOWER THORACIC REGION
1. **Patient position:** seated, with the feet on the floor.
2. **Physician position:** Standing behind the patient and to the side of the motion barriers.
3. **Technique:**
   a. The physician places one arm over the patient's shoulder on the side of the motion barriers. He may use either his axilla or his forearm.
   b. The patient is flexed or extended to the motion barrier. Extension may be achieved by

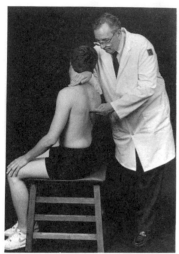

Figure 9-21. Muscle energy treatment for a flexion type II somatic dysfunction of the middle and lower thoracic region. The barriers to extension have been engaged, with right rotation and side-bending of the patient.

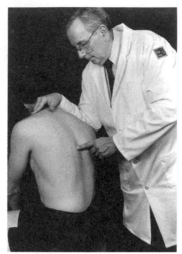

Figure 9-22. Muscle energy treatment for an extension type II somatic dysfunction of the middle and lower thoracic region. The barriers to flexion have been engaged, with right rotation and side-bending of the patient.

asking the patient to sit up straight or to stick his belly out (Fig. 9-21). Flexion is achieved by having the patient slump forward (Fig. 9-22). Motion should be to the involved segment.

c. Using his axilla or arm, the physician side-bends the patient and rotates him into the motion barriers at the involved segment.

d. If the dysfunction is low enough that side-bending unbalances the patient, a translatory force in the opposite direction will aid in keeping both buttocks on the table.

e. The patient then side-bends or rotates toward the freedom of motion. The physician provides a resistance with his arm. This is held for 3 to 4 seconds.

f. The patient relaxes, and the new motion barriers are engaged.

g. The process is repeated twice more.

h. A passive stretch is given.

COUNTERSTRAIN TECHNIQUES
Eileen L. DiGiovanna
Lillian Somner

As in other areas of the body, when counterstrain treatment is used in the thoracic spine, the positions for treating tender points, corresponding to vertebral segment dysfunctions, are held for 90 seconds. The patient is returned to neutral position slowly and without active engagement of his muscles.

Anterior Tender Points
Figure 9-23 shows the locations of the anterior tender points for the thoracic spine. All anterior tender points are treated in flexion.

Figure 9-23. Locations of anterior tender points, thoracic spine.

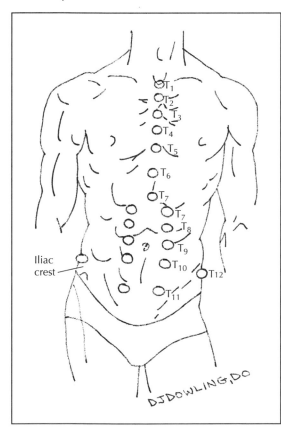

UPPER THORACIC SPINE (T1–T4)
1. **Patient position:** supine. The head and upper torso rest on the physician's knee so that the upper thoracic spine is flexed to the desired level.
2. **Physician position:** standing at the head of the table and resting his knee on the table. One hand monitors the tender point.
3. **Technique:** Pure flexion is usually all that is necessary. However, some slight side-bending and rotation modification may help localize and reduce the point tenderness (Fig. 9-24).

MIDTHORACIC SPINE (T5–T8)
Midthoracic dysfunctions may require such marked flexion that flexion of the upper body alone may not be sufficient. Flexion may be increased if the patient's hips are bent and the spine is allowed to flex from the lumbar area into the lower thoracic area.

1. **Patient position:** supine, upper body supported by pillows, hips bent to 90 degrees, with lower legs resting on the physician's knee.
2. **Physician position:** side of table, one foot on the table with the knee bent, supporting the patient's lower legs.
3. **Technique:** Patient is flexed up by bringing the knees toward the abdomen while monitoring the tender point. When tenderness is relieved, the position is held for 90 seconds (Fig. 9-25).
4. **Modifications:**
   a. The technique may be performed with the patient in a lateral recumbent position with hips and knees flexed; the physician flexes the patient's torso until the tender point is relieved.
   b. Another alternative is similar to that used for the upper thoracics, with the upper back supported by the physician's knee.

LOWER THORACIC SPINE (T9–L1)
1. **Patient position:** supine, with knees and hips flexed and supported by the physician's knee. A pillow may be placed under the hips and upper back to aid flexion if necessary.

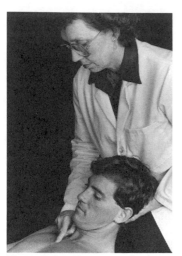

Figure 9-24. Counterstrain treatment of anterior tender points, upper thoracic spine.

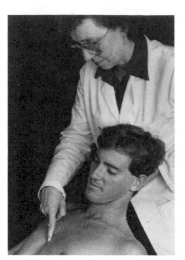

Figure 9-25. Counterstrain treatment of anterior tender points, midthoracic spine.

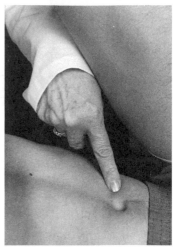

Figure 9-26. Counterstrain treatment of anterior T10 tender point, knees rotated to side of dysfunction.

2. **Physician position:** standing at the side of the table next to the side of the tender point, one foot on the table and supporting the patient's legs.

3. **Technique:** The patient's knees and hips are flexed and the physician supports the patient's thighs on her thigh. Pressure is applied cephalad as the knees are rotated toward the side of dysfunction (Fig. 9-26).

Posterior Tender Points

Figure 9-27 shows the locations of the posterior tender points. All posterior tender points are treated in extension with the patient prone. The patient's position varies only so that motion may be localized to a given point.

UPPER THORACIC SPINE (T1–T2)
1. **Patient position:** prone, with arms at his side.
2. **Physician position:** standing on the side of the patient opposite the tender point.
3. **Technique:** One hand supports the patient's chin; the other hand monitors the tender point on the opposite side of the spinous process. The head and neck are extended to the involved segment (Fig. 9-28). Rotation and side-bending will be away from the point.

Figure 9-27. Location of posterior tender points, thoracic spine.

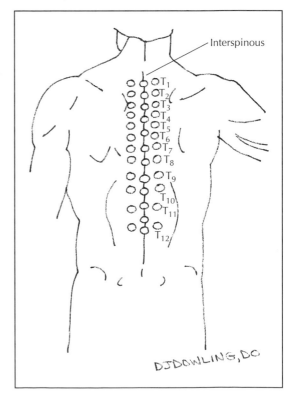

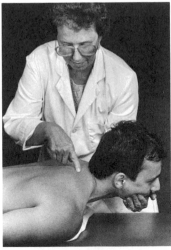

Figure 9-28. Counterstrain treatment of posterior tender points, upper thoracic spine.

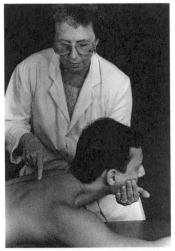

Figure 9-29. Counterstrain treatment of posterior tender points, midthoracic spine. Tender point is right; slight rotation is induced to the left.

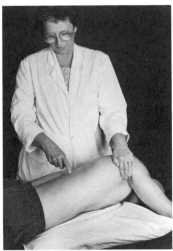

Figure 9-30. Counterstrain treatment of posterior tender points, lower thoracic spine.

MIDTHORACIC SPINE (T3–T5)
1. **Patient position:** same as above, except the arms are extended over the head.
2. **Physician position:** same as above.
3. **Technique:** same as above (Fig. 9-29) with slight rotation.

LOWER THORACIC SPINE (T6–L2)
1. **Patient position:** prone, arms extended above head.
2. **Physician position:** as above. The cephalic (with respect to the patient) hand supports the patient's axilla on the side of the tender point.
3. **Technique:** Rotation and side-bending are induced through pull on the axilla to the opposite side and cephalad, with care not to irritate the skin and other tissue. Extension may be facilitated by placing pillows under the patient's chest (Fig. 9-30).
4. **Variation:** The physician may use the pelvis to increase the rotation of a spinous process that is already rotated to one side. This relieves a tender point directly on the spinous process.

FACILITATED POSITIONAL RELEASE
Stanley Schiowitz

Thoracic Region Techniques
SUPERFICIAL MUSCLE HYPERTONICITY,
LEFT POSTERIOR REGION OF T7 VERTEBRA
1. **Patient position:** seated.
2. **Physician position:** standing behind and to the left of the patient.
3. **Technique:**

a. The physician places his right index finger on the site of the dysfunction.
b. The physician's left arm is placed on the patient's left shoulder with the elbow at the lateral aspect to allow direction and control of the patient's motion. The physician's forearm rests behind the patient's neck.

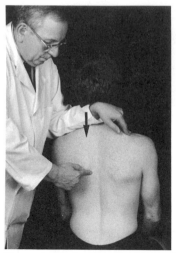

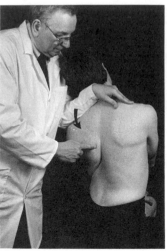

Figure 9-31. Facilitated positional release treatment for dorsal superficial muscle hypertonicity: application of compression at the left cervicothoracic junction.

Figure 9-32. Facilitated positional release treatment for dorsal superficial muscle hypertonicity: with side-bending and backward bending added.

c. The patient is instructed to sit up straight until the thoracic kyphosis flattens slightly.
d. If necessary, the patient is told to push his chest out until backward bending is created up to the monitoring finger, for further flattening of the thoracic spine.
e. The physician applies compression with his forearm near the patient's neck. The vector of force is aimed straight down parallel to the spine (Fig. 9-31).
f. Maintaining the backward bending and compression, the physician creates side-bending down to the monitoring finger by pressing down with his left arm (Fig. 9-32).
g. The position is held for 3 seconds, then released; the dysfunction is reevaluated.

SOMATIC DYSFUNCTION (T7 E Sl Rl)
1. **Patient position:** seated.
2. **Physician position:** standing behind and to the left of the patient.
3. **Technique:**
   a. The physician's monitoring finger is at the posterior transverse process.
   b. The physician's left arm is placed on the patient's left shoulder with the elbow at the lateral aspect to allow direction and control of the patient's motion. The physician's forearm rests behind the patient's neck.

c. The patient is instructed to sit up straight until the thoracic kyphosis flattens slightly.
d. If necessary, the patient is told to push his chest out until backward bending is created up to the monitoring finger, for further flattening of the thoracic spine.
e. The physician applies compression with his forearm near the patient's neck. The vector of force is aimed straight down parallel to the spine.
f. Maintaining the backward bending and compression, the physician creates side-bending down to the monitoring finger by pressing down with his left arm, to increase extension and add rotation to the left side-bending component.
g. The position is held for 3 seconds, then released; the dysfunction is reevaluated.

To treat a flexion dysfunction (T7 FSl Sl), flexion of spine is added after the compressive forced is applied. Side-bending and rotation are introduced to the left down to the dysfunction.

THORACIC DYSFUNCTION, PATIENT PRONE (T3 E Sr Rr)
1. **Patient position:** prone.
2. **Physician position:** standing beside the table, opposite the side of the dysfunction.

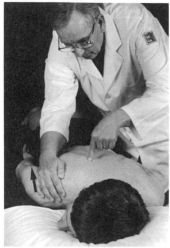 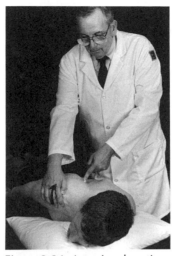

Figure 9-33. Facilitated positional release treatment for T3 extension dysfunction (T3 F. Sr Rr), patient prone. The physician applies a downward and parallel pull, creating compression and side-bending.

Figure 9-34. A torsional motion is added, turning the shoulder upward and creating compression, extension, side-bending, and rotation.

3. **Technique:**

   a. The physician places the index finger of his cephalic hand (with respect to the patient) at the posterior transverse process of T3. With the patient prone, mild flattening of the thoracic kyphosis is usually created. If not, a pillow is placed under the patient's head and neck.

   b. With his caudal hand, the physician grasps the patient's shoulder over the acromion process. With his hand on the superior aspect of the shoulder girdle, he pulls the shoulder, parallel to the table and toward the patient's feet, until force is felt at the monitoring finger (Fig. 9-33). This creates right side-bending.

   c. Maintaining this force, the physician straightens up, thereby pulling the patient's shoulder backward off the table, creating right rotation.

   d. These combined motions create compression, extension, side-bending, and rotation up to the monitoring finger (Fig. 9-34).

   e. The position is held for 3 seconds, then released; the dysfunction is reevaluated.

HIGH-VELOCITY, LOW-AMPLITUDE THRUSTING TECHNIQUES
Barry S. Erner
Paula D. Scariati

This section describes high-velocity, low-amplitude thrusting techniques for treating somatic dysfunctions of the thoracic spine by region—upper, middle, and lower spine. For most of the techniques the patient is supine; a variation is illustrated in which the patient is seated.

Upper Thoracic Somatic Dysfunction (T1–T3)
1. **Patient position:** supine.
2. **Physician position:** standing at the side of the table opposite the side of the posteriorly rotated transverse process.
3. **Technique:**
   a. The patient places his clasped hands behind his neck and approximates his elbows.
   b. The physician palpates the restricted segment and rests its posterior transverse process on the thenar eminence of his thrusting hand.
   c. With his other hand, the physician grasps the patient's elbows and rolls the patient's body over his thenar eminence.
   d. The physician exerts a rapid anteroposterior

thrust through the patient's arms onto the transverse process resting on his thenar eminence (Fig. 9-35).

Midthoracic Somatic Dysfunction
1. **Patient position:** supine.
2. **Physician position:** standing at the side of the table opposite to the side of the dysfunction.
3. **Technique:**
   a. The patient crosses his arms over his chest. The upper arm is the arm on the side of the posterior transverse process.
   b. The physician palpates the restricted segment and rests its posterior transverse process on the thenar eminence of his thrusting hand (Fig. 9-36).
   c. With his other hand, the physician grasps the patient's elbows and rolls the patient's body onto his thenar eminence.
   d. The physician exerts a rapid downward thrust through the patient's arms into the transverse process resting on his thenar eminence (Fig. 9-37).

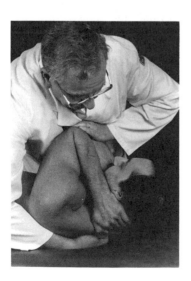 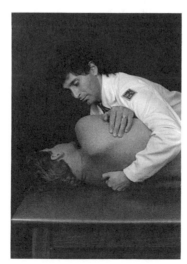

Figure 9-35. High-velocity, low-amplitude thrusting technique for upper thoracic somatic dysfunction.

Figure 9-36. Hand placement for midthoracic high-velocity, low-amplitude thrusting technique.

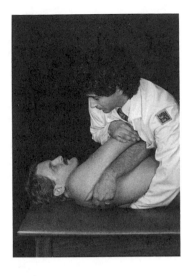 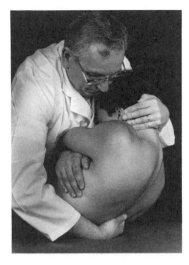

Figure 9-37. Downward thrust on midthoracic segment.

Figure 9-38. High-velocity, low-amplitude thrusting technique for somatic dysfunction of a lower thoracic segment.

Lower Thoracic Somatic Dysfunction

1. **Patient position:** supine.
2. **Physician position:** standing at the side of the table opposite to the side of the posteriorly rotated transverse process.
3. **Technique:**
   a. The patient crosses his arms over his chest. The upper arm is the arm on the side of the posterior transverse process.
   b. The physician palpates the restricted segment and rests its posterior transverse process on the thenar eminence of his thrusting hand.
   c. With his other hand, the physician grasps the patient behind the shoulders and "hugs" him, creating and localizing flexion down to the restricted segment.
   d. The physician rolls the patient over his thenar eminence and exerts a rapid thrust, creating a vector force through the posterior transverse process (Fig. 9-38).

Alternative Techniques for Thoracic Somatic Dysfunction

ALTERNATIVE 1

1. **Patient position:** on the table reclined with back supported by the physician's knee.
2. **Physician position:** standing at the head of the table, with one knee on the table.
3. **Technique:**
   a. The physician places his knee under the posterior transverse process of the restricted segment.
   b. The patient is instructed to reach back and grasp his hands together around the physician's waist.
   c. The physician grasps the patient beneath the scapulae bilaterally and exerts an upward cephalad traction force. Simultaneously, the physician rolls the patient over his knee (Fig. 9-39).

ALTERNATIVE 2

1. **Patient position:** seated on a stool, feet flat on the floor.
2. **Physician position:** standing behind the patient.
3. **Technique:**
   a. A pillow is placed between the patient's spine and the physician's knee for comfort.
   b. The patient is instructed to interlock his fingers behind his neck.
   c. The physician localizes the rotated transverse process with his knee (with the right knee for a right-sided lesion).
   d. The physician grasps the patient's forearms by sliding his arms underneath the patient's armpits and resting on the dorsal surface of the patient's wrists.
   e. The physician exerts an upward cephalad force while simultaneously rolling the patient's spine over his knee (Fig. 9-40).

Figure 9-39. Alternative high-velocity, low-amplitude thrusting technique for somatic dysfunction of the thoracic spine, patient supine.

Figure 9-40. Alternative high-velocity, low-amplitude thrusting technique for somatic dysfunction of the thoracic spine, patient seated.

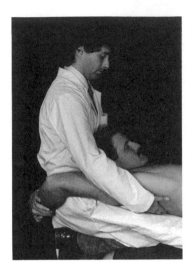
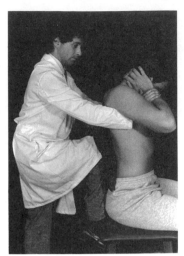

EXERCISE THERAPY
Stanley Schiowitz
Albert R. DeRubertis

The thoracic region is much more complex than the cervical region. It consists of the thoracic spine, rib cage, shoulder girdle, and the intricate musculature that accompanies the functioning of each of the above. Prescribing exercise treatment for dysfunctions of any of these areas should include recognition of their interdependence. Pain and limited motion in one segment can be secondary to dysfunction of another.

Regional motions and functions can be divided as follows:

1. Thoracic spine: forward bending, backward bending, rotation, side-bending.
2. Scapula: elevation, protraction, retraction, rotation.
3. Ribs: individual ribs have rotary elevating or depressing motions. The entire thorax, however, expands in the anteroposterior plane (pump handle motion) and in the frontal plane (bucket handle motion).

Regional Stretch
FORWARD BENDING
1. **Patient position:** seated, with back upright.
2. **Instructions:**
   a. Drop your head forward, allowing its weight to create forward bending.
   b. Allow the forward bending to continue gradually into the thoracic region, from the first thoracic vertebra down. Do not create pain.
   c. To increase stretch, maintain your body in its position of forward bending, drop both hands between your legs, and reach for the floor (Fig. 9-41). Do not change or increase your forward-bending position.
   d. Hold for 5 to 15 seconds, then slowly return to upright position.
   e. Relax, rest, and repeat.

BACKWARD BENDING
1. **Patient position:** seated, with back upright and hands at sides.

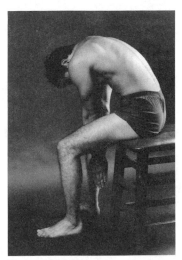

Figure 9-41. Thoracic stretch, forward bending.

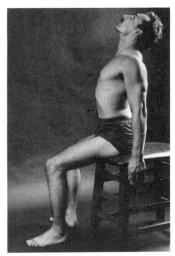

Figure 9-42. Thoracic stretch, backward bending.

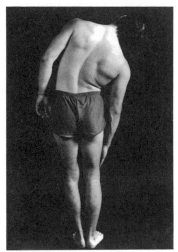

Figure 9-43. Thoracic stretch, side-bending.

2. **Instructions:**
   a. Drop your head backward, allowing its weight to create backward bending.
   b. Allow the backward bending to continue into the thoracic region.
   c. To increase stretch, push out your chest and abdomen and point your hands downward and backward toward the floor (Fig. 9-42). Do not change or increase your backward bending position.
   d. Hold for 5 to 15 seconds. Slowly return to the upright position.
   e. Relax, rest, and repeat.

SIDE-BENDING
1. **Patient position:** standing, back upright, hands at sides.
2. **Instructions:**
   a. Tilt your head, neck, and thoracic region to the right as you walk your right hand down your right leg toward the floor (Fig. 9-43).
   b. To increase stretch, raise your left arm over your head and try to touch the top of your right shoulder.
   c. Hold for 5 to 15 seconds. Slowly return to the upright position.
   d. Relax, rest, and repeat.
   e. To stretch the left side laterally, reverse the instructions.

ROTATION
1. **Patient position:** seated, facing backward, on an armless chair, with legs straddling the seat.
2. **Instructions:**
   a. Fold your arms in front of your chest, each hand holding the opposite elbow.
   b. Slowly turn your head, then your neck, and then your back to the right, as far as possible without pain. Do not change your seated position.
   c. To increase stretch, with your right hand pull your left elbow toward the right, increasing the rotary motion (Fig. 9-44).
   d. Hold for 5 to 15 seconds. Slowly return to the starting position.
   e. Relax, rest, and repeat.
   f. To stretch in left rotation, reverse the instructions.

Upper Back Stretch
PASSIVE STRETCH
1. **Patient position:** seated.
2. **Instructions:**
   a. Raise your left elbow to shoulder level and place that hand over your right shoulder.
   b. Place your right hand on your left elbow and gently push it toward your back (Fig. 9-45). This will create a passive left upper back stretch.

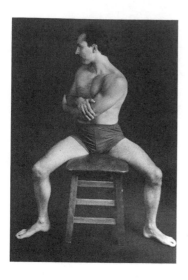

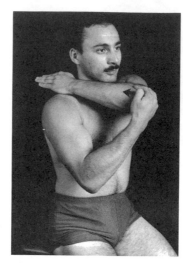

Figure 9-44. Thoracic stretch, rotation.

Figure 9-45. Passive upper back stretch, patient seated.

c. Maintain at maximum painless stretch for 5 to 15 seconds. Return to starting position.

d. Relax, rest, and repeat.

e. To stretch the right side, reverse the instructions.

ACTIVE STRETCH

Exercise 1

1. **Patient position:** prone, forehead touching the table.

2. **Instructions:**

a. Abduct shoulders to 90 degrees and bend elbows to 90 degrees. Hands, elbows, and arms rest on the table (or floor).

b. Simultaneously raise both upper extremities

Figure 9-46. Active upper back stretch, patient prone.

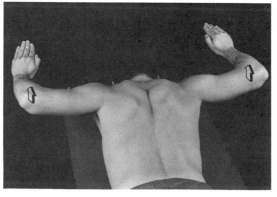

off the table, including the hands, elbows, and arms (Fig. 9-46).

c. Hold for 5 to 15 seconds.

d. Return arms to table, relax, rest, and repeat.

Note: Modifying the degree of shoulder abduction will change the area of the back that is stretched.

Exercise 2

1. **Patient position:** prone, forehead touching the table.

2. **Instructions:**

a. Place both arms, elbows straight and palms down, raised over your head.

b. Simultaneously raise both upper extremities off the floor, including the hands, elbows, and arms (Fig. 9-47).

c. Hold for 5 to 15 seconds.

d. Return arms to table, relax, rest, and repeat.

Exercise 3

1. **Patient position:** sitting, with back upright.

2. **Instructions:**

a. Stretch both arms over your head, with fingers interlocked.

b. Press both arms backward.

c. Tilt your upper body to one side (Fig. 9-48). Hold for 5 seconds, then tilt upper body to other side.

d. Return to starting position. Relax, rest, and repeat.

Figure 9-47. Active upper back stretch, patient prone.

Figure 9-48. Active upper back stretch, patient seated.

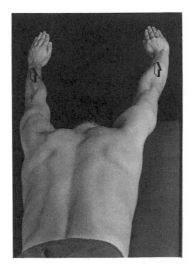
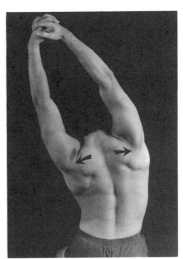

KYPHOSIS
Exercise 1
1. **Patient position:** supine, knees flexed, with a small pillow under the midthoracic region.
2. **Instructions:**
   a. Clasp your hands behind your neck.
   b. Try to touch the shoulder blades together at the midline (Fig. 9-49).
   c. Hold for 5 to 15 seconds.
   d. Relax, rest, and repeat.

Exercise 2
1. **Patient position:** same as in previous exercise.
2. **Instructions:**
   a. Bring both arms fully extended over your head.
   b. Press your forearms and elbows down toward the table (Fig. 9-50).
   c. Hold for 5 to 15 seconds.
   d. Relax, rest, and repeat.

Exercise 3
1. **Patient position:** seated, back upright.
2. **Instructions:**
   a. Hold broomstick or pole at each end, your hands facing forward.
   b. Raise the pole over your head.
   c. Tuck in your chin and, holding your neck in a fixed position, bring the pole down between your shoulder blades (Fig. 9-51).
   d. Hold for 5 to 15 seconds. Return to starting position.
   e. Relax, rest, and repeat.

Scapular Motions
ELEVATION STRETCH (SHRUG)
1. **Patient position:** standing, back upright, arms extended down at sides.
2. **Instructions:**
   a. Raise your shoulders straight up, trying to touch them to your ears (Fig. 9-52).

Figure 9-49. Stretch for kyphosis.

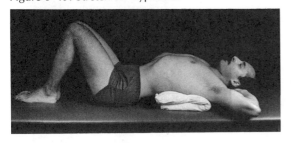

Figure 9-50. Stretch for kyphosis.

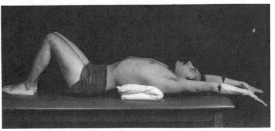

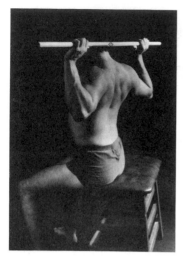

Figure 9-51. Stretch for kyphosis, with pole.

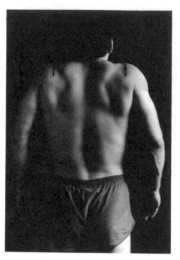

Figure 9-52. Scapula elevation stretch (shrug).

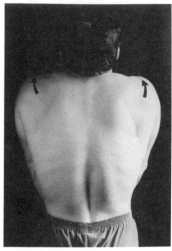

Figure 9-53. Scapula protraction.

b. Hold for 5 to 15 seconds.

c. Slowly return to starting position.

d. Slowly relax, rest, and repeat.

PROTRACTION STRETCH

1. **Patient position:** standing, back upright, arms extended at sides.
2. **Instructions:**
   a. Raise your shoulders straight up, trying to touch your ears.
   b. Roll your shoulders forward, separating the shoulder blades (Fig. 9-53).
   c. Hold for 5 to 15 seconds.
   d. Slowly relax, rest, and repeat.

RETRACTION STRETCH

1. **Patient position:** standing, back upright, arms extended at sides.
2. **Instructions:**
   a. Raise your shoulders straight up, and try to touch your ears.
   b. Roll your shoulders backward, trying to bring the shoulder blades together (Fig. 9-54).
   c. Hold for 5 to 15 seconds.
   d. Slowly relax, rest, and repeat.

The previous two exercises can be modified to create increased strength and stretch. Perform the shrug maneuver; then, with your shoulders elevated, proceed into the anterior and posterior shoulder roll.

ROTATION

1. **Patient position:** standing, back upright.
2. **Instructions:**
   a. Place both hands on your shoulders and raise your arms away from the body (abduct) to 135 degrees (Fig. 9-55).
   b. Maintain this raised position.
   c. Hold for 5 to 15 seconds.
   d. Relax, rest, and repeat.

Thorax

PECTORAL MUSCLE STRETCH

1. **Patient position:** standing, facing a corner, with hands on adjacent walls and feet away from the wall.
2. **Instructions:**
   a. Drop your body forward, supported by your hands. This will bring the shoulder blades together and create pectoral muscle stretch (Fig. 9-56).
   b. Hold this position for 5 to 15 seconds.
   c. Return to starting position, relax, rest, and repeat.

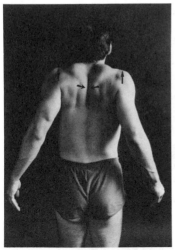

Figure 9-54. Scapula retraction.

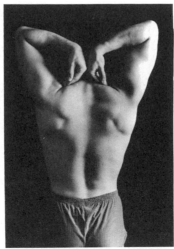

Figure 9-55. Scapula rotation.

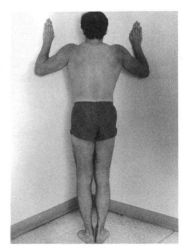

Figure 9-56. Pectoral muscle stretch.

INSPIRATION RIB STRETCH

1. **Patient position:** supine, both knees bent, feet on table, entire spine flattened.
2. **Instructions:**
   a. Raise both fully extended arms off the floor, while breathing in deeply (Fig. 9-57).
   b. Hold this position for 4 to 5 seconds.
   c. Lower both arms to floor as you slowly breathe out.
   d. Relax, rest, and repeat.

INSPIRATION RIB ISOMETRICS

1. **Patient position:** supine, both knees bent, feet on table, hands on sides of the rib cage.
2. **Instructions:**
   a. Inhale deeply while pressing firmly against your rib cage (Fig. 9-58). Try to prevent lateral chest expansion.
   b. Hold this position for 4 to 5 seconds.
   c. Exhale while you maintain your hand pressure.
   d. Relax, rest, and repeat.

EXPIRATION ABDOMINAL STRETCH

1. **Patient position:** supine, hips and knees flexed to 90 degrees, feet supported by chair.
2. **Instructions:**
   a. Place both hands on your upper abdomen and breathe out slowly while contracting the abdominal muscles.
   b. Press both hands firmly down on abdomen to create forced exhalation (Fig. 9-59).
   c. Maintain firm hand pressure on abdomen as you slowly inhale, resisting abdominal stretch.
   d. Hold full inhalation 4 to 5 seconds.
   e. Relax, rest, and repeat.

ABDOMINOTHORACIC STRETCH

1. **Patient position:** supine, knees bent, feet on floor, both hands over head, elbows bent to 90 degrees.

Figure 9-57. Inspiration rib stretch.

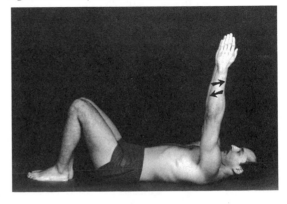

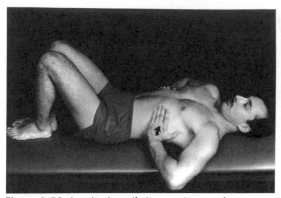

Figure 9-58. Inspiration rib isometric stretch.

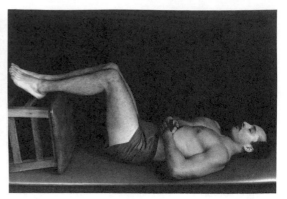

Figure 9-59. Passive abdominal expiration stretch.

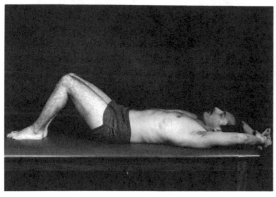

A   B

Figure 9-60. Abdominothoracic stretch. **(A)** Abdominal inspiration with expansion of the abdominal cavity. **(B)** As air is transferred to the thoracic cage, the abdominal muscles are contracted and the chest cavity is expanded.

2. **Instructions:**
   a. Inhale deeply. Try to use the abdomen only, with maximum abdominal muscle stretch (Fig. 9-60A).
   b. Close your throat to prevent the escape of air.
   c. Transfer the air to your upper chest by con-tracting your abdominal muscles. Your rib cage should rise (Fig. 9-60B).
   d. Hold this position for 4 to 5 seconds. Release the air.
   e. Relax, rest, and repeat.

10

Evaluation of the Lumbar Spine

FUNCTIONAL ANATOMY AND BIOMECHANICS
Stanley Schiowitz

The five lumbar vertebrae are separated from one another by intervertebral disks. The combined unit of the vertebrae and disks, in the upright position, forms the anteroposterior lordotic lumbar spinal curve.

Osteology

The lumbar vertebral bodies are larger than the thoracic vertebral bodies. They are wider transversely than in the anteroposterior dimension and are higher in front than in back, creating a posterior body wedge. In conjunction with a similar intervertebral disk shape, the wedge shape of the lumbar vertebral bodies helps maintain lumbar lordosis.

The spinous processes of the lumbar vertebrae are large, quadrangular, and directed dorsally in a horizontal plane. The transverse processes are long, thin, and directed laterally in a horizontal plane. In contrast to the different planar relationships of the thoracic vertebral structures, in the lumbar spine the spinous process, transverse processes, and vertebral body all lie at the same spinal level.

The fifth lumbar vertebra differs from those above it in having a larger body, thicker and shorter transverse processes, and a smaller spinous process; it is also markedly higher in its anterior aspect. The largest number of congenital defects occur at the level of the fifth lumbar vertebra.

The superior articular facets of the lumbar vertebrae are concave and face primarily medially and backward. They are rotated 45 degrees from the sagittal plane toward the frontal plane. The inferior articular facets are convex and face laterally and forward. The superior and inferior articular facets of the contiguous lumbar vertebrae fit into each other, forming zygophyseal joints.

Many variations of articular facets occur in the lumbar region, notably at the lumbosacral articulation. These variations include sagittal plane rotations of 0 to 90 degrees, a horizontal planar orientation, and facet asymmetries. These variants contribute to low back instability, disk disease, and somatic dysfunction.

Intervertebral Motion

All individual vertebral motions follow the rules of coupled motions:

1. Flexion and extension are coupled with a ventrad-dorsad translatory slide in the sagittal plane.

An Osteopathic Approach to Diagnosis and Treatment, second edition
Eileen L. DiGiovanna and Stanley Schiowitz
Lippincott–Raven Publishers, Philadelphia © 1997.

2. Lateral flexion is coupled with a contralateral translatory slide in the frontal plane.
3. Rotation is coupled with disk compression in the horizontal plane.

The motions of flexion and extension are greatest at all levels, as influenced by the vertical sagittal orientation of the facets. There is a small degree of lateral flexion present that is always accompanied by very limited rotation. The convex-concave articular shapes mandate the combined roll-and-slide motion.

Somatic Dysfunction

Group curves are common in the lumbar region and are usually secondary to thoracic scoliosis or to sacral base unleveling. Single-segment intervertebral somatic dysfunctions involve restricted motion in all three planes: however, rotation is the primary motion most commonly restricted. This rotation restriction is accompanied by ipsilateral lateral flexion.

Somatic dysfunctions are commonly diagnosed by monitoring the rotary motions of the lumbar transverse processes.

Intervertebral Disks

A healthy disk consists of a jellylike substance, the *nucleus pulposus*, surrounded by a fibrotic ring, the *annulus fibrosis*. The annulus comprises a series of collagen fibers that are firmly attached to their superior and inferior vertebral endplates. The fibroelastic mesh is formed by concentric circumferential lamellae. The collagen fibers of the lamellae lie at a 65-degree angle from the vertical, and their vertical orientation alternates in successive lamellae. This anatomical arrangement allows the disk to undergo rotary motions and shearing forces while still maintaining a restrictive stability. The nucleus moves in a direction opposite to vertebral motion, creating pressure on the annulus and a normalizing feedback mechanism.

The lumbar intervertebral disks sustain the most degenerative changes and dysfunctions of all the spinal disks, with the possible exception of the C5-C6 disk. It is thought that sitting postures in which the lumbar spine is flexed cause more fluid to be expressed from the lumbar disks than do erect postures. Restriction of this motion by extensive standing, fusion, degenerative arthritis, or spinal motion restriction of any cause is postulated to reduce nutrient flow to the disks and hasten lumbar disk degeneration. Degenerative changes result in loss of tissue elasticity, loss of restrictive stability, depressed feedback mechanisms, and loss of disk height. The relationships of the superior to inferior articular facets become abnormal. The ligaments connecting the vertebrae and disks become lax, and there is a greater tendency toward dysfunction.

Neurology

The lumbar plexus lies within the posterior part of the psoas major muscle and in front of the transverse processes of the lumbar vertebrae. It consists of the ventral rami of the first, second, third, and part of the fourth lumbar nerves.

The spinal cord ends at about the level of the second lumbar vertebra. Lower nerve roots run caudally and laterally to exit from the intervertebral foramina. Diskogenic herniation disturbs the nerve root of the lower vertebra involved. Therefore, an L5-S1 herniated disk will cause dysfunction of the first sacral nerve root.

Herniated disks are most common in the lower lumbar region because of narrowing of the posterior longitudinal ligament, the increased incidence of degenerative disk disease, ligament laxity, and excessive stress placed on the disks in this location. At a minimum, the clinician should be able to recognize the symptoms of L4, L5, and S1 nerve root dysfunctions. Dysfunction of the L4 nerve causes diminution in the patellar reflex, reduction of strength in the quadriceps and anterior tibialis muscles, and cutaneous sensation changes on the medial aspect of the leg and foot. Dysfunction of the L5 nerve does not affect a reflex but does impose a loss of strength of the first toe in dorsiflexion, loss of strength of the extensor hallucis muscle, and cutaneous sensation changes on the side of the leg and top of the foot. Dysfunction of the S1 nerve causes diminution in the Achilles reflex, a reduction of strength in the peroneus longus and brevis muscles, and sensation changes on the lateral aspect of the foot.

Myology

The erector spinae is a large muscle group lying at each side of the vertebral column. It originates at the sacrum and continues through to the cervical region. At the lumbar region it is divided, medially to laterally, into the spinalis, longissimus, and iliocostalis muscles. Bilateral muscle contraction causes extension of the vertebral column. Unilateral contraction causes ipsilateral extension and side-bending.

The multifidus and rotatores muscles are small muscles of the back lying deep to the erector spinae. They function primarily as postural muscles, with control of individual vertebral motions. Bilateral contraction creates local extension, and unilateral contraction causes lateral flexion with contralateral rotation.

The quadratus lumborum is a lateral muscle attached to the 12th rib, iliac crest, and vertebral column. Its rib attachment allows it to function with respiration by fixing the last rib and assisting in stabilizing the origin of the diaphragm. Bilateral contraction creates extension; unilateral contraction causes extension with ipsilateral side-bending.

The synergistic action of the abdominal muscles creates forward bending. External oblique contraction creates rotation to the opposite side; internal oblique contraction creates rotation to the same side. The combined actions of the abdominal muscles provide a coordinated mechanism for controlling dangerous torque, bending, and shear stresses in the lumbar spine. Their normal functioning is essential to the maintenance of the spinal mechanism.

The iliopsoas muscle plays an important role in the function and stability of the lumbar region. It is composed of two muscles. The psoas major originates from the anterior surfaces and lower borders of the transverse processes of all the lumbar vertebrae by five digitations, each extending from the body of the two vertebrae and their intersegmental disks, starting from the 12th thoracic vertebra and ending at the fifth lumbar vertebra. The muscle descends along the pelvic brim, passes behind the inguinal ligament and in front of the capsule of the hip joint, and ends in a tendon that receives, on its lateral side, nearly the whole of the fibers of the iliacus. The psoas major inserts into the lesser trochanter of the femur. The iliacus muscle originates from the superior two thirds of the concavity of the iliac fossa, from the inner lip of the iliac crest, from the ventral sacroiliac and iliolumbar ligaments, and from the upper, lateral surface of the sacrum. In front, it reaches as far as the anterosuperior and anteroinferior iliac spines,

and receives some fibers from the upper part of the capsule of the hip joint. It inserts into the lateral side of the tendon of the psoas major, which inserts into the lesser trochanter of the femur.

From above, the iliopsoas flexes the thigh on the pelvis; from below, it flexes the trunk forward by bilateral contraction. Unilateral contraction creates lateral trunk flexion with a pelvic shift to that side.

The iliopsoas remains in constant activity in the erect posture and prevents hyperextension of the hip joint in a standing subject. An increase in lumbar lordosis while standing erect causes increased activity of the psoas and low back instability and dysfunction.

The cardinal signs of iliopsoatic dysfunction in the standing and supine positions are as follows:

1. Standing: hip and knee flexion and pelvic tilt on the side of the dysfunction, a positive Trendelenburg sign, and a typical psoatic stance and gait.
2. Supine: exaggerated lumber lordosis and a positive Thomas test.

Somatic dysfunction of the lumbar region that is related to iliopsoas contracture usually occurs at the upper lumbar vertebral levels.

In the pelvis, these muscles create a supportive mechanism for the abdominal viscera, the psoas shelf, as they traverse the pubic bones in their descent to the lesser trochanters. Any somatic dysfunction that changes this structural relationship can cause visceral symptoms and pathology. Anterior sacral or pelvic tilt, psoas contracture, abdominal muscle weakness, pregnancy, wearing of high heels, poor posture, and somatosomatic reflexes can all increase the stress of the viscera onto the abdominal wall, which in turn can lead to diaphragmatic hernia, inguinal and femoral hernias, retroverted uterus, renal and visceral ptosis, and syndromes such as dysmenorrhea, menorrhagia, polyuria, constipation, and colitis.

The iliopsoas muscle also plays an important role in the synergistic activities of the muscles of the low back in maintaining a normal lumbosacral angle and proper postural balance.

LUMBOSACRAL ANGLE
(FERGUSON'S ANGLE)
The lumbosacral angle is the angle formed, in the lateral upright position, by extending the line of

inclination of the sacrum as it meets a line parallel to the ground. This angle is normally between 25 and 35 degrees. A major portion of low back pain is attributable to an increased lumbosacral angle. The greater the angle, the greater is the inclination and the higher the shear stress placed on the lumbosacral joint and its attachments. In addition, the increased angle increases lumbar lordosis.

Factors that can influence the lumbosacral angle are obesity, pregnancy, abdominal muscle weakness, wearing of high heels, foot pronation. Achilles valgus, atypical lumbosacral facets, spondylolisthesis, diminished disk height, ligamentous weakness, organic kyphoscoliosis, poor posture, occupation, somatotype, heredity, psoatic dysfunction, anterior sacral/pelvic tilt, and somatic dysfunction.

An increased lumbosacral angle changes the articular relationships, as the inferior lumbar facets slide caudally on their matched superior sacral facets.

SYNERGISTIC ACTION OF THE MUSCLES
IN MAINTAINING LUMBAR CURVATURES
The abdominal muscles support and assist in the flattening of the lumbar lordosis. The psoas mus-cles pull on the vertebrae and anterior pelvis, increasing the lumbar lordosis. The gluteus maximus and hamstrings pull on the posterior pelvis, decreasing the lumbar lordosis. The erector spinae muscles and the abdominal muscles assist in flattening the lumbar lordosis.

Lumbar-Pelvic Rhythm
When a subject bends forward to touch the floor, combined motions of the lumbar vertebrae, pelvis, and hip joints are put into play. The individual vertebrae flex on each other, straightening the lumbar lordosis and sometimes causing a mild reversal of that curve. Simultaneously, a secondary pelvic rotation motion occurs around the axis of the hip joints as the hip joints move posteriorly in the horizontal plane. These are smooth, interrelated motions, both in total forward bending and in its reversal, straightening up.

In evaluating gross body movement, the physician must examine all three aspects of lumbosacral rhythm. It is common to relate all forward-bending restrictions to lumbar dysfunction. This assumption is not correct. Hip joint or pelvic dysfunctions are often at fault.

MOTION TESTING
Lisa R. Chun

Thoracolumbar Regional Motion Testing
1. **Patient position:** standing with his weight evenly distributed and feet placed 4 to 6 inches apart and parallel.
2. **Physician position:** kneeling directly behind the patient, his eyes level with the lumbar region.
3. **Hand position:** on the iliac crests and monitoring the anterior superior iliac spines.
4. **Evaluation:**
   a. The physician notes the limitation of motion, the progression from thoracic through the lumbar spine, the fluidity with which the motion is achieved, and the symmetry or asymmetry created.
   b. Rotation of the lumbar spine is usually no more than 5 degrees in each direction. The test is more for thoracic than for lumbar rotation.
   c. Pelvic rotation will occur with this technique; however, it can be minimized by monitoring at the anterior superior iliac spine (ASIS).
5. **Techniques:**
   Forward bending:
   a. The patient is instructed to slowly bend forward as if to touch his toes; the knees remain locked (Fig. 10-1).
   b. Forward bending is continued until movement is felt at the anterosuperior iliac spines, at which time the patient is instructed to stop.
   c. The physician determines the angle created by the anterior displacement in a sagittal plane of the spinous process of the first tho-

racic vertebra from a position of neutral to one of flexion. The angle of flexion normally approximates 105 degrees.

d. The patient is instructed to return to a neutral standing position.

Backward bending:

a. The patient is instructed to slowly bend backward toward the physician (Fig. 10-2). The movement should be mainly from the waist up.

b. Once motion is felt at the anterior superior iliac spines, the patient is instructed to stop bending backward.

c. The physician determines the angle created by the posterior displacement of the first thoracic spinous process from a position of neutral to one of extension. The normal angle of extension is approximately 60 degrees.

d. The patient is instructed to return to a neutral standing position.

Side-bending:

a. The patient is instructed to slowly slide one hand down the lateral aspect of the ipsilateral leg without deviating into lumbar flexion or extension and without flexing or hyperextending the knee (Fig. 10-3).

b. The side-bending motion is continued until movement of the contralateral iliac crest is felt by the physician, at which time the patient is instructed to stop side-bending.

c. The physician determines the angle created by the lateral displacement in the frontal plane of the first thoracic spinous process from a position of neutral to one of side-bending. The normal angle of side-bending is approximately 40 degrees.

d. The patient is instructed to return to a neutral standing position.

e. Repeat procedure for the other side of the body.

f. The physician compares right side-bending with left side-bending.

Rotation:

a. The patient is instructed to turn his body, from the waist up, to one side, while keeping his feet firmly on the ground with the knees straight (Fig. 10-4).

b. This motion is continued until movement is felt at the contralateral anterior superior iliac spine, at which time the patient is instructed to stop rotation.

c. The physician determines the angle created by the posterior displacement of the lateral tip of the posteriormost acromion process from a position of neutral to one of rotation. The normal angle of rotation is approximately 40 degrees.

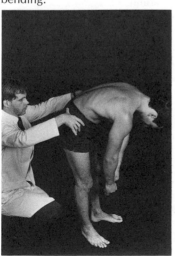

Figure 10-1. Thoracolumbar regional motion testing: forward bending.

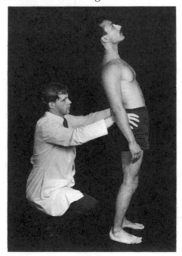

Figure 10-2. Thoracolumbar regional motion testing: backward bending.

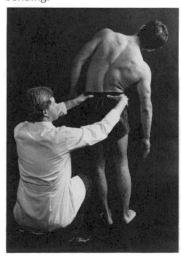

Figure 10-3. Thoracolumbar regional motion testing: side-bending.

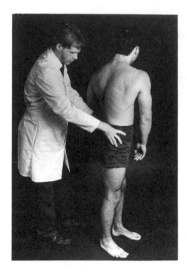
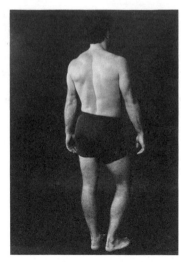

Figure 10-4. Thoracolumbar regional motion testing: rotation.

Figure 10-5. Lateral lumbar flexion: hip drop test.

d. The patient is instructed to return to a neutral standing position.
e. The procedure is repeated for the other side of the body.
f. The physician compares right rotation to left rotation.

Lateral Lumbar Flexion: Hip Drop Test

1. **Patient position:** standing relaxed, facing forward, with weight evenly distributed over feet, feet placed 4 to 6 inches apart.
2. **Physician position:** facing the patient's back, his eyes level with the lumbar region.
3. **Technique:**
   a. The patient is instructed to bend one knee, keeping the corresponding foot on the ground and keeping the other knee straight (Fig. 10-5).
   b. The patient should allow the compensatory shift in body weight distribution.
   c. The physician notes the degree of lumbar side-bending and the degree of curve created, as measured by the drop in the iliac crest.
   d. The patient's is instructed to return to a neutral standing position.
   e. The procedure is repeated with the patient bending the other knee.
   f. The physician compares right side-bending with left side-bending. Side-bending is most restricted to the side of greatest iliac crest lowering.

Intersegmental Motion Testing

See intersegmental motion testing for the thoracic spine. Similarities in patient position, physician position, and technique exist. Modify the hand position to palpate the lumbar vertebrae.

INTERSEGMENTAL MOTION TESTING: ALTERNATIVE TECHNIQUE

1. **Patient position:** varies according to motion being tested. *Rotation:* prone, with arms on the table. *Flexion, extension*, and *side-bending*: lateral recumbent, with both hips and knees flexed and on the table, head supported.
2. **Physician position:** standing at the side of the table facing the patient.
3. **Hand position:** varies according to motion being tested. *Rotation:* monitoring fingers are placed on the transverse processes of the lumbar vertebra to be examined. *Side-bending*: monitoring fingers are placed on the transverse processes of the lumbar vertebra to be examined and of the vertebra above it. *Flexion and extension*: monitoring finger is between the spinous processes of the vertebra to be tested, as well as the one above it.
4. **Technique:**
   Rotation:
   a. The physician assesses the symmetry or asymmetry of both soft tissue and bone at the transverse processes of the vertebra being examined.
   b. The physician applies a firm, equal pressure

in a ventral direction on the transverse processes of the vertebra being assessed.

c. The ease of ventral motion of one transverse process indicates a rotation to the contralateral side. For example, if the right transverse process moves more freely ventrally than the left, the left transverse process is rotated posteriorly. The vertebra is rotated left.

d. The procedure is repeated at each lumbar level.

e. The physician compares rotation between levels.

Rotation, patient laterally recumbent:

a. The physician flexes the patient's hips and knees until motion is felt at the spinous processes.

b. The physician leans into the patient's knees once this flexion position is attained.

c. Using the patient's knees as a fulcrum, the physician side-bends the lumbar spine by raising the patient's ankles to the ceiling (Fig. 10-6).

d. Side-bending is created until motion is felt at the monitoring finger.

e. The physician assesses the relationship created between the vertebra being monitored and the one above it. The physician should also note if there is a change in position of the monitored vertebra between the neutral position and side-bending.

f. Posterior protrusion (rotation) of the upper process indicates a type II somatic dysfunction, according to Fryette's second principle of physiologic motion of the spine. Ventral

rotation of the upper transverse process indicates a type I somatic dysfunction, according to Fryette's first principle of physiologic motion of the spine.

g. The procedure is repeated for each lumbar vertebra.

h. The physician compares the motions at various levels.

Flexion-extension, patient laterally recumbent:

a. The physician creates flexion by moving the patient's legs and knees toward the patient's abdomen.

b. Motion is created only until it is felt at the monitoring finger.

c. The physician induces extension by moving the patient's legs and knees away from the patient's abdomen and applying axial compression through the patient's femurs.

d. Motion is created only until it is felt at the monitoring finger.

e. Each vertebra is assessed in both flexion and extension before continuing to the next vertebral level.

f. Ease of flexion with a barrier to extension indicates a flexion dysfunction.

g. The procedure is repeated for all lumbar vertebrae.

Rotoscoliosis Motion Testing

1. **Patient position:** prone.

2. **Physician position:** standing at the side of the table with his dominant eye over the midline of the patient's body. The physician's eyes should be as horizontal to the examining surface as is possible.

3. **Hand position:** monitoring fingers are placed on the transverse processes of the vertebra being examined.

4. **Technique:**

a. Each vertebra is assessed in all three positions before the next vertebra is evaluated.

b. The monitoring fingers remain in contact with the patient's skin until all positions have been assessed for one vertebra.

c. After the motions of one vertebra have been compared in all three positions, the physician compares the anteroposterior symmetry or asymmetry of that vertebra with the symmetry or asymmetry of the other lumbar vertebrae.

Figure 10-6. Intersegmental motion testing: rotation, patient recumbent, alternative technique.

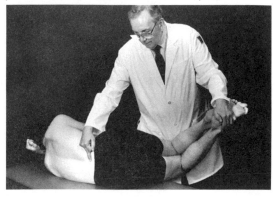

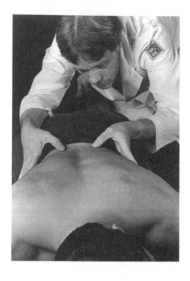

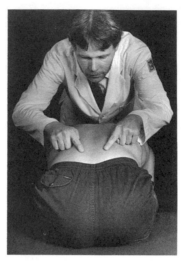

Figure 10-7. Lumbar rotoscoliosis testing in neutral position.

Figure 10-8. Lumbar rotoscoliosis testing in flexion.

d. **Neutral:**
  i. With the patient prone, the physician determines the anteroposterior symmetry or asymmetry of a vertebra by comparing the corresponding right and left transverse processes (Fig. 10-7).
  ii. The physician then continues to the next positional motion testing.
e. **Flexion:**
  i. The patient is seated with his feet firmly and equally supported.
  ii. The patient is instructed to bend forward, allowing the arms to fall between the knees.

iii. This flexion motion is discontinued when motion is felt at the monitored transverse processes.
iv. The physician determines the anteroposterior symmetry or asymmetry of the corresponding transverse processes (Fig. 10-8).

f. **Hyperextension:**
  i. The patient is prone.
  ii. The patient hyperextends the lumbar spine by placing either his elbows on the table or his hands on the table with his elbows extended (Fig. 10-9).
  iii. Extension is created until motion is felt at the transverse processes of the monitored vertebra.
  iv. The physician determines the anteroposterior symmetry or asymmetry of the corresponding transverse processes.

Figure 10-9. Lumbar rotoscoliosis testing in extension.

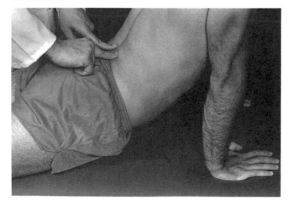

References

Adams MA, Hutton HC. 1983. The effect of posture on the fluid content of lumbar intervertebral discs. Spine 8(6):665–671.

Bogduk N, Twomey T. 1987. Clinical Anatomy of the Lumbar Spine. Edinburgh: Churchill Livingstone.

Cailliet R. 1968. Low Back Syndrome, 2nd ed. Philadelphia: F.A. Davis.

Farfan HF. 1975. Muscular mechanism of the lumbar spine and the position of power and efficiency. Orthop Clin North Am 6(1):135–144.

Farfan JF, Sullivan JD. 1967. The relation of facet orientation to intervertebral disc failure. Can J Surg 10:179.

Jayson IV. 1976. The Lumbar Spine and Back Pain, 3rd ed. Edinburgh: Churchill Livingstone.

Jones L. 1955. The Postural Complex. St. Louis: Charles C Thomas.

Kapanji IA. 1974. The Physiology of the Joints. Vol 3. The Trunk and the Vertebral Column. Edinburgh: Churchill Livingstone.

Michele AA. Iliopsoas. St. Louis: Charles C Thomas.

Schiowitz S, DiGiovanna E, Ausman P. 1983. An Osteopathic Approach to Diagnosis and Treatment. Old Westbury: New York College of Osteopathic Medicine of the New York Institute of Technology.

Warwick R, Williams PL. 1973. Gray's Anatomy, 35th British ed. Philadelphia: W.B. Saunders.

Weisel SW, Bernini P, Rothman RH. 1982. The Aging Lumbar Spine. Philadelphia: W.B. Saunders.

White AA, Panjabi MM. 1978. Biomechanics of the Spine. Philadelphia: J.B. Lippincott.

11

Treatment of the Lumbar Spine

MYOFASCIAL TECHNIQUES

Toni Spinaris
Eileen L. DiGiovanna

The principles of myofascial treatment were discussed in Chapter 5. This section describes the application of passive, active direct, and active indirect techniques to the lumbar region.

Passive Technique (Prone)

1. **Patient position:** prone.
2. **Physician position:** standing at the side of the table, opposite the side to be treated.
3. **Technique:**
   a. The physician places the thumb of one hand parallel to the paravertebral muscle on the side opposite where she is standing, between the muscle and spinous processes. She reinforces the thumb by placing the thenar eminence of her other hand on top of it (see Figs. 9-1 and 9-2).
   b. She pushes the muscle away from the spinous processes, keeping her elbows straight and using body weight to move the muscle.
   c. The stretch is held a few seconds, allowing the muscle to relax, and then slowly released.
   d. The stretch is repeated several times. The thumb and reinforcing hand may be moved

up and down the spine to stretch various portions of the muscle.

ALTERNATE PRONE TECHNIQUE

1. **Patient and physician positions** remain the same.
2. **Technique:**
   a. The stretch is made using the heel of the cephalad hand, which is pushing the muscle away from the spinous processes.
   b. The caudad hand grasps the anterior superior iliac spine (ASIS) on the far side and rotates the pelvis by pulling the ASIS up and toward the physician. This provides an additional stretch on the lumbar muscles.

Passive Technique (Lateral Recumbent)

1. **Patient position:** Lying on side with muscles to be treated uppermost and knees and hips slightly flexed for balance.
2. **Physician position:** Standing at the side of the table facing the patient.
3. **Technique:**
   a. The physician grasps the upper paravertebral muscles with the fingers of both hands.

An Osteopathic Approach to Diagnosis and Treatment, second edition
Eileen L. DiGiovanna and Stanley Schiowitz
Lippincott–Raven Publishers, Philadelphia © 1997.

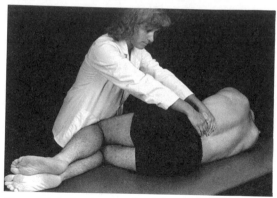

Figure 11-1. Passive myofascial technique applied to the lumbar spine, patient recumbent.

b. Keeping the elbows straight, the physician leans back and stretches the muscles by pulling them perpendicularly away from the spinous processes (Fig. 11-1).
c. This stretch is held for several seconds and then slowly released.
d. This may be repeated several times, with the physician moving the hands up and down the spine to stretch various parts of the muscle.

ALTERNATE LATERAL RECUMBENT
TECHNIQUE
1. **Patient and physician positions** remain the same. This technique will add a longitudinal stretch to the perpendicular one being performed above.
2. **Technique:**
   a. The physician grasps the muscle as above. She then places her cephalad forearm on the patient's shoulder and her caudad forearm on the patient's iliac crest.
   b. As she pulls the muscle perpendicularly, she adds a longitudinal stretch by pushing the shoulder and iliac crests with her forearms to separate them.

Active Direct Techniques
1. **Patient position:** Recumbent on his side, with the affected muscles down.
2. **Physician position:** Standing at the side of the table facing the patient.
3. **Technique:**
   a. The physician grasps the patient's ankles and

raises them off the table, stretching the involved muscles (those close to the table) (Fig. 11-2).
b. The patient is instructed to push his ankles down toward the table and to hold this for several seconds.
c. The physician exerts a resistive force equal to the patient's contraction, causing it to be isometric.
d. The patient relaxes and the physician induces further side-bending by raising the ankles further.
e. The process may be repeated several times to relax the muscles.
f. The physician may localize the area being treated by flexing the patient's hips. Approximately 90 degrees of hip flexion will bring maximum contraction to the lower lumbar spine. Greater flexion will bring maximum contraction further up the lumbar spine.

MODIFICATION
1. **Patient position:** recumbent on his side with the affected muscles up away from the table. Hips and knees are flexed.
2. **Physician position:** standing at the side of the table facing the patient.
3. **Technique:**
   a. The physician grasps the patient's ankles and lowers his legs below the level of the table top (Fig. 11-3).
   b. The patient is asked to push his ankles toward the ceiling. This causes contraction of the uppermost muscles.

Figure 11-2. Active direct myofascial lumbar technique, patient recumbent.

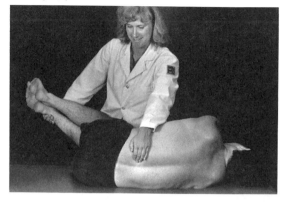

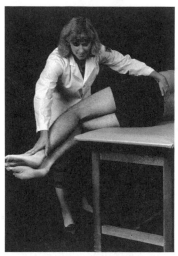

Figure 11-3. Modified active direct myofascial lumbar technique.

c. The physician provides an isometric resistive force for several seconds; then the patient is allowed to relax.

Active Indirect Techniques

1. **Patient position:** recumbent on his side with affected muscles down toward the table. Hips and knees are flexed.

2. **Physician position:** standing at the side of the table facing the patient.
3. **Technique:**
   a. The physician grasps the patient's ankles and lowers them off the table below the level of the table top.
   b. The patient is instructed to push his ankles up toward the ceiling. This causes contraction of the uppermost muscles (those antagonistic to the involved muscle).
   c. The physician provides an isokinetic resistance (resistive force that allows the ankles to move against that resistance).
   d. This process may be repeated several times. This procedure uses contraction of the antagonist muscles to relax the agonist muscle by reciprocal inhibition.

MODIFICATION

The above technique may be modified to treat the uppermost muscles by raising the ankles toward the ceiling and having the patient push down toward the floor. The legs are allowed to move against an isokinetic resistance. The patient is now contracting the muscles closest to the table to relax the uppermost muscles by reciprocal inhibition. A passive stretch may be added at the end of either of these techniques.

MUSCLE ENERGY TECHNIQUES
Sandra D. Yale
Nancy Brous

The principles of muscle energy treatment were discussed in Chapter 5. This section describes the application of techniques to group curves and single-segment dysfunctions in the lumbar spine. In all of these techniques the patient lies on his side on the table or in a modified Sims position, the transverse processes of the segment being treated up or down, according to the precise technique.

Type I Neutral (Group) Curves

1. **Patient position:** lateral recumbent with concavity toward the table; therefore, the posteriorly rotated transverse processes are up.
2. **Physician position:** standing at the side of the table facing the patient.
3. **Technique:**
   a. The physician monitors the apex of the curve with one hand.

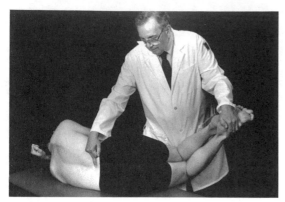

Figure 11-4. Muscle energy treatment for a type I curve, convex right.

b. The physician flexes the patient's hips to 90 degrees.
c. The physician side-bends the lumbar spine to the apex by elevating the patient's ankles with the nonmonitoring hand (Fig. 11-4).
d. The patient is then instructed to push his feet toward the floor for 3 seconds.
e. The physician provides resistance, producing a static contraction.
f. The patient is asked to relax.
g. The physician further elevates the patient's legs until motion is felt at the new barrier.
h. The procedure is repeated three times.
i. A passive stretch is added.

Type II Somatic Dysfunction (Single-Segment Dysfunction)
FLEXED SOMATIC DYSFUNCTION
1. **Patient position:** lying on the table in a lateral recumbent position. The posteriorly rotated transverse process to be treated faces down, toward the table.
2. **Physician position:** standing at the side of the table facing the patient.
3. **Technique:**
   a. The physician instructs the patient to lie on his side with the posterior transverse process down.
   b. The physician stands facing the patient and monitors the somatic dysfunction with one hand at the interspinous region.

c. With the other hand the physician flexes the patient's hips and knees until motion is felt at the level below the dysfunction (i.e., at L2 on L3).
d. The patient straightens his lower leg and the physician extends it until motion is felt at the same level. The flexed upper leg is "locked" in place with the dorsum of the foot of the top leg placed in the popliteal space of the lower leg by the physician.
e. The physician changes hands so that the caudal (with respect to the patient) hand is now monitoring the involved segment.
f. With his other hand the physician grasps the patient's lower arm and pulls it upward, causing rotation of the torso, until motion is felt at the level of the restriction.
g. Further rotation and localization are achieved by directing the patient to use his top hand to grasp the table edge behind his back.
h. The physician places his cephalic hand on the patient's shoulder.
i. The patient is instructed to take a deep breath, then exhale. Thereafter the patient is directed to reach farther down the table edge. The physician places light pressure against the patient's shoulder and more precisely localizes the somatic dysfunction.
j. The physician again switches hands and uses his cephalic hand to monitor the level of the restriction.
k. The physician grasps the ankle of the patient's upper leg and elevates it until the lumbar spine side-bends to the motion barrier.
l. The patient pushes his elevated foot down toward the table while the physician maintains resistance, producing a static contraction (Fig. 11-5).
m. After 3 seconds, the patient is asked to relax.
n. The physician then increases extension, sidebending, and rotation into the new motion barriers by again elevating the patient's upper ankle.
o. The procedure is repeated three times.
p. A passive stretch is given.

Variation: The patient is instructed to push the upper knee upward rather than the foot down.

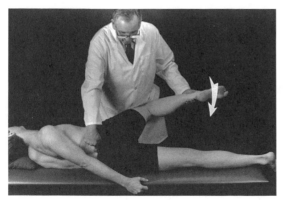

Figure 11-5. Muscle energy treatment for a flexed somatic dysfunction.

EXTENDED SOMATIC DYSFUNCTION

1. **Patient position:** lying on the table in a lateral recumbent position. The posteriorly rotated transverse process to be treated faces up. The patient is then placed in the modified Sims position.
2. **Physician position:** standing at the side of the table facing the patient.
3. **Technique:**
   a. The patient is instructed to lie on his side with the posterior transverse process up.
   b. The physician faces the patient and monitors the somatic dysfunction with his cephalic hand.
   c. The physician flexes the patient's knees and

hips until motion is felt at the area of somatic dysfunction.
   d. The physician switches monitoring hands so that the caudal (with respect to the patient) hand is on the somatic dysfunction.
   e. Rotation is achieved by placing the patient in the lateral Sims position.
   f. Additional rotation is induced by having the patient inhale, then exhale and simultaneously reach toward the floor.
   g. The physician pushes down on the shoulder with his cephalic hand until the torso is rotated down to the monitored segment, exaggerating the Sims position.
   h. The patient's legs are lowered off the side of the table to create lumbar side-bending up to the restricted area (Fig. 11-6A).
   i. Since this position is uncomfortable for the patient, the physician may either place a pillow under the patient's lower knee or sit behind the patient and put his thigh between the patient's legs and the table (Fig. 11-6B). (This position requires the physician to change the hand monitoring.)
   j. The patient pushes his feet toward the ceiling while the physician resists, creating an isometric contraction, which is held for 3 seconds.
   k. The patient relaxes. The physician engages a new motion barrier by further lowering the patient's legs.
   l. The procedure is repeated three times.
   m. A passive stretch is given.

Figure 11-6. Muscle energy treatment for an extended somatic dysfunction. **(A)** Physician standing. **(B)** Physician seated.

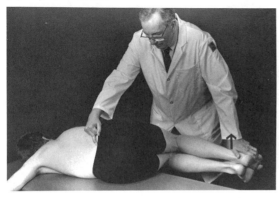

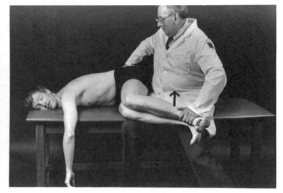

A   B

Summary of Muscle Energy Techniques for Lumbar Somatic Dysfunction

Extension Somatic Dysfunctions: S.U.E.
S: Lateral Sims position.
U: Posterior process is up.
E: Extension somatic dysfunction.

Flexion Somatic Dysfunctions: F.D.R.
F: Flexion somatic dysfunction.
D: Posterior process is down.
R: Lateral recumbent position.

COUNTERSTRAIN TECHNIQUES
Eileen L. DiGiovanna

Many of the counterstrain techniques for lumbar somatic dysfunctions are facilitated by slight rotation of the patient's thighs or hips, and by resting some part of the patient's leg on the physician's thigh or knee. Anterior tender points are treated with the patient supine, posterior tender points with the patient prone.

Anterior Tender Points

Figure 11-7 shows the locations of the anterior lumbar tender points.

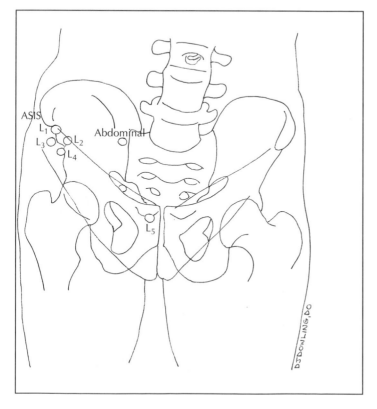

Figure 11-7. Anterior lumbar tender point locations.

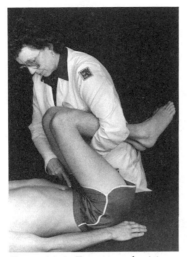

Figure 11-8. Treatment for L1 lumbar tender point, L1.

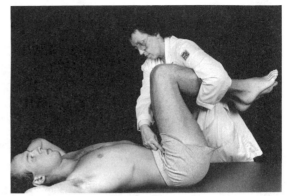

Figure 11-9. Treatment for L2 lumbar tender point, L2.

L1 TENDER POINT (MEDIAL TO ANTERIOR SUPERIOR ILIAC SPINES)

1. **Patient position:** supine.
2. **Physician position:** standing next to the table on the side of the tender point.
3. **Technique:**
   a. The patient's upper body is propped up on pillows.
   b. Both knees are flexed and rotated toward the tender point. Because the lower body is rotated, this position is equivalent to upper body rotation away from the tender point (Fig. 11-8).
   c. The hips are side-bent toward the tender point.
   d. The patient's legs may be supported on the physician's thigh if desired.

Note: The L1 tender point is treated in the same manner as the tender points corresponding to vertebrae T9–T12.

L2 TENDER POINT

1. **Patient position:** supine.
2. **Physician position:** standing at the side of the table opposite the tender point, which is located on the inferior medial surface of the anterior inferior iliac spine.
3. Both thighs are rotated 60 degrees away from the tender point, with side-bending away (Fig. 11-9).

ABDOMINAL L2 TENDER POINT

The abdominal L2 tender point is found 2 inches lateral to the umbilicus. The treatment is the same as for the anterior inferior iliac spine tender point except that the thighs are rotated toward the tender point (the equivalent of rotation away from the tender point at the vertebral level) (Fig. 11-10).

L3, L4 TENDER POINTS

1. **Patient position:** supine.
2. **Physician position:** standing at the side of the table on the side of the tender point, with one foot on the table.
3. **Technique:**
   a. The patient's hips and knees are flexed. His legs rest on the physician's thighs.
   b. The spine is side-bent away from the tender point with slight rotation toward the tender point.

L5 TENDER POINT

1. **Patient position:** supine.
2. **Physician position:** standing at the side of the table next to the tender point, which is on the pubic ramus. Her foot is on the table.

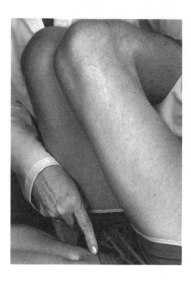

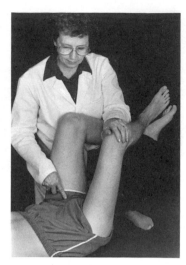

Figure 11-10. Treatment for abdominal lumbar tender point.

Figure 11-11. Treatment for anterior L5 tender point.

3. **Technique:**
   a. The patient's hips and knees are flexed. His legs rest on the physician's thighs.
   b. The far ankle is crossed over the one closer to the physician. The knees are dropped slightly apart (Fig. 11-11).

c. There is side-bending away from the tender point and slight rotation toward it.

Posterior Tender Points

Figure 11-12 shows the locations of the posterior tender points.

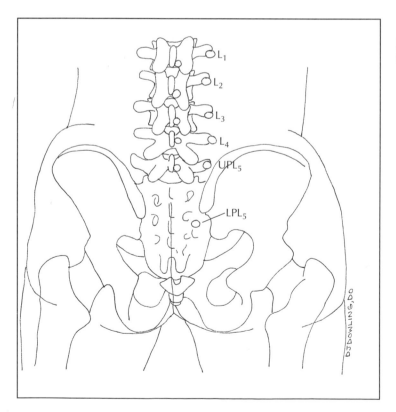

Figure 11-12. Posterior lumbar tender point locations.

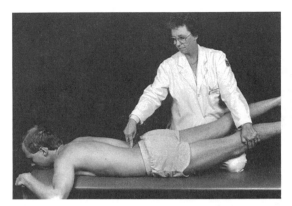

Figure 11-13. Counterstrain treatment for posterior lumbar tender points, spinous process.

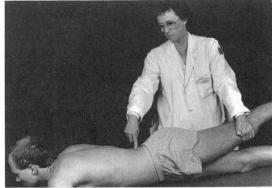

Figure 11-14. Counterstrain treatment for posterior transverse process lumbar tender points with rotation introduced.

L1–L5 TENDER POINTS (SPINOUS OR TRANSVERSE PROCESS)

1. **Patient position:** prone.
2. **Physician position:** standing at the side of the table.
3. **Technique:**
   a. The extended leg is elevated, extending the lumber spine. Both legs may be used.
   b. If the tender point is near the midline, this position may be sufficient. It is best if the physician stands on the same side as the leg being elevated (Fig. 11-13).
   c. If the tender point is over the transverse process, some rotation may be necessary. This is best done with the physician standing at the side opposite the tender point. The leg is elevated and adducted over the other leg enough to cause rotation at the vertebral level being treated. External rotation of the thigh assists this process (Fig. 11-14).

L3, L4, L5 UPPER POLE TENDER POINTS

The L3 to L5 vertebrae also have tender points on the lateral buttocks. The L5 tender point is superior to the posterior inferior iliac spines. These tender points are treated in a manner similar to that described for tender points on the transverse processes. The leg is elevated and adducted. It may rest on the operator's knee, which is placed on the table.

L5 LOWER POLE TENDER POINT

1. **Patient position:** prone.
2. **Physician position:** seated on a stool at the side of the table next to the tender point.

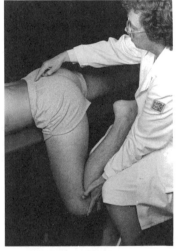

Figure 11-15. Counterstrain treatment for lower pole L5 tender point.

3. **Technique:**
   a. The patient's leg is dropped off the table with the knee and hip flexed. The hip is slightly rotated internally.
   b. While supporting the patient's leg, the physician pushes the knee toward the table, adducting the thigh (Fig. 11-15).
   c. Treatment is monitored at the tender point just medial to the posterior inferior iliac spine and just inferior to it.

FACILITATED POSITIONAL RELEASE
Stanley Schiowitz

Lumbar Region Techniques
SUPERFICIAL MUSCLE HYPERTONICITY,
LEFT LOW BACK

1. **Patient position:** prone, with a pillow under the abdomen. The pillow should be large enough to cause flattening of the lumbar lordosis.
2. **Physician position:** standing at the left side of the table. The physician's left index finger monitors the site of tissue tension.
3. **Technique:**
   a. The physician places his left knee on the table beside the patient's left ilium.
   b. With his right hand the physician slides the patient's legs toward the left side of the table, producing side-bending of the patient's lumbar spine around the physician's left knee. Side-bending is continued until tissue motion is felt by the left (monitoring) index finger (Fig. 11-16).
   c. The physician releases the patient's legs, crosses the patient's right leg over the left at the ankle, and then places his right hand under the patient's right thigh. The physician grasps the patient's right thigh medially, extends it posteriorly, and externally rotates it until motion is felt by the left (monitoring)

index finger in the area of tissue tension. A torsional motion is created up to the monitoring finger.
   d. This position is held for 3 seconds, then released; the dysfunction is reevaluated.

SOMATIC DYSFUNCTION (L4 E Sl Rl)

1. **Patient position:** prone, with a pillow under the abdomen. A second pillow is placed between the patient's left thigh and the table. This both protects the patient's thigh and acts as a fulcrum for motion.
2. **Physician position:** standing at the left side of the table.
3. **Technique:**
   a. The physician monitors the left transverse process of the L4 vertebra with his left index finger.
   b. The physician grasps the patient's left lower leg or ankle with his right hand.
   c. The patient's left leg is brought into abduction until motion is felt at the monitoring finger; then internal rotation up to the monitoring finger is added.
   d. The patient's left leg is then pushed toward the floor until motion is felt by the physician's monitoring finger (Fig. 11-17).

Figure 11-16. Facilitated positional release treatment for the left low back, superficial muscle hypertonicity.

Figure 11-17. Facilitated positional release treatment for a lumbar extension somatic dysfunction.

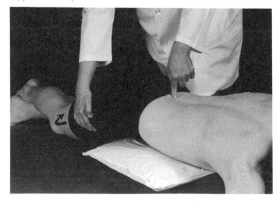

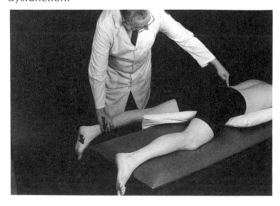

e. The position is held until the physician feels articular release. This usually occurs in 3 to 4 seconds.

f. The position is released and the patient is returned to neutral position. The dysfunction is reevaluated.

SOMATIC DYSFUNCTION (L4 F Sr Rr)
1. **Patient position:** prone, with a pillow placed under the abdomen.
2. **Physician position:** sitting at the right side of the table, facing the patient's head. The physician's left lateral thigh and knee are beside the table.
3. **Technique:**
   a. The physician monitors the transverse process of L4 on the right side with one finger of the left hand.
   b. The physician drops the patient's flexed right knee and thigh off the table over his left thigh.
   c. The physician grasps the patient's knee with the right hand and flexes the patient's hip until motion is felt at the monitored transverse process.
   d. The physician pushes the patient's right knee toward the table, into adduction, using his knee and thigh as a fulcrum, until motion is felt at the monitored transverse process.
   e. With his right hand, the physician turns the patient's knee in a circular direction, creating internal rotation of the hip (Fig. 11-18).
   f. This position is held until the physician feels articular release.
   g. This position is held for 3 seconds, then released; the dysfunction is reevaluated.

LUMBAR DISKOGENIC PAIN SYNDROME
This technique is useful for patients with radicular pain, bulging disks, stenosis, or herniations, or for patients after laminectomy. Treatment is described for a right-sided dysfunction.
1. **Patient position:** prone, with a pillow placed under the abdomen.
2. **Physician position:** seated at the right side of the table, facing the patient's head. The physician's thighs and knees are parallel to the table. The physician monitors the disk space to be treated with one finger of the left hand.
3. **Technique:**
   a. The patient's right hip and thigh are flexed

and the thigh is placed over both of the physician's legs, allowing the knee to flex down toward the floor.

b. The physician places his right hand on the patient's right shin or ankle.

c. The physician raises his right foot off the floor, raising the patient's thigh, until motion is felt at the monitoring finger.

d. The physician pushes his right knee laterally against the back of the patient's knee, creating a traction force that is monitored by his finger.

e. With his right hand, the physician turns the patient's right leg down toward the floor, creating a rotary motion of the thigh and hip, with the knee acting as the fulcrum (Fig. 11-19).

f. Mild tension is maintained at the monitoring finger until motion is felt. The physician will feel a release of tissue tension in 3 to 5 seconds.

g. The physician releases the position, returns the leg to the table, and reevaluates the dysfunction.

   Note: This treatment may be applied to both sides for optimum results.

Tissue Texture Dysfunctions of the Piriformis and Gluteal Muscles
1. **Patient position:** prone, with a pillow placed under the abdomen.
2. **Physician position:** sitting beside the table on the side of the dysfunction (right), facing toward the patient's head. The physician's left thigh and knee are beside the table.
3. **Technique:**
   a. The physician monitors the tissue to be treated with one finger of the left hand.
   b. The physician drops the patient's flexed right knee and thigh off the table over his left thigh.
   c. The physician holds the patient's knee with his right hand, gently flexing the patient's hip until motion is felt at the monitoring finger.
   d. The physician pushes the patient's right knee toward the table (adduction), using his left knee and thigh as a fulcrum, until motion is felt at the monitoring finger.
   e. With his right hand, the physician turns the

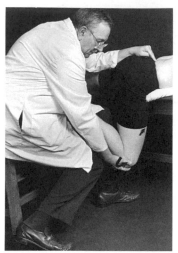

Figure 11-18. Facilitated positional release treatment for a lumbar flexion somatic dysfunction.

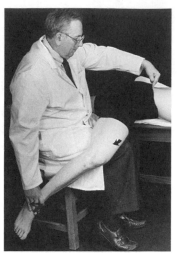

Figure 11-19. Figure 11-19. Facilitated positional release treatment for lumbar diskogenic pain syndrome.

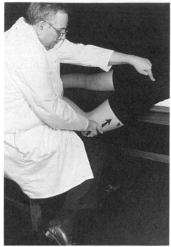

Figure 11-20. Facilitated positional release treatment for tissue texture dysfunctions in the gluteal region.

patient's knee in a circular direction, producing internal rotation of the hip, until motion is felt at the monitoring finger.

f. With his right hand, the physician pushes the patient's knee dorsally toward his monitoring finger, producing a mild compressive force (Fig. 11-20). There should be an immediate release of tissue tension.

g. The position is held for 3 seconds, then released; the dysfunction is reevaluated.

HIGH-VELOCITY, LOW-AMPLITUDE THRUSTING TECHNIQUES

Barry S. Erner
Paula D. Scariati

This section describes high-velocity, low-amplitude thrusting techniques for treating somatic dysfunctions of the lumbar spine.

Lumbar Somatic Dysfunction

1. **Patient position:** lateral recumbent, with the posteriorly rotated transverse process up.
2. **Physician position:** standing facing the front of the patient.

3. **Technique:**
   a. The physician uses one hand to monitor the posteriorly rotated transverse process at all times while positioning and treating the patient.
   b. The physician flexes the hip and knee of the patient's superior leg until he feels motion in his monitoring hand. He then hooks the patient's foot in the popliteal fossa of the inferior leg, which is resting on the table in an extended position.

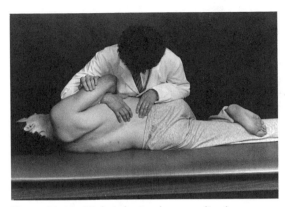

Figure 11-21. High-velocity, low-amplitude treatment of the lumbar region.

c. The physician rotates the patient's torso in the same direction as the posteriorly rotated transverse process by pulling on the patient's underneath arm. Rotation is induced down to but not including the vertebral segment of the somatic dysfunction.

d. The physician places the forearm of his thrusting arm over the patient's superior iliac crest and maintains finger monitoring of the dysfunction.

e. The physician places his other arm beneath the patient's upper arm and stabilizes the patient's lateral torso and rib cage.

f. The patient inhales deeply and exhales.

g. The physician exerts a rapid rotary thrust at the end of exhalation. This is achieved by rotating the patient's pelvis forward and toward the table (Fig. 11-21).

Alternative Technique

LEG OFF TABLE

1. **Patient position:** lateral recumbent position with the posteriorly rotated transverse process up.

2. **Physician position:** standing facing the front of the patient.

3. **Technique:**

   a. The method is the same as in the technique just described, except that the patient's superior leg is dropped off the table into full hip flexion. This leg is then locked between the physician's legs and maintained in full hip flexion.

   b. Localization and thrust are the same as in the first technique.

POSTERIOR TRANSVERSE PROCESS DOWN

1. **Patient position:** lateral recumbent with posterior transverse down.

2. **Physician position:** standing at the side of the table facing the front of the patient.

3. **Technique:**

   The technique is exactly the same as for the posterior transverse process except that the dysfunctional vertebra will be moved on the one below it, whereas in the first technique the dysfunctional vertebra was moved on the one above it. The monitoring must still be done at the site of the posterior process.

EXERCISE THERAPY

Stanley Schiowitz
Albert R. DeRubertis

Low back pain is the single most common cause of work absenteeism in the United States. Some 70% to 80% of adults suffer from low back pain at some time in their lives. It is important that primary care physicians understand low back structural biomechanics because they will regularly encounter patients with low back pain.

A comprehensive therapeutic approach includes exercises designed to establish and maintain musculoskeletal structural integrity. A simple approach is to evaluate the lumbar lordosis, the structures involved in its formation, and the muscles that act synergistically to maintain it.

The three questions to be answered are:

1. Is the anteroposterior lumbar curve flattened or exaggerated?

2. Do the individual vertebrae move freely?

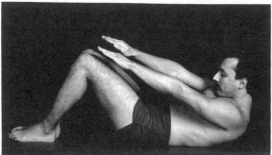

Figure 11-22. Upper abdominal strengthening exercise.

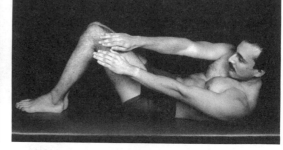

Figure 11-23. Rotary abdominal strengthening exercise.

3. Do the muscles involved require stretching (extensibility) or strengthening (contractility)?

The muscles involved in creating low back pain are usually the erector spinae, the gluteus maximus, the hamstrings, the iliopsoas, and the abdominals. With the exception of the abdominals and occasionally the back extensors, these muscles require stretching. Regional motion testing may demonstrate restriction caused by muscle contraction. Specific testing for motion, stretch, and strength should be employed.

The exercises described in this chapter are based on the above approach. Many serve more than one function.

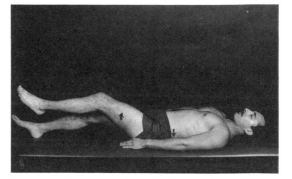

Figure 11-24. Lower abdominal strengthening exercise, one leg raised.

Abdominal Muscles

UPPER ABDOMINAL
STRENGTHENING EXERCISE
1. **Patient position:** supine, hips and knees flexed, feet on floor, arms extended.
2. **Instructions:**
   a. Roll your head, neck, and upper back off the floor.
   b. Try to touch your knees with your hands (Fig. 11-22).
   c. Hold this position for 5 to 15 seconds. Slowly lower your body to the floor.
   d. Relax, rest, and repeat.

ROTARY ABDOMINAL
STRENGTHENING EXERCISE
1. **Patient position:** supine, hips and knees flexed, feet on floor, arms extended.

2. **Instructions:**
   a. Roll your head, neck, and upper back off the floor.
   b. Try to touch your left knee only with both hands, creating a body twist (Fig. 11-23).
   c. Hold this position for 5 to 15 seconds. Slowly lower your body back to floor.
   d. Relax and rest.
   e. Repeat by trying to touch your right knee.

LOWER ABDOMINAL
STRENGTHENING EXERCISES
Exercise 1
1. **Patient position:** supine on floor, both knees slightly bent, heels on floor.
2. **Instructions:**
   a. Tighten your abdominal muscles and maintain your back flat against the floor.
   b. Raise your left leg off the floor 6 to 8 inches. Maintain both knees in their slightly flexed position (Fig. 11-24).

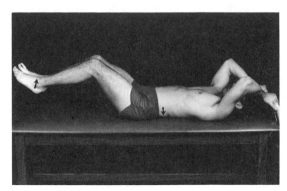

Figure 11-25. Lower abdominal strengthening exercise, both legs raised.

c. Hold this position for 5 to 15 seconds.
d. Slowly lower the left leg to the floor.
e. Relax, rest, and repeat by raising your right leg.

Exercise 2

1. **Patient position:** supine on floor, both hands over head and firmly holding onto a solid structure.
2. **Instructions:**
   a. Tighten your abdominal muscles, keeping your back flat against the floor.
   b. Flex both knees to 45 degrees. Now raise both feet 6 to 8 inches off the floor (Fig. 11-25).

c. Hold this position for 5 to 15 seconds.
d. Slowly lower both feet to the floor.
e. Relax, rest, and repeat.

Lower Back Muscles

STRETCH

Exercise 1

1. **Patient position:** seated on edge of chair, both feet flat on floor.
2. **Instructions:**
   a. Cross both arms in front of your chest.
   b. Let your body bend forward between your legs. Let the body weight create low back stretch (Fig. 11-26).
   c. Hold for 5 to 15 seconds.
   d. Return slowly to the upright position. Relax, rest, and repeat.
      Caution: This can create vertigo and hypotension.

Exercise 2

1. **Patient position:** seated on the floor or a table with both legs extended.
2. **Instructions:**
   a. Lean forward and grasp your shins with each hand.
   b. Pull your trunk into further forward bending by bringing your hands down your legs (Fig. 11-27).

Figure 11-26. Lower back muscle stretch, seated on chair.

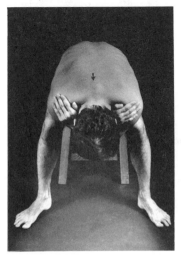

Figure 11-27. Lower back muscle stretch, seated on floor.

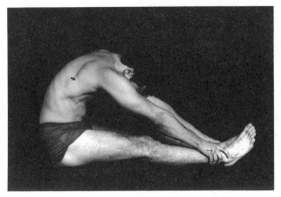

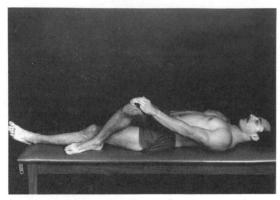

Figure 11-28. Lower back muscle rotary stretch, legs extended.

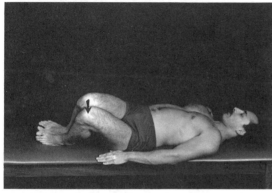

Figure 11-29. Lower back muscle rotary stretch, hips and knees bent.

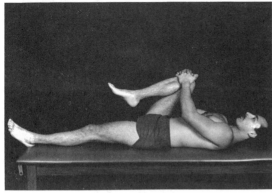

Figure 11-30. Gluteus maximus active muscle stretch.

c. Feel stretch in the lower back. Hold for 5 to 15 seconds. Slowly return to the starting position.

d. Relax, rest, and repeat.

ROTARY STRETCH

Exercise 1

1. **Patient position:** supine, arms and legs extended.

2. **Instructions:**

   a. Bend your right knee up, cross it over your left leg, and place the right foot flat on the floor, close to the left knee.

   b. Grasp your right knee with your left hand and slowly pull it toward the left side of the floor. Keep your shoulders flat on the floor (Fig. 11-28).

   c. This will create a right low back rotary stretch. Hold for 5 to 15 seconds.

   d. Release right knee, relax, and repeat.

   e. For left low back rotary stretch, reverse the knee and hand instructions.

Exercise 2

1. **Patient position:** supine, both hips and knees bent, feet together and flat on the floor.

2. **Instructions:**

   a. Using your left foot as a fulcrum, pivot both knees to the left. Allow the weight of the legs to create a right low back rotary stretch (Fig. 11-29).

   b. Keep your shoulders flat on the floor. Do not use muscular contraction to increase stretch.

   c. Hold at maximum relaxed stretch for 5 to 15 seconds. Return knees to starting position.

   d. Relax, rest, and repeat.

   e. For left rotary stretch, reverse the instructions.

Gluteus Maximus Muscles

ACTIVE STRETCH

1. **Patient position:** supine, both knees bent, feet on floor.

2. **Instructions:**

   a. Bring your right knee up to your chest as far as possible and grasp with both hands. At the same time fully extend your left leg (Fig. 11-30).

   b. Hold for 5 to 15 seconds.

c. Reverse the procedure by bringing your left knee up to your chest and fully extending your right leg.

d. Hold this position for 5 to 15 seconds. Return to starting position.

e. Relax, rest, and repeat.

PASSIVE STRETCH

1. **Patient position:** supine, arms at sides, knees bent, feet on floor.

2. **Instructions:**

a. Bring your right knee to your chest. Clasp both your hands over that knee.

b. Passively and slowly, pull your right knee to your chest (Fig. 11-31). Hold this position for 5 to 15 seconds.

c. Return to starting position; repeat with other knee.

d. Repeat, flexing both hip and knees to chest at one time.

   Note: If you have knee dysfunction, clasp both hands on the posterior thigh near the popliteal region.

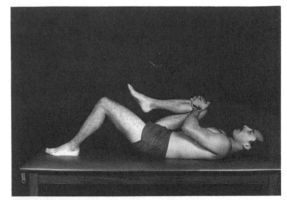

Figure 11-31. Gluteus maximus passive muscle stretch.

Lumbar Spine

LUMBAR FLATTENING (PELVIC TILT TO DECREASE LORDOSIS)

1. **Patient position:** supine, arms above head, both knees bent, feet on floor.

2. **Instructions:**

a. Tighten your abdominal muscles and your buttocks at the same time.

b. Flatten your back firmly against the floor. Roll your pelvis backward if necessary to achieve full flattening (Fig. 11-32).

c. Hold this position for 5 to 15 seconds.

d. Relax, rest, and repeat.

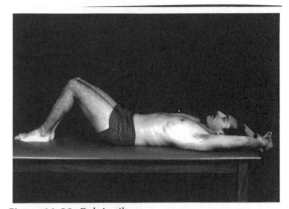

Figure 11-32. Pelvic tilt.

CAT BACK—LUMBAR FLEXIBILITY

1. **Patient position:** hands and knees on the floor, back up, fully lengthened and straight.

2. **Instructions:**

a. **Flexion:**

   i. Drop your head down between your arms, looking toward your thighs.

   ii. Arch your back upward and try to bring your pelvis toward your head (Fig. 11-33).

   iii. Try to achieve full back flexion with reversal of lumbar lordosis.

   iv. Hold this position for 5 to 15 seconds, return to starting position.

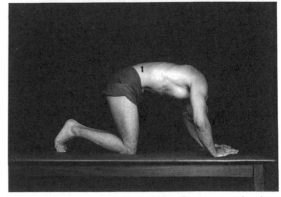

Figure 11-33. Lumbar flexibility—flexion (cat back).

v. Relax, rest, and then do the following extension exercise.

b. **Extension:**

i. Bring your head back into full head and neck extension.

ii. Arch your back down toward the floor. Try to bring your buttocks toward your head.

iii. Try to achieve full back extension, exaggerating the lumbar lordosis (Fig. 11-34).

iv. Hold this position for 5 to 15 seconds. Return to starting position.

v. Relax, rest, and repeat the entire exercise.
   Note: Try to maintain your abdominal muscles in a flattened, mildly contracted position throughout the exercise.

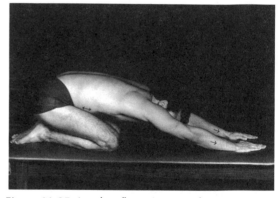

Figure 11-34. Lumbar flexibility—extension (cat back).

LUMBAR FLATTENING

1. **Patient position:** kneeling, buttocks resting on heels.

2. **Instructions:**

a. Bring both fully extended arms forward. Touch both palms to floor, bringing your chest parallel to floor.

b. Contract your abdominal muscles while pushing both arms forward. This should bring your chest against your knees (Fig. 11-35).

c. Maintain maximum stretch for 5 to 15 seconds. Return to starting position.

d. Relax, rest, and repeat.

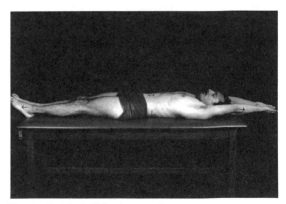

Figure 11-35. Lumbar flattening stretch.

FULL BODY STRETCH (FLATTEN
ALL CURVES)

1. **Patient position:** supine, arms fully extended overhead, legs fully extended downward.

2. **Instructions:**

a. Stretch your arms overhead and your legs downward. Point your toes into plantar flexion.

b. Tighten your abdominal muscles and flatten your lumbar spine.

c. Tuck in your chin and flatten your cervical spine (Fig. 11-36).

d. Hold this position for 5 to 15 seconds.

e. Relax, rest, and repeat.

Figure 11-36. Full body stretch.

Anterior Pelvic Muscle Stretch

1. **Patient position:** prone, legs extended, arms at sides.

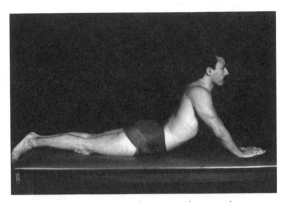

Figure 11-37. Anterior pelvic muscle stretch.

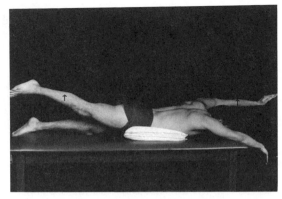

Figure 11-38. Back extensor muscle strengthening, left arm and right leg raised.

2. **Instructions:**
   a. Place both hands, palms down, on the floor at shoulder level.
   b. Raise your upper body off the floor by fully extending your arms. Keep your upper thighs on the floor (Fig. 11-37).
   c. Allow your abdomen and pelvis to sag (stretch) toward the floor. Your body weight will perform the necessary stretch.
   d. Hold this position for 5 to 15 seconds. Lower your body to the floor.
   e. Relax, rest, and repeat.

Back Extensor Muscle Strengthening

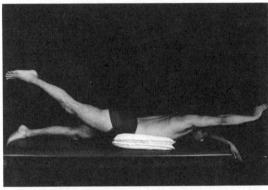

Figure 11-39. Back extensor muscle strengthening, right arm and right leg raised.

1. **Patient position:** prone, arms fully extended upward, legs fully extended downward. Two pillows are placed under the abdomen.
2. **Instructions:**
   a. Raise your left arm and right leg up off the floor, fully extended (Fig. 11-38). Hold for 5 seconds. Lower and repeat with your left arm and right leg.
   b. Raise your right arm and right leg off the floor, fully extended. (Fig. 11-39). Hold for 5 seconds. Lower and repeat with your left arm and left leg.
   c. Raise both arms, fully extended, off the floor (Fig. 11-40). Hold for 5 seconds. Lower. Now raise both legs fully extended off the floor (Fig. 11-41).
   d. Raise all four fully extended extremities off the floor simultaneously (Fig. 11-42). Hold for 5 seconds. Lower.
   e. Relax, rest, and repeat the entire exercise.

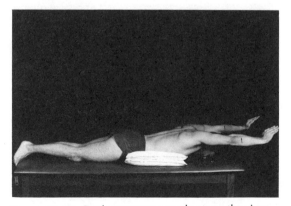

Figure 11-40. Back extensor muscle strengthening, both arms raised.

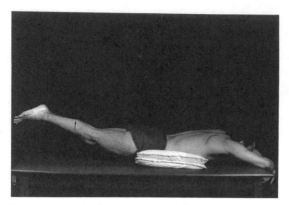

Figure 11-41. Back extensor muscle strengthening, both legs raised.

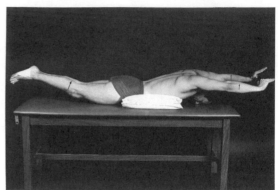

Figure 11-42. Back extensor muscle strengthening, all extremities raised.

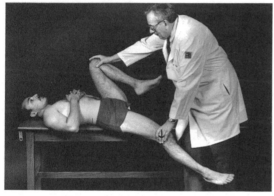

Figure 11-43. Psoas muscle stretch, assisted.

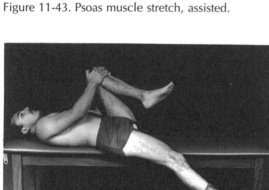

Figure 11-44. Psoas muscle stretch, unassisted.

Hip Flexor Stretch

PSOAS—ASSISTED

1. **Patient position:** supine on edge of table or bed, so that side to be stretched can drop off toward the floor (right side).
2. **Instructions:**
   a. Bend your left hip and knee to chest and hold them with both hands. Keep your low back flat on the table.
   b. Drop your right leg off the table toward floor.
   c. The assistant holds the left hip and knee in full flexion, while gently pushing down on the right thigh, creating stretch (Fig. 11-43).
   d. Hold maximum painless stretch for 5 to 15 seconds. Return both legs to the table in full extension.
   e. Relax, rest, and repeat.

PSOAS—UNASSISTED

1. **Patient position:** supine on edge of table or bed, so that side to be stretched can drop off toward the floor (right side).
2. **Instructions:**
   a. Bend your left hip and knee to chest. Hold them firmly against your chest. Keep your low back flat on the table.
   b. Drop your right leg off the table toward the floor. Allow its weight to create stretch.
   c. For additional stretch, a 3 to 5 pound weight can be added at the ankle (Fig. 11-44).
   d. Hold the maximum painless stretch for 5 to 15 seconds. Return both legs to the table in full extension.
   e. Relax, rest, and repeat.

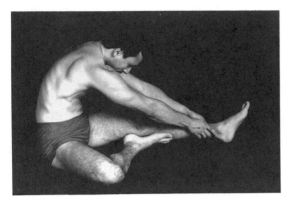

Figure 11-45. Hamstring muscle stretch, seated.

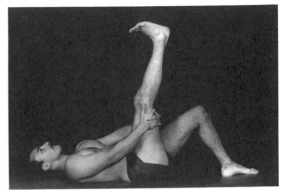

Figure 11-46. Hamstring muscle stretch, supine.

Hamstring Stretch

SEATED STRETCH

1. **Patient position:** seated with the back upright and the left leg in full extension. The right leg is bent so that the right foot is touching the left thigh.
2. **Instructions:**
   a. Bend forward from your hips. Place both hands on your left leg until you feel stretch (left-sided).
   b. Hold this position; then walk your hands farther down the left leg to increase the stretch to maximum (Fig. 11-45).
   c. Hold this position for 5 to 15 seconds. Return to the upright position.
   d. Relax, rest, and repeat.
   e. To stretch the right side, reverse instructions.

SUPINE STRETCH

1. **Patient position:** supine, hips and knees flexed, both feet flat on the floor.
2. **Instructions:**
   a. Flex the hip to be stretched toward your chest. Then extend that leg fully toward the ceiling. Bend your toes down toward your body. Hold in maximum painless stretch.
   b. Bring both hands or a towel around and behind the extended knee or thigh. Slowly pull your thigh toward your chest. Maintain full leg extension (Fig. 11-46).
   c. Hold this position for 5 to 15 seconds. Return to the original position.
   d. Relax, rest, and repeat.
   e. To stretch the other side, reverse instructions.

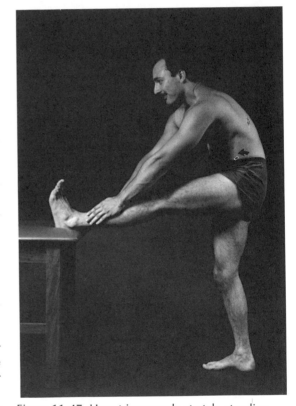

Figure 11-47. Hamstring muscle stretch, standing.

STANDING STRETCH

1. **Patient position:** standing near a table or other firm support. Support must be of sufficient height to allow stretch.

2. **Instructions:**
   a. Place the heel of the foot to be exercised on the support. Keep the knee fully extended.
   b. With both hands on your leg, slowly bend forward from your hips until you feel maximum painless stretch in the back of your raised leg (Fig. 11-47).
   c. Hold for 5 to 15 seconds, increasing the painless stretch as tolerated. Return leg to floor.
   d. Relax, rest, and repeat.

   e. To stretch the other side, reverse instructions.

Reference

Mitchell FL Jr, Moran PS, Pruzzo NT. 1979. An Evaluation and Treatment Manual of Osteopathic Muscle Energy Procedures. Valley Park, Mo: Mitchell, Moran, and Pruzzo.

12

Evaluation of the Pelvis and Sacrum

FUNCTIONAL ANATOMY AND BIOMECHANICS
Stanley Schiowitz

Anatomy

The pelvis consists of two innominate bones that meet at the midline anteriorly and end posteriorly in a wedge-shaped opening that is filled by the sacrum. This completes the overall ring shape of the pelvis.

Each innominate bone consists of three bones, the ilium, ischium, and pubes which fuse in late adolescence to form one bone. On the lateral surface of the innominate is the acetabulum, which articulates with the head of the femur to create the hip joint.

The sacrum is a large bone in the shape of an inverted triangle that is formed by the fusion of the five sacral vertebrae. It is inserted between the two innominate bones in the upper, posterior aspect of the pelvic cavity. The upper aspect of the sacrum—the base of the triangle—articulates with the fifth lumbar vertebra, creating, with the L5 intervertebral disk, the lumbosacral articulation. The weight of the upper body is transmitted through the sacrum, innominate bones, and acetabulum to the femurs, then down to the feet and the supporting surface.

In the upright position the sacrum lies in an oblique plane, running from above downward in an anteroposterior direction. Its anterior surface is concave. Its posterior surface is convex and contains the palpable spinous tubercles. The sacrum contains the sacral canal, in which are located the cauda equina and four sacral foramina: these apertures provide passageway for the ventral and dorsal rami of the first four sacral spinal nerves. Bilaterally the sacrum has auricular surfaces that articulate with the innominate bones to form the sacroiliac joints.

The sacroiliac articulations are kidney-shaped and convex ventrally. The sacral and iliac articulations seem to match in a crescent-shaped, convex-concave arrangement, but this is not true for the joints' entire bony relationship. Horizontal sections from various levels of the sacroiliac articulation show that the convex-concave relationship exists only at the upper and middle portions. In the lower portion the relationship is variously described as a flattened, planar joint or a reverse, concave-convex relationship (Fig. 12-1); anatomists differ in their descriptions of the sacroiliac articulations.

Occasionally the right and left sacroiliac articulations do not mirror each other in the same body. It is generally agreed that the midarticulation has the greatest convex-concave relationship, promoting joint stability and flexion-extension motions.

An Osteopathic Approach to Diagnosis and Treatment, second edition
Eileen L. DiGiovanna and Stanley Schiowitz
Lippincott–Raven Publishers, Philadelphia © 1997.

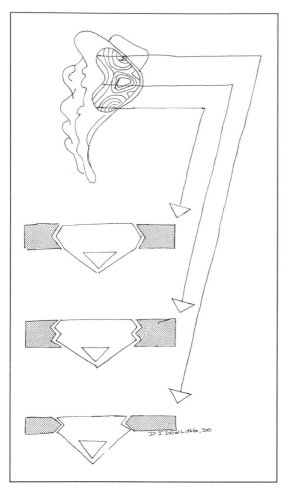

Figure 12-1. Sacroiliac articulation configurations as seen at different sacral levels.

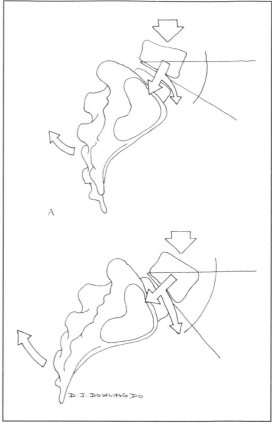

Figure 12-2. An increase in the lumbosacral angle creates a greater anterior vector force, which increases the lumbosacral strain.

This is usually found at the level of the second sacral vertebra.

The multiple forms and contours found at any sacroiliac articulation account for the diversity of motions of this joint. The joint is held together by its ligaments. There are no direct muscular attachments from the sacrum to the ilium.

Pelvic Motions

The pelvis moves as a single unit whose gross motions are initiated by the motions of other body segments. Rotation, side-bending, and forward and backward bending are all related to the hip or trunk motions. In addition, there are patterns of movement between the sacrum and the ilium, and patterns of movement at the pubic articulation.

Review of some everyday activities will demonstrate their effect on the pelvic structures. In the standing position, body weight is transmitted through the fifth lumbar vertebra to the sacrum, where the force vector splits in two. One force vector drives the sacrum into its articulation, and the other rotates the sacrum anteriorly. The greater the lumbosacral angle, the greater is the anterior vector force, which in turn increases the lumbosacral strain (Fig. 12-2).

During the act of walking, the ilium on the side of the stance leg is elevated, while the ilium on the swing side is tilted down, and rotated toward the stance leg. This creates pubic shear and torsion (Fig. 12-3, *top*). The stance leg, from heel strike to toe-off, is associated with a close-packed hip joint

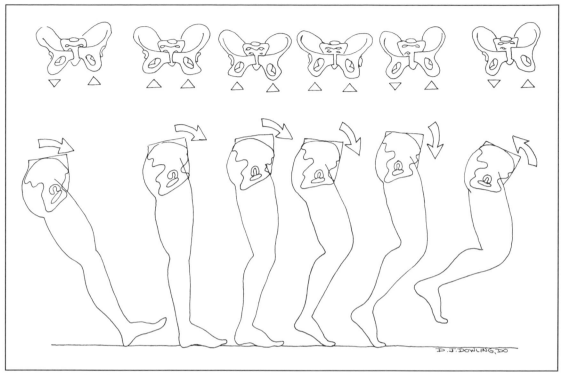

Figure 12-3. Pubic shear and torsion in walking (*top*), corresponding to the position of the weight-bearing ilium as the stance leg moves from heel strike to toe-off (*bottom*).

articulation and causes anterior rotation of the ilium (Fig. 12-3, *bottom*). The body weight shifts to the side of the stance leg, creating lateral flexion stress of the sacrum. The one-legged weight stress produces unilateral stance leg sacroiliac joint locking, allowing the creation of the oblique axis (Mitchell, 1965). This in turn permits sacral torsional motion.

Respiratory motions create sacral flexion/ extension (Sutherland, 1936). Flexion and extension of the sacrum create pressure on the ilia that is transmitted to the pubic articulation.

The three principal kinds of motions that occur in the pelvis are sacral motions on the ilium, ilial motions on the sacrum, and pubic motions. Each is described below.

SACRAL MOTION ON THE ILIUM
The sacral motions on the ilium and the axes on which they occur, are as follows:

1. Sacral flexion and extension are caused by respiratory motion and occur on a superior transverse axis, also known as the respiratory axis, that is located at the level of the articular processes of the second sacral segment.
2. Sacral flexion and extension are transmitted as force vectors through the lumbar spine to the middle transverse axis, located at the level of the second sacral body.
3. Rotation of the sacrum occurs on a vertical axis.
4. Lateral flexion of the sacrum occurs on an anteroposterior axis.
5. Torsional motions of the sacrum occur on a right or left oblique axis, located from the superior end of the articular surface of one side to the inferior end of the articular surface of the other side.

The axes of sacral motion on the ilium are shown in Figure 12-4.

The coupled motions of rotation and lateral bending of the sacrum are variable, depending somewhat on how those movements are initiated. According to Kappler, sacral rotation induced by lumbar spinal rotation occurs in the same direc-

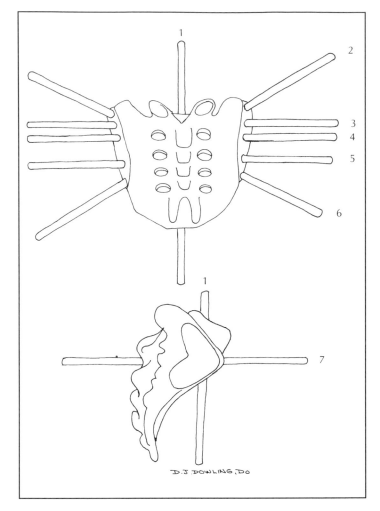

Figure 12-4. Axes of motion of the sacrum on the ilia. *1*, vertical axis; *2*, right oblique axis; *3*, respiratory axis; *4*, sacroilial axis; *5*, iliosacral axis; *6*, left oblique axis; *7*, anteroposterior axis.

tion as the lumbar spinal rotation, but lateral flexion of the sacrum occurs to the opposite side. When lateral sacral flexion is induced by lateral flexion of the lumbar spine, sacral rotation may occur to either side.

ILIAL MOTIONS ON THE SACRUM
The motions of the ilium on the sacrum, and the axes on which these movements occur, are as follows.

1. Anteroposterior rotation of the ilium on the sacrum occurs on the inferior transverse axis, located at the inferior pole of the lower sacral articulation (Fig. 12-5).

2. Ilial translatory motions on the sacrum occur in a superoinferior direction (Fig. 12-6).
3. Ilial translatory motions on the sacrum occur in an anteroposterior direction (Fig. 12-7).

PUBIC MOTIONS
The pubic motions, shown in Figure 12-8, are as follows:

1. Caliper motion (flexion-extension of sacrum).
2. Torsional motion (swing-tilt of swing leg).
3. Superoinferior translatory motion (one-legged weightbearing).

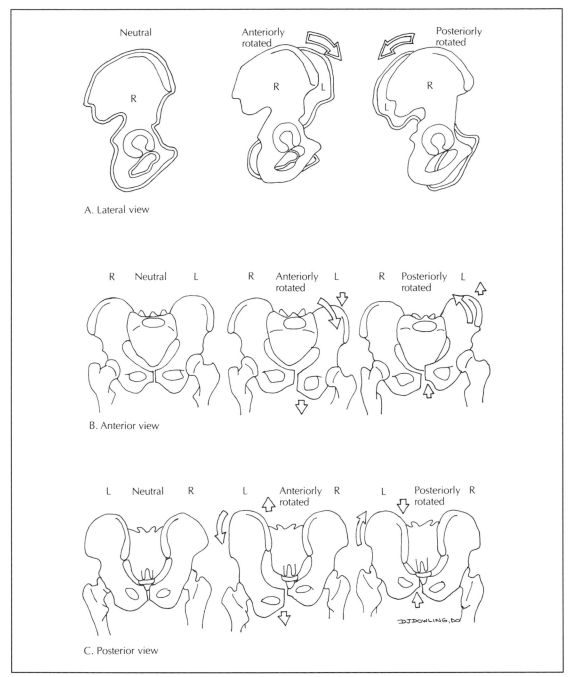

Figure 12-5. Anteroposterior rotation of the innominate on the sacrum. The directions are named for left-sided movement in this illustration.

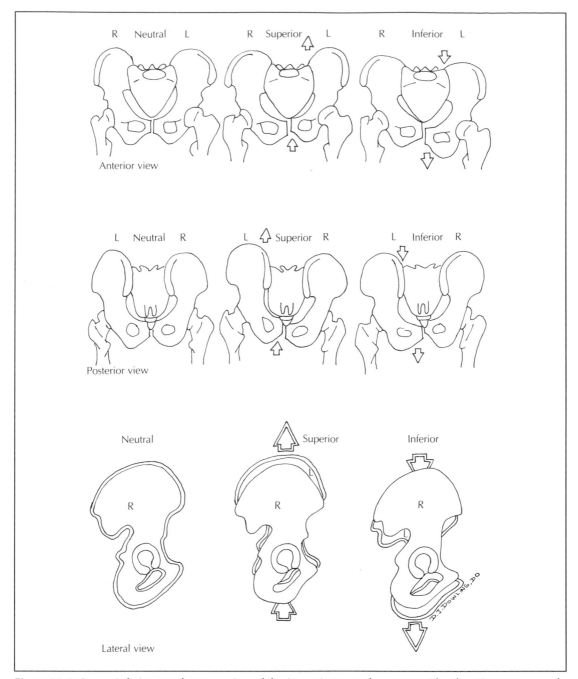

Figure 12-6. Superoinferior translatory motion of the innominate on the sacrum. The directions are named for left-sided movement.

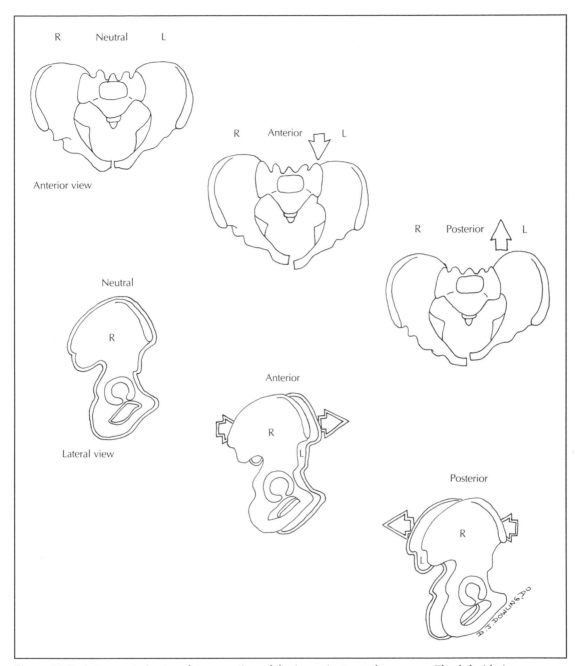

Figure 12-7. Anteroposterior translatory motion of the innominate on the sacrum. The left side is illustrated.

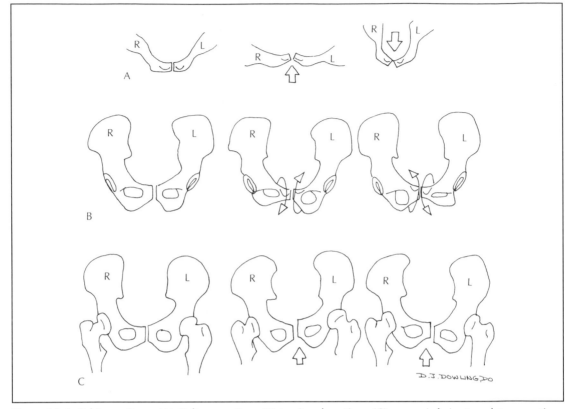

Figure 12-8. Pubic motions. **(A)** Caliper motion, **(B)** torsional motion, **(C)** superoinferior translatory motion.

The Pelvis During Pregnancy

During vaginal delivery, the sacrum undergoes a process called *nutation* (nodding) that facilitates delivery. In nutation the sacrum flexes at its middle transverse axis. This diminishes the anteroposterior diameter of the pelvic brim. At the same time the iliac bones approximate, narrowing the transverse diameter of the pelvic brim, and the ischial tuberosities separate, widening the pelvic outlet (Fig. 12-9).

The patient's position and the stress involved, when added to the laxity of the ligaments at delivery, can create sacroiliac dysfunctions. These dysfunctions worsen and are locked into malposition as the ligaments regain their normal rigidity post partum. Dysfunction can be prevented after delivery by holding the hip in internal rotation as each leg is removed from the lithotomy position and placed flat on the table.

Pelvic Somatic Dysfunctions

Pelvic somatic dysfunctions are of the following types:

1. Primary pubic dysfunctions are superior-inferior or abducted-adducted dysfunctions.
2. Dysfunctions of motion created by the sacrum moving on the ilium are commonly unilateral anterior sacral dysfunctions or oblique torsional sacral dysfunctions.
3. Dysfunction created by the ilium moving on the sacrum usually involves anteroposterior ilial rotation or superoinferior ilial shear.

These dysfunctions may be difficult to diagnose individually since many of the motion functions and diagnostic findings overlap. Specific treatment of a specific dysfunction is most effective. However, because of the firm ligamentous attachments of this articulation, nonspecific treatment may be equally as effective.

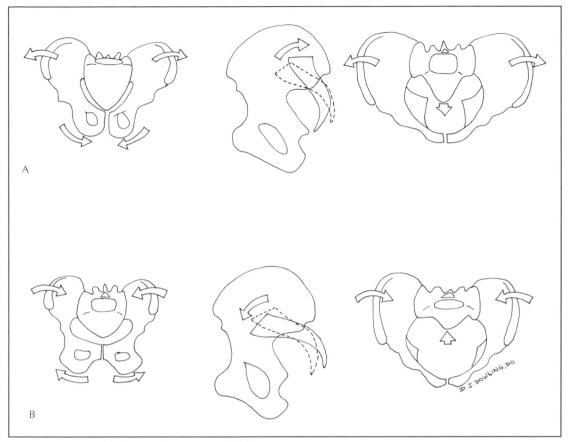

Figure 12-9. Sacral relations during vaginal delivery. **(A)** Counternutation, **(B)** nutation.

EXAMINATION AND MOTION TESTING
Dennis J. Dowling

Patient Standing
1. **Patient position:** standing, barefoot, with the feet parallel and six to eight inches apart.
2. **Physician position:** kneeling behind the patient with his eyes approximately at the level of the iliac crests and the posterior superior iliac spines (PSIS).

STATIC EXAMINATION (FIG. 12-10)
1. **Technique:**
   a. Iliac crests: The physician places his hands on the patient's iliac crests and evaluates the symmetry of heights of the two crests.

b. Posterior superior iliac spines: A landmark for the PSIS is usually visible as a skin dimple indicating the location of attachment of the deep fascia. The physician places his thumbs at these locations, hooks his thumbs beneath the PSIS, and compares heights.

c. Gluteal folds: The physician observes directly these folds, which delineate the lower border of the gluteus maximus muscle, and compares heights. A variation in height may indicate the influence of habitual patterns, postural imbalances, leg length differences, neurologic dysfunction, or other factors.

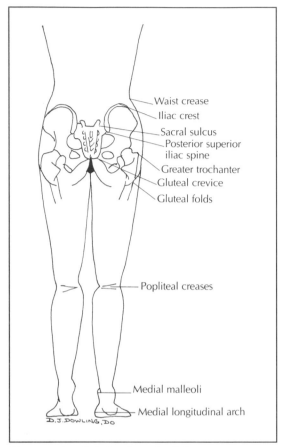

Figure 12-10. Relationship of pelvic structures on static examination, patient standing.

2. **Other findings:** The physician may also examine asymmetry of the popliteal creases, the greater trochanters of the femurs, the medial malleoli, and the medial longitudinal arches of the feet.

MOTION TESTING (STANDING
FLEXION TEST)
1. **Technique:**
   a. The physician places his thumbs at the inferior aspect of the PSIS.
   b. The patient is directed to bend forward from the waist and reach with his hands toward his toes, without bending his knees (Fig. 12-11).
   c. As the patient is flexing forward, the physi-

cian observes the movement of the PSIS as the ilium moves on the sacrum.
   d. Flexion of the spine carries the base of the sacrum anteriorly and motion is introduced into the sacroiliac joint. A certain amount of play occurs before the movement of the sacrum carries the ilium into anterior rotation, which in turn causes the PSIS to rise superiorly.
   e. Restriction on one side causes the iliosacral joint to lock prematurely on that side, causing the PSIS to elevate sooner and probably farther than the PSIS on the other side. This is considered a positive test result.
   f. A positive test indicates iliosacral somatic dysfunction on the ipsilateral side.
2. **Variations:**
   a. The PSIS may initially be at different heights. Asymmetry may indicate somatic dysfunction but does not determine which side is involved.
   b. Placement of a wooden shim under the foot on the same side as the lower PSIS, until both PSIS are at the same level, facilitates diagnosis.
   c. Proceed with test as outlined above.

Patient Seated—Seated Flexion Test
1. **Patient position:** seated on a stool, both feet flat on the floor and the arms resting comfortably on the thighs.
2. **Physician position:** kneeling behind the patient with his eyes at the level of the iliac crests.

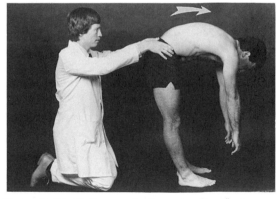

Figure 12-11. Static examination, standing flexion test.

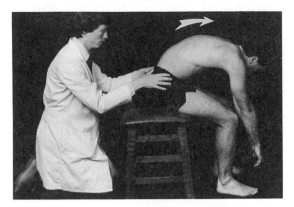

Figure 12-12. Static examination, seated flexion test.

MOTION TESTING (SEATED FLEXION TEST)
1. **Technique:**
   a. The physician places his thumbs at the inferior aspect of the PSIS.
   b. The patient is directed to bend forward from the waist and reach toward the floor (Fig. 12-12).
   c. As the patient bends forward, the physician observes the movement of the PSIS, indicating movement of the sacrum on the ilium.
   d. In the seated position the innominate is initially locked in place via the ischial tuberosity. The sacroilial portion of the joint becomes involved as the sacrum engages the ilium, which rotates anteriorly with sacral flexion, elevating the PSIS bilaterally.
   e. Restriction on one side causes the sacroiliac joint to lock prematurely. The ilium and PSIS begin and carry through excursion sooner and probably farther than on the contralateral side. This is considered a positive test result.
   f. A positive test indicates sacroiliac somatic dysfunction on the ipsilateral side.
2. **Variations:** An uneven PSIS level may be related to such factors as wallets, clothing restriction, twisting of the torso, or other influences.

Patient Supine
1. **Patient position:** supine.
2. **Physician position:** varies according to the region examined.

STATIC EXAMINATION
1. Pubic tubercles
   a. The pubic tubercles are located on the ante-rior superior aspects of the pubic bones (Fig. 12-13). The pubic symphysis is located medially.
   b. The patient is more comfortable if he voids before the examination.
   c. The physician places the palm of one hand flat on the patient's lower abdomen.
   d. The physician gently slides this hand downward until the pubic bones are located.
   e. The tubercle positions are located by placing the pads of the index fingers gently on the cephalic aspect.
   f. The physician brings his eyes directly over the pubic region and evaluates the position of his index fingers relative to each other.
   g. Asymmetry of position indicates a pubic dysfunction. The diagnosis is named according to the side on which the standing flexion test is positive, and according to the relative position of the pubic tubercle involved.
2. Anterior superior iliac spines (ASIS)
   a. The ASIS is a bony protuberance on the anterior portion of the ilium (Fig. 12-14).
   b. The physician places the pads of his thumbs under the ASIS bilaterally.
   c. With his eyes directly over the pelvic region, the physician evaluates the position of the ASIS (superior/inferior, ventral/dorsal) relative to each other.
   d. Asymmetry of position may indicate ilial dysfunction. The diagnosis is named accord-

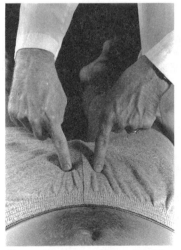

Figure 12-13. Location of pubic tubercles.

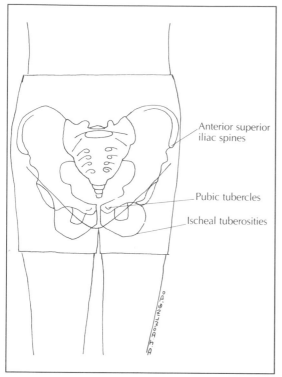

Figure 12-14. Relationship of anterior superior iliac spines to other pelvic structures.

ing to the side on which the standing flexion test is positive.

3. Medial malleoli
   a. The physician stands at the foot of the table and places his thumbs under the distal ledge of the medial malleoli (Fig. 12-15).
   b. The physician evaluates the relative positions of the malleoli (caudal/cephalad).
   c. The side of the dysfunction is determined by the side of the positive standing flexion test.

MOTION TESTING

1. Innominate (ilial) rocking
   a. The physician stands on the side of the table, facing toward the patient's head.
   b. The physician places his thenar and hypothenar eminences against the ASIS.
   c. A gentle but firm rocking motion against the ASIS is directed along planes that are roughly sagittal (Fig. 12-16). Each ASIS should be examined alternately.
   d. The physician allows the ilia to recoil anteriorly against gentle pressure.
   e. Ease of motion in anterior and posterior directions is noted as the innominates are rocked.
   f. The diagnosis is made by noting the resistance to motion.

2. Iliosacral dysfunction: Leg lengthening or shortening
   a. The physician stands at the foot of the table.
   b. The patient flexes his knees and places his feet flat on the table.

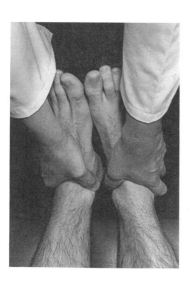

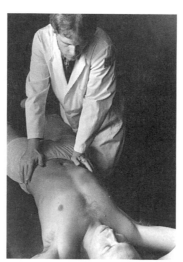

Figure 12-15. Medial malleoli.

Figure 12-16. Innominate rocking.

Figure 12-17. Hip reflexion with external rotation and extension of the hip and knee.

Figure 12-18. Hip flexion with internal rotation and extension of the hip and knee.

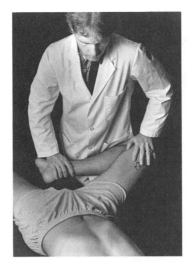
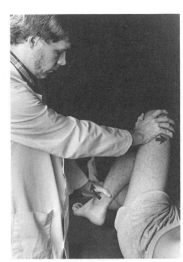

c. The patient elevates his buttocks off the table, then lowers them onto the table.
d. The physician extends the patient's legs to their full length and notes the relative position of the medial malleoli.
e. The physician then:
   i. Fully flexes one of the patient's hips and knees.
   ii. Externally rotates and abducts the hip (Fig. 12-17).
   iii. Firmly extends the patient's leg.
   iv. Compares the change in position of the ipsilateral medial malleolus in relation to the contralateral medial malleolus.
   v. Fully flexes the ipsilateral hip and knee.
   vi. Internally rotates and adducts the hip (Fig. 12-18).
   vii. Firmly extends the patient's leg.
   viii. Compares the change in position of the ipsilateral medial malleoli relative to each other.
   ix. Repeats the procedure for the other leg.
f. The physician notes the total excursion of each medial malleolus during the procedure.
g. A smaller amplitude of malleolar excursion on one side indicates dysfunction of the iliosacral joint on that side.
   Note: The physician should flex both sides equally. Inequality of motion testing may produce erroneous results.
h. The action of flexion, along with internal/external rotation, changes the orientation of the ilium relative to the sacrum if there is no

restriction. Extension maintains this change in relationship. If the iliosacral joint is restricted, hip flexion induces posterior rotation of the ilium, which causes posterior movement of the sacral base. Little or no change occurs at the joint, as indicated by the small total excursion of the medial malleolus.

Patient Prone
1. **Patient position:** prone.
2. **Physician position:** varies according to the region examined.

STATIC EXAMINATION
1. Posterior superior iliac spines
   a. The physician stands at the side of the table and faces toward the patient's head.
   b. The physician places his thumbs on the inferior slope of each PSIS and, viewing them directly from above, notes their relative orientation (superior/inferior, ventral/dorsal).
   c. The dysfunction is named according to the side on which the standing flexion test is positive.
2. Sacral sulci
   a. The physician stands at the side of the table and faces toward the patient's head.
   b. The physician places his thumbs on each PSIS.
   c. The physician hooks his thumbs medially along the PSIS and into the sacral sulci (Fig. 12-19).

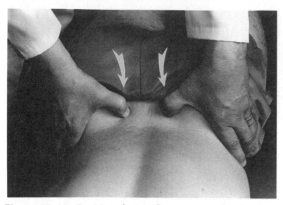

Figure 12-19. Position for evaluating sacral sulci.

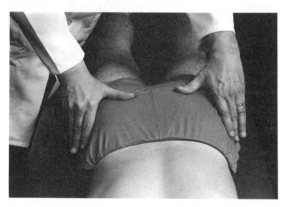

Figure 12-20. Position for evaluating inferior lateral angles.

d. The physician evaluates the relative depth of the sulci by two means:
  i. By palpating the depth of each sulcus by thumb position.
  ii. By lowering his eyes to the level of the sulci for visual evaluation of depth.
3. Inferior lateral angles
  a. The inferior lateral angles are bony protuberances located lateral to the sacral hiatus. They outline the inferior lateral aspect of the sacrum.
  b. The physician may locate the inferior lateral angles by palpating down the length of the sacral crest to the hiatus and then moving his thumbs laterally to the inferior lateral angles (Fig. 12-20).
  c. The position of the inferior lateral angles may be evaluated in two orientations:

  i. Posterior/anterior
    (a) The physician places his thumbs on the surface of the sacrum at the inferior lateral angles.
    (b) He lowers his eyes to the level of the sacrum.
    (c) The relative positions of inferior lateral angles are described as anterior or posterior.
  ii. Superior/inferior
    (a) The physician places his thumbs along the lower edges of the inferior lateral angles.
    (b) He views the sacrum from above.
    (c) The positions are described as superior or inferior.
       Note: Because of sacral structure and the types of movement available, the inferior lateral angles exhibit pairing in these positions: **posterior and inferior,** and **anterior and superior.**
4. Medial malleoli
  a. The physician places his thumbs on the underside of the medial malleoli and evaluates their relative position (Fig. 12-21).
  b. Asymmetry of the malleoli is named according to the side on which the standing flexion test is positive.

MOTION TESTING
1. Sacral mobility
  a. The physician stands at the side of the table and faces toward the patient's head.
  b. The physician places his palms on the patient's inferior lateral angles and the fingertips at the sacral sulci (Fig. 12-22).
  c. The physician directs a force cephalad from the inferior lateral angles into the sacroiliac joint on the same side. Force should not be directed obliquely because this may give erroneous findings.
  d. A positive test indicating dysfunction consists of a decrease in joint play on one or both sides and restriction of sacral motion.
2. Spring test
  a. The physician stands at the side of the table facing across the patient's body.
  b. The physician places his hands transversely across the patient's lumbar spine.
  c. Gentle pressure is exerted downward through the lumbar spine (Fig. 12-23).

Figure 12-21. Evaluation of medial malleoli, patient prone.

Figure 12-22. Sacral motion testing, patient prone.

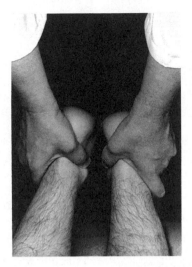
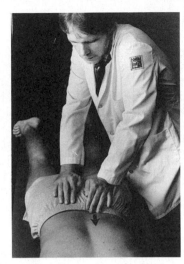

d. A positive test consists of a steel-like resistance to the exerted force. In a normal response some play is transmitted through the spine.

3. Sacral mobility, respiratory motion
   a. The physician stands at the side of the table facing across the table.
   b. The physician's cephalad hand is placed over the sacrum with the thenar and hypothenar eminences at the sacral base and the fingertips at the apex. The other hand is placed over the first hand. The physician should stand comfortably with elbows flexed (Fig. 12-24).
   c. The patient takes a deep breath. The sacral base moves posteriorly in response to inspiration.
   d. The physician monitors sacral motion during exhalation, with attention to asymmetric movement.

Figure 12-24. Test for sacral mobility during respiration.

Figure 12-23. Spring test, patient prone.

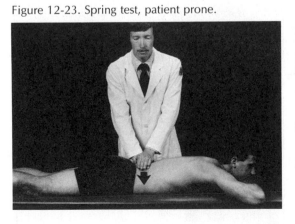
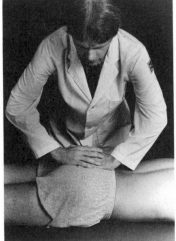

ILIOSACRAL SOMATIC DYSFUNCTION DIAGNOSIS
Michael J. DiGiovanna

Somatic dysfunction at the sacroiliac joint can occur through one of two general mechanisms. A force can be exerted on the sacroiliac joint cephalad through a lower extremity, in which case the dysfunction is termed *iliosacral*. The dysfunctional force can also be exerted on the sacroiliac joint caudad through the spine, in which case the dysfunction is termed *sacroiliac*. The dysfunctions considered in this section are related to the iliosacral mechanism of injury and therefore are dysfunctions of the ilium moving on the sacrum, whereby the sacrum becomes a fixed point.

Primary iliosacral somatic dysfunctions are classified according to a system in which dysfunction is defined as unopposed freedom of motion in one of the planes of motion of the ilia moving on the sacrum. The ilium moving on the sacrum produces anterior and posterior rotation of the ilium about a slightly oblique axis (posterior to anterior, medial to lateral) that passes approximately through the ipsilateral S2 vertebral foramen, a small amount of superior and inferior glide, and anterior and posterior glide along approximately sagittal planes. The dysfunctions that arise in ilial motion on the sacrum therefore are anterior and posterior rotation dysfunctions, and superior and inferior innominate shear dysfunctions.

One other problem that must be sought at the time of evaluation for iliosacral somatic dysfunction is the short leg syndrome. Although short leg syndrome may be of congenital, traumatic, or postoperative origin and thus not a true somatic dysfunction, it can cause a wide variety of iliosacral and sacroiliac somatic dysfunctions. The diagnostic tests used during the physical examination are similar to those used for iliosacral diagnosis, and may be employed here. These tests were described in the previous section.

Some iliosacral somatic dysfunctions are due to various injuries or chronic conditions. The shear phenomenon, specifically superior, has occasionally been related to falls in which the individual lands on one ischial tuberosity or leg. The upwardly directed force is sufficient to induce an iliosacral somatic dysfunction.

Determination of Iliosacral Somatic Dysfunction

The first step in the evaluation of iliosacral somatic dysfunction is to determine if such a dysfunction is present. The test used to determine the presence of iliosacral somatic dysfunction is the standing flexion test. This test was outlined earlier in this chapter (see Examination and Motion Testing). If positive, it should determine not only the presence of iliosacral somatic dysfunction but also the side of the dysfunction. Many of the tests described in this section can lead to one of two diagnoses; a positive standing flexion test will determine the side of the dysfunction.

If the iliac crests are of different height, the short leg syndrome should be considered, whether or not the standing flexion test is positive. If the anterior and posterior superior iliac spines (ASIS, PSIS) are more inferior on the same side as the inferior iliac crest, an even stronger suspicion of short leg syndrome should exist. Similar findings may be noted in cases of innominate shear.

A short leg can arise not only from differences in length between the femurs and tibias, but also from knee, ankle, and foot problems. Apparent differences in leg length may also be due to muscle imbalance, so a course of stretching and relaxation of the muscles likely to have an impact on leg length should be employed. In addition, ilial rotations may give rise to apparent leg length differences. These observations underscore the importance of correcting all somatic dysfunctions and musculoskeletal imbalances before diagnosing short leg syndrome. A more definitive diagnosis can be made with standing postural radiography. Treatment of short leg syndrome may be necessary to prevent further recurrence of existing iliosacral or sacroiliac somatic dysfunctions.

Criteria for Diagnosing Iliosacral Somatic Dysfunctions

1. Anterior ilial rotation
   a. PSIS: higher on involved side.
   b. ASIS: lower on involved side.

c. Sacral sulcus: appears shallower on ipsilateral side.
d. Standing flexion test: positive on ipsilateral side.
e. Leg may appear longer on ipsilateral side.
f. Sacral inferior lateral angles appear even.
2. Posterior ilial rotation
   a. PSIS: lower on involved side.
   b. ASIS: higher on involved side.
   c. Sacral sulcus: appears deeper on ipsilateral side.
   d. Standing flexion test: positive on ipsilateral side.
   e. Leg may appear shorter on ipsilateral side.
   f. Sacral inferior lateral angles appear even.
3. Superior innominate shear
   a. PSIS: higher on involved side.
   b. ASIS: higher on involved side.
   c. Sacral sulci: approximately equal depth.
   d. Standing flexion test: positive on ipsilateral side.
   e. Leg may appear shorter on ipsilateral side.
   f. Sacral inferior lateral angles appear even.
4. Inferior innominate shear
   a. PSIS: lower on involved side.
   b. ASIS: lower on involved side.
   c. Sacral sulci: approximately equal depth.
   d. Standing flexion test: positive on ipsilateral side.
   e. Leg may appear longer on ipsilateral side.
   f. Sacral inferior lateral angles appear even.

SACROILIAC SOMATIC DYSFUNCTION DIAGNOSIS
Michael J. DiGiovanna

The various methods of diagnosing sacroiliac somatic dysfunction can be categorized according to the physiologic motions of the sacroiliac articulation. These motions are the following:

1. **Flexion:** the sacral base moves anteriorly (Fig. 12-25A).
2. **Extension:** the sacral base moves posteriorly (Fig. 12-25C).
   Flexion and extension occur about an axis perpendicular to the sagittal plane.
3. **Rotation:** the sacrum rotates around a vertical axis perpendicular to the horizontal plane (Fig. 12-26).
4. **Lateral flexion:** the sacrum rotates around an anteroposterior axis perpendicular to the coronal plane (Fig. 12-27).
   Somatic dysfunction can occur in any one or a combination of these motions.
5. **Torsional motion** around diagonal axes, either forward or backward. By definition, a left diagonal axis runs from the superior end of the left articulation to the inferior end of the right articulation. A right diagonal axis runs from the superior end of the right articulation to the inferior end of the left articulation (Fig. 12-28).
   The sacrum may rotate forward on the left axis (left on left torsion) or backward (right on

left torsion). It may rotate forward on the right axis (right on right torsion) or backward (left on right torsion) (Fig. 12-29).

Diagnostic Test for Sacroiliac Somatic Dysfunctions
1. **Seated flexion test**
   a. **Interpretation:** The posterior superior iliac spine (PSIS) on the side of the dysfunction rises higher than the PSIS on the contralateral side. This test differentiates sacroiliac from iliosacral dysfunctions.
2. **Palpation of sacral sulci**
   a. **Interpretation:** The thumb that depresses further into the sacral sulcus indicates the side of the deep sacral sulcus.
3. **Palpation of inferior lateral angles (ILAs)**
   a. **Interpretation:** The side on which the physician's thumb is more posterior, according to palpation and visual observation, is the posterior inferior lateral angle. The more inferior ILA may be determined in similar fashion. Because of sacral biomechanics, the more posterior inferior lateral angle will also be the more inferior.
4. **Lumbar spring test:** Spring is defined as any amount of give in the forward direction, or as

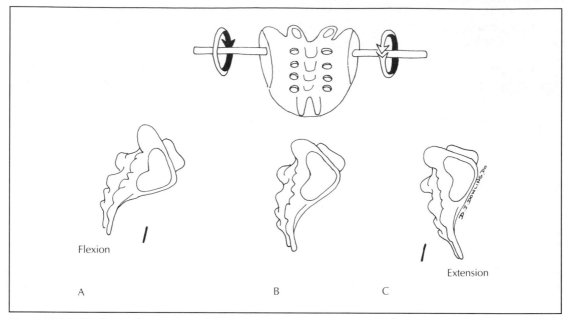

Figure 12-25. Flexion and extension of the sacrum. **(A)** Flexion, **(B)** neutral, **(C)** extension.

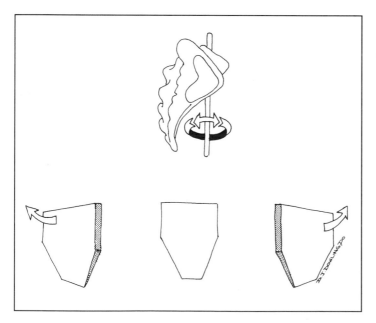

Figure 12-26. Rotation of the sacrum.

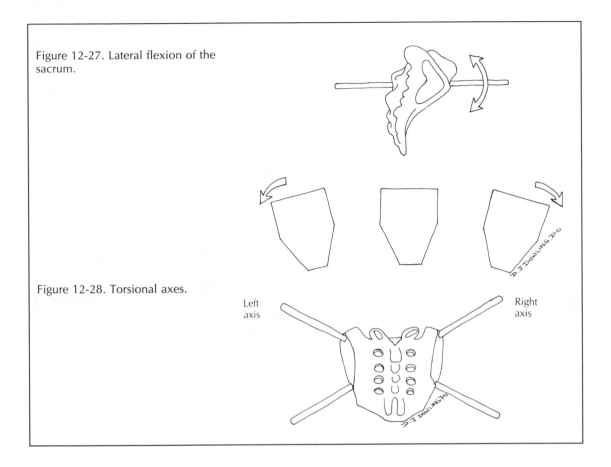

Figure 12-27. Lateral flexion of the sacrum.

Figure 12-28. Torsional axes.

the lumbar vertebrae moving into extension. A positive test result is defined as no spring in the lumbar spine in the setting of a backward sacral torsion.

Findings on the above tests are written down in the order in which the tests were performed. The findings can then be more easily used to adduce the somatic dysfunction.

Types of Dysfunctions
1. Forward sacral torsions (see Fig. 12-29A & D)
   a. Left on left sacral torsion
   b. Right on right sacral torsion
2. Backward sacral torsions (see Fig. 12-29B & C)
   a. Left on right sacral torsion
   b. Right on left sacral torsion
3. Unilateral sacral flexions
   a. Left unilateral sacral flexion
   b. Right unilateral sacral flexion

4. Bilateral sacral flexion dysfunction
5. Bilateral sacral extension dysfunction

To diagnose a sacral somatic dysfunction on this list, the physician must adhere to a particular set of criteria. These criteria will be described below in terms of the anatomic nature of the dysfunction that leads to the diagnostic findings.

SACRAL TORSION
Sacral torsions occur around an oblique axis (see Fig. 12-29). In naming a sacral torsion, the direction of rotation of the side of the sacral base that undergoes motion is designated first, followed by the axis around which the torsional motion occurs.

The direction of rotation on axis torsions may be forward or backward. A forward sacral torsion is either a left-on-left or a right-on-right sacral torsion. These are considered forward torsions in that one side of the sacral base moves anteriorly. In a

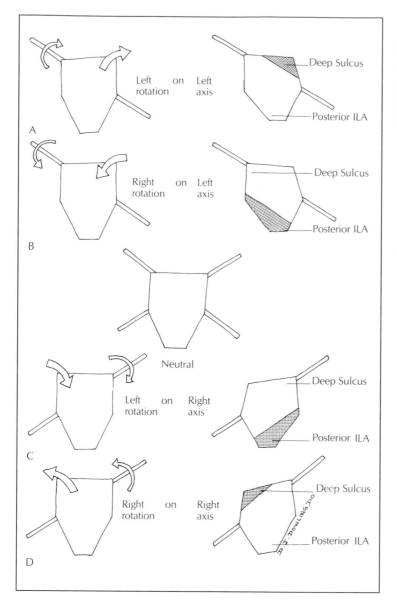

Figure 12-29. Sacral torsion. **(A)** Left rotation of sacrum on left oblique axis. **(B)** Right rotation of sacrum on left oblique axis. **(C)** Left rotation of sacrum on right oblique axis. **(D)** Right rotation of sacrum on right oblique axis.

backward sacral torsion, one side of the sacral base moves posteriorly, producing either a left-on-right or a right-on-left sacral torsion. In sacral torsions, the direction of rotation will cause a slight amount of side-bending in the same direction as rotation.

Forward Sacral Torsions
In forward sacral torsions, the sides of the deep sacral sulcus and the inferior/posterior inferior lateral angles are opposite and the lumbar spring test is negative (a good amount of spring is present in

the lumbar spine). Since the base of the sacrum is moving forward (anteriorly), no locking of the lumbar vertebrae occurs; hence the negative lumbar spring test.

1. **Left-on-left sacral torsion**
   Deep sulcus: right.
   PSIS: even.
   Inferior/posterior ILA: left
   Seated flexion test: positive right.
   Sacral restriction: right.

Figure 12-30. Unilateral sacral flexion.

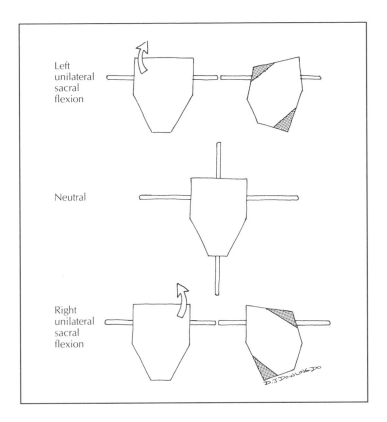

Sacral mobility: right base anterior and to the
  left.
2. **Right-on-right sacral torsion**
   Deep sulcus: left.
   PSIS: even.
   Inferior/posterior inferior lateral angle: right.
   Seated flexion test: positive left.
   Sacral restriction: left.
   Sacral mobility: left base anterior and to the
     right.

Backward Sacral Torsions
In backward sacral torsions the sides of the deep
sacral sulcus and the inferior/posterior inferior lateral angles are opposite and the lumbar spring test
is positive. There is little or no spring in the lumbar spine because of the locking that has occurred
with the sacral base moving backward and engaging the lumbar vertebrae.

1. **Left-on-right sacral torsion**
   PSIS: even.
   Deep sulcus: right.
   Inferior/posterior ILA: left.

Sacral restriction: left.
Sacral mobility: left base posterior and to the
  left.
2. **Right-on-left sacral torsion**
   PSIS: even.
   Deep sulcus: left.
   Inferior/posterior ILA: right.
   Seated flexion test: positive right.
   Sacral restriction: left.
   Sacral mobility: right base posterior and to the
     right.

UNILATERAL SACRAL FLEXIONS
In a unilateral sacral flexion the sacrum rotates
around a midsagittal axis, with side-bending occurring in the opposite direction. The side of the
deep sacral sulcus is ordinarily the same side as
the inferior/posterior inferior lateral angle. The
lumbar spring test is negative (good motion) (Fig.
12-30).

1. **Left unilateral sacral flexion**
   Deep sulcus: left.
   Inferior/posterior ILA: left.

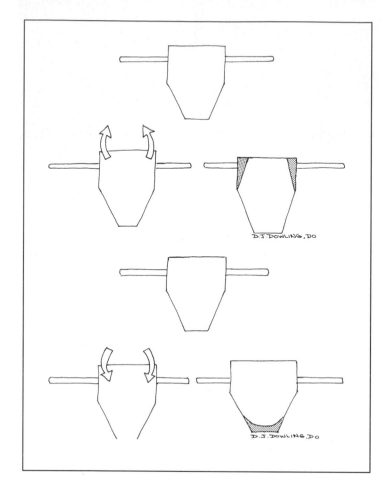

Figure 12-31. Bilateral sacral flexion dysfunction.

Figure 12-32. Bilateral sacral extension dysfunction.

Seated flexion test: positive left.
Sacral restriction: left.
Sacral mobility: left base anterior.

2. **Right unilateral sacral flexion**
   Deep sulcus: right.
   Inferior/posterior ILA: right.
   Seated flexion test: positive right.
   Sacral restriction: right.
   Sacral mobility: right base anterior.

BILATERAL SACRAL DYSFUNCTIONS

In bilateral sacral dysfunctions, the dysfunction occurs in one of the normal motions of the sacrum, flexion or extension. There is no difference in the depth of the sacral sulci or in the level of the inferior lateral angles. The amplitude of motion is de-creased in the direction opposite to the dysfunc-tion (Figs. 12-31, 12-32).

1. **Bilateral sacral flexion dysfunction**
   Sacral motion is decreased bilaterally on mo-tion testing.
   The sacrum flexes but is restricted in extension.
   The lumbar spring test is normal, since flexion (anterior motion) of the sacrum does not lock the lumbar vertebrae.
   Seated flexion is symmetrically positive.

2. **Bilateral sacral extension dysfunction**
   Sacral motion is decreased bilaterally on mo-tion testing.
   The lumbar spring test is positive, since exten-sion (backward motion) of the sacrum does lock the lumbar vertebrae.

PUBIC SOMATIC DYSFUNCTION DIAGNOSIS
Michael J. DiGiovanna

Somatic dysfunctions that occur at the pubic symphysis may be either primary pubic dysfunctions or secondary to ilial dysfunctions. Although pain is usually a poor indicator of dysfunction, the pubic symphysis is one area where pain is a fairly reliable indicator. Patients with primary or secondary pubic dysfunctions will present with midline groin pain. Other, nonmusculoskeletal causes of pain such as urinary tract infections and inguinal hernias must be ruled out.

Four dysfunctions are possible at the pubic symphysis: superior pubes, inferior pubes, abducted pubes, and adducted pubes. The last two dysfunctions are also known as an open pubic dysfunction and a closed pubic dysfunction, respectively. The distinction as to whether one pube is inferior or the other pube is superior is made on the standing flexion test. This test determines the side of the dysfunction, defined as the side on which the posterior superior iliac spine rides superiorly with trunk flexion.

Interpretation of Palpatory Findings

With the index finger in the midline over the pubic symphysis, the physician looks for the normal space between the pubic rami. If the space appears larger than normal, a pubic abduction (opened) dysfunction is present. If the space between the pubic rami appears narrower than normal, a pubic adduction (closed) dysfunction is present. Only through the experience of multiple palpations of pubic symphyses can appreciation of the normal width of the pubic symphysis be obtained.

With the index fingers on the pubic tubercles, the physician assesses the cephalic-caudal relationship of each to the other. The diagnosis is based on the results of the standing flexion test. If the standing flexion test is positive on one side and that same side appears to have a pubic ramus lower than the other, an inferior pubic dysfunction is present. Conversely, if a pubic ramus appears more cephalad on the same side as the standing flexion test, a superior pubic dysfunction is present.

References

Bourdillon JF. 1987. A torsion free approach to the pelvis. Manual Med 3(1):20–23.

Dowling DJ. 1985. An Illustrated Guide to OMT of the Neck and Trunk. Self-published.

Fryette HH. 1959. Principles of Osteopathic Technic. Carmel, CA: Academy of Applied Osteopathy.

Greenman PE. 1986. Innominate shear dysfunction in the sacroiliac syndrome. Manual Med 2:114–121.

Kapandji IA. 1974. The Physiology of the Joints. Vol III. The Trunk and Vertebral Column. New York: Churchill Livingstone.

Kappler, R. 1975. Lecture notes. Chicago: College of Osteopathic Medicine.

Kennedy, Hall. 1975. Unilateral sacroiliac dysfunction. 1975 Yearbook of Selected Osteopathic Papers. Ed: Ruth Hewitt. Colorado Springs: American Academy of Osteopathy.

Kidd R. 1988. Pain localization with the innominate up slip dysfunction. Manual Med 3(3):103–105.

Larson NJ. 1984. Physiologic movement of the Sacrum. Read before the Chicago College of Osteopathic Medicine, February 1984.

Mitchell FL. 1965. Structural pelvic function. 1965 Year Book of Selected Osteopathic Papers, Vol II. pp 178–199. M. Barnes, Ed. Carmel, Calif: Academy of Applied Osteopathy.

Mitchell FL Jr, Moran PS, Pruzzo NT. 1979. An Evaluation and Treatment Manual of Osteopathic Muscle Energy Procedures. Valley Park, Mo: Mitchell, Moran, and Pruzzo Associates.

Moore KL. 1980. Clinically Oriented Anatomy. Baltimore: Williams & Wilkins.

Northup TL. 1943. Sacroiliac lesions primary & secondary. Academy of Applied Osteopathy Year Book. 1943–44, pp 53–54. Ann Arbor: Academy of Applied Osteopathy.

Schiowitz S, DiGiovanna EL, Ausman PJ. 1983. An Osteopathic Approach to Diagnosis and Treatment. Old Westbury, NY: New York College of Osteopathic Medicine.

Schwab WA. 1965. Principles of manipulative treatment: The low back problems. Academy of Applied Osteopathy 1965 Yearbook of Selected Osteopathic Papers, Vol II, pp 65–69. M. Barnes, Ed. Carmel, Calif: Academy of Applied Osteopathy.

Sutherland WG. 1936. The Cranial Bowl. Mankato, MN: Free Press.

Warwick R, Williams PL. 1973. Gray's Anatomy, 35th British Edition. Philadelphia: W.B. Saunders.

13

Treating Dysfunctions of the Innominate

MUSCLE ENERGY TECHNIQUES FOR ILIAC DYSFUNCTIONS

Lisa R. Chun

This section describes muscle energy techniques for anterior and posterior iliac dysfunctions and for superior and inferior innominate shear.

Anterior Iliac Dysfunction

1. **Patient position:** prone; the hip and knee on the ipsilateral side of the dysfunction are flexed and hanging off the edge of the table.
2. **Physician position:** standing on the same side of the table as the dysfunction, facing the patient. The physician supports the patient's flexed leg by placing the sole of the patient's foot against the physician's extended leg.
3. **Hand position:** one hand monitors the dysfunctional sacroiliac joint while also stabilizing the sacrum. The other hand grasps and supports the patient's flexed knee.
4. **Technique:**
   a. The physician flexes both the hip and the leg on the side of the dysfunction until motion is felt at the sacroiliac joint. This position is maintained by the physician.
   b. The patient is instructed to attempt to straighten the flexed leg by pushing the sole

of the foot into the physician's extended leg, using 5 to 10 pounds of force.
   c. The physician resists this motion, causing an isometric contraction (Fig. 13-1).
   d. After 3 to 5 seconds, the patient is instructed to stop the attempt and relax.
   e. The physician allows the patient to relax, while supporting the lower extremity.
   f. Once the tissue under the monitoring finger is relaxed, the physician engages the new motion barrier by flexing both the hip and the leg on the dysfunctional side until motion is felt at the involved sacroiliac joint.
   g. Repeat steps b through f twice more.
   h. The physician places the flexed lower extremity into a neutral midline position.
   i. The physician reevaluates the dysfunction.
   j. Treatment may be repeated if indicated.

Posterior Iliac Dysfunction

1. **Patient position:** prone, with extended lower extremities on the table.
2. **Physician position:** standing on the side of the table opposite the dysfunction, facing the patient.

An Osteopathic Approach to Diagnosis and Treatment, second edition
Eileen L. DiGiovanna and Stanley Schiowitz
Lippincott–Raven Publishers, Philadelphia © 1997.

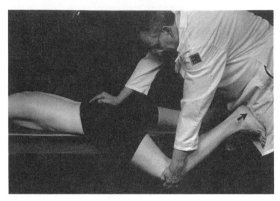

Figure 13-1. Muscle energy technique for anterior iliac dysfunction, patient prone.

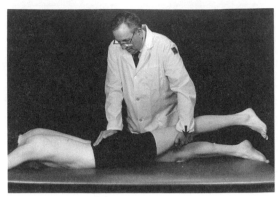

Figure 13-2. Muscle energy technique for posterior iliac dysfunction, patient prone.

3. **Hand position:** cephalic hand monitors the dysfunctional sacroiliac joint while stabilizing the patient's ilium. The caudal hand grasps the patient's leg above the knee on the dysfunctional side.
4. **Technique:**
   a. The physician engages the restricted motion barrier by extending the lower extremity on the dysfunctional side until motion is felt at the sacroiliac joint.
   b. The physician maintains this position.
   c. The patient is instructed to attempt to bring the extended lower extremity down toward the table, using 5 to 10 pounds of force.
   d. The physician resists this motion, causing an isometric contraction (Fig. 13-2).
   e. After 3 to 5 seconds, the patient is instructed to stop the attempt and to relax.
   f. The physician allows the patient to relax while maintaining the extension of the lower extremity.
   g. Once tissue of the sacroiliac joint is felt to loosen, the physician engages the new motion barrier by repositioning the involved lower extremity into extension until motion is felt at the dysfunctional sacroiliac joint.
   h. Steps b through g are repeated twice more.
   i. The physician places the extended lower extremity into a neutral midline position.
   j. The physician reevaluates the status of the dysfunction.
   k. Treatment may be repeated if indicated.

Superior Innominate Shear

1. **Patient position:** supine, with lower extremities extended and resting on the table.
2. **Physician position:** standing at the foot of the table, facing the patient.
3. **Hand position:** both hands grasping the distal portions of the tibia and fibula on the side of the dysfunction proximal to the ankle joint.
4. **Technique:**
   a. The physician abducts and extends the involved lower extremity until the loose-packed position of the sacroiliac joint is identified.
   b. The physician maintains this position.
   c. The physician internally rotates the involved lower limb until a close-packed position of the hip joint is felt by the physician.
   d. The physician applies a continuous long axis traction on the involved lower limb while maintaining the lower limb in extension, abduction, and internal rotation (Fig. 13-3).
   e. The patient is instructed to breathe deeply three or four times while the physician maintains traction on the lower limb position.
   f. After three or four complete respirations, the patient is instructed to cough forcibly, at which time the physician tugs sharply along the long axis of the involved limb.
   g. The physician places the involved limb into a neutral midline position.
   h. The physician reevaluates the status of the dysfunction.
   i. Treatment may be repeated if indicated.

Figure 13-3. Muscle energy technique for superior innominate shear.

Figure 13-4. Muscle energy technique for inferior innominate shear.

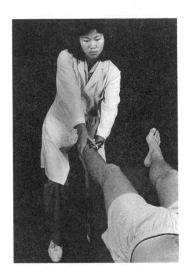
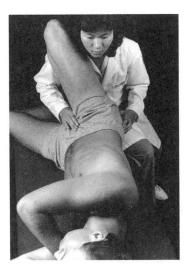

Inferior Innominate Shear

1. **Patient position:** lateral recumbent, with dysfunctional side up. The ipsilateral lower extremity, as the dysfunction, is flexed and placed on the physician's shoulder.
2. **Physician position:** sitting on the table behind the patient.
3. **Hand position:** one hand placed on both the pubic and ischial rami of the dysfunctional side, the other hand placed on both the ischial tuberosity and the posterior inferior iliac spine of the dysfunctional side.
4. **Technique:**
   a. With the patient relaxed, the physician laterally distracts the innominate bone.
   b. Maintaining this position, the physician then applies a cephalad force upon the pubic and ischial rami, ischial tuberosity, and posterior

inferior iliac spine of the dysfunctional side (Fig. 13-4).
   c. The physician then instructs the patient to inhale deeply and exhale completely.
   d. The physician maintains the cephalad force on the distracted innominate during the inspiratory phase of the patient's respiratory cycle.
   e. During the expiratory phase of the patient's respiratory cycle, the physician increases the cephalad force on the distracted innominate.
   f. Steps c through e are repeated twice more.
   g. The physician slowly releases the innominate and positions the patient's involved leg into a neutral midline position.
   h. The physician reevaluates the status of the dysfunction.
   i. Treatment may be repeated if indicated.

HIGH-VELOCITY, LOW-AMPLITUDE THRUSTING TECHNIQUES FOR ILIAC DYSFUNCTIONS
Barry S. Erner

This section describes high-velocity, low-amplitude thrusting techniques for dysfunctions of the posterior and anterior iliac. The patient assumes a lateral recumbent position with the side of dysfunction facing up or down.

Posterior Ilial Somatic Dysfunction

1. **Patient position:** lateral recumbent position with somatic dysfunctional side facing up.
2. **Physician position:** standing, facing the front of the patient.
3. **Technique:**
   a. The physician flexes the hip/knee of the patient's superior leg until motion is felt at the lumbosacral angle, then places the foot of this flexed leg in the popliteal fossa of the inferior leg.
   b. Using the patient's lower arm, the physician rotates the patient's torso away from the table until all spinal rotation up to the lumbosacral angle is removed.
   c. The physician places his other forearm over the patient's superior ilium.
   d. The physician exerts a rapid rotational for-

ward thrust through the dysfunctional ilium (Fig. 13-5).

Anterior Ilial Somatic Dysfunction

1. **Patient position:** lateral recumbent position with somatic dysfunction side up.
2. **Physician position:** standing, facing the front of the patient.
3. **Technique:**
   a. The physician flexes the hip of the patient's superior leg until motion is felt at the lumbosacral angle. This leg is then dropped off the table.
   b. The physician rotates the patient's torso by pulling on the lower arm until all spinal rotation up to the lumbosacral angle is removed, then maintains this position with his cephalad arm.
   c. The physician places the forearm of his caudal arm over the patient's inferior iliac crest.
   d. The physician exerts a rapid, rotational, slightly downward thrust through the dysfunctional ilium following the long axis of the femur (Fig. 13-6).

Figure 13-5. High-velocity, low-amplitude thrusting technique for a posterior ilial somatic dysfunction.

Figure 13-6. High-velocity, low-amplitude thrusting technique for an anterior ilial somatic dysfunction.

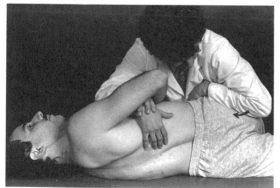

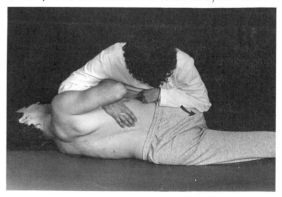

MUSCLE ENERGY TECHNIQUES FOR PUBIC DYSFUNCTIONS
Lisa R. Chun

This section describes muscle energy techniques for treating somatic dysfunctions of the pubes (inferior and superior), and for open (abduction) and closed (adduction) pubic dysfunctions. The patient begins each treatment supine, often with the hips and knees flexed.

Inferior Pubic Dysfunction
1. **Patient position:** supine; hip and leg on the side of the dysfunction are flexed.
2. **Physician position:** sitting on or standing at the same side of the table as the dysfunction, facing the patient.
3. **Hand position:** monitoring finger on the anterior superior iliac spine of the dysfunctional side, other hand placed in a fist (palm up) on the ischial tuberosity of the dysfunctional side. The fist also rests on the table.
4. **Technique:**
   a. The physician places the patient's flexed knee onto the anterior aspect of her shoulder.
   b. The physician flexes the patient's involved hip until motion is felt at the monitoring finger.
   c. The patient is instructed to attempt to straighten the flexed hip using 5 to 10 pounds of force.
   d. The physician resists this force, creating static contraction, while applying a cephalic force on the involved ischial tuberosity with the fist (Fig. 13-7).
   e. After 3 to 5 seconds, the patient is instructed to discontinue the attempt and to relax.
   f. The physician allows the patient to relax, while maintaining both hip flexion and the cephalic force at the ischial tuberosity.
   g. Once the tissue under the physician's monitoring finger is felt to relax, the physician engages the new restricted motion barrier by repositioning the involved hip into flexion until motion is felt under the monitoring finger.
   h. Steps c through g are repeated twice more.
   i. The physician places the flexed lower extremity into a neutral, midline position.
   j. The physician reevaluates the status of the dysfunction.
   k. Treatment may be repeated if indicated.

Figure 13-7. Muscle energy technique for inferior pubic dysfunction.

Figure 13-8. Muscle energy technique for superior pubic dysfunction.

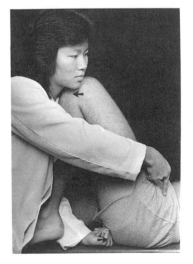
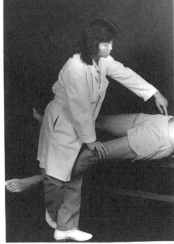

Superior Pubic Dysfunction

1. **Patient position:** supine, lower extremity on side of the dysfunctional side extended and hanging off the edge of the table.
2. **Physician position:** standing on the same side of the table as the dysfunction, facing the patient. The physician's legs are used to support the patient's hanging leg.
3. **Hand position:** monitoring finger on the anterior superior iliac spine contralateral to the dysfunctional side, other hand on the thigh of the patient's hanging leg.
4. **Technique:**
   a. The physician extends the patient's involved side of the pelvis by pressing down on the patient's thigh.
   b. This extension is created only until motion is felt under the monitoring finger.
   c. The patient is instructed to attempt to raise the extended leg to the ceiling using 5 to 10 pounds of force.
   d. The physician resists this force, creating an isometric contraction (Fig. 13-8).
   e. After 3 to 5 seconds, the patient is instructed to stop the attempt and to relax.
   f. The physician allows the patient to relax, while maintaining the same degree of hip extension.
   g. Once the tissue under the monitoring finger is felt to loosen, the physician engages the new motion barrier by repositioning the involved hip into extension until motion is felt under the monitoring finger.
   h. Steps c through g are repeated twice more.
   i. The physician places the extended hip into a neutral position.
   j. The physician reevaluates the status of the dysfunction.
   k. Treatment may be repeated if indicated.

Abduction (Open) Pubic Dysfunction

1. **Patient position:** supine, hips flexed and knees flexed to 90 degrees; lying closer to one side of the table than the other.

2. **Physician position:** standing at the side of the table to which patient is closest and facing the patient.
3. **Technique:**
   a. The physician wraps her arms around the patient's flexed knees and draws them against herself.
   b. The patient is instructed to attempt to spread his knees apart with maximal force.
   c. The physician resists this force, creating static contraction.
   d. After 3 to 5 seconds, the patient is instructed to relax.
   e. The physician allows the patient to relax, while maintaining the position attained.
   f. Steps b through e are repeated twice more.
   g. The physician reevaluates the status of the dysfunction.
   h. Treatment may be repeated if indicated.

Adduction (Closed) Pubic Dysfunction

1. **Patient position:** supine, hips flexed and knees flexed to 90 degrees.
2. **Physician position:** standing at the side of the table facing the patient.
3. **Hand position:** the physician's forearm is placed between the patient's knees. One hand is on the medial aspect of one of the patient's knees, with the elbow joint on the medial aspect of the other knee.
4. **Technique:**
   a. The patient is instructed to attempt to bring his knees together with a maximal force.
   b. The physician's forearm resists this attempt by acting as a solid bar.
   c. After 3 to 5 seconds, the patient is instructed to relax.
   d. The physician allows the patient to relax while maintaining the position attained.
   e. Steps a through d are repeated twice more.
   f. The physician reevaluates the status of the dysfunction.
   g. Treatment may be repeated if indicated.

HIGH-VELOCITY, LOW-AMPLITUDE THRUSTING TECHNIQUES FOR PUBIC DYSFUNCTIONS

Barry S. Erner

This section describes high-velocity, low-amplitude (HVLA) thrusting techniques for treating a superior position of the pubic tubercle and pubic restriction.

Superior Pubes

1. **Patient position:** supine.
2. **Physician position:** standing at the side of the table, on the same side as the dysfunction.
3. **Technique:**
   a. The physician flexes the patient's knee/hip on the side of the dysfunction and rests the patient's ankle/calf on his shoulder.
   b. The physician makes a tight fist with his treating hand.
   c. The physician places his fist against the ischial tuberosity on the side of the pubic dysfunction.
   d. The physician exerts a rapid cephalad/clockwise thrust through the ischium (Fig. 13-9).

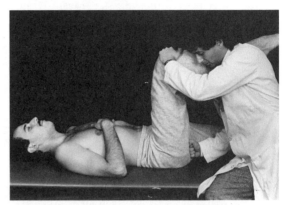

Figure 13-9. HVLA treatment for a superior pubic dysfunction.

Alternate Technique to Treat Pubic Restriction

1. **Patient position:** supine.
2. **Physician position:** standing at the side of the table.
3. **Technique:**
   a. The physician flexes, abducts, and externally rotates the patient's legs bilaterally.
   b. The patient's feet are placed with the soles approximated.
   c. The physician exerts a quick downward thrust through the patient's knees bilaterally, symmetrically, and simultaneously (Fig. 13-10).

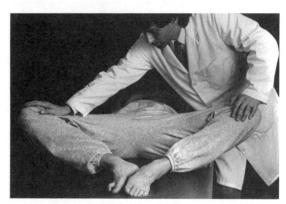

Figure 13-10. An alternate HVLA treatment technique for pubic restriction.

References

Greenman PE. 1986. Innominate shear dysfunction in the sacroiliac syndrome. Manual Med 2:114–121.

Schiowitz S, DiGiovanna E, Ausman P. 1983. An Osteopathic Approach to Diagnosis and Treatment. Old Westbury, NY: New York College of Osteopathic Medicine of the New York Institute of Technology.

14 Treating Sacral Dysfunctions

MUSCLE ENERGY TECHNIQUES
Lisa R. Chun

This section describes muscle energy techniques for unilateral sacral flexion dysfunctions and dysfunctions of forward and backward sacral torsion.

Unilateral Sacral Flexion Dysfunction

1. **Patient position:** prone, arms hanging off the sides of the table.
2. **Physician position:** standing at the same side of the table as the dysfunction.
3. **Hand position:** the heel of the caudal hand is on the caudal edge of the inferior lateral angle (ILA) of the sacrum on the side to be treated. The middle or index finger of that hand is placed in the sacral sulcus.
4. **Technique:**
   a. The physician abducts the lower extremity of the involved side until motion is felt at the sacral sulcus being monitored.
   b. The physician maintains the abduction while introducing internal rotation.
   c. Internal rotation is continued until motion is felt at the sacral sulcus being monitored. This position of abduction and internal rotation is maintained.
   d. Using the hand on the patient's sacrum and

an extended elbow, the physician applies a constant force at the posterior inferior lateral angle down toward the table and cephalad (Fig. 14-1). The force applied is more cephalad.
   e. The patient is instructed to inhale deeply and to hold his breath.
   f. The physician increases the pressure on the inferior lateral angle during the inspiratory phase.
   g. The patient is instructed to exhale completely.
   h. The physician maintains the cephalad force on the posterior inferior lateral angle during the expiratory phase.
   i. Steps e through h are repeated twice more.
   j. At the end of the last expiratory phase, an additional cephalad thrust may be provided by the physician on the posterior inferior lateral angle.
   k. The physician places the abducted and internally rotated leg into a neutral midline position.
   l. The physician reevaluates the status of the dysfunction.
   m. Treatment may be repeated if indicated.

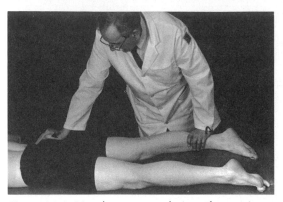

Figure 14-1. Muscle energy technique for treating unilateral sacral flexion dysfunction.

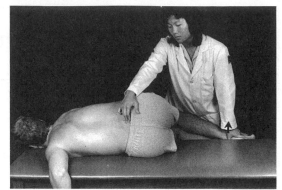

Figure 14-2. Muscle energy technique for treating forward sacral torsion dysfunction.

Forward Sacral Torsion Dysfunction

1. **Patient position:** Sims position (lateral recumbent position with upper torso prone and hips and knees flexed), with the axis of the dysfunction down toward the table. The patient's arms hang off the sides of the table.
2. **Physician position:** standing at the side of the table facing the patient.
3. **Hand position:** monitoring finger(s) at the lumbosacral junction. The other hand is used to engage the motion barriers. To facilitate engagement of the restricted motion barriers, the hand monitoring the lumbosacral junction is switched.
4. **Technique:**
   a. The physician flexes the patient's hips until motion is felt at the lumbosacral junction.
   b. The physician maintains this position by leaning into the patient's knees.
   c. The patient is instructed to inhale deeply and exhale completely. During the exhalation, the patient is instructed to reach for the floor with the upper arm.
   d. The physician assists the patient in this rotational move by pressing the patient's shoulder toward the floor until motion is felt at the lumbosacral junction.
   e. To achieve rotation, steps c and d may have to be repeated.
   f. Once rotational motion is felt at the monitoring finger(s), the side-bending component of the treatment is engaged by lowering the feet off the table.
   g. While maintaining flexion, the physician,

using the patient's knees as a fulcrum, applies downward pressure on the patient's ankle (Fig. 14-2).
   h. The patient's lower legs may have to be sidebent over the edge of the table.
   i. Once motion is felt at the lumbosacral junction, the position is maintained.
   j. The patient is instructed to attempt to raise his ankles to the ceiling using 5 to 10 pounds of force.
   k. The physician isometrically resists this attempt.
   l. After 3 to 5 seconds, the patient is instructed to stop the attempt and to relax.
   m. Once the tissue of the lumbosacral junction is felt to loosen, the physician reengages the restricted motion barriers by repeating steps c through j.
   n. Repeat steps k through m twice more.
   o. The physician places the patient into a neutral position.
   p. The physician reevaluates the status of the dysfunction.
   q. Treatment may be repeated if indicated.

Backward Sacral Torsion Dysfunction

1. **Patient position:** lateral recumbent position with the axis of the dysfunction down toward the table; knees flexed.
2. **Physician position:** standing at the side of the table facing the patient's anterior.
3. **Hand position:** monitoring finger at the lumbosacral junction. The other hand is used to en-

gage the restricted motion barriers. To facilitate engagement of the restricted motion barriers, the hand monitoring the lumbosacral junction is switched during the procedure.

4. **Technique:**
   a. The physician flexes the patient's hips and knees until motion is felt at the monitoring finger(s).
   b. The physician maintains this position by leaning into the patient's upper knee.
   c. The patient is instructed to straighten his lower leg.
   d. The physician hooks the foot of the patient's upper leg onto the straightened lower leg.
   e. While still leaning on the patient's upper knee, the physician moves the patient's lower thigh into extension.
   f. Hip extension is continued until motion is felt at the lumbosacral junction.
   g. The physician maintains this position by placing the forearm of her monitoring hand on the patient's hip.
   h. The physician grasps the lower arm, on which the patient is lying, and pulls directly up toward the ceiling, thereby rotating the patient's torso backward.
   i. The patient is then instructed to reach his top arm behind him and grasp the edge of the table.
   j. The patient is instructed to inhale deeply.
   k. The patient is instructed to exhale completely and simultaneously to reach down the edge of the table. At the end of the exhalation, the patient grasps the edge of the table.
   l. The physician may facilitate this motion by pressing the patient's upper shoulder back toward the table and caudad while the patient is exhaling.
   m. For this rotation motion to be felt at the lumbosacral junction, steps k and l may have to be repeated. This is continued only until motion is felt at the monitoring fingers. Once motion is felt, the position is maintained.
   n. The physician lowers the patient's upper leg below the table until motion is felt at the lumbosacral junction.
   o. Once motion is felt, this position is maintained.
   p. The patient is instructed to attempt to bring the ankles toward the ceiling using 5 to 10 pounds of force.
   q. The physician isometrically resists this attempt.
   r. After 3 to 5 seconds, the patient is instructed to stop the attempt and to relax.
   s. The physician allows the patient to relax while maintaining the above position.
   t. Once the tissue at the lumbosacral junction is felt to loosen, the physician reengages the restricted motion barriers by repeating steps j through o.
   u. Steps p through t are repeated twice more.
   v. The physician places the patient into a neutral position.
   w. The physician reevaluates the status of the dysfunction.
   x. Treatment may be repeated if indicated.

TECHNIQUE MODIFICATION: BACKWARD SACRAL TORSION DYSFUNCTION

1. **Patient position:** as above.
2. **Physician position:** as above.
3. **Technique:**
   a. Steps a through m in the above technique are performed.
   b. The patient is instructed to attempt to push his flexed knee up to the ceiling using 5 to 10 pounds of force.
   c. The physician isometrically resists this attempt with her hand on the side of the patient's flexed knee. The physician should feel a contraction under her monitoring fingers. If no contraction is felt, the physician repositions the involved hip and knee using flexion or extension. Once a contraction is felt by the monitoring fingers, the treatment has been localized to the lumbosacral junction.
   d. After 3 to 5 seconds, the patient is instructed to stop the attempt and to relax the involved lower extremity while maintaining the above position.
   e. Once the tissue at the lumbosacral junction is felt to loosen, the physician reengages the restricted motion barriers by repeating steps j through m of the previous test.
   f. Steps b through e of this section are repeated twice more.
   g. The physician places the patient into neutral position.
   h. The physician reevaluates the status of the dysfunction.
   i. Treatment may be repeated if indicated.

COUNTERSTRAIN TECHNIQUES FOR THE SACRUM AND PELVIS
Eileen L. DiGiovanna

Anterior Tender Points

There are three significant tender points generally related to the pelvis or sacrum: the low ilium sacroiliac anterior sacral tender point, located on the superior surface of the ramus of the pubes; the iliacus tender point, located in the lower quadrant of the abdomen and deep in the fossa (often a tender point of concern in dysmenorrhagic women); and the inguinal ligament tender point, located on the inguinal ligament at its attachment to the pubes (Fig. 14-3). Techniques for treating each of these tender points are described below.

LOW ILIUM SACROILIAC ANTERIOR SACRAL
TENDER POINT
1. **Patient position:** supine.

2. **Physician position:** standing at either side of the table.
3. **Technique:**
   a. The thigh is flexed to about 40 degrees.
   b. Both thighs may be flexed with the legs resting on the physician's thigh, as in the treatment of the lumbar tender point (Fig. 14-4).

ILIACUS TENDER POINT
1. **Patient position:** supine.
2. **Physician position:** standing at the side of the table near the tender point, with one foot on the table.
3. **Technique:**
   a. Both of the patient's legs are flexed with the legs resting on the physician's thigh.

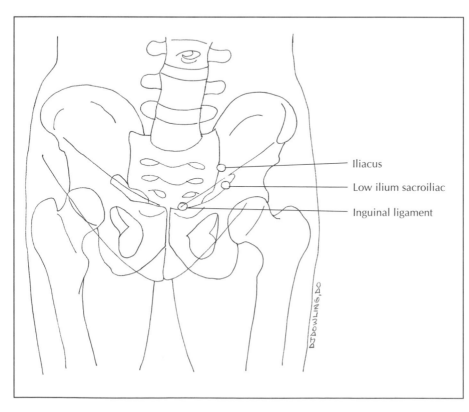

Figure 14-3.
Anterior pelvic
tender points.

Iliacus

Low ilium sacroiliac

Inguinal ligament

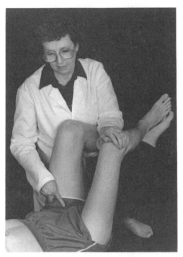

Figure 14-4. Counterstrain treatment for low ilium sacroiliac anterior sacral tender point.

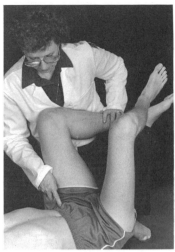

Figure 14-5. Counterstrain treatment for an iliacus tender point.

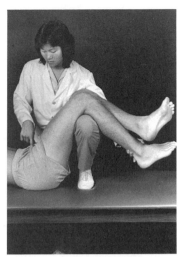

Figure 14-6. Counterstrain treatment for an inguinal ligament tender point.

   b. The ankles are crossed and the knees are dropped apart. This motion externally rotates the thighs (Fig. 14-5).

INGUINAL LIGAMENT TENDER POINT
1. **Patient position:** supine.
2. **Physician position:** standing at the side of the table opposite the tender point, with her foot on the table.
3. **Technique:**
   a. The patient's legs are flexed and rested on the physician's thigh.
   b. The leg nearest the physician is crossed at the knee over the further leg.
   c. The lower leg is internally rotated by the physician pushing laterally on the ankle (Fig. 14-6).

Posterior Tender Points
The locations of the posterior tender points are shown in Figure 14-7.

PIRIFORMIS TENDER POINT
This is the tender point most commonly associated with sacral dysfunctions and is frequently involved in sciatic radiation of pain because of its close association with the sciatic nerve. It is located in the muscle body.

1. **Patient position:** prone, with involved leg dropped off the side of the table.
2. **Physician position:** seated at the side of the dysfunction.
3. **Technique:**
   a. The patient's hip and knee are flexed.
   b. The leg is externally rotated and abducted, and may be rested on the physician's lap (Fig. 14-8).
   c. The movement of flexion and external rotation may be modified to achieve maximal softening of the piriformis.

MIDPOLE SACRAL TENDER POINT
This tender point is palpated by pushing medially on the lateral side of the sacrum at the midpoint between the posterior superior iliac spine (PSIS) and apex.

1. **Patient position:** prone.
2. **Physician position:** standing or sitting at the side of the table next to the tender point.
3. **Technique:**
   a. The leg is abducted straight laterally.

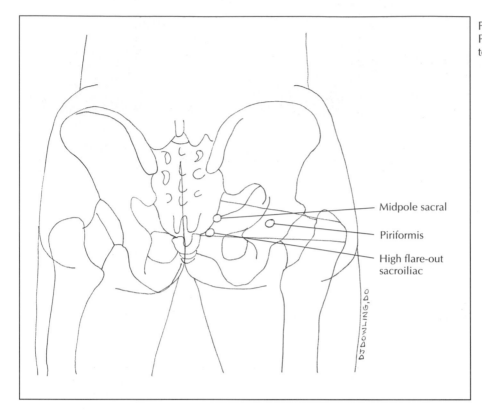

Figure 14-7.
Posterior pelvic
tender points.

Midpole sacral

Piriformis

High flare-out
sacroiliac

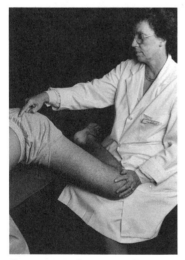

Figure 14-8. Counterstrain
treatment for a piriformis tender
point.

b. Occasionally the thigh must be extended or flexed, although this is not usual (Fig. 14-9).

HIGH FLARE-OUT SACROILIAC
TENDER POINT

This tender point, about 4 inches below and medial to the PSIS, is frequently associated with coccygodynia.

1. **Patient position:** prone.
2. **Physician position:** standing at the side of the table.
3. **Technique:**
    a. The leg nearest the tender point is extended (Fig. 14-10).
    b. Some adduction may be needed, and occasionally external rotation of the thigh is needed. This may be accomplished by standing on the side opposite the tender point, reaching across the thigh, adducting, and externally rotating while extending the leg.

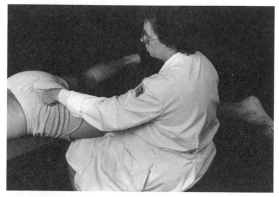

Figure 14-9. Counterstrain treatment for a midpole sacral tender point.

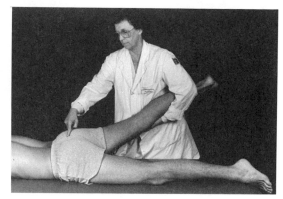

Figure 14-10. Counterstrain treatment for a high flare-out sacroiliac tender point.

HIGH-VELOCITY, LOW-AMPLITUDE THRUSTING TECHNIQUES

Barry S. Erner
Dennis J. Dowling

Anterior Sacral Flexion

1. **Patient position:** prone.
2. **Physician position:** standing at the same side of the table as the side of the dysfunction.
3. **Technique:**
   a. The physician places the thenar eminence of his treating hand over the inferior lateral angle of the dysfunctional side of the sacrum.
   b. The physician extends and internally rotates the patient's leg on the side of the dysfunction. The leg is then abducted until motion is felt by the palpating hand.
   c. The patient is instructed to take a deep breath and hold it.
   d. The physician exerts a downward pressure over the sacrum at the inferior lateral angle, creating relative extension.
   e. At the end of inspiration, the physician exerts a quick downward thrust with his thenar eminence over the inferior lateral angle (Fig. 14-11).

Anterior Sacral Flexion/Sacral Torsion

1. **Patient position:** supine.
2. **Physician position:** standing on the same side as the sacral deep sulcus.

Figure 14-11. High-velocity, low-amplitude thrusting technique for anterior sacral flexion dysfunction.

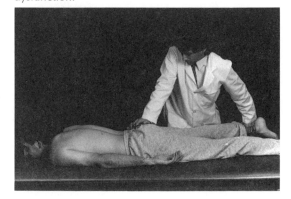

3. **Technique:**
   a. The physician side-bends the patient's legs away from the deep sulcus side.
   b. The physician side-bends the patient's torso away from the deep sulcus side. (The patient is now in a "C" position. Both the physician and the deep sulcus are at the apex.)
   c. The patient is instructed to clasp his hands behind his neck.
   d. The physician places the thenar eminence of his caudad hand on the patient's anterior superior iliac spine (ASIS) on the side opposite to the deep sulcus.
   e. The physician places his cephalad hand over the patient's opposite shoulder. (The hand can be placed over this arm and then between the forearm and upper arm with the back of the physician's hand resting on the patient's sternum.)
   f. To help stabilize the patient, the physician may place his cephalad knee next to the patient's shoulder.

   g. The physician uses his cephalad hand to rotate the patient toward the physician.
   h. The physician's hand holds the patient's ASIS and resists its tendency to lift from the table during the rotation.
   i. The rotation can be timed with exhalation by the patient.

References

Greenman PE. 1986. Innominate shear dysfunction in the sacroiliac syndrome. Manual Med 2:114–121.

Jones L. 1981. Strain and Counterstrain. Colorado Springs: American Academy of Osteopathy.

Moran PS, Pruzzo NA, et al. 1973. An Evaluation and Treatment Manual of Osteopathic Manipulative Procedures. Vol I. The Postural Structural Model. Kansas City: Institute for Continuing Education in Osteopathic Principles.

Schiowitz S, DiGiovanna E, Ausman P. 1983. An Osteopathic Approach to Diagnosis and Treatment. Old Westbury, N.Y.: New York College of Osteopathic Medicine of the New York Institute of Technology.

15

Locomotion and Balance

THE FUNCTIONAL, BIOMECHANICAL, AND CLINICAL SIGNIFICANCE OF GAIT

Stanley Schiowitz

The first scientific observations of gait were probably made by Hippocrates and Aristotle. As clinicians, we continue that tradition by observing patients walking every day and by selecting certain characteristics for assessment.

The examiner focuses on asymmetric movement while viewing the patient from the front, side, or back. Asymmetric movements are characterized by reduced or excessive displacements or by a change in the speed of movement during parts of the gait cycle. Asynchronous movement in the sagittal plane is best observed from the side, and coronal plane dysfunction is best observed from the front or rear.

To use gait fully as a diagnostic tool, the clinician should be aware of the patient's normal gait parameters—his usual speed, step length, and step rate. A variation in any one of these parameters will affect the others.

Kinematics of Gait

Physiologic, efficient locomotion entails translation of the body's center of gravity through space along a path requiring the least expenditure of energy. The center of gravity is constantly being dis-

placed beyond the body's base of support. The resulting loss of balance is corrected by moving one lower extremity forward to change the base of support. Repetition of this pattern on alternating legs creates the walking cycle.

The normal walking cycle is divided into two phases—stance phase, when the foot is on the ground, and swing phase, when it is moving forward. Sixty percent of the normal cycle is spent in stance phase. Of this 60%, 25% is in double stance. The remaining 40% of the walking cycle is in swing phase.

Stance phase is divided into the following segments: heel strike, foot flat, midstance, and push-off or toe-off. Swing phase is divided into acceleration, midswing, and deceleration.

The average width of the base of gait, as measured from heel to heel, is between 2 and 4 inches. The average length of a step is 15 inches, with a cadence of 90 to 120 steps per minute. The feet are usually in slight abduction.

The forces acting in gait are gravity, muscle contraction, and momentum. Muscle contraction generally initiates motion; gravity and momentum then add their contributions. According to Winter and Robertson, during swing phase, gravity, mus-

An Osteopathic Approach to Diagnosis and Treatment, second edition
Eileen L. DiGiovanna and Stanley Schiowitz
Lippincott–Raven Publishers, Philadelphia © 1997.

cle contraction, and knee acceleration cause the shank to rotate. In the first half of the swing, gravity and momentum contribute 80% of the force, while in the second half of the swing, muscles contribute 80% of the force.

The counterpressure of the ground against the feet is the force that propels the body. We are not usually aware of the earth's thrust. However, in soft snow, sand, or mud this thrust is reduced, necessitating increased muscular activity and energy used to maintain forward locomotion. Friction between the foot and the ground is essential for transmission of the ground's pressure. The friction must be sufficient to counterbalance the horizontal vector component of force. The greater the horizontal force, the greater is the dependence on friction. The corollary holds true: on icy streets, small, almost vertical steps are taken.

Walking is initiated through the complex interplay of neural mechanisms, muscular activity, and biomechanical forces. The triceps surae relaxes, permitting forward inclination of the body ahead of the center of gravity. The line of the center of gravity, which is midway between the feet and anterior to the ankle joint, moves toward the swing limb in a posteroanterior direction. As the swing limb prepares for toe-off, the center of gravity shifts to the stance side. The weight is balanced on the stance leg to allow forward propulsion of the swing limb.

Both phases of gait are in operation simultaneously, alternating sides at the completion of each cycle. The swing phase leg rotates the pelvis toward the stance side, with concomitant rotation of the spine to the swing side. The hip joint flexes with this swing action. The knee joint flexes during the first half and extends during the second half of the swing, while the ankle and foot are dorsiflexed.

On the stance side, the hip joint extends, accompanied by muscular contraction that prevents dropping of the pelvis toward the swing side. The knee joint is in slight flexion at the moment of foot contact, or heel strike, after which the knee is extended.

The foot and ankle in this segment, from heel strike to full weight-bearing, is in plantar flexion of the ankle. The foot then converts to a rigid lever for transferring the body weight to the forefoot for push-off. At this time the heel rises rapidly and the foot everts, causing increased external rotation of the leg with hyperextension of the metatarsophalangeal joints at the end of the propulsive phase. The clinical significance of the mechanics of the subtalar joint (as used in the stance phase) cannot be overemphasized. The slightest disturbance will cause noticeable dysfunction.

A definite sequence is observed in weight-bearing on the osseous tripod of the foot: the weight passes from the heel to the fifth metatarsal head and then across the metatarsal heads to the big toe. Any change in pressure on one of these points will be accompanied by a change in the normal sequence of motion and weight-bearing at other points. Calluses usually develop at these sites.

The normal walking cycle in the lower extremities is accompanied by regular motions of the shoulders, arms, and head. Their actions are part of any clinical evaluation. When the pelvis on the swing side moves forward, the shoulder on that side drops back. Therefore, the opposite arms and legs swing in tandem.

The action of the arm in the anteroposterior plane reduces rotation of the shoulders, which directly aids in keeping the head forward. Arm swing balances the rotation of the pelvis. These motions are in direct proportion to each other. If the arms do not swing, the upper trunk will rotate in the same direction as the pelvis.

Gait Efficiency

Efficiency of gait can be considered in terms of the translatory movement of the body's center of gravity through a smooth undulating pathway of low amplitude. The center of gravity in the erect, motionless human is just anterior to the second sacral vertebra. In walking it is displaced both vertically and horizontally, describing a sinusoidal curve.

Vertical displacement of the center of gravity occurs twice during the cycle from heel strike to heel strike of the same foot. The total amount of vertical displacement is about 1.8 inches. The summits occur at 25% and 75% of the cycle. At the midpoint of the gait cycle (double weight-bearing), the center of gravity is at its lowest point.

Saunders, Inman, and Eberhart have proposed six major determinants of gait for the maintenance of mechanical efficiency:

1. **Pelvic rotation.** The pelvis rotates on the swing side, approximately 4 degrees on either side of the central axis. Since the pelvis is a semi-rigid

structure, this rotation occurs alternately at each hip joint as the hip passes from relative internal rotation to external rotation during stance phase.

2. **Downward pelvic tilt.** The pelvis tilts downward in the coronal plane on the swing side. The alternate angular displacement is 5 degrees at the stance hip joint, creating relative adduction of the extremity in stance and relative abduction in swing.

3. **Knee flexion of the swing leg.**

These three determinants of gait—pelvic rotation, pelvic tilt, and swing knee flexion—all act by flattening the vertical arc through which the center of gravity is moving. Pelvic rotation elevates the extremities of the arc, while pelvic tilt and knee flexion depress its summit.

4, 5. **The combined actions of the foot, ankle, and knee of the stance leg** constitute the fourth and fifth determinants of gait. These actions help maintain a smooth pathway for the translatory motion of the center of gravity. A first arc occurs at heel strike when the ankle rotates from dorsiflexion to plantar flexion, with the heel functioning as the fulcrum. A second arc occurs with rotation of the foot, with the forepart of the foot functioning as the fulcrum. This occurs with heel rise. Both arcs are accompanied by stance knee flexion, which maintains a level center of gravity.

6. **Displacement of center of gravity.** Displacement of the center of gravity over the weightbearing extremity aids in maintaining body balance as the swing leg is lifted from the ground. The relative adduction of that hip, along with the tibiofemoral angle, reduces the amount of lateral displacement necessary for balance. The center of gravity deviates laterally about $1\frac{3}{4}$ inches. Thus, deviation of the center of gravity is almost equivalent in horizontal and vertical planes.

Pelvic Motion

The pelvis is not a rigid structure. It has an anterior articulation at the symphysis pubis and two articulations with the sacrum.

As the pelvis rotates and tilts, a torsional effect develops at the symphysis pubis. This is created because every part of the pelvis is moving at a different linear velocity. Measuring the displacement of rotation and tilt of the lateral edge of the right innominate from the fixed left hip will show

that the angular velocity is constant from every part of the left and right innominates, but the linear velocity, and therefore the distance traveled, increases from left to right. Thus the combined motions of rotation and tilt occur at different speeds of linear displacement for different parts of the pelvis and create a torsion at the symphysis pubis with every step taken.

The sacrum moves with the innominate and undergoes the same rotation, tilt, and lateral shift as does the innominate, but not at the same speed. When swing of the right leg initiates rotation of the right innominate toward the left, with right innominate tilt and left lateral shift, the sacrum will move on its vertical axis and rotate to the left, with right sacral flexion. Simultaneously the center of gravity in the horizontal plane shifts to the left, producing left sacral lateral flexion. The vertical center of gravity moves to the superior pole of the left sacroiliac, locking the articulation into a mechanical position that establishes movement of the sacrum on the left oblique axis. This sets the pattern so the sacrum can torsionally turn to the left (Mitchell, 1965). Walking creates the mechanics of oblique sacral motion without dysfunction, or, in the above example, a left-on-left sacral torsional motion (Fig. 15-1).

During these motions, the lumbar spine rotates to the right and flexes laterally to the left, compensating for the right sacral flexion created by pelvic rotation toward the left with right pelvic tilt.

Asymmetric Motion

In the perfectly balanced, symmetric human, the joint motions of gait have little or no effect on the body's structural integrity. However, asymmetry develops in virtually everyone and causes constant small structural stress situations that can lead to somatic dysfunctions.

What happens to symmetry of gait in short leg syndrome? What happens to the comparative reversals of motions of lumbar rotation and lateral flexion if scoliosis is present? Radiographs of patients with low back problems often show lateral flexion, rotation deformity of one lumbar vertebra on the one below it. The intervertebral disk is wedged and spondylytic changes are present, yet the site has not sustained previous specific trauma. This condition is very likely produced by the constant stress of gait on a localized somatic dysfunction.

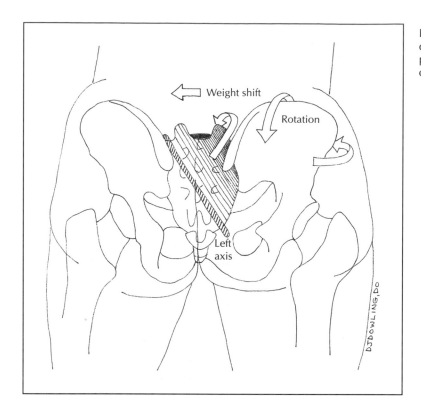

Figure 15-1. Pelvic determinants of normal gait, posterior view. Shown is left-on-left sacral torsional motion.

Structural deformities should be treated, even if asymptomatic, while the subject is young. This will prevent some of the constant microtraumas that occur with daily locomotion, and will prevent symptomatic dysfunction in later life.

Neurologic Gait Patterns

Analysis of gait is the most important test in neurology and one of the least performed. The following points should be noted in this evaluation: the position of the body, movement of the legs, position and movement of the arms, distance between the feet, both in forward direction (stride) and in lateral direction (width), regularity of movements, ability to walk in a straight line, ease of turning, and ease of stopping. Along with these observations, the examiner should note any changes in the six major determinants of gait.

Following are descriptions of several neurologic gait patterns.

Hemiplegic gait. In hemiplegic gait the leg is usually stiff, with loss of flexion at the hip and knee joints. The patient leans to the affected side and throws the whole leg outward from the body before bringing it back toward the trunk, producing a circumduction movement. The shoe is dragged against the floor, and there is usually an accompanying affected arm that does not swing but is held in fixed position against the abdomen with the elbow flexed.

High steppage gait. High steppage gait can be divided into two characteristic patterns. In the first pattern the toe touches the floor first, with a foot drop due to paralysis of pretibial or peroneal muscles. The leg is raised high by abnormal knee and hip flexion. The toe touches the ground first, followed by a slapping noise as the foot strikes the floor.

In the second pattern the heel touches the floor first because of loss of sense of position. The high steppage gait is bilateral, with ataxia and side-to-side reeling. The heel touches the floor first and a stomp of the foot is heard. Romberg's sign is present, caused by a dysfunction of the afferent portion of peripheral nerves or posterior roots.

Carcinoma, diabetic neuropathy, tabes dorsalis, Friedreich's ataxia, subacute combined degeneration of the cord, compression lesions of the posterior columns, and multiple sclerosis that affects the posterior columns may all produce a high steppage gait.

Shuffling gait. Shuffling gait can be described as small, flat-footed shuffling steps: the foot does not clear the ground. In parkinsonism, rigidity, tremor, paucity of movement, shuffling with haste, and difficulty in starting, stopping, or turning are noted. The patient is in flexion, with lack of extension movements at the hips, knees, and elbows. The thorax and pelvis rotate in the same direction in swing phase. The amplitude of vertical excursions of the head is lessened in forward motion. The first noticeable motor signs in parkinsonism may be a nonrhythmic pattern with random or poorly timed activity of the arms in gait.

The shuffling gait seen in arteriosclerosis is due to loss of confidence and equilibrium. The patient stands erect, takes small shuffling steps with a wide base, and seems to stare at a distant point. Turning is achieved through a series of small steps made by one foot, the other foot acting as a pivot.

Ataxic gait. Ataxic gait is a reeling, unsteady gait with a wide base and a tendency to fall toward the side of the lesion. Vertigo may accompany ataxia. It may be found in cerebellar disease, multiple sclerosis, and sometimes myxedema. Ataxic gait must be differentiated from drunken and staggering gait, in which the subject reels, totters, tips forward and backward, and may lose balance and fall. This gait is seen in alcohol or barbiturate poisoning, drug reaction, polyneuritis, or general paresis.

Scissors gait. In scissors gait the legs are adducted, crossing alternately in front of one another. Both lower limbs are spastic, and there is spasm of the adductor muscles at the hip joints, often accompanied by pronounced compensatory motions of the trunk and upper extremities. Bilateral upper motor neuron lesions, advanced cervical spondylosis, or multiple sclerosis may produce this gait pattern.

Waddling gait. Waddling gait can be described as rolling from side to side. The pelvic rotation and tilt on the swing side are increased (penguin walk). Muscular dystrophy with weakness of hips, exaggerated lordosis, and pot-bellied posture can produce this gait.

Hysterical gait. Hysterical gait may simulate any paralysis or may be bizarre. There may be inability to walk, but in bed the subject may lose the characteristic spasticity.

When outlining therapy for the neurologic patient, the clinician must discuss all problems with him. Many of these patients hope that osteopathic manipulation will cure their problems, and they must be advised of the limitations of the expected results. Some have, as a secondary complaint, severe pain and dysfunction of the low back area. These symptoms can be greatly relieved. Some have asymptomatic somatic dysfunctions of the upper cervical vertebrae, which should be treated.

Musculoskeletal Gait Patterns

Several musculoskeletal gait patterns are described below.

Antalgic gait. Antalgic gait is characterized by a short stance phase and a rapidly executed swing phase: the patient tries to avoid standing on a painful extremity. Most musculoskeletal dysfunctions of gait are antalgic. The physician must evaluate where the pain is located. A simple question such as, When you put your weight on that foot, where does it hurt? may assist in accurate diagnosis.

Gluteus medius gait. A gluteus medius gait is characterized by a shift of the body toward the deficient side, indicating a weakness of that gluteus medius muscle. It can be evaluated by finding a Trendelenburg sign in the upright position.

Gluteus maximus gait. In gluteus maximus deficiency, the trunk and pelvis are hyperextended backward over both hips to maintain the center of gravity behind the involved hip joint.

Short lower extremity. In short lower extremity, the pelvis and trunk depress in stance phase.

Elevated pelvis gait. In elevated pelvis gait, there is a hiking or elevation of the pelvis on the swing side if that hip or knee joint has motion limitation from any cause.

Congenital hip dislocation. Congenital dislocation of the hip creates a waddling gait.

Osteoarthrosis gait. Severe osteoarthrosis of the hip or knee joints will produce the scissors gait.

Foot problems. Any dysfunction of the foot may alter normal mechanics. These could include Morton's foot (neuroma), corns, calluses, bunions, hallux rigidus, plantar warts, or poorly fitting shoes. If plantar flexion is absent, there is no push-off and the heel and forefoot come off the floor together.

Pediatric Gait Patterns

Pediatric musculoskeletal problems should be evaluated and treatment instituted before the onset of weight-bearing. Equinus, calcaneus valgus, pronation, flatfoot, tibial torsion, metatarsal varus, clubfoot, and congenital dislocation of the hips should all be diagnosed and treated properly before the child begins to walk.

In one study, 64% of limping children with no history of gait dysfunction or trauma had primary involvement of the hip joint. Most cases were due to transient synovitis and resolved with rest. Many children with hip-related gait dysfunction have had a recent upper respiratory tract infection. Other causes include osteitis, rheumatic fever, rheumatoid arthritis, and Perthes' disease.

Gait Patterns in Low Back Dysfunction

An initial diagnosis of somatic dysfunction may often be made by evaluating the patient's gait. The most obvious problems are those relating to low back dysfunction.

A psoas dysfunction secondary to lumbar vertebral osteopathic somatic dysfunctions will produce the typical psoatic limp. The patient bends forward and toward the side of the dysfunction, and that hip will be in abduction. The somatic dysfunction is usually found in the upper lumbar area. Neglecting this site and treating the lower back or sacroiliac articulation is usually a futile effort.

Unilateral erector spinae contraction will cause lateral flexion to the side of contraction, scoliosis with convexity to the opposite side, and extension of the spine. The patient walks with a stiff back, with no lumbar rotation or flexion. The spinal areas involved are usually at the fourth or fifth lumbar and first sacral segments. An acute anterior sacrum dysfunction on the same side may also be present. If findings include a raised iliac crest height, lumbar scoliotic convexity, and sciatic pain distribution, all on the same side, the prog-

nosis for a speedy recovery is often good. If the pain is on the other side, the cause may be a prolapsed disk or some other serious pathologic condition, and both physician and patient may be in for a difficult time.

Gait Patterns in Lower Extremity Dysfunction

Sciatica is associated with an antalgic, erector spinae gait pattern as the patient tries to avoid weight-bearing on the affected side. A common somatic dysfunction pattern in these patients comprises unilateral sacral flexion and flexion of the fifth lumbar vertebra, with rotation and side-bending to the painful side, accompanied by trigger points at the piriformis, gluteus maximus, and gluteus medius muscles.

Observation of an asymmetric pelvic swing or tilt noted should be followed by a hip drop test. The findings on this test often concur with the gait observations, pointing toward lumbar lateral flexion restriction.

Somatic dysfunctions involving the lower extremity usually manifest with an antalgic gait. The clinician can use observation to determine the area involved, but then must depend on palpation and motion testing to establish the diagnosis.

The skill of observation can be improved if the physician is aware of the alterations of motion commonly produced by localized somatic dysfunction. At the hip joint, look for limitation in internal and external rotation in the swinging lower extremity. In the knee joint, there will be a restriction of femoral medial rotation on the tibia when attempting a close-packed position in extension of the stance lower extremity. At the ankle, the subtalar joint will be limited in eversion-inversion as the leg rotates internally-externally in stance phase. Lateral weight-bearing of the foot will shift toward the medial arch, with cuboid dysfunction during stance phase.

POSTURAL IMBALANCE AND LIFT THERAPY
Eileen L. DiGiovanna
Joseph A. DiGiovanna

Human bipedal posture has made balance extremely important to musculoskeletal function. In the erect human, gravity pulls on all parts of the body. Although a column of vertebrae stacked evenly on top of each other would have been well balanced given little motion, anteroposterior curves developed in the spine to promote flexibility and increase strength. The transitions between spinal curves are well suited to meet the force of gravity. Correct posture is essential to keep the force of gravity centered on those vertebrae designed for this function.

Few persons are totally symmetric, and therefore postural imbalance is a significant source of musculoskeletal problems.

The body has certain automatic compensatory mechanisms that tend to right the body and maintain it in a state of equilibrium. For example, if, while standing, the left leg is lifted off the ground, the body's center of gravity will automatically move to the right, and the spine will shift and curve in the frontal plane to maintain the body in balance. Similarly, if the arms are held in front of the body, the spine will shift and curve in the sagittal plane, increasing lumbar lordosis to maintain balance. If a weight is held in the outstretched arms, the lordosis will exaggerate further to maintain body equilibrium. Thus, the body will make any adjustments necessary to maintain its balance and upright posture.

Numerous conditions can produce asymmetry in body mechanics and lead to functional postural imbalance. They include:

1. Trauma
2. Degenerative processes
3. Habit or occupation
4. Genetic tendencies
5. Mental attitude
6. Pregnancy
7. Obesity
8. Loss of muscle tone
9. Disease processes such as osteoporosis and polio
10. Congenital anomalies

Short Leg Syndrome
A source of postural imbalance in a large percentage of the "normal" population is the short leg syndrome. In 1977, Myron Beal reported the results of some studies on the short leg syndrome; included in his review were two earlier studies performed by Pearson et al. on rural schoolchildren in 1947 and 1949. In the 1947 study, of 736 children, 410 had a difference of 0.5 mm in the lengths of the two legs, 152 had a difference of 5 to 10 mm, and 32 had a difference of 10 to 15 mm. The 1949 study, done on 710 students, found that 385 had a leg length difference of 0.5 mm, 194 a difference of 5 to 10 mm, and 17 a difference of 10 to 15 mm. Beal also reported on a study by Denslow that was done on asymptomatic young male students: 146 had a leg length difference of 5 to 10 mm, 28 a difference of 10 to 15 mm, 1 a difference of 15 to 20 mm, and 2 a difference of 20 mm.

The frequency of short leg syndrome is higher in persons with low back pain than in persons without low back pain, and the patients tend to be older.

DIAGNOSIS
I. History
The patient commonly reports bending over and feeling pain in the back, or feeling as though the back had locked. The patient may notice that he wears out one shoe faster than the other, or that one pant leg or shirt sleeve seems longer than the other.

Screening for scoliosis is often required by the school system and may allow early recognition of a postural problem.

Physical Examination
Scoliosis is often discovered during a routine physical examination. It must be determined if the scoliosis is due to a short leg (nonstructural or functional) or is developmental or congenital in origin (structural). A structural examination for asymmetry may yield important clues to solving the problem. A difference in leg length is assessed by measuring with a tape measure from the ante-

rior superior iliac spines to the medial malleolus of each leg.

Radiologic Assessment

Once the diagnosis of short leg is suspected, the patient may be further evaluated with standing postural radiographs of the low back and femoral heads. These films are made with the patient standing erect, toes pointing forward and the feet approximately 6 inches apart. Equilibrium must be maintained as much as possible. A level floor is essential.

The iliac crests, sacral base, and femoral heads are measured bilaterally. This may be done with use of a specially gridded film or by use of a *T*-square to draw horizontal lines. The most important measurement is the sacral base (Fig. 15-2).

Normally the lumbar spine is convex on the side of the short leg as the spine side-bends back toward the midline. Occasionally a compensatory curve will develop in the thoracic spine in the opposite direction from that in the lumbar spine. Sacral base leveling with straightening of the scoliotic curve is the goal of therapy.

Various types of unleveling of the femoral heads and sacral base may be found, as follows:

1. Parallel unleveling: sacral base unleveling equal and on the same side as the low femoral head.
2. Femoral head unleveling greater than sacral base unleveling: both low on same side.
3. Sacral base unleveling greater than femoral head unleveling: both low on same side.
4. Femoral head unleveling without sacral tilt.
5. Sacral base tilt without a short leg.
6. Sacral base low on one side with short leg on the opposite side.
7. Sacral base low on one side, lumbar spine convex on the side of the long leg.

PHYSICAL MANIFESTATIONS

A short leg has numerous effects on the body. The sacral base tilts toward the side of the short leg. The iliac crest is generally low on the short leg side. The lumbar spine develops a convexity toward the side of the short leg, and once the problem has existed for sufficient time, a compensatory curve will develop in the thoracic spine. The shoulder will be low on one side, depending on whether or not a secondary thoracic curve is present; the scapula will be low on the same side as the shoulder. The cervical angle will be more acute as the head is tilted toward the midline.

Asymmetric tensions are palpable in the paravertebral muscles. The muscles on the side of the convexity are stretched and those on the side of the concavity are shortened. There is usually a gapping of the medial knee compartment on the side of the short leg and an approximation of the medial knee compartment on the side of the longer leg. Stress is also created in the hip and ankle joints of the long leg.

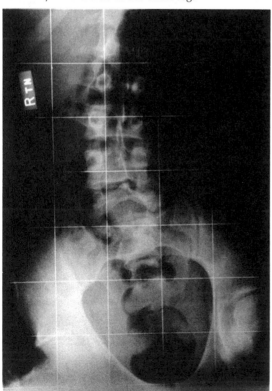

Figure 15-2. Postural radiograph showing short right leg with marked sacral base unleveling. Note spinal convexity on the side of the short leg.

TREATMENT

1. **Osteopathic manipulative treatment:**
   a. Relaxes and stretches contracted muscles
   b. Corrects somatic dysfunctions
   c. Increases mobility
   d. Normalizes tissues
2. **Exercises:** Exercises should be designed to stretch and tone the asymmetric muscles.

3. **Lift therapy:** A lift placed in the heel of the shoe on the side of the short leg lifts the short leg and corrects the postural imbalance. The lift should be made of a firm, comfortable substance such as leather, cork, or hard rubber. Foam rubber is not satisfactory because it flattens, and height cannot be correctly measured.

When a heel lift is prescribed, the patient must be informed of the need to wear the lift at all times when walking. Once he is out of bed in the morning, he must wear shoes or slippers with the lift. The strain on the back is too great if the lift is worn only occasionally. The only exception is when walking on sand, where the surface is soft, giving, and already uneven.

When considering whether or not to prescribe a heel lift, several factors must be considered:

1. **Sacral base unleveling:** determined by radiographic assessment. Sacral base unleveling rather than femoral head heights has been deemed most significant. Most osteopathic physicians are of the opinion that anything over a quarter inch should be lifted. In certain cases, even an eighth inch should be treated.
2. **Length of time present:** The period may be short, as in the case of a fractured lower extremity, or longer, as in the case of a developmental shortening.
3. **Amount of compensation:** includes such factors as the degree of side-bending and rotation of the spine, wedging of vertebrae, and alteration of facets. Generally, the longer the condition has been present, the more compensation will have occurred.

David Heilig has developed a formula useful for determining the amount of lift to be used:

$$\text{Lift required} = \frac{\text{Sacral base unleveling}}{\text{Duration} + \text{Compensation}}$$

$$L = \frac{SBU}{D + C}$$

Duration is graded on a scale of 1 to 3:

$$1 = 1\text{--}10 \text{ years}$$

$$2 = 10\text{--}30 \text{ years}$$

$$3 = \text{over } 30 \text{ years}$$

Compensation is graded on a scale of 0 to 2:

$$0 = \text{side-bending without rotation}$$

$$1 = \text{rotation toward the convexity}$$

$$2 = \text{wedging, altered facets}$$

Except in the very young or in cases of acute shortening, it is best to begin by adding half the total difference. In older persons or in cases of greater compensation, it is best to start with no more than one-eighth inch. The lift is slowly increased over time, with manipulative treatment used to aid in adaptation to the lift. After the lift has been worn for a period of time and the patient is comfortable with it, the postural study should be repeated with the lift in place to determine if the correction is adequate.

If the lift is more than one-quarter-inch thick, it will have to be added to the outside of the heel. Lifts may also be added to orthotic devices. If the total lift required is greater than one-half inch, half the amount of heel lift will have to be added to the sole of the shoe as well. For example, if one-half inch is added to the heel, one-quarter inch should be added to the sole.

Before adding a lift it is important to ascertain that short leg is not due to a pronated foot on one side. In this case, an orthotic device to correct the pronation will probably correct the leg shortening.

Correcting a shortened extremity will correct many other postural defects, since it is the key to many musculoskeletal abnormalities. Besides correction of the postural deficits mentioned in the structural evaluation, a whole shift of body weight will occur. The pelvis will shift back to the midline, realigning the center of gravity and the weight-bearing portions of the body. The new position will affect the biomechanics of the entire musculoskeletal system.

References

Adams RD, Victor M. 1985. Principles of Neurology. New York: McGraw-Hill.

Basmajian JV. 1987. Muscles Alive, 4th ed. Baltimore: Williams & Wilkins.

Beal M. 1977. The short leg problem. J Am Osteopath Assoc 76(10):745–751.

Bickerstaff RE. 1968. Gait. In: Neurological Examination in Clinical Practice, 2nd ed. Oxford: Blackwell Scientific Publications.

Cailliet R. 1968. Foot and Ankle Pain. Philadelphia: F.A. Davis.

———. 1981. Low Back Pain Syndrome, 3rd ed. Philadelphia: F.A. Davis.

Forssberg H, Grillner S, Rossignol S. 1977. Phasic gain control of reflexes from the dorsum of the paw during spinal locomotion. Brain Res 132:121–139.

Heilig D. 1978. Principles of lift therapy. J Am Osteopath Assoc 77(6):466–472.

Henszinger RN. 1977. Limp. Pediatr Clin North Am 24: 723–730.

Hoppenfeld S. 1976. Physical Examination of the Spine and Extremities. New York: Appleton-Century-Crofts.

Illingworth CM. 1978. 128 limping children with no fracture, sprain, or obvious cause. Clin Pediatr 17: 139–142.

Kappler RE. 1973. Role of psoas mechanism in low-back complaints. J Am Osteopath Assoc 72(8):794–801.

———. 1982. Postural balance and motion patterns. J Am Osteopath Assoc 81(9):598–606.

Mann RA, Hagy JL, White V, et al. 1979. The initiation of gait. J Bone Joint Surg [Am] 61:232–239.

Merrifield HH. 1971. Female gait patterns in shoes with different heel heights. Ergonomics 14:411–417.

Michelle AA. 1962. Iliopsoas. St. Louis: Charles C Thomas.

Mitchell FL. 1965. Structural pelvic function. In: Academy of Applied Osteopathy, 1965 Year Book. Vol II.

Morris JM. 1977. Biomechanics of the foot and ankle. pp. 178–199. Carmel, Calif: The Academy of Applied Osteopathy. Clin Orthop Rel Res 122:10–17.

Murray MP, Sepoc SB, Gardner GM, et al. 1978. Walking patterns of men with parkinsonism. Am J Phys Med 57:278–294.

Rasch PJ, Burke RK. 1978. Kinesiology and Applied Anatomy, 6th ed. Philadelphia: Lea & Febiger.

Roaf R. 1977. Posture. Orlando, Fla: Academic Press.

Saunders JB, Inman VT, Eberhart HD. 1953. The major determinants in normal and pathological gait. J Bone Joint Surg [Am] 35:543–558.

Schwartz RP, Heath AL, Misiek W, et al. 1933. Kinetics of Human Gait. Rochester, NY: University of Rochester Medical Society.

Simon RB. 1979. A neurologic screening exam in six minutes. Diagnosis 1(1):44–58.

Smidt GL. 1974. Methods of studying gait. Phys Ther 54: 13–17.

Soderberg GL, Dostal WF. 1978. Electromyographic study of three parts of the gluteus medius muscle during functional activities. Phys Ther 58:691–696.

Strachan WF. 1941. Lateral imbalance and the use of lifts. J Am Osteopath Assoc 41:190–192.

Wells KF, Luttgens K. 1976. Kinesiology, 6th ed. Philadelphia: W.B. Saunders.

Winter DA, Robertson DGE. 1978. Joint torque and energy patterns in normal gait. Biol Cybernet 29: 137–142.

Zarrugh MY, Radcliff CW. 1979. Computer generation of human gait kinematics. J Biomech 12:99–111.

Zohn DA, Mennell JMcM. 1987. Musculoskeletal Pain: Diagnosis and Physical Treatment. Boston: Little, Brown.

16

Evaluation of
the Thorax

APPLIED ANATOMY AND BIOMECHANICS
Dennis J. Dowling

Anatomic Relationships

LANDMARKS

On palpation, several landmarks may be noted and their relations to specific ribs established. The 1st rib is attached to the manubrium of the sternum just inferior to the clavicle anteriorly: posteriorly, it is cephalad to the superior border of the scapula. The 2nd rib articulates with both the manubrium and the body of the sternum at the sternal angle anteriorly. Posteriorly, the 3rd rib is located at approximately the median aspect of the spine of the scapula. The costal cartilage of the 7th rib attaches to the sternal body and xiphoid process ventrally, and the angle of the rib rests near the tip of the scapula's inferior angle. The cartilage of the 10th rib is palpated at the lowest aspect of the thoracic cage in the midclavicular line. The 12th rib is almost horizontal and is found by palpating in the soft tissues posteriorly above the iliac crests.

STRUCTURE

The ribs are often classified as true or false. The cartilage of the true ribs, the 1st through 7th ribs, attaches to the sternum. The false ribs, ribs 8 through 12, are further divided into vertebrochondral ribs (8th through 10th ribs) and floating ribs. The cartilage of the vertebrochondral ribs unites with the cartilage of the 7th ribs. The floating ribs lack cartilage and float freely.

Typical Ribs

The 3rd through 9th ribs are typical ribs. The round, knoblike rib head is followed by the neck and tubercle, a body that arcs at the region of the rib angle, and a distal concavity where the cartilage attaches. The body of a typical rib is thin and flat, with interior and exterior surfaces and a costal groove on the inferior edge.

Each rib head has two facets for articulation with the body of the next superior vertebra and the same-numbered vertebral body. These articulations jointly constitute the costovertebral articulation. The tubercle articulates with the transverse process of the same vertebra via a facet and is known as the costotransverse articulation.

Atypical Ribs

The 1st, 2nd, 10th, 11th, and 12th ribs are considered atypical ribs. The 1st rib is flat, has the greatest curvature and the shortest length of all the ribs, and has no angle or costal groove. Its superior surface has grooves for passage of the subclavian vessels and elevations for the attachment of the anterior and middle scalene muscles. The single facet

An Osteopathic Approach to Diagnosis and Treatment, second edition
Eileen L. DiGiovanna and Stanley Schiowitz
Lippincott–Raven Publishers, Philadelphia © 1997.

of the head articulates with the body of the T1 vertebra.

The 2nd rib is similar to the 1st but longer and not as flat. The two demifacets on the rib head articulate with the T1 and T2 vertebrae.

The 10th rib is typical in every respect expect its costovertebral articulation. The single articular facet on the head forms a joint with the facet on the body of the T10 vertebra.

The 11th and 12th ribs have neither neck nor tubercles. As in the 10th rib, the heads have single facets corresponding to facets on the same-numbered vertebral bodies. The ventral ends float freely. The 12th rib does not possess a costal groove.

A second, overlapping classification system for ribs is that of "true" and "false" ribs. True ribs are ribs 1 through 7, while 10 through 12 are False. All True ribs attach directly to the sternum via the sternochondral joints. Ribs 8 through 10 "piggyback" with their cartilage onto the cartilage of the 7th rib. This collection then forms the common costal cartilage. The remaining ribs have no cartilage.

Supporting Structures
The clavicle is located at the anterosuperior aspect of the thoracic cage. Its medial end articulates with the manubrium and the cartilage of the first rib.

Even though the clavicle and its component joints are considered shoulder in function, they are important during respiration. As the occiput can be considered C_o, the clavicle can be thought of as Rib_o. It must remain mobile during each phase of respiration for the rib cage, especially the 1st rib, to function properly.

The sternum is composed of three parts: the xiphoid, body, and manubrium. The lateral edges of the sternum are scalloped for the attachment of costal cartilage.

The posterior portion of the thoracic cage and much of its motion are defined by the shape of the thoracic vertebrae. The bodies of the thoracic vertebrae have costal facets for articulation with the heads of the ribs. The long, thick, transverse processes have facets on their bulbous tips for articulation with the rib tubercles.

ARTICULATIONS
The **sternoclavicular joint,** one of the true joints of the shoulder girdle, may affect rib cage motion either primarily, via the manubrium and ligamentous attachments to the costal cartilage, or secondarily, because of the position of the upper extremity.

The **costovertebral joint** is the articulation of the rib head with the bodies of one or two vertebrae. For a typical rib, the costovertebral joint includes the bodies of the vertebra at the same level and the vertebra immediately above, the annulus fibrosus of the intervening disk, and the costal facets. It is a synovial joint with a single capsule. The facets of the costovertebral joint are slightly convex and form an angle that fits into the depression formed by the vertebral facets and the disk. Several ligaments are associated with the costovertebral joint, including the interosseous ligament and the superior, intermediate, and inferior bands of the radiate ligament.

The **costotransverse articulation** is likewise a simple synovial joint surrounded by a capsule. Three ligaments—the superior, posterior, and interosseous costotransverse ligaments—connect the transverse process to the neck of the tubercle. The superior costotransverse ligament also connects the transverse process to the neck of the next lower rib.

Together, the costotransverse and costovertebral joints form a complex coupled joint. An imaginary line drawn between the two articulations is the axis that defines the direction of rib motion (Fig. 16-1).

The **costochondral region** of a rib consists of a concave pit on the end of the bony portion, to which is attached the cone-shaped cartilage.

The **sternochondral articulation** is formed by the costal cartilage and the triangular notches of the sternum. Small synovial joints are present. The apex of each notch faces medially, with an anteroposterior axis that allows freedom of motion along the coronal plane. The joints are supported by radiate ligaments.

MUSCLES
The major muscle of inspiration is the diaphragm, which is responsible for at least 60% of the generated thoracic cage pressure change. The muscular portion inserts onto the xiphoid process, the lower six ribs, and the upper lumbar vertebrae. All of these muscular portions converge on the aponeurotic central tendon (Fig. 16-2).

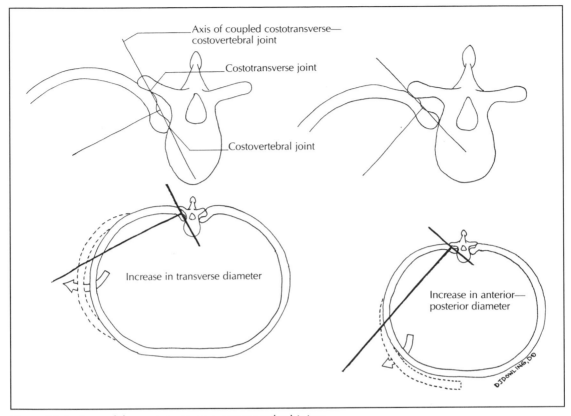

Figure 16-1. Axes of the costotransverse-costovertebral joints.

The diaphragm is a dome-shaped muscle with two lateral hemidiaphragms whose shape is influenced by the viscera. In addition to inspiration and expiration, the diaphragm is important in micturition, defecation, parturition, circulation of blood, lymphatic pumping, and speech.

Other inspiratory muscles include the external intercostals, the levator costarum, and the so-called secondary or accessory muscles. In truth, these muscles are used whenever inhalation occurs. In conditions such as asthma or emphysema, they become more pronounced as their percentage of inhalation increases. The accessory muscles are called into action for forced inspiration, such as is needed during exercise, or in pathologic states, including attacks of asthma. These auxiliary inspiratory muscles include the sternocleidomastoid, the scalenes, the serratus posterior superior, the pectoralis, the inferior fibers of the serratus anterior, the latissimus dorsi, and the superior fibers of iliocostalis muscles.

Expiration is primarily produced by recoil of the diaphragm and the energy stored in the costal cartilage. The sternocostalis and internal intercostalis muscles are also involved. The accessory expiratory muscles include the rectus abdominis, external oblique, internal oblique, transversus abdominis, serratus posterior inferior, transversus thoracic, pyramidalis, subcostalis, quadratus lumborum, iliocostalis, longissimus, and latissimus dorsi muscles (the latissimus may play a role in either expiration or inspiration, depending on the fixed position of the arm).

INNERVATION

The vertebral region is supplied primarily by dorsal rami, and the ventral rami form the 11 pairs of intercostals and the pair of subcostals. They begin in the intercostal space, then enter the costal groove of the 1st through 11th ribs at the level of the angle. The intercostals connect to the sympathetic chain via the rami communicantes. The

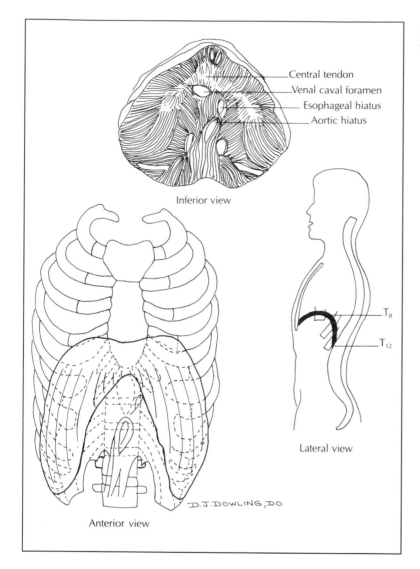

Central tendon
Venal caval foramen
Esophageal hiatus
Aortic hiatus

Inferior view

T_8

T_{12}

Lateral view

D.J. DOWLING, DO

Anterior view

Figure 16-2. The thoracic diaphragm.

sympathetic trunks are located anterior to the heads of the ribs.

The diaphragm is innervated by the phrenic nerve, which consists of the ventral rami of the third, fourth, and fifth cervical nerves. Sensory input is also conducted through the phrenic nerve, with contributions from the intercostals.

Biomechanics
MUSCULAR ACTION
During inspiration, the diaphragm descends as it contracts. Movement is checked by the stretching of the mediastinal contents and by resistance of the abdominal organs. Simultaneous descent and contraction of the diaphragm decreases intrathoracic pressure and thereby increases the volume of the thoracic cavity. As the central tendon becomes fixed, continued contraction of the muscular fibers causes elevation of the lower ribs. Elevation of the upper ribs is assisted by the sternum.

Diaphragmatic movement increases the thoracic volume in three dimensions. Depression of the central tendon alters the vertical dimension, elevation of the ribs increases the transverse dimension, and elevation of the sternum and upper ribs

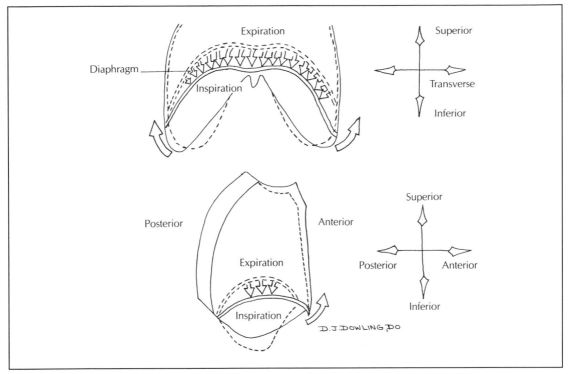

Figure 16-3. Diameter changes that occur during diaphragmatic motion.

changes the anteroposterior dimension (Fig. 16-3). Both the external intercostals and the levator costarum assist in inspiration by elevating the ribs.

The sternocostalis and internal costalis muscles depress the ribs during expiration. The accessory expiratory muscles can be divided into abdominal muscles, thoracic cage muscles, and thoracolumbar muscles. The abdominal muscles strongly depress the thoracic floor and increase intraabdominal pressure. Thoracic cage muscles such as the serratus posterior inferior act directly on rib attachments to draw the ribs downward. The thoracolumbar muscles also depress the ribs and possibly the scapula.

RIB MOTION

The axis formed by the coupled costovertebral and costotransverse joints determines the primary direction of rib movement. This is influenced by the angle between the vertebral body and the transverse process and by the distance between the costal articulations with the vertebra. The axes of the ribs permit three basic types of motion: bucket handle, pump handle, and caliper motion (Fig. 16-4).

Bucket handle motion. The handle on a bucket is fixed at both ends. The axis is closer to a sagittal plane in the lower ribs. With one end of the bucket handle fixed at the vertebral end, the majority of the rib elevation occurs through upward excursion of the lateral portion. This motion increases the transverse diameter of the rib cage.

Pump handle motion. The term *pump handle motion* is derived from the similarity between the rib motion and that of an old-fashioned water pump. One end is fixed, and the free end describes an arc. The costovertebral-costotransverse axis of the upper ribs lies close to the coronal plane. As the ribs move about this axis, they increase the anteroposterior diameter of that portion of the rib cage.

Mixed pump and bucket handle motion. The costovertebral-costotransverse axis for the middle ribs lies at a roughly 45-degree angle to the sagittal and coronal planes. The motion of these ribs is of a mixed pump and bucket handle type with an

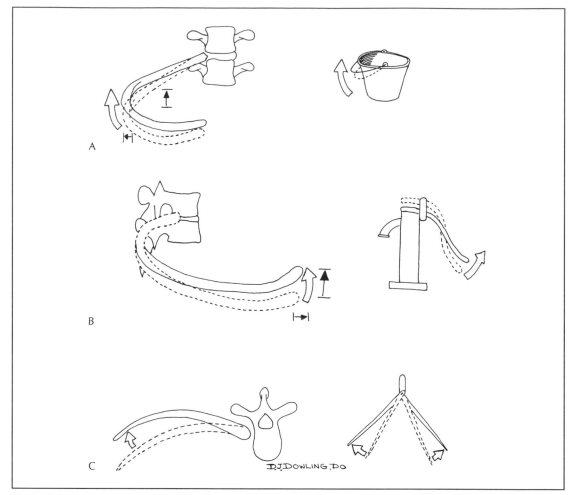

Figure 16-4. Rib motions: **(A)** bucket handle motion, **(B)** pump handle motion, **(C)** caliper motion.

increase in both the transverse and anteroposterior dimensions.

Caliper motion. The 11th and 12th ribs have only costovertebral articulations. Since there are no transverse process limitations, the motion of these ribs is caliperlike along a horizontal plane. This motion produces slight changes in both the anteroposterior and the transverse dimensions.

ANTEROPOSTERIOR SHAPE CHANGES

During inhalation, the 1st through 10th ribs elevate. The sternum moves upward and forward. The small amount of motion possible at the sternal angle—since it is usually a symphysis—allows the angle to flatten. The upper ribs move farther forward than the lower ribs because of the greater pump handle motion that occurs in this region.

COSTAL CARTILAGE ELASTICITY

The costal cartilage is hyaline. It is basically unossified embryonic cartilaginous rib and contributes significantly to thoracic cage mobility. During inspiration, the sternum has a greater superior excursion than the ribs. The ribs initially move inferiorly relative to the sternum. Since the cartilage is basically fixed at the sternal end, it twists along the long axis and behaves as a torsion rod and stores potential energy. As the diaphragm relaxes and ascends, this energy is released as the cartilage recoils (Fig. 16-5).

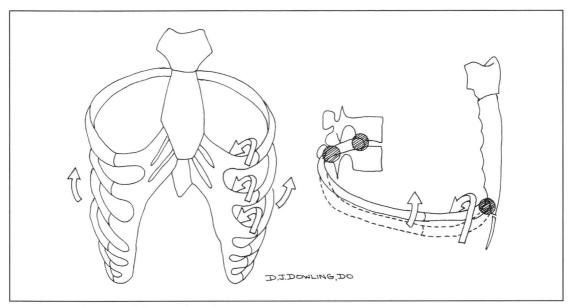

Figure 16-5. Elasticity of the costal cartilage.

Osteopathic Diagnosis

Palpation and visual observation are used during osteopathic examination. Knowledge of the structure and biomechanics of the area under evaluation is integral to this process. Somatic dysfunctions restrict motion of the thoracic cage and its components. The bucket handle and pump handle movements may be limited when examined at the greatest extent of inspiration and expiration. Asymmetric excursion and difficulty in movement imply restriction of the region examined.

The Lymphatic System
Dennis J. Dowling

The Immune System

The immune system is actually a multiorgan system that prevents damage from microorganisms and also maintains homeostasis. It includes first-line defenses which act as barriers and filtration mechanisms to reduce or eliminate incursion by particles and infectious agents.

During the act of inhalation, air brought in through the nostrils is filtered through follicles, humidified by mucus, and brought into the pharynx past the adenoidal and tonsilar lymphatic tissues. Offensive materials such as dust and bacteria become solubilized and subjected to the bacteriostatic properties of mucus and saliva. If they manage to make it as far as the bronchi, an escalatorlike action of the lining cilia brings some of these materials back up to the posterior pharynx, where they can be swallowed and subjected to the acids and enzymes of the stomach. Other components that escape this process might be consumed by scavenger cells called *macrophages*. If they still persist, the body may recognize them and send weapons known as antibodies to deal with recognized antigens.

The skin is a first line of defense for excluding bacterial and viral infection. Most often, it takes a breakdown in the skin's integrity to lead to infection via this route. Practically each of the body's fluids has some bacteriostatic properties to reduce proliferation in anticipation of a more directed response. Perspiration contains lactic and fatty acids known to have this potential. Aberrant cell production, such as cancer, is also recognized and, for the most part, removed.

Thermostatic changes regulated by the central nervous system may actually be a basic attempt to reduce replication of microorganisms. Fever as a symptom shows evidence that there is invasion and response. Temperature gradients of a certain level inhibit protein synthesis. The problem in infection is not that there is a fever. The patient may suffer when it doesn't occur when it should, is dangerously high, changes too quickly, or remains elevated inappropriately after the infection has been adequately managed. Generally, the very old, the very young, or immune-impaired persons tend to show these difficulties.

Modern medical pharmacological interventions have been very effective in facilitating the body's immune response. Medication augments the efficiency of the response *but rarely replaces it*. Almost all of the antibiotics and antiviral agents used, especially on an outpatient basis, are bacteriostatic in function. They inhibit further replication of the number of organisms, and thus allow the body to mount its own defenses to fight and destroy the invaders. When these systems are absent or overwhelmed, more destructive and dangerous bacteriocidal agents may prove helpful. In some cases, more harm comes from the side effects of these medications than the good accomplished.

When operating optimally, the body is an integrated machine capable of defending and repairing itself. These activities are dependent on each of neurological, endocrinological, hematological, respiratory, urological, gastrointestinal, and vascular systems. The importance of the immune system in its more specific functions has implications for the constant health of the individual.

Lymphatics
FUNCTION
The two primary functions of the lymphatic system are filtering of particulate matter before it enters the vascular system and development and delivery of components to combat foreign substances. It is selective for particulate size and returns the nearly 200 grams of protein that leak out through capillary filtration every 24 hours.

COMPONENTS
Lymph, a clear, transparent, watery substance, is produced primarily by the liver and gastrointestinal tract and contains fat, fatty acids, glycerol, amino acids, glucose, and other substances. These substances may give the lymph a more milklike appearance. When produced by other regions, it is a filtrate of excess fluid drained away from the arterial ends of capillaries by lymph vessels. Normal lymphatic flow is approximately 2 liters per day for the entire body. In combating foreign substances, the immune function of the lymphatic system relies on the phagocytic action of scavenger cells such as macrophages and competent cells such as the lymphocytes, which have varied function. Some interact directly with foreign intrusions, while others, the B lymphocytes, produce antibodies as a means of unlocking or weakening the invaders' defenses.

STRUCTURE
The structure of the system consists of lymph nodes and channels. The channels usually transverse at least two nodes. Since not all of these are in use at any given time, there is a tremendous reserve capacity. Flow along these channels is unidirectional, controlled by a valvular system. Sections between valves contract in sequential reaction to distension, further promoting one-way flow. Some of the larger vessels are also selective in the amount and size of the material they contain. Both a deep and superficial system of vessels exist, with each servicing specific regions. The deep system (Fig. 16-6) drains the structures of the thorax, abdomen, pelvis, and perineum. The channels and their affiliated nodes surround major organs and vasculature and join into larger vessels until they unite with either the right lymphatic duct or the thoracic duct. The superficial lymphatic vessels (Fig. 16-7) drain the skin and other musculoskeletal structures and are located with their nodal components near veins and travel through the superficial fasciae. Again, the direction of flow is from the periphery to the core, with drainage symmetrically occurring toward the cervical, axillary, and inguinal regions and thereafter to the deeper system. The thoracic duct, the largest of all lymphatic channels, is also under some direct neural influence from the sympathetic system.

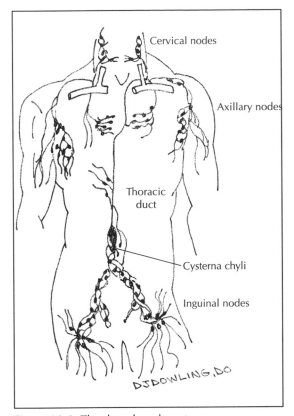

Figure 16-6. The deep lymph system.

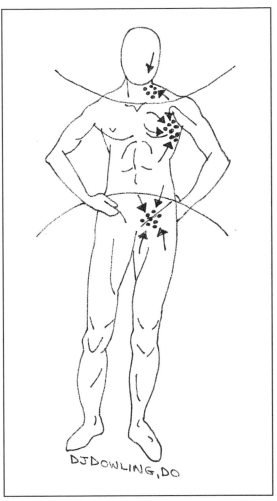

Figure 16-7. Symmetric drainage of the skin by the superficial lymph system.

FLOW
In the generally healthy individual, the abdominal lymphatics are responsible for most of lymphatic fluid production. Paradoxically, increased pressure on these vessels causes them to initially open rather than close. Intraluminal distension also creates some of the flow along with reactive contraction of the vessels. Intestinal motility, by direct pressure on the vessels and by increased production of the lymphatic fluid, produces flow.

DIAPHRAGM
The major pump of the lymphatic system is muscular activity, with the diaphragm acting as the primary engine. As the diaphragm descends into the abdominal cavity during inhalation, intraabdominal pressure is increased, thereby creating increased pressure on the vessels and other lymphatic tissue such as the nodes. The contents of the relatively large pleural lymphatic nodes are pressured by the expanding pleural sacs to empty their contents. This causes the contents to be propulsed along in a cephalad direction toward the subclavian veins. Elevation of the diaphragm during exhalation lowers the intraabdominal pressure and creates a pressure gradient for more fluid to be drawn into the abdominal vessels. Increase in respiratory capacity therefore increases the function and efficiency of the system.

SKELETAL MUSCLE
Skeletal muscular activity is the other major pump of the lymphatic system. The intermittent action of contraction and relaxation during physical activity produces a change in interstitial pressure,

increasing flow by compression, especially against the influence of gravity, from the periphery toward the trunk. Even passive activity such as massage or manipulation alters the pressure on the smaller lymphatic vessels.

DYSFUNCTION

Impaired function of either of these muscular pumps, the diaphragm or skeletal muscle, leads to stasis of the lymphatic system. Restricted thoracic cage motion, as is often seen in chronic conditions such as asthma, emphysema, bronchitis, and acute respiratory illness, handicaps adequate function. This would act locally in the lungs as well as systemically. Peripheral edema is often seen in states of impaired musculoskeletal activity, especially when the other means of drainage, the venous system, is blocked, stiff, damaged, or weakened. This is found most frequently in the lower extremities but can be observed in other gravity-dependent regions such as the sacrum and buttocks in a patient in a prolonged supine position.

PRESSURES

As a system of tubes, the lymphatic vessels are closed endothelial tubes that are permeable to fluids and high molecular compounds. Four major pressures act to mobilize fluids into and out of the lymphatic capillary:

1. *Capillary pressure* moves fluids out through the capillary membranes.
2. *Interstitial fluid pressure* moves fluid inward when the pressure is positive and outward when negative.
3. The *plasma colloid osmotic pressure* causes osmosis of fluid inward through the membrane.
4. Osmosis outward through the membrane is caused by *interstitial fluid colloid osmotic pressure.*

NODES

Lymph nodes vary in size and are aggregates of lymphatic tissue. Kidney bean–shaped, each consists of a cortex containing germinal centers and an inner medulla. Reticuloendothelial cells are located along trabeculae connective tissue and act as a filtration system for particulate matter. An efferent lymph vessel exits at the hilum along with a vein and is accompanied by an artery. An afferent lymph vessel enters on the convex side through the capsule.

SPLEEN

The spleen is the largest of all lymphatic tissues and rests against the lower ribs (9 through 11), the diaphragm, the stomach, and the left kidney in the left hypochondral region. A parenchyma of red and white pulp is surrounded by a capsule of fibrous connective tissue that contains efferent lymphatics, blood vessels, nerves, and some smooth muscle. The red pulp is a cordal and sinusoidal system concerned primarily with the production of blood products. The white pulp, which is lymphoid tissue, produces thymus-dependent T lymphocytes and B lymphocytes and plasma cells. The latter components produce the humeral antibody component of the immune system, and the T lymphocytes are involved in the cell-mediated arm of the system.

The vasculature consists of the splenic artery, the largest branch from the celiac trunk, and the splenic vein, which unites with the mesenteric vein to form the portal vein. Five percent of the blood volume per minute enters the spleen.

Normally, the spleen sequesters one third of the available platelet pool and approximately 40 to 50 ml of erythrocytes. These latter elements may either be immature cells or aged or abnormal red blood cells. As a preparation site for newly produced cells, the surface area is increased by pitting and the cells are converted to normally functioning biconcave disks. Embryologically, the spleen is responsible for the production of fetal hemoglobin and retains some potential for extramedullary hematopoiesis throughout life. Besides removing the effete, less functioning cells, the spleen also clears microorganisms and particulate matter. It produces jellylike substances called *opsonins*, which may cover certain particles or organisms. These amalgams are then more easily destroyed by the liver or macrophages. The spleen is more efficient than the liver at removing antigen/antibody complexes and poorly opsonized material.

Splenic activity can be influenced by several factors. The shape of the spleen can be compressed by a distended stomach or a full colon. Several times per minute, the descent of the diaphragm pushes the spleen further inferiorly, and in intense activities such as exercise, it increases both the rate and the extent of splenic compression. Sympathetic stimulation causes contraction of the capsule, which causes further expulsion of blood and other contents into the circulation. During times of injury, this can act as an autotransfusion process, with the delivery of erythrocytes to compensate for loss and platelets to begin some of the bandaging process. The immunological components can be propelled to reach a site of active or potential infection.

INFECTION

In response to infection, the lymphatic tissue reacts much in the way a corporation might to increased demand. Production of immunocompetent cells and destruction of the invading organisms or substances are increased. Lymphoid tissue that is previously nonpalpable may hypertrophy. Upper respiratory infections frequently have findings of lymphadenopathy in the cervical chain lymph nodes. Inguinal lymph node adenopathy may be noted in cases of urinary or pelvic infection. Enlargement of the spleen, splenomegaly, occurs during mononucleosis. Because it is usually covered by the stomach and the costal cartilage, a palpable spleen is a cardinal finding of this viral infection. The spleen may also become enlarged when the marrow is unable to further undertake hematopoiesis. The primitive production of fetal hemoglobin can be reestablished and may help maintain the blood's oxygen-carrying capacity in spite of idiopathic anemia. The liver may increase in size from infection or other toxic influence. Hepatitis, or inflammation of the liver, frequently results in hepatomegaly. Subsequent to infection, it may be quite some time before the lymphatic tissue regresses to its previous size, if at all.

Historical Perspective

I have successfully treated many cases of pneumonia, both lobar and pleurotic, by convecting the ribs at their spinal articulations . . . I carefully adjust the misplaced ribs . . .
— Andrew Taylor Still

SPANISH FLU

The Spanish flu pandemic of 1917—19 has been called by some in the pre-HIV age as "the last great plague." The middle estimate of the worldwide death toll was approximately 20 million lives. Perhaps as many as 500 million people suffered the illness commonly known as "grippe." Although other plagues had higher death rates, in terms of shear numbers, the Spanish flu pandemic is cred-

ited as one of the worst, if not the worst. In the United States one person in every four (approximately 20 million cases) fell ill with the flu.

The symptoms were similar to that experienced with other flu epidemics, but the especially virulent nature of the illness and the complications that ensued, especially susceptibility to subsequent pneumonia, raised both the morbidity and mortality. One out of four American soldiers who perished in the time of World War I actually died from this one-two combination. In the United States, close to 500,000 people are estimated to have finally died as a result of the disease or the postflu pneumonia. Insurance companies estimated that 13% of the deaths were due directly to influenza and 87% resulted from the combination with pneumonia. In some communities along the Atlantic seaboard estimates were as high as a 50% risk of dying after pneumonia.

A disease that had previously been called "the old man's friend" was indiscriminate in regards to the delivery of death as most city morgues were grossly overwhelmed. There was no panic until it was almost over. The course was insidious, and after some time various cities and communities banned sports events and public gatherings and fined people for spitting, and the Red Cross undertook to manufacture fifty thousand flu masks.

A survey conducted by the *Journal of the American Osteopathic Association* in 1919 revealed that 1,350 osteopathic physicians reported 43,500 well-defined cases. Out of these, only 160 deaths were noted, with 10 of them attributed to pneumonia. The rate of cases of pneumonia following influenza was 1 out of 16 cases, while insurance companies typically reported 1 out of 2. At the mortality rate reported by osteopathic physicians, an estimate of potentially 73,500 deaths versus the 500,000 otherwise reported can be inferred. In other words, there was an apparent 2.5% mortality rate for allopathy compared to a 0.37% rate for osteopathy.

At least one distinguishing intervention was the attention of the osteopathic profession toward maximizing respiratory function, raising the ribs, mobilizing restricted spinal regions, and increasing vascular and lymphatic flow. Otherwise, descriptions of treatment by individual osteopathic physicians are not much different than those of their allopathic colleagues. It is possible that some potentially harmful interventions were also attempted, but in the majority of cases, the pharmacologic and other therapeutic approaches were similar.

OSTEOPATHIC RESEARCH
Other investigators over the years have studied the effect of osteopathic manipulation on the immune system. Castilio and Ferris-Swift studied the effect of manipulation in the splenic region on blood indices. They found an average increase of 2,000 in the leukocyte count in 80% of the cases with a right shift and an increase in the opsonic index in as many cases. The bacteriolytic power of the serum was found to be increased in 68% of the subjects, and a decrease in the erythrocyte count was found in 75% of the cases.

Watson and Percival examined pneumonia mortality rates in children at comparable inner-city hospitals. Children treated for bronchopneumonia with manipulation at Los Angeles County Osteopathic Hospital had a 10.66% mortality rate, versus 29.6% at an allopathic hospital. Lobar pneumonia had essentially the same mortality rate, with findings of 11.2% versus 10.8% for the respective hospitals.

Measel studied antibody response following manipulation twice daily for a week combined with administration of a polyvalent pneumococcal vaccine. The study subjects showed a significant increase in antibody response to many of the subserotypes when compared to matched control subjects. An unpublished study by this author found a trend toward increased white blood cell count in the majority of treated subjects as compared to controls within 1 hour after treatment. There was a significant increase in the lymphocyte absolute number and an insignificant decrease in hemoglobin as measured at an independent laboratory.

Some of the effect attributed to the manipulative interventions has been discussed as demargination. A significant percentage of hematological cells actually lie against vessel walls as a reserve. Activities such as exercise lead to increased flow. It appears that these cells, the large majority of which are immunocompetent and mature, are then "knocked off" and delivered into the blood stream. Even if this were the only effect, it would still be an improvement over the stagnation that occurs in patients unable to move or exercise themselves.

TREATMENT
Much of the treatment performed historically within the osteopathic profession has been thoracic pumping. Other means of lymphatic pumping include pectoral traction, rib raising, effleurage, Dalrymple pedal pumping, cervical lymphatic drainage, and splenic and hepatic pumping. Air sinus drainage techniques performed about the face are used in conjunction with the other techniques to help promote the production and clearance of watery mucus from the upper respiratory region. The most efficient approach is to first treat the central components, thereby freeing drainage into the larger lymphatic structures, and thereafter work outward toward the periphery.

CONTRAINDICATIONS
Some of the techniques may be limited or inappropriate, depending on the patient's medical condition. Splenomegaly, hepatitis, pneumothorax, osteoporosis, pyelonephritis, thrombotic phenomenon, and recent surgery may preclude the use of thoracic manipulation for fear of further complications. Anemia, pregnancy, and a history of neoplastic processes are relative contraindications. There has not been any proof that such manipulations promote metastasis by increasing circulation. In fact, an argument could be made that the presentation of neoplastic cells to bodily organs that can develop seek-and-destroy components for abnormal tissue may be beneficial. However, caution must be exercised in this regard. The same holds true if there is an abscess or other localized infection. Sometimes it is wiser to allow the body to wall off and deal with an invader than it is to break the compartment and allow further spread.

Cardiac and respiratory conditions most likely will benefit from this therapy. However, care must be taken to develop interventions that facilitate improvement without compromising other considerations. Thoracic pumping may increase respiratory capacity and fluid dynamics, but to one experiencing the sensation of extreme chest pressure, the benefits may be outweighed by the psychological considerations. As in all cases of manipulative or other interventions, decisions are best developed when a diagnosis is made and indications and contraindications are evaluated.

EVALUATION OF THE THORAX
Eileen L. DiGiovanna

There are several reasons for evaluating the thorax during a structural examination. The status of the rib cage is an important clue to the status of the respiratory mechanism. Free motion of the ribs is necessary for full expansion of the lungs. Conversely, pulmonary diseases cause secondary changes in rib motion.

The ribs may also be a source of chest wall or upper back pain. Rib dysfunction may result in shoulder, arm, or neck pain. Finally, rib dysfunctions may be primary or secondary to thoracic spine dysfunction.

Observation of the chest wall will reveal any asymmetry, the typical barrel chest of chronic pulmonary diseases, increased or decreased rate of respiration, or the degree to which the patient uses abdominal versus thoracic breathing.

The thorax is palpated to detect static asymmetries as well as asymmetries or restrictions of rib motion. Static asymmetries represent anterior or posterior ribs. Palpation for static asymmetries is particularly helpful when localized pain is due to rib dysfunction. Ribs may be palpated along the posterior thorax at the angle of the ribs with the patient prone. A posterior rib on palpation appears to lie more posteriorly than the rib above or below it. Posterior ribs are frequently due to posterior rotation of the transverse process with which the rib articulates. As with any somatic dysfunction, there will be associated tissue changes in the area of the rib head.

Palpation along the sternal border anteriorly will reveal ribs that have moved anteriorly, a common cause of anterior chest wall pain. Rib dysfunction on the left side may be mistaken by the patient for cardiac pain. Tenderness and tissue changes may be palpated along the sternal border at the costochondral junction.

Palpation of the anterior chest wall may disclose elevated or depressed ribs. In the case of a depressed rib, the space between it and the rib below will be narrowed, while the space between it and the rib above will be widened. These differences are reversed for an elevated rib: the space between it and the rib above will be narrowed, while the space between it and the rib below is widened. A single rib or a group of ribs may be elevated or depressed. Motion testing is necessary for diagnosis, as the findings on static palpation may be misleading.

Diagnostic Terminology
Various authors use different terms to describe rib dysfunctions. Some common terms are:

1. Anterior or posterior ribs
2. Elevated or depressed ribs
3. Ribs in a position of inspiration or expiration (inhalation or exhalation dysfunctions)
4. Ribs restricted in inspiration or expiration (inhalation or exhalation restrictions)

When reading literature, note whether the author states that a rib is in a *position of inspiration* (elevated) or *restricted* in inspiration (depressed). An inspiration restriction denotes a rib that does not move into a position of inspiration but is held in a depressed or expiratory position. Inspiratory and expiratory restrictions are restrictions of motion of the rib on its respiratory axis; that is, during inspiration the anterior portion of the rib is elevated and during expiration the rib is depressed.

Evaluation of the First Rib
The first rib is unlike the other ribs because of its attachments to the scalene muscles and its functional relationship to the clavicle. It is customarily palpated at three sites:

1. The posterior superior surface, through the trapezius
2. The anterior superior surface in the depression behind the clavicle
3. The anterior articulation just below the clavicle at the sternal border

The technique for motion testing of the first rib is described below.

1. **Patient position:** supine.
2. **Physician position:** seated at the head of the table.

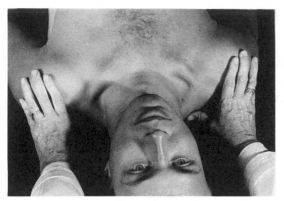

Figure 16-8. Position for evaluating the first rib.

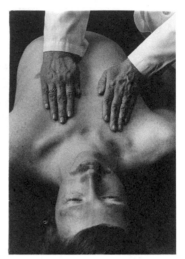

Figure 16-9. Pump handle
motion testing of the upper ribs.

3. **Technique:**
   a. The physician places her thumbs or finger
      pads on the anterior surface in the supracla-
      vicular depression and evaluates the static
      position of the first ribs. Is one rib higher than
      the other?
   b. Tissue texture and muscle tone over the rib
      are examined for abnormalities.
   c. The physician places her thumbs on the pos-
      terior surface just anterior to the trapezius
      and springs the ribs lightly, evaluating the
      resistance of the ribs (Fig. 16-8). If resistance
      is felt when the rib is sprung, that rib is dys-
      functional.
   d. The physician evaluates rib motion by plac-
      ing her thumbs or finger pads on the antero-
      superior surface of the first ribs and asking
      the patient to make a full inspiratory and ex-
      piratory effort.
   e. **Significance:**
      i. If one rib stops moving before the other rib
         during inspiration, that rib has an *inspira-
         tory restriction.*
      ii. If one rib stops moving before the other rib
          during exhalation, that rib has an *expira-
          tory restriction.*

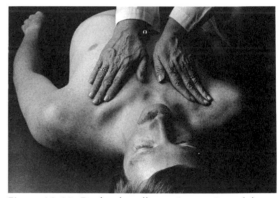

Figure 16-10. Bucket handle motion testing of the
upper ribs.

Gross Motion Testing of the Ribs

This section describes a general screening test for
evaluating motion of groups of ribs.

1. **Patient position:** supine.
2. **Physician position:** standing at the side of the
   table, facing the patient's head.

3. **Technique:**
   a. **Upper ribs (1–3)**
      i. Pump handle motion
         a) The physician places her fingers flat
            along the sternal border bilaterally, with
            the fingertips touching the inferior sur-
            face of the clavicle (Fig. 16-9).
         b) Motion is evaluated as the patient in-
            hales and exhales deeply.
      ii. Bucket handle motion
         a) The physician places her fingers flat on
            the upper chest wall and at a 45-degree
            angle to the sternal border, with the
            index finger lying just below clavicle
            (Fig. 16-10).

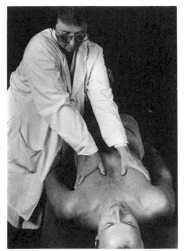

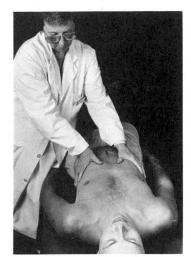

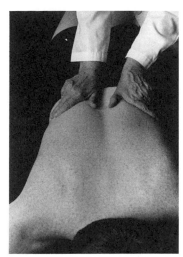

Figure 16-11. Gross motion testing of the middle ribs.

Figure 16-12. Gross motion testing of the lower ribs.

Figure 16-13. Gross motion testing of ribs 11 and 12.

b) Motion is evaluated in full inhalation and exhalation.

b. **Middle ribs (4–7)**
   i. The physician places her thumbs along the sternal border with the tips toward the patient's head.
   ii. The fingers are placed laterally along the middle ribs, each finger covering one rib (Fig. 16-11).
   iii. As the patient inhales and exhales fully,
      a) Evaluate pump handle motion with the thumbs.
      b) Evaluate bucket handle motion with the fingers.
   iv. In a female patient it may be preferable to evaluate pump handle and bucket handle motions individually by placing the fingers along the sternal border first and then along the ribs at the midaxillary area.

c. **Lower ribs (8–10)**
   i. The physician places her thumbs along the costochondral border and spreads the fingers along the ribs laterally (Fig. 16-12).
   ii. The evaluation of the lower ribs follows that for the middle ribs.

d. **Ribs 11 and 12**
   These ribs are evaluated with the patient prone. Their caliper-type motion is evaluated.
   i. The physician forms a C with her thumb and second and third fingers. The thumb

is placed at the area of the rib heads and the fingers along the ribs (Fig. 16-13).
   ii. Rib motion is evaluated in full inhalation and exhalation.
   iii. **Significance:**
      a) If a group of ribs stops moving on one side before the other during inhalation, one or more ribs in that group have an inhalation restriction. The restriction may be of pump handle motion, bucket handle motion, or both.
      b) If a group of ribs stops moving on one side before the other during exhalation, one or more ribs in that group have an exhalation restriction. The restriction may be of pump handle motion or bucket handle motion.
      c) Occasionally bilateral restrictions may be present. Their identification requires knowledge of normal rib excursions, which comes with experience and concentration on full ranges of motion.

Individual Rib Motion Testing

The individual ribs are tested in the manner just described for each level of ribs, but only one rib on each side is tested and compared. Individual ribs may be tested if one rib is painful or if restriction of motion is found on gross motion testing. If a group inhalation restriction has been found, usually the top rib in the group is responsible for the restriction. If a group exhalation restriction has been found, usually the lowest rib in the group is responsible.

Evaluation of the Sternum

Because of the close association of the sternum with the ribs, the sternum must be evaluated when respiratory excursion appears limited. The sternum is evaluated by placing the thumb of one hand on the manubrium and the other thumb on the body of the sternum (Fig. 16-14). By applying pressure with each thumb alternately, the physician can determine if sternal motion is free at the angle of Louis.

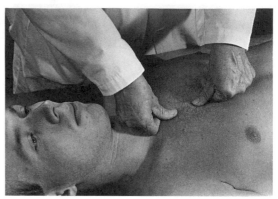

Figure 16-14. Evaluation of the sternum.

Evaluation of the Clavicle

Evaluation of the clavicle is discussed in Chapter 19 (Diagnosis and Treatment of the Upper Extremity—The Shoulder Girdle). Because of the close relationship between the clavicle and the first rib, when first or second rib restriction is found, the clavicle must be evaluated.

THE DIAPHRAGM
Paula D. Scariati

The major muscles of respiration are the diaphragm, the internal and external intercostal muscles, the parasternal muscles, and the scalenes. Abdominal muscles that participate in respiration include the external and internal oblique muscles and the transverse and rectus abdominis muscles. The diaphragm generates two thirds of the inspiratory effort. Nevertheless, a person with a paralyzed diaphragm may still have good respiratory function.

The diaphragm is composed of muscular portions and an aponeurotic portion, the *central tendon.* The muscular portion is divided into three parts, based on origin:

1. Sternal part
   Origin: posterior aspect of the xiphoid process of the sternum
   Insertion: central tendon
2. Costal part (forms the right and left hemidiaphragms)
   Origin: internal surface of the inferior six ribs at their costal margins

Insertion: central tendon
3. Lumbar part
   Origin: arises from the lumbar vertebrae via two crura and arcuate ligaments
   a. Left crus: attaches to L1–L2 and the associated intervertebral disk on the left side of the aorta.
   b. Right crus: attaches to L1–L3 and the associated intervertebral disks on the right side of the aorta.
   c. Median arcuate ligament: unites the medial side of the two crura. It passes over the anterior surface of the aorta and gives origin to some of the fibers of the right crus.
   d. Medial arcuate ligament: a thickening of the anterior layer of thoracolumbar fascia over the superior part of the psoas major muscle. It forms a fibrous arch from the crus of the diaphragm to the transverse process of L1.
   e. Lateral arcuate ligament: a thickening of the anterior layer of thoracolumbar fascia

over the superior part of the quadratus lumborum muscle. It forms a fibrous arch that runs from the transverse process of L1 to the 12th rib.

Embryology

The splanchnic mesenchyme surrounding the laryngotracheal tube forms the connective tissue, cartilage, muscle, and the blood and lymphatic vessels of the lung. The diaphragm, the dome-shaped, musculotendinous partition between the thoracic and abdominal cavities, originates in four different structures: (1) the *septum transversum,* which develops into the central tendon of the diaphragm in the adult, (2) the *pleuroperitoneal membranes*, which form a part of the musculature of the main part of the diaphragm, (3) the *dorsal mesentery of the esophagus,* which contributes to the formation of the crura of the diaphragm, and (4) the *body wall,* which contributes to the peripheral portions of the diaphragm and forms the costodiaphragmatic recesses, giving the diaphragm its dome shape.

Structure, Function, and Innervation of the Diaphragm and Associated Muscles

The central tendon is a strong, C-shaped aponeurosis that is the insertion site for all the muscular fibers of the diaphragm. The middle portion of the central tendon lies just inferior to the heart and fuses with the fibrous pericardium here.

The motor innervation of the diaphragm is provided by the phrenic nerve, which originates in nerve roots C3–C5. During embryogenesis, the diaphragm migrates caudad relative to the vertebral column. The sensory innervation of the diaphragm is mainly provided by the phrenic nerve, with intercostal nerves providing sensory innervation to the fringes of the diaphragm that develop from the lateral body wall.

The function of the diaphragm is to contract during inspiration. This causes the dome of the diaphragm to move inferiorly and compress the abdominal viscera (through increased intraabdominal pressure). Intrathoracic pressure decreases as a consequence of the increased volume of the thoracic cavity. Air is drawn into the lungs; venous and lymphatic motion are facilitated.

All of the structures that pierce the diaphragm are affected by the integrity of the muscle. The three main apertures in the diaphragm allow passage of the venae cavae, esophagus, and aorta. The right phrenic nerve passes via the vena caval foramen. The superior epigastric vessels pass through the sternocostal hiatus. The musculophrenic vessels pass near the ninth costal cartilage. The subcostal nerves and vessels pass posterior to the lateral arcuate ligament. The sympathetic trunk passes posterior to the medial arcuate ligament. Splanchnic nerves pierce the crura. The hemiazygous vein passes through the left crus.

Because of its varied origins and insertions, the diaphragm acts in a number of ways during inspiration. The **crural diaphragm** contracts and moves the central tendon caudad, increasing intraabdominal pressure and pushing the abdominal wall outward. Simultaneously, it contributes to decreasing the intrapleural pressure and inflating the lungs. The **costal diaphragm** has a similar action, but as it exerts a caudal force on the central tendon, it concomitantly exerts a cephalic force on the costal margin. Thus it both expands the rib cage and assists in lung inflation with abdominal motion.

Increased intraabdominal pressure secondary to diaphragmatic contraction also acts to expand the rib cage. This is achieved by the transmission of abdominal pressure through an area of apposition of the costal diaphragm to the inner surface of the lower rib cage.

The different actions of the crural and costal portions of the diaphragm on respiratory effort indicate that the tension developed by one portion of the muscle is not transmitted to the other portion. Thus these muscles are linked mechanically in parallel at the start. However, as lung volumes increase, the costal and crural parts become linked in series. Thus, with progressive hyperinflation, the diaphragm becomes a less effective force generator because its costal and crural parts develop the same tensions; they then have the same action.

RIB CAGE MUSCLES DURING RESPIRATION
In addition to the diaphragm, the rib cage muscles contribute to respiration. The parasternal muscles act to decrease the angle between the upper border of the ribs and the sternum. Because the ribs are fixed in their anteroposterior positions by bony attachments, these muscles facilitate the bucket handle motion of the rib cage. The primary action of the scalene muscles is to elevate the first and

second ribs by decreasing the angle between the upper border of the rib and the vertebral column, thus facilitating the pump handle motion of the ribs.

Normally, the parasternals and scalenes contract with the diaphragm. If the diaphragm were to contract alone, it would displace the abdomen more than the rib cage. Working together, these forces counterbalance each other and vary according to position (e.g., erect versus supine) and postural compliance (e.g., kyphosis with decreased rib compliance).

INTERACTING SYSTEMS OF CONTROL

The anatomical and mechanical events described are often regulated by and interact with other systems of control, including neural control, humoral influences, and mechanical factors such as the mucous coat of the respiratory passageways, cilial clearance, and the muscle and cartilage incorporated into the various parts of the respiratory passageways.

Physiology

Inhaled air passes through the nose and pharynx and is distributed to the lungs by way of the trachea, bronchi, and bronchioles. The trachea is the first-generation respiratory passageway; the right and left main-stem bronchi are second-generation passageways. Each division thereafter constitutes another generation. After passing through 20 to 25 generations of airways, inhaled air reaches the alveoli, where exchange of oxygen and carbon dioxide takes place.

The process of respiration can be divided into four events:

1. **Pulmonary ventilation,** defined as the inflow and outflow of air between the atmosphere and the alveoli
2. **Diffusion** of oxygen and carbon dioxide between the lungs and the alveoli
3. **Transport** of oxygen and carbon dioxide in the blood and body fluids to and from the cells
4. **Regulation** of ventilation

In pulmonary ventilation, the lungs move in two planes: (1) up and down, facilitated by diaphragmatic contraction, and (2) anteriorly-posteriorly, facilitated by rib motion. Normal, quiet breathing

entails mostly motion in the vertical plane. Maximal respiratory efforts recruit anteroposterior lung motion, which increases lung volume by 20%.

During inspiration, intraalveolar pressure becomes negative with respect to the atmospheric pressure. This effect is secondary to diaphragmatic contraction, and air is drawn into the lungs. Expiration is passive. Intraalveolar pressures increase and air flows out.

In normal, quiet respiration, the chest wall always tends to expand, whereas the lungs tend to collapse. This recoil tendency of the lungs is due to two factors:

1. Elastic fibers in the lung which are stretched and in response tend to shorten (the stretch reflex).
2. Surface tensions caused by intermolecular attractions between the surface molecules of alveolar fluid. This tension is countered to a great extent by lung surfactant.

Under resting conditions, a negative pressure of about 4 mm Hg is required to keep the lung expanded. This is known as the pleural pressure or the lung recoil pressure.

Compliance is defined as the expansibility of the lungs and the thorax. The muscles of respiration use energy to expand the lungs and the thoracic cage around the lungs during respiration.

The interactions of respiration are far greater than the musculo-osseous-thoracic interactions described here. The ability to manipulate the muscle, fascia, bone, and the cranial rhythmic impulse allows the osteopathic physician to address respiratory dysfunctions at a variety of levels.

References

Castilio Y, Ferris-Swift L. 1934. The effect of direct splenic stimulation on the cells and the antibody content of the blood stream in acute infectious diseases. The College Journal, Kansas City College of Osteopathy and Surgery 18(7).

———, Ferris-Swift L. 1932. Effects of splenic stimulation in normal individuals on the actual and differential blood cell count and the opsonic index. Kansas City College of Osteopathy and Surgery Bulletin 16: 10–16.

Cathie AG. 1965. Physiologic motions of the spine as related to respiratory activity. In: Academy of Applied

Osteopathy—1965 Yearbook. Carmel, Calif: Academy of Applied Osteopathy.

Chiles HL. Editorial: a new survey of public health. J Am Osteopath Assoc 1(19):227–230.

Galewaler JE. 1969. Motion, the lymphatics and manipulation. J Am Osteopath Assoc 69:247–254.

Guyton AC. 1986. Textbook of Medical Physiology, 7th ed. Philadelphia: W.B. Saunders.

Kapandji IA. 1974. The Physiology of the Joints. Vol III. Edinburgh: Churchill Livingstone.

Kohn GC, ed. 1995. Encyclopedia of Plague and Pestilence. New York: Facts on File.

Langley L, Telford IR, Christensen JB. 1980. Dynamic Anatomy and Physiology, 5th ed. New York: McGraw-Hill.

Measel JW. 1982. The effect of the lymphatic pump on the immune response: I. Preliminary studies on the antibody response to pneumococcal polysaccharide assayed by bacterial agglutination and passive hemagglutination. J Am Osteopath Assoc 82:28–31.

———. 1982. Introduction: thoughts on osteopathic practice and infectious diseases. Osteopath Ann 10(3): 92–94.

Moore KL. 1985. Clinically Oriented Anatomy, 2nd ed. Baltimore: Williams & Wilkins.

———. 1988. The Developing Human: Clinically Oriented Embryology, 4th ed. Philadelphia: W.B. Saunders.

Pansky B. 1984. Review of Gross Anatomy, 5th ed. New York: Macmillan.

Robbins SL, ed. 1984. Pathologic Basis of Disease, 3rd ed. Philadelphia: W.B. Saunders.

Sabiston DC. 1986. Textbook of Surgery: The Biological Basis of Modern Surgical Practice. Philadelphia: W.B. Saunders.

Schiowitz S, DiGiovanna E, Ausman P. 1983. An Osteopathic Approach to Diagnosis and Treatment. Old Westbury, NY: New York College of Osteopathic Medicine.

Tacker EE. 19xx. Spanish influenza—what and why? J Am Osteopath Assoc 2(19):270–273.

Watson JO, Percival EN. 19xx. Pneumonia research in children at Los Angeles County Osteopathic Hospital. J Am Osteopath Assoc 39(3):153–159.

Webster GV. 19xx. Subdiaphragmatic drainage. J Am Osteopath Assoc 1(28):145.

Williams G. 1960. Virus Hunters. New York: Alfred A. Knopf.

Zink JG, Lawson WB. 1978. The role of pectoral traction in the treatment of lymphatic flow disturbance. Osteopath Ann 6(11):439–496.

17

Treatment of
the Thoracic Cage

MUSCLE ENERGY TECHNIQUES FOR THE RIBS
Eileen L. DiGiovanna

Muscle energy treatment of the ribs is used to correct inspiratory and expiratory restrictions. Each treatment entails the following general principles:

1. Patient contracting a muscle to move a rib
2. Patient providing respiratory assistance
3. Force applied by physician to assist motion

Techniques are described separately for the 1st rib, the 2nd through 10th ribs, and the 11th and 12th ribs.

Inspiratory Restrictions
FIRST RIB: PUMP HANDLE MOTION
1. **Patient position:** supine.
2. **Physician position:** standing at the side of the table, facing the patient's head.
3. **Technique:**
   a. The patient places his hand, palm up, on his forehead.
   b. The physician reaches under the patient with her near hand and grasps the posterosuperior surface of the first rib with her fingers.
   c. The physician places her other hand, palm down, on top of the patient's hand.
   d. The patient is asked to raise his head off the table and simultaneously take a deep breath.

e. As the patient lifts his head, the physician resists motion by pressing down on the patient's hand and simultaneously pulling caudad on the back of the rib (Fig. 17-1).
   f. Repeat the above steps three times.
4. Three mechanisms have aided in moving the rib in an elevated, or inspiratory, pump handle motion:
   a. Patient's contraction of the anterior scalene elevated the rib, since the head is fixed.
   b. The deep inspiration assisted the rib into a position of inspiration.
   c. The physician's pull on the posterior part of the rib flipped the anterior part upward.

FIRST RIB: BUCKET HANDLE MOTION
1. **Patient position:** supine, with his head turned 40 degrees from the midline, toward the rib being treated.
2. **Physician position:** standing at the side of the table, facing the patient's head.
3. **Technique:**
   a. The technique is as for treating the pump handle motion of the first rib, except that the middle scalene muscle, which attaches more laterally, instead of the anterior scalene muscle is used (Fig. 17-2).

An Osteopathic Approach to Diagnosis and Treatment, second edition
Eileen L. DiGiovanna and Stanley Schiowitz
Lippincott–Raven Publishers, Philadelphia © 1997.

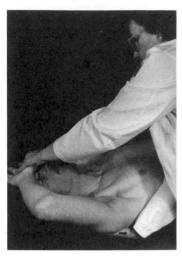

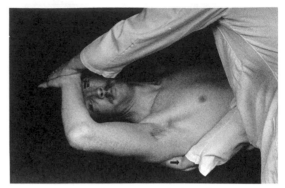

Figure 17-2. Muscle energy technique for treatment of inspiratory restriction of the first rib (bucket handle motion).

Figure 17-1. Muscle energy technique for treatment of inspiratory restriction of the first rib (pump handle motion).

RIBS 2–10: PUMP HANDLE MOTION

1. **Patient position:** supine.
2. **Physician position:** standing at the side of the table, facing the patient's head.
3. **Technique:**
   a. The patient places his hand, palm up, on his forehead.
   b. The physician reaches behind the patient with her near hand and grasps the supero-posterior part of the rib being treated.
   c. The physician places her hand on top of the patient's hand.
   d. The patient is instructed to lift his hand toward the ceiling. The physician provides resistance (Fig. 17-3).
   e. At the same time, the physician pulls down on the posterior rib and the patient inhales deeply.
4. In this technique, the patient uses the serratus anterior muscle to elevate the anterior part of the rib as the physician pulls down on the posterior rib to aid elevation at the anterior part.

RIBS 2–10: BUCKET HANDLE MOTION

1. **Patient position:** supine.
2. **Physician position:** standing at the side of the table, facing the patient's head.
3. **Technique:**
   a. The technique is the same as for treating the pump handle motion of these ribs, except

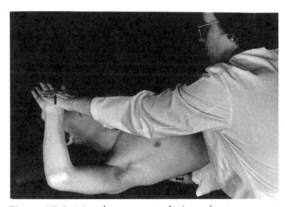

Figure 17-3. Muscle energy technique for treatment of inspiratory restriction of the 2nd through 10th ribs (pump handle motion).

that the patient is instructed to move his arm up and out at a 45-degree angle. The lateral part of the serratus will then elevate the lateral part of the ribs to improve the bucket handle motion.

RIBS 11 AND 12

1. **Patient position:** prone.
2. **Physician position:** standing at the side of the table, opposite the rib being treated.
3. **Technique:**
   a. The patient's legs are pulled toward the physician.
   b. The patient's arm on the involved side is placed above his head.
   c. The physician grasps the anterior inferior iliac spines and rotates the pelvis.

d. The palm of the physician's opposite hand is placed over the involved rib(s).

e. The patient is asked to inhale deeply.

f. As the patient inhales, the physician pushes laterally on the rib, separating it from its articulation to allow the breath to carry it into inhalation (see Fig. 17-6).

Expiratory Restrictions

RIB 1: PUMP HANDLE MOTION

1. **Patient position:** supine.

2. **Physician position:** standing or seated at the head of the table.

3. **Technique:**

   a. The patient's neck is bent forward.

   b. The physician places her thumb on the rib between the two heads of the sternocleidomastoid muscle.

   c. The patient inhales, then exhales completely.

   d. The physician presses down on the rib, following it into exhalation.

   e. The physician holds the rib down as the patient takes a shallow breath and exhales again.

RIB 1: BUCKET HANDLE MOTION

1. **Patient position:** supine, with the head side-bent slightly toward the affected rib.

2. **Physician position:** standing or seated at the head of the table.

3. **Technique:** The technique is the same as for treating expiratory restriction of the pump handle motion of the first rib, except that the physician's thumb is placed lateral to the sternocleidomastoid muscle.

RIBS 2–5: PUMP HANDLE MOTION

1. **Patient position:** supine.

2. **Physician position:** standing or seated at the head of the table.

3. **Technique:**

   a. The physician places her fingers on the superior surface of the costal cartilage of the rib being treated and the one below it.

   b. The patient's neck is bent forward fully.

   c. The patient exhales fully as the physician encourages the rib to move into a position of expiration.

   d. The physician holds down the rib as the patient inhales, then moves it farther into expi-

Figure 17-4. Muscle energy technique for treatment of expiratory restriction of the second through fifth ribs (pump handle motion).

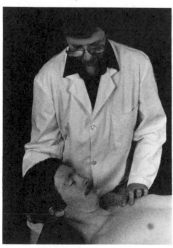

Figure 17-5. Muscle energy technique for treatment of expiratory restriction of the 6th through 10th ribs (bucket handle motion).

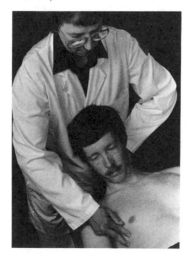

Figure 17-6. Muscle energy technique for treatment of expiratory restriction of the 11th and 12th ribs (arm at side for treating expiratory restrictions and above head for inspiratory restrictions).

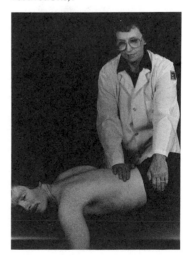

ration as the patient exhales forcefully (Fig. 17-4).

Note: The intercostal muscles are thus used to pull down on the ribs as the physician forces them down with her finger.

RIBS 2–5: BUCKET HANDLE MOTION
1. **Patient position:** supine, with the shoulders and neck side-bent toward the affected side.
2. **Physician position:** standing or seated at the head of the table.
3. **Technique:** The technique is the same as for treating pump handle motion expiratory restriction of ribs 2–5, except that the physician's fingers are placed in the midaxillary line above and below the rib being treated.

RIBS 6–10: PUMP HANDLE MOTION
1. **Patient position:** supine, with the shoulders lifted up by the physician's hand placed between the scapulae or with the upper back resting on the physician's thigh. The upper trunk is thus bent forward.
2. **Physician position:** standing at the head of the table, supporting the patient.
3. **Technique:**
   a. The rib is forced into expiration as the patient exhales forcefully.

b. The rib is held down during inhalation.
c. The maneuver is repeated twice more.

RIBS 6–10: BUCKET HANDLE MOTION
1. **Patient position:** same as for treating pump handle motion, except that the upper trunk is side-bent toward the affected rib as well as forward bent (Fig. 17-5).
2. **Physician position:** standing at the head of the table, supporting the patient.
3. **Technique:** same as for treating pump handle motion.

RIBS 10–12
1. **Patient position:** prone.
2. **Physician position:** at the side of the table, opposite the involved rib.
3. **Technique:**
   a. The patient's legs are pulled toward the physician.
   b. The patient's arm remains at his side (the only position difference from the treatment of inspiratory restrictions).
   c. The physician grasps the anterior inferior iliac spine and pulls it posteriorly.
   d. With the thenar eminence on the involved rib, the physician pushes it away from its articulation as the patient exhales forcefully (Fig. 17-6).

COUNTERSTRAIN TECHNIQUES FOR THE RIBS
Eileen L. DiGiovanna

This section describes counterstrain techniques for tender points of the anterior and posterior ribs. In most of these techniques the patient's head or thorax is bent to the side, with additional rotation into or away from the tender point.

Anterior tender points represent depressed ribs (inhalation restrictions), and posterior tender points represent elevated ribs (exhalation restrictions). Note that ribs generally need to be held 120 seconds rather than the usual 90 seconds.

Anterior Tender Points
RIBS 1 AND 2 (DEPRESSED)
The locations of the tender points of the anterior rib cage are shown in Figure 17-7. The tender point for the first rib is lateral to the sternum, at the level of the angle of Louis, just below the sternoclavicular joint. The tender point for the second rib is in the midclavicular line at the level of the second rib interspace.
1. **Patient position:** supine.

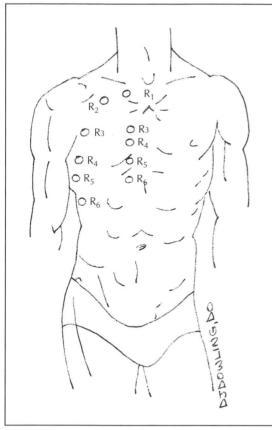

Figure 17-7. Tender point locations, anterior rib cage.

2. **Physician position:** standing at the patient's side near the head of the table.
3. **Technique:**
   a. The tender point is monitored with the physician's finger.
   b. The patient's head is slightly flexed, rotated, and side-bent toward the tender point (Fig. 17-8).
   c. Slightly more flexion is required for the second rib than for the first.
   d. When the point is no longer tender, the position is held for 120 seconds. The patient is slowly returned to neutral.

RIBS 3–6 (DEPRESSED)
The anterior tender points for the third through sixth ribs lie along the anterior axillary line on the ribs, or more medially along the sternal border at the rib interspaces.
1. **Patient position:** seated on the table.
2. **Physician position:** standing behind the patient.
3. **Technique:**
   a. The physician places her foot on the table opposite the side of the tender point and drapes the patient's arm over her thigh.
   b. The physician moves her thigh laterally so that the patient, who is leaning on the thigh, side-bends to the side of the tender point.
   c. The patient is asked to curl his legs onto the table toward the side of the tender point (Fig. 17-9).

Figure 17-8. Counterstrain technique for a depressed first rib.

Figure 17-9. Counterstrain technique for somatic dysfunction of ribs 3–6 (depression).

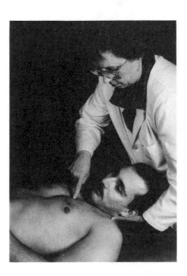

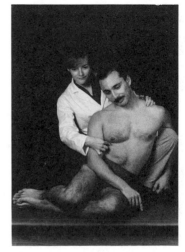

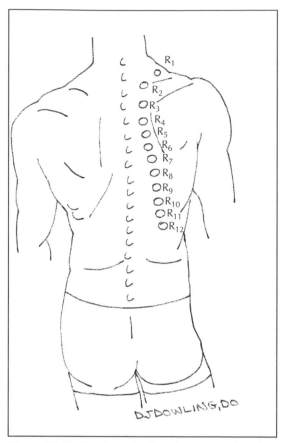

Figure 17-10. Tender point locations, posterior rib cage.

d. The free arm may be crossed over the patient's lap.
e. When the point is no longer tender, the position is held for 120 seconds. The patient is then slowly returned to a neutral position.

Posterior Tender Points

The posterior tender points lie along the angles of the ribs. Their locations are shown in Figure 17-10.

RIB 1 (ELEVATED)
1. **Patient position:** seated.
2. **Physician position:** standing behind the patient.
3. **Technique:**
   a. The physician places her foot on the table on the side of the tender point and drapes the patient's arm over her thigh.
   b. The patient leans on the physician's thigh, which is moved laterally, causing elevation of the first rib.
   c. The head is side-bent toward the tender point. It is then bent forward or backward, whichever gives maximal softening of the tissues (Fig. 17-11).

Figure 17-11. Counterstrain technique for an elevated first rib.

Figure 17-12. Counterstrain technique for elevation of the second through eighth ribs.

Figure 17-13. Lateral view of counterstrain technique for elevated ribs.

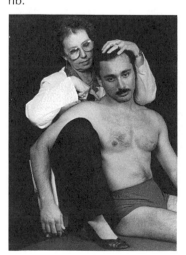
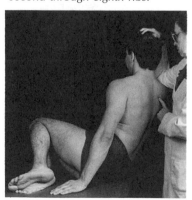
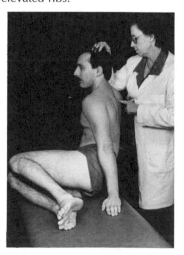

RIBS 2–8 (ELEVATED)
1. **Patient position:** seated.
2. **Physician position:** standing.
3. **Technique:**
   a. The physician places her foot on the table on the side of the tender point and drapes the patient's arm over her thigh.
   b. The thigh is moved laterally with the patient leaning on it, further elevating the ribs on that side.
   c. For upper ribs the head is side-bent and rotated away from the tender point.
   d. For lower ribs the patient is asked to curl his legs onto the table on the side opposite the tender point (Figs. 17-12, 17-13).
   e. The arm may be placed behind the patient.
   f. When the point is no longer tender, the position is held for 120 seconds. The patient is then returned to a neutral position.

FACILITATED POSITIONAL RELEASE
Stanley Schiowitz

Rib Techniques
FIRST RIB DYSFUNCTION
1. **Patient position:** supine.
2. **Physician position:** standing beside the table, on the side of the dysfunction.
3. **Technique:**
   a. The physician places his caudal (with respect to the patient) hand over the patient's rib with the fingers on the posterior aspect of the first rib (right hand on right rib). The hand placement may be modified laterally to treat tissue only, or at the costovertebral junction to obtain first thoracic articular release.
   b. The physician bends the patient's elbow and places his left hand on the patient's flexed elbow, and then brings the humerus up to 90 degrees of flexion.
   c. The physician pushes down on the patient's elbow directly toward his monitoring fingers (Fig. 17-14).
   d. Maintaining this compression, the physician adds internal rotation of the shoulder joint. This is accomplished by placing the patient's right forearm on the ventral aspect of the physician's right forearm and turning the patient's forearm outwards by a caudal motion of the physician's forearm. This should create tissue release or articular motion.
   e. The position is held for 3 seconds.
   f. Maintaining the compressive torsional force, the physician brings the patient's arm toward the midline (adduction), and then circumducts the arm down to the table top until the arm is along the patient's side (Fig. 17-15).

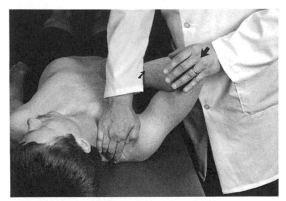

Figure 17-14. Facilitated positional release treatment for first rib dysfunction: application of compression with internal rotation of shoulder.

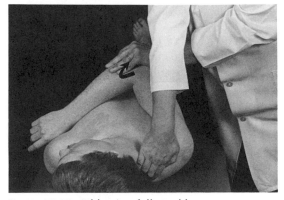

Figure 17-15. Adduction followed by circumduction to release the arm.

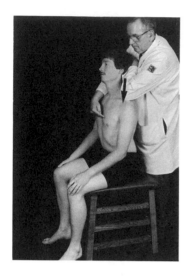

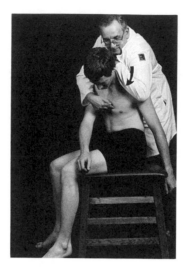

Figure 17-16. Facilitated positional release treatment for anterior rib cage dysfunction: application of compression at the cervicothoracic junction.

Figure 17-17. Facilitated positional release treatment for anterior rib cage dysfunction, with forward bending, side-bending, and rotation added.

g. The position is released and the dysfunction reevaluated.

ANTERIOR RIB CAGE AND COSTOCHONDRAL DYSFUNCTIONS
Example: Fourth, Left, Costochondral Dysfunction
1. **Patient position:** seated.
2. **Physician position:** standing behind the patient.
3. **Technique:**
   a. The physician places his right hand around the front of the patient with the index finger on the dysfunction.
   b. The physician's left hand is on the patient's cervicothoracic junction, with the left arm resting on the superior aspect of the patient's shoulder and his elbow over the acromiom process.
   c. The patient is instructed to sit up straight until the thoracic kyphosis flattens slightly.
   d. The physician applies compression at the cervicothoracic junction and left shoulder, directly toward the floor (Fig. 17-16). (Do not allow forward bending.)
   e. Maintaining the compressive force, the physician bends the patient's body forward up to the monitoring finger. (The patient may be told to drop his head forward.)
   f. The physician adds left side-bending until motion is felt at the monitoring finger. Rotation may have to be added (Fig. 17-17).

g. The position is held for 3 seconds, then released; the dysfunction is reevaluated.

DORSAL RIB DYSFUNCTIONS
Use the technique as described in Chapter 9, the section titled "Thoracic Dysfunction, Patient Prone," by modifying the placement of your monitoring finger so that it is on the articulation of the rib and the transverse process involved.

LATERAL RIB DYSFUNCTIONS
Example: Fifth Right Rib
1. **Patient position:** seated.
2. **Physician position:** standing on the patient's right side. Initially he is oriented approximately 90 degrees away from the patient (his back near the patient's right shoulder).
3. **Technique:**
   a. The physician places his left axilla over the patient's right shoulder as close to the cervicothoracic junction as possible.
   b. The physician uses his left hand to grasp the patient's right elbow. The patient's elbow is flexed and the shoulder is brought to approximately 45 degrees of flexion and abduction.
   c. The physician uses his right index finger to monitor the dysfunction.
   d. The patient is instructed to sit up straight.
   e. The physician adds a compressive force from his axilla down onto the patient's shoulder parallel to the spine.

f. A slight force is also added from the patient's right elbow up toward the shoulder.

g. By further adding pressure on the shoulder, side-bending is introduced down to the monitoring finger.

h. Rotation toward the physician's monitoring finger is introduced. If tissue tension increases, rotation away may be attempted.

i. The position is held for 3 seconds, then released; the dysfunction is reevaluated.

HIGH-VELOCITY, LOW-AMPLITUDE THRUSTING TECHNIQUES FOR THE RIBS
Barry S. Erner

Posterior Rib Head Somatic Dysfunction

1. **Patient position:** supine.
2. **Physician position:** standing at the side of the table opposite the side of the dysfunction.
3. **Technique:**
   a. The patient crosses the arm closest to the physician over his chest and grasps his opposite shoulder. With his far arm, the patient reaches across and grasps the opposite iliac crest (Fig. 17-18).
   b. The physician places the thenar eminence of his localizing hand under the posterior rib head being treated.
   c. The physician rests his other hand over the anterior chest wall, stabilizing the rib cage.
   d. After the patient has exhaled completely, the

physician exerts a rapid thrust through the patient's crossed arms toward his thenar eminence, which is resting on the posterior rib head dysfunction (Fig. 17-19).

Note: As with high-velocity, low-amplitude thrusting techniques of the thoracic spine, flexion of the spine down to the segment of dysfunction may be necessary for rib dysfunctions lower in the thorax. Flexion is achieved by the physician grasping the patient behind the shoulders with his nonlocalizing hand, then flexing the patient to create localization down to the necessary point.

Upper Rib Somatic Dysfunction (Ribs 1–4)

This technique is used for restricted motion at the costovertebral junction.

1. **Patient position:** prone.
2. **Physician position:** standing at the side of the table, opposite the dysfunction.
3. **Technique:**
   a. The patient cups his chin with the palm of his hand on the same side as the rib dysfunction.
   b. The elbow is moved cephalad as far as possible.
   c. The patient's head is rotated into the motion barrier.
   d. The physician crosses his hands, placing one hand over the rib head dysfunction and the other on the side of the patient's occiput on the same side as the somatic dysfunction. Downward tension is exerted with the thrusting hand.
   e. The physician exerts rotational and lateral flexion forces on the patient's head, creating

Figure 17-18. Patient position for high-velocity, low-amplitude thrusting technique for a posterior rib head somatic dysfunction.

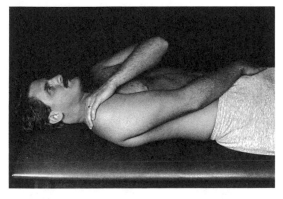

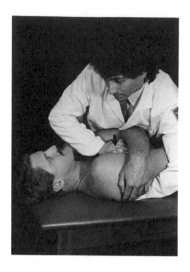

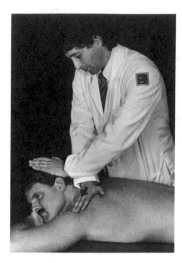

Figure 17-19. High-velocity, low-amplitude thrusting technique for a posterior rib head somatic dysfunction.

Figure 17-20. High-velocity, low-amplitude thrusting technique for upper rib somatic dysfunction, patient prone.

a locking at the cervicothoracic spinal junction.

f. Additional rotation and lateral flexion are induced by the physician until spring is noted under the hand placed over the rib head somatic dysfunction.

g. The physician exerts a rapid thrust on the dysfunctional rib. The force vector exaggerates the lateral cephalic springing motion noted in f (Fig. 17-20).

Note: No thrust should be applied to the patient's head or neck.

Figure 17-21. Alternative technique for treatment of upper rib somatic dysfunction, patient prone.

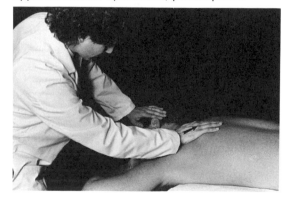

Alternative Technique

1. **Patient position:** prone.
2. **Physician position:** standing at the head of the table, facing the patient.
3. **Technique:**
   a. The patient cups his chin with the palm of his hand on the same side as the rib dysfunction.
   b. The physician's hand placement is the same as previously described, except that the hands are not crossed.
   c. The localization and thrust are medial-caudal (Fig. 17-21).

First Rib Somatic Dysfunction (Expiratory Restriction)

1. **Patient position:** sitting on a stool or the treatment table, feet flat on floor.
2. **Physician position:** standing behind the patient with his knee and hip flexed and placed on the stool opposite the side of the rib dysfunction.
3. **Technique:**
   a. The patient drapes his arm on the side opposite the dysfunction over the physician's flexed knee.
   b. The patient leans on the physician's knee, allowing his torso to become limp.
   c. The patient places his arm on the same side as the rib dysfunction between his legs.
   d. The physician flexes the cervical spine laterally toward the dysfunction until all the

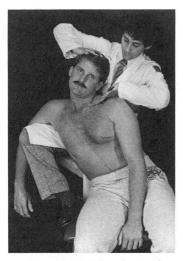

Figure 17-22. High-velocity, low-amplitude thrusting technique for a first rib somatic dysfunction.

slack is removed from the cervicothoracic junction.

e. The physician places his thrusting hand with the metacarpophalangeal border (between the thumb and index finger) in the crease created by the patient's neck and the trapezius muscle.

f. The physician simultaneously applies a downward and medial thrust while rapidly exaggerating full cervical spine lateral flexion (Fig. 17-22).

RIB-RAISING TECHNIQUES
Eileen L. DiGiovanna

In certain pulmonary diseases it is helpful to loosen tenacious mucus and to articulate the ribs to improve their motion. Rib-raising techniques achieve both these goals as the physician purposefully elevates groups of ribs. This section describes a few of these techniques.

THE BEDRIDDEN PATIENT
This technique is especially useful for the patient who is unable to sit up, for a weakened, sick patient, or for a comatose patient.
1. **Patient position:** supine.
2. **Physician position:** standing or seated at the side of the table or bed.
3. **Technique:**
   a. The physician places her hands, palm up, on the bed, with her fingers under the patient's rib cage, at the costovertebral junction.
   b. With the wrist as a fulcrum, the physician uses her fingers to raise and lower the ribs (Fig. 17-23), separating the articular surfaces.
   c. This process is repeated up and down the thorax.

Rib Raising and Thoracic Pump in the Bedridden Patient
1. **Patient position:** supine.
2. **Physician position:** standing at the head of the table or bed.
3. **Technique:**
   a. The patient raises her arms above her head

Figure 17-23. Rib raising in the bedridden patient.

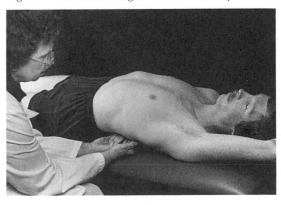

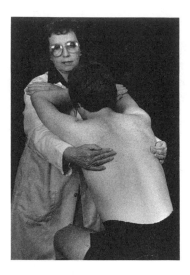

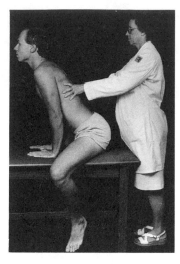

Figure 17-24. Rib raising for the seated patient.

Figure 17-25. Alternate approach to rib raising in the seated patient.

and clasps her hand behind the physician's thighs.

b. As the physician rocks back and forth, doing the thoracic pump, the patient's chest is elevated through the pull on her arms.

Pectoral Pull

1. **Patient position:** supine.
2. **Physician position:** seated or standing at the head of the bed or table.
3. **Technique:**
   a. The physician grasps the anterior axillary folds bilaterally.
   b. As the patient inhales, the physician exerts a cephalad traction on the pectoralis muscles. This is released during exhalation. This creates both a rib-raising and a pumping action to the thorax.

The Seated Patient

This technique is applicable to patients who are able to sit upright, and especially to patients who have difficulty breathing and prefer to be upright.

1. **Patient position:** seated on the edge of the bed or on a chair.
2. **Physician position:** standing in front of the patient.
3. **Technique:**
   a. The patient crosses his arms in front of him with the elbows resting on the physician's upper arms.

b. The physician reaches behind the patient's back, with the fingers of each hand grasping a group of ribs (Fig. 17-24).
c. The physician rocks back while pressing down on the posterior ribs. At the same time the patient falls forward onto his arms, which elevates the anterior rib cage.
d. The physician repeats this maneuver rhythmically, moving her hands up and down the thoracic spine.
e. The patient may assist in the treatment by inhaling deeply as the physician rocks back and exhaling fully as the physician moves forward.

Alternative Technique

1. **Patient position:** seated straddling the table.
2. **Physician position:** standing behind the patient.
3. **Technique:**
   a. The physician places the thumbs of each hand pointing toward the spine and spreads her fingers over the ribs bilaterally.
   b. The patient places his hands on the table in front of him.
   c. The physician pushes forward on the rib cage as the patient inhales and leans forward between his arms (Fig. 17-25).
   d. This maneuver is repeated rhythmically as the physician moves her hands up and down the thorax.
   e. The patient's inhalation elevates the ribs anteriorly as the physician depresses them posteriorly.

LYMPHATIC PUMP
Eileen L. DiGiovanna

Movement of the lymph depends on muscular movement and changes in intrathoracic pressures. A bedridden patient loses considerable muscular motion. Since the movement of lymph is necessary to carry immune cells and phagocytes to their sites of action, aid should be given to patients who have decreased active motion. One of the best ways the osteopathic physician can help such a patient is with some form of lymphatic pump.

Thoracic Pump
PATIENT PASSIVE
This technique may be used in comatose patients or patients who are too weak to aid in treatment.
1. **Patient position:** supine.
2. **Physician position:** standing at the head of the table or bed.
3. **Technique:**
   a. The physician places her hands on either side of the patient's anterior chest wall with her fingers pointing toward the patient's feet. The heel of the physician's hand just touches the inferior border of the clavicle (Fig. 17-26).
   b. For a female patient, the physician's hands may point toward the midline and slightly overlap on top of the sternum.
   c. The physician maintains her elbows in a locked position.
   d. The physician leans her body weight forward, gently compressing the patient's chest. Care should be taken that the pressure is not too great.
   e. The physician initiates a rhythmic motion by rocking back and forth, compressing and releasing. The motion should cause the patient's feet to move.
   f. The rhythmic movement is continued for 2 or 3 minutes.

PATIENT RESPIRATORY ASSIST
This technique uses the patient's respiration to assist, through sudden intrathoracic pressure changes, the movement of lymph through the thoracic duct and cysterna chyli.

1. **Patient position:** supine.
2. **Physician position:** standing at the head of the table or bed.
3. **Technique:**
   a. The physician's hands are placed on the patient's chest in the same manner as in the previous technique.
   b. The patient is instructed to inhale deeply, then exhale slowly. At the end of exhalation, the patient is told to inhale deeply.
   c. As the patient inhales and exhales, the physician's hands follow the respiratory motion.
   d. At the end of exhalation, the physician gently compresses the chest and provides a resistance to the patient's next inhalation.
   e. When the physician feels the patient is using force to inhale, she quickly releases the resistance. The patient will gasp with a sudden intake of air.

Pedal Pump (Dalrymple Technique)
In some patients it is difficult to use the thoracic pump. Some difficulties that might preclude its use include the following:

1. The physician cannot get to the head of the bed.
2. The patient may be on a respirator or may have tubes or wires in the thorax.
3. The patient may be too osteoporotic for pressure to be applied to the chest.
4. The patient may have had chest trauma or surgery.

In these instances, a pedal pump rather than a thoracic pump may be used to mobilize lymph. The technique described below should not be used in patients suspected of having phlebothrombosis or who are at high risk of clot formation.

1. **Patient position:** supine.
2. **Physician position:** standing at the foot of the table or bed.

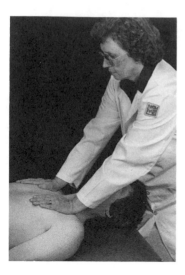 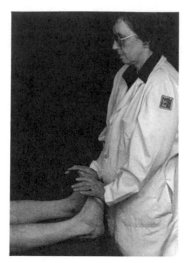

Figure 17-26. Thoracic pump for lymphatic drainage.

Figure 17-27. Pedal pump for lymphatic drainage.

3. **Technique:**
  a. The physician grasps the patient's feet by placing her hands on the dorsum or on soles of the feet.
  b. The patient's feet are pumped up and down so that the leg muscles are used to move the lymph (Fig. 17-27).
  c. This technique should produce a gentle rocking of the body.

References

Jones L. 1981. Strain and Counterstrain. Colorado Springs, Colo: American Academy of Osteopathy.
Mitchell F Jr., Moran P, Pruzzo N. 1979. An Evaluation and Treatment Manual of Osteopathic Muscle Energy Procedures. Valley Park, Mo: Mitchell, Moran and Pruzzo Associates.

18

The Upper Extremity

THE SHOULDER
Eileen L. DiGiovanna

Functional Anatomy

The shoulder is the articulation between the head of the humerus and the glenoid fossa of the scapula. It is the most mobile joint in the body as well as the most unstable. The glenohumeral articulation functions within the setting of the shoulder girdle. The shoulder girdle consists of three bones (the clavicle, humerus, and scapula), three true, synovial joints (glenohumeral, sternoclavicular, and acrominoclavicular), two functional joints, two accessory joints, and the muscles that move the three bones.

SYNOVIAL JOINTS

The sternoclavicular joint has sellar articular surfaces, frequently with an interposed meniscus. This joint affords movement of the clavicle in a frontal and horizontal plane as well as rotation on its long axis.

The acromioclavicular joint is a plane joint. Occasionally there is an intraarticular plate between the surfaces. The acromioclavicular joint permits motion of the clavicle in an anteroposterior or cephalic-caudal direction, as well as rotation. More motion is possible at the lateral end of the clavicle because of the crank shape of the bone.

The glenohumeral joint allows greater freedom of motion than any other joint in the body. The humeral head is convex and has a larger surface area than the concave glenoid fossa on which it moves. The humeral head slides along the surface of the fossa and rolls in various angular motions.

The capsule of the glenohumeral joint is loose and pleated. The ligaments, which are merely thickenings in the capsule, provide little support. Most of the support of the joint is provided by the rotator cuff muscles, which snug the head into the fossa. These muscles include the supraspinatus, infraspinatus, teres minor, and subscapular muscles.

FUNCTIONAL JOINTS (PSEUDOJOINTS)

The two functional joints in the shoulder girdle are the suprahumeral joint and the scapulothoracic joint. Both figure prominently in shoulder biomechanics and pathology. The suprahumeral joint is formed by the articulation of the head of the humerus with the coracoacromial arch, composed of the acromium, the coracoid process, and the ligament between them. Articulation occurs during abduction. At rest, there is a space in the joint through which pass the tendon of the long head of the biceps, the supraspinatus muscle and supraspinatus tendon, the subacromial bursa, and the capsule—all important and sensitive structures.

An Osteopathic Approach to Diagnosis and Treatment, second edition
Eileen L. DiGiovanna and Stanley Schiowitz
Lippincott–Raven Publishers, Philadelphia © 1997.

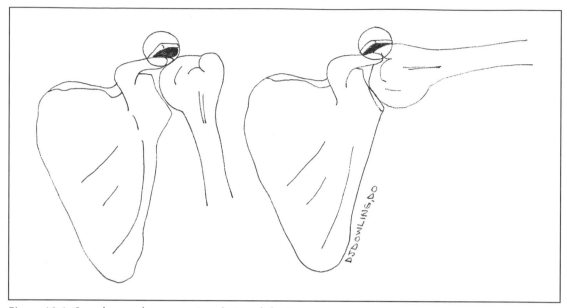

Figure 18-1. Suprahumeral compression during abduction.

These soft tissues are compressed during abduction around 90 degrees (Fig. 18-1). Internal rotation of the humerus causes impingement to occur at about 60 degrees. During external rotation, the head of the humerus glides posteriorly and impingement does not occur until 120 degrees of abduction. For this reason, persons with habitually slouched shoulders and internally rotated arms are more prone to degenerative processes such as tendinitis and bursitis.

The second functional joint is the scapulothoracic joint. Because muscle and fascia lie between the articulating surfaces, it is not a true joint.

ACCESSORY JOINTS

The accessory joints are the costosternal joints anteriorly, especially those of the first and second ribs, and the costovertebral joints posteriorly. The accessory joints are not anatomically involved in the shoulder joint or shoulder girdle, but dysfunction of these joints can interfere with free shoulder motion.

Motion of the Shoulder Bones

HUMERUS

The humerus moves in the following ways:

1. **Flexion** to 180 degrees.

2. **Extension** to 45 degrees.
3. **Abduction** to 180 degrees, placing the arm in the same position as flexion to 180 degrees.
4. **Adduction,** achieved with slight flexion or extension to clear the trunk.
5. **Horizontal flexion and extension,** after the arm has been abducted to 90 degrees.
6. **Internal and external rotation** around the long axis of the humerus, for a total of 180 degrees.
7. **Circumduction,** a combination of movements causing the arm to describe an irregular cone.

SCAPULA

The motions of the scapula are the following:

1. **Elevation,** upward and parallel to the spine, and **depression,** a return from elevation (Fig. 18-2).
2. **Abduction** or **protraction** away from the spine, which is combined with a lateral tilt around the thorax (Fig. 18-3).
3. **Adduction** or **retraction,** moving closer to the spine (Fig. 18-4).
4. **Upward or forward tilt,** turning on a horizontal axis so that the posterior surface faces upward and the inferior angle protrudes. This motion is accompanied by a longitudinal axis rotation of the clavicle (Fig. 18-5).

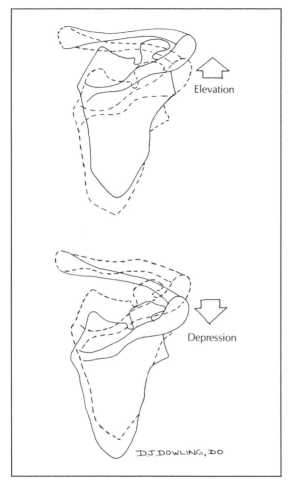

Figure 18-2. Elevation and depression of the scapula.

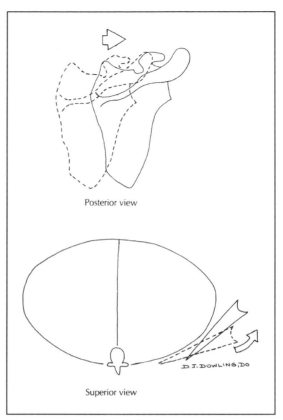

Figure 18-3. Scapular abduction (protraction).

5. **Upward and downward rotation** in relation to the glenoid fossa's elevation or depression: a frontal plane rotation (Fig. 18-6).

The glenoid fossa rotates upward during abduction, and this movement accomplishes several important functions:

1. The humerus impinges on the acromion at 90 degrees. To prevent impingement and permit abduction to 180 degrees, the scapula must rotate.
2. The fossa moves under the head of the humerus and increases the stability of the joint when the arm is elevated, preventing a downward dislocation.

3. The fibers of the deltoid, attached from the scapula to the humerus, contract to abduct the arm to 90 degrees, at which point they are maximally contracted. As the fossa rotates upward, it maintains the deltoid in position for maximal contraction.

JOINT RHYTHMS AND MECHANISMS
The scapulohumeral rhythm is a free-flowing and synchronous movement of the scapula and humerus. During abduction, the scapula rotates as the humerus elevates. For every 15 degrees of abduction, humeral elevation accounts for 10 degrees and scapular rotation for 5 degrees. Dysfunction of humeral elevation or of scapular rotation can disturb this rhythm and interfere with shoulder function. Dysfunction of clavicular motion can also interfere with this rhythm.

Glenohumeral movement requires a synchronous posterior downward glide of the humeral

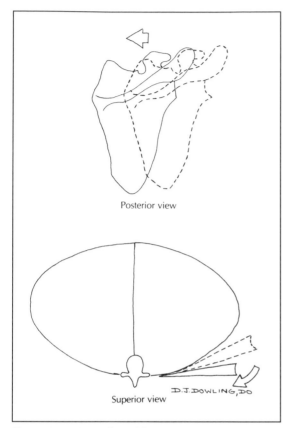

Figure 18-4. Scapular adduction (retraction).

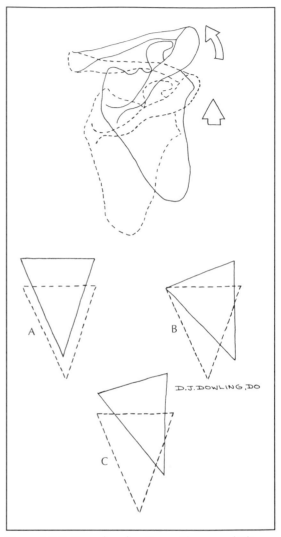

Figure 18-5. Scapular elevation with upward tilt:
(A) pure elevation, (B) pure tilt, (C) coupled
motions.

head during abduction to prevent impingement on
the coracoacromial arch. This necessitates an external rotation of the humerus to turn the greater
tuberosity away from the arch.

Another mechanism indirectly involved in
shoulder function is the bicipital mechanism. The
tendon of the long head of the biceps passes
through a groove between the greater and lesser
tuberosities of the humerus and attaches to the
rim of the glenoid. The tendon glides through the
groove whenever the humerus is moved. Contraction of the muscle does not move the tendon. Biceps tendinitis, capsulitis, or adhesions may prevent free gliding of the tendon and interfere with
normal motions.

The clavicle moves during most shoulder activity. Dysfunctions in clavicular motion can interfere with normal shoulder movement.

Evaluation of the Shoulder

Observation is the first step in evaluating the
shoulder. The physician should look for a smooth
contour and symmetry between the two shoulders. Blemishes or signs of trauma should be
noted.

The shoulder should then be palpated. This is
best done by the physician standing behind the
patient. Symmetry, smoothness of contour, swelling, and tenderness should be noted.

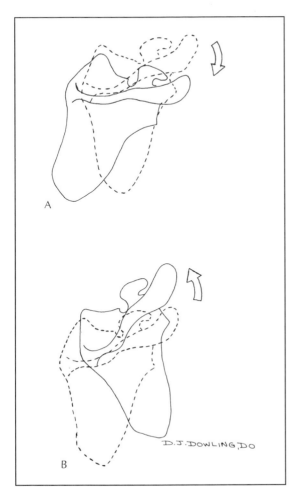

Figure 18-6. Rotation of the scapula: (A) downward, (B) upward.

The range of motion should be tested passively and actively, with any restrictions noted. A general motion screening is done by asking the patient to raise both arms slowly and touch the backs of his hands over the head. The physician observes scapular motion and symmetry of shoulders, elbows, and wrist angles.

The Apley scratch test is a good method to test active range of motion. The patient is instructed to reach across his chest, over the shoulder, and touch the opposite scapula. Then he reaches behind his back and touches his opposite scapula. Finally, he reaches behind his head and touches the opposite scapula. These maneuvers test all the ranges of motion in the shoulder joint.

Muscle strength and sensation should be tested. There are no specific reflexes at the shoulder. These are found at the elbow.

TESTS FOR SHOULDER DYSFUNCTION
Several specific tests may be used to detect shoulder dysfunction: these are described below.

Arm drop test. The patient's arm is elevated to 90 degrees of abduction and released. If there is a tear in the rotator cuff muscles, the arm will drop. If the tear is partial, by tapping on the arm the physician will cause it to drop.

Apprehension test. This test is for a chronically dislocating shoulder. The arm is abducted, extended, and externally rotated. At the point where the shoulder is about to dislocate, the patient will appear apprehensive.

Yergason test. The Yergason test is performed to assess the stability of the biceps tendon in the bicipital groove. The physician applies traction to the elbow and externally rotates the arm. The patient attempts to internally rotate the arm against resistance. If the tendon is unstable in the groove, it will pop out with a snap, and the patient will experience pain (Fig. 18-7).

All patients with chronic shoulder problems must be evaluated for dysfunctions of the cervical spine, upper thoracic spine, and upper ribs.

Shoulder Pathology

TENDINITIS
The two tendons of the shoulder most commonly involved by an inflammatory process are those of the long head of the biceps and the supraspinatus tendon. Both pass through the suprahumeral space and are compressed during abduction of the shoulder.

The tendons lack adequate circulation at the area where a gap occurs between vessels entering the tendon from the muscle and vessels entering from the bone. This area is known as the *critical zone.* The critical zone is also the most likely site of deposition of calcium in calcific tendinitis. About 90% of nontraumatic shoulder pain is due to tendinitis.

BURSITIS
Although bursitis is a common diagnosis in shoulder pain, only a small percentage of shoulder pain is actually due to bursitis. The most commonly affected bursa is the subacromial bursa, because

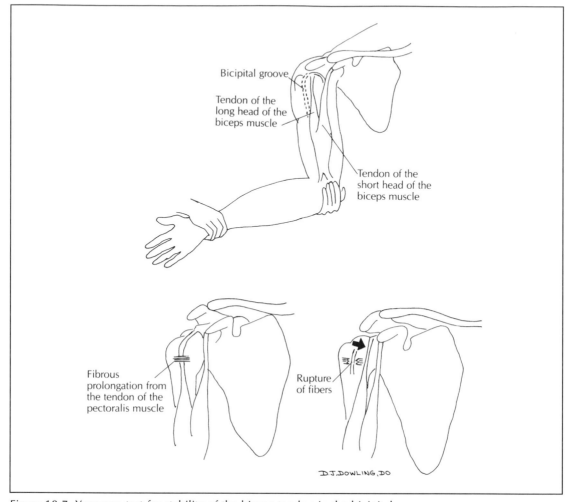

Figure 18-7. Yergason test for stability of the biceps tendon in the bicipital groove.

of its location in the suprahumeral space. Occasionally, a calcium deposit in a tendon will rupture through into the bursa, leading to calcific bursitis.

FROZEN SHOULDER

Also known as adhesive capsulitis, frozen shoulder results from prolonged immobilization of the shoulder. Frozen shoulder may result from application of a splint or sling, or from failure to move the shoulder because of pain from trauma or an inflammatory process in the shoulder. Inflammatory and fibrous changes occur in all the periarticular soft tissues. The range of motion of the shoul-

der can be markedly restricted, with abduction and internal rotation usually the most affected. Patients should be instructed to exercise the shoulder. Complete immobilization should not be continued for more than 48 hours. Prevention is the best treatment.

ARTHRITIS

Any type of arthritis may involve any of the shoulder girdle joints. The sternoclavicular joint is most commonly affected.

TRAUMA

The shoulder sustains trauma from direct blows, from falls on an outstretched arm, or from twisting injuries. Fractures commonly involve the clavicle. The neck of the humerus is another common site of fracture.

The humeral head may dislocate from the fossa since support of this joint is so poor. Anterior dislocations, under the clavicle or under the coracoid, are the most common. Posterior dislocations are less common but are more difficult to evaluate without radiography. In both fractures and dislocations, the physician must be alert to nerve compression or vascular compromise, since many important nerves and muscles lie in this area.

Occasionally the biceps tendon is unstable in its groove, usually when the transverse ligament has been damaged by trauma or worn by repeated microtrauma. The tendon then will snap out of the groove on certain motions, such as the Yergason test.

ACROMIOCLAVICULAR SEPARATION

Following a blow to the acromion, the scapula may torque around the coracoid and tear ligaments at the acromioclavicular joint, producing acromioclavicular separation. The injury may be graded as first degree, second degree, or third degree, depending on the amount of ligamentous injury. Acromioclavicular separation is best diagnosed with radiographs of the patient holding a weight in his hand to pull the acromion away from the end of the clavicle.

SOMATIC DYSFUNCTION

Most articular somatic dysfunctions of the shoulder occur at the sternoclavicular or acromioclavicular joints. These dysfunctions are characterized by pain at the involved joint and restricted motion in one or more of the planes of joint motion.

THE ELBOW
Eileen L. DiGiovanna

Functional Anatomy

The elbow links the forearm with the upper arm and, in concert with the shoulder, allows motion of the hand through space. The elbow functions as a ginglymus or hinge joint. It is formed by the articulation of the proximal ends of the radius and ulna with the distal end of the humerus.

The motions observed in the elbow joint are flexion, extension, and rotation (supination and pronation). Flexion and extension are the only motions that involve the true elbow joint. Flexion may be active or passive. Active flexion ends at about 145 degrees and is primarily limited by opposition of the contracting muscles of the arm and forearm. The range of passive flexion is slightly larger as the muscles relax and are flattened. Bony opposition and tension in the triceps and posterior capsular ligaments also limit flexion. The primary flexor muscle is the biceps brachii, which is assisted by the brachialis and the brachioradialis.

Extension of the elbow from the anatomic position is limited (5 to 10 degrees) by contact of the olecranon process with the fossa, tension in the anterior ligament, and resistance of anterior muscles. The triceps brachii is the only elbow muscle that functions in extension. Since most elbow extension is accomplished by gravity, the triceps functions primarily against resistance.

Besides flexion and extension, the forearm can rotate around its longitudinal axis. Rotation involves the superior radioulnar joint of the elbow and the inferior radioulnar joint, which lies above the wrist. These motions are observed with the forearm flexed to 90 degrees.

Supination is the rotary motion that turns the palm of the hand toward the ceiling; pronation is the rotary motion that turns the palm toward the floor. In neutral rotation the palm faces medially with the thumb up. The total range of rotation is about 180 degrees.

During supination, the interosseous membrane between the radius and ulna becomes taut. Supination involves the supinator and biceps muscles; pronation involves the pronator quadratus and pronator teres. The pronators are less powerful than the supinators.

When the arm is in the anatomic position, the upper arm and the forearm form an angle at the elbow, with the forearm directed away from the body in a valgus position. This is known as the *carrying angle* and is normally greater in women than in men (10 to 15 degrees in women, 5 degrees in men). If the carrying angle exceeds 15 degrees, it is called *cubitus valgus*. A decrease is known as *cubitus varus* or "gunstock" deformity.

Evaluation

The elbow should be examined first by observation. The carrying angle should be noted, as should any swelling, which may be diffuse or localized to the olecranon bursa posteriorly. Signs of old or new trauma should be noted, such as scars, abrasions, bruises, and the like.

The soft tissues and bony structures are then palpated to evaluate the integrity of the bones and the presence of any swelling, tenderness, masses, asymmetries, or crepitus. The ulnar nerve may be palpated in the groove between the medial epicondyle and the olecranon. The physician checks for scar tissue around the nerve that might compromise it. The Tinel test (tapping the nerve gently) may disclose a neuroma. The olecranon bursa should not be palpable unless it is filled with fluid or thickened.

Range of motion should be checked actively and passively. Both muscle strength and sensation should be tested.

There are three reflexes of the upper extremity, all deep tendon reflexes:

1. **Biceps reflex:** elicited by tapping the biceps tendon in the antecubital fossa: tests primarily C5.
2. **Brachioradialis reflex:** elicited by tapping the tendon on the lateral aspect of the lower forearm above the wrist: tests C6.
3. **Triceps reflex:** elicited by tapping the triceps tendon on the posterior arm just above the olecranon: tests C7.

Although these are upper extremity reflexes, they are tests for cervical nerve root dysfunction.

It may be necessary to test the elbow for ligamentous stability. This is done by placing first a valgus stress and then a varus stress on the elbow, using one hand as a fulcrum and the other as an opposing force.

Elbow Pathologies

EPICONDYLITIS

Epicondylitis is a common elbow problem, generally called tennis elbow if the lateral epicondyle is involved and golfer's elbow if the medial epicondyle is involved. This is an overuse syndrome that is associated with any activity that requires repetitive pronation and supination, such as gripping a tennis racquet, golf club, screwdriver, or doorknob. The wrist extensor muscles are involved in lateral epicondylitis. Tennis elbow is tested by having the patient make a fist and hold it in extension while the physician tries to force it into flexion. A positive test will reproduce the patient's pain over the lateral epicondyl.

Whenever the elbow is evaluated the shoulder and wrist should be examined as well, since symptoms may be referred.

SOMATIC DYSFUNCTION

The most common articular somatic dysfunction at the elbow involves the head of the radius. Restriction in anterior or posterior motion is tested by moving the radial head in an anteroposterior direction. This condition often mimics the pain of tennis elbow. The anterior slide of the radial head is coupled with supination-flexion, and the posterior slide with pronation-extension.

THE WRIST AND HAND
Eileen L. DiGiovanna

Functional Anatomy

THE WRIST

The wrist or carpus is the distal articulation of the radius and the articular disk with the proximal row of carpal bones. The disk joins the ulna and the radius and lies between the ulna and the proximal row of carpal bones. Laterally to medially, these bones are the scaphoid (navicular), lunate, and the triquetrum. A small bone, the pisiform, lies slightly anterior to the triquetrum.

A midcarpal joint lies between the proximal and distal rows of carpal bones. The distal row is made up of the trapezium, the trapezoid, the capitate, and the hamate. The third functional joint at the wrist is the distal radioulnar joint.

The wrist moves in two planes. In the *sagittal plane* it flexes to approximately 85 degrees and extends to approximately 45 degrees. Flexion and extension appear to occur around more than one axis. In the *coronal plane* the wrist moves into abduction (radial deviation) and adduction (ulnar deviation). Abduction is about 15 degrees and adduction 45 degrees.

Pronation and supination occur at the radioulnar joint and, combined with flexion, extension, abduction, and adduction, permit circumduction so that the hand can lie in any plane.

The wrist is moved by four groups of muscles:

1. **Flexor carpi ulnaris:** flexes the wrist and adducts the hand.
2. **Extensor carpi ulnaris:** extends the wrist and adducts the hand.
3. **Flexor carpi radialis and palmaris longus:** flex the wrist and abduct the hand.
4. **Extensor carpi radialis longus and brevis:** extend the wrist and abduct the hand.

The bodies of these muscles lie close to the elbow, and the corresponding tendons are long, passing down the forearm to attach to the wrist.

The carpal bones form an arch spanned by the flexor retinaculum. The concavity of the arch lies on the palmar surface between the bones and the transverse ligament (the flexor retinaculum) and is called the *carpal tunnel*. Through this tunnel pass the tendons of the wrist and finger flexors and the median nerve. It is the site of origin of the thenar and hypothenar muscles.

Another tunnel, the tunnel of Guyon, is formed by the ligament attaching the hook of the hamate and the pisiform. Through this tunnel pass the ulnar nerve and artery.

On the lateral aspect of the wrist is a small depression known as the anatomic snuffbox. The floor of the snuffbox is the scaphoid or navicular bone. It lies distal to the radial styloid and becomes prominent when the thumb is forcefully extended. It is bounded by the abductor pollicis longus, the extensor pollicis brevis, and the extensor pollicis longus tendons.

THE HAND

The human hand is prehensile to a degree not attained in other species. Only in man can the thumb be brought into opposition with each of the other fingers. This is a remarkable organ of sense, capable of measuring thickness and distance as well as perceiving light touch and temperature. The delicate movements of the hand allow grasping and fine movements.

The hand consists of five metacarpal bones that articulate proximally with four carpal bones in the distal row. The second and third metacarpals remain relatively fixed while the first, fourth, and fifth move around this fixed segment. The five metacarpals articulate distally with the proximal phalanges of the fingers. These are usually considered hinge joints. They permit flexion-extension, abduction, adduction, and circumduction.

An extensor tendon lies along the dorsal aspect of each joint, and there are fibrocartilaginous plates over the palmar surface, known as palmar or volar plates. These plates lie between the joint and the flexor tendons.

Each finger, except the thumb, has a proximal and a distal interphalangeal joint. Since there are only two bones in the thumb, there is only one joint. The interphalangeal joints are hinge joints, allowing flexion and extension and some axial rotation.

The skin over the palm of the hand is thicker than over the dorsum and is firmly attached to the fascia at the palmar creases. This permits the hand to grasp objects securely. Also important to grasp is the ability of the hand to change shape to conform to the object being grasped. It can flatten and spread out to conform to a flat surface or it can form a hollow cuplike depression.

The muscles of the fingers lie in the forearm. The tendons cross the wrist with the wrist muscle tendons. The flexor muscles cross the palm through numerous fibroosseous tunnels. The extensor tendons pass along the dorsum of the hand through fewer tunnels. The flexor and extensor muscles are all extrinsic muscles.

Intrinsic muscles include the interosseous and lumbrical muscles. In addition to assisting with flexion and extension, they abduct and adduct the fingers.

At the base of the thumb on the palmar surface is the thenar eminence, which is made up of the intrinsic muscles of the thumb: the adductor pollicis, opponens pollicis, abductor pollicis brevis, and flexor pollicis brevis. These muscles are innervated by the median nerve. The thenar eminence atrophies when the median nerve is trapped, as in carpal tunnel syndrome.

On the medial aspect of the palm, at the base of the fifth digit, is the hypothenar eminence, which contains three muscles: the flexor digiti minimi, abductor digiti minimi, and opponens digiti minimi.

PREHENSILE MOTIONS OF THE HAND

According to Kapandji, there are six ways in which the hand can grasp objects: the thumb is involved in four kinds of prehensile motions.

1. **Prehension by terminal opposition** is the finest and most precise form of grasp. The tip of the finger pad or fingernail makes contact when the thumb and index finger grasp a thin object.
2. **Prehension by subterminal opposition** is the most common form of grasp. The object is held between the pads of the thumb and index fingers.
3. In **prehension by subterminolateral opposition,** the pad of the thumb holds an object, such as a coin, pressed against the radial surface of the first phalanx of the index finger.
4. **Palmar prehension** is used to grasp heavy, relatively large objects. The entire hand is wrapped around the object. The thumb opposes the force of the other four fingers.
5. **Prehension by digitopalmar opposition** entails grasp of a small-diameter object by the fingers pressing against the palm. The thumb is not involved.
6. **Prehension between lateral aspects of the fingers** is exemplified by holding a cigarette. This grip is weak, and the object must be small. The thumb is not involved.

Evaluation

OBSERVATION

The hand should be observed while in use, such as while unbuttoning a shirt, and at rest. At rest the hand should lie in slight flexion. The fingers should be counted.

Any joint or soft tissue swelling should be noted. Infection may spread rapidly through the soft tissues of the hand. Fusiform swelling of the proximal interphalangeal joints is indicative of rheumatoid arthritis. Discrete bony nodules on the

distal interphalangeal joints are called Heberden's nodes and are indicative of osteoarthritis.

The arthritides may cause painful swelling of the hand and wrist joints and may result in specific deformities. A "swan's neck" deformity occurs when the proximal interphalangeal joint is hyperextended and the distal interphalangeal joint is flexed. Various joints may sublux, and ulnar deviation may develop.

If the tendon of the extensor digitorum communis avulses from the base of the middle phalanx, the proximal interphalangeal joint will hyperflex and the distal interphalangeal joint will extend, producing the "boutonniere" deformity. A mallet finger is one in which the distal interphalangeal joint is flexed and will not extend because of avulsion of the distal insertion of the extensor digitorum communis.

The nails should be inspected for clubbing, color (abnormal pallor or cyanosis), or infection around the edges (paronychia). Any atrophy of the thenar or hypothenar areas should be noted.

PALPATION

The wrist and hand joints should be palpated for swelling, asymmetries, temperature changes, and tenderness. The skin of the wrist and hand should be evaluated for temperature and moisture changes. Calluses should be noted. The anatomic snuffbox may be palpated. In case of trauma, any tenderness in this area should be noted, since the navicular is the most commonly fractured of the carpal bones.

The tunnels across the dorsum of the wrist should be palpated for swelling or tenderness. The volar tunnels should be similarly evaluated. Ganglia may occur in the tendon sheaths.

RANGE OF MOTION

All joints should be put through their passive range of motion and the patient asked to demonstrate active range of motion. The digits are evaluated together and individually. The fingers and thumb should be flexed and extended, and finger abduction and adduction should be tested. When the patient touches the thumb to the tip of each of the other fingers, the wrist should flex, extend, abduct, and adduct.

MUSCLE STRENGTH TESTING

A general screening of hand strength is to ask the patient to squeeze two or three of the examiner's

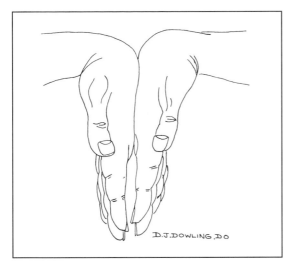

Figure 18-8. Phalen's test.

fingers. If a weakness is found, each finger flexor is tested individually. The extensors are checked by trying to force the fingers into flexion.

To test the intrinsic muscles, the patient spreads his fingers while the examiner tries to close them. Then the patient tries to close his fingers against the examiner's resistance.

The pinch mechanism is tested by having the patient form an O with his thumb and index finger as the examiner hooks his fingers into the O and tries to pull it apart.

Wrist flexion and extension strength should be tested with the hand made into a fist.

SENSATION TESTING

The peripheral nerves may be tested by sensation testing the following sites:

1. **Radial nerve:** dorsum of web space between thumb and index finger
2. **Median nerve:** tip of index finger
3. **Ulnar nerve:** tip of fifth finger

The dermatome levels are the following:

1. C6: thumb and index finger and lateral palm
2. C7: middle finger
3. C8: fourth and fifth fingers and medial palm

SPECIAL TESTS

Bunnel-Littler test. This test evaluates the tightness of the intrinsic muscles of the hand. The meta-

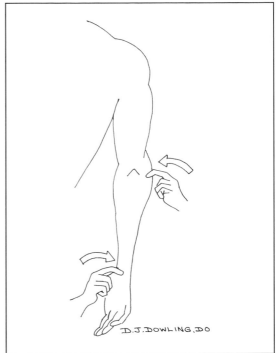

Figure 18-9. Tinel sign of the wrist and elbow.

carpophalangeal joint is held in extension and the patient tries to move the proximal interphalangeal joint into flexion. If the proximal interphalangeal joint does not flex, then the intrinsic muscles are tight or the joint capsule is contractured. The metacarpophalangeal joint is rested briefly, then retested. If the proximal interphalangeal joint still cannot flex, the problem is in the joint capsule.

Allen test. This test evaluates functioning of the medial and ulnar arteries. Occlude the two arteries and have the patient open and close his fist. The palm should be pale. Release one artery and the hand should flush. Repeat with the other artery.

Phalen's test. This test is for carpal tunnel syndrome. The patient flexes the wrists and presses the backs of his hands together. He holds this position for a minute. In carpal tunnel syndrome this will produce pain or paresthesias in the affected hand (Fig. 18-8).

Tinel sign. By tapping over the volar carpal ligament, pain or paresthesias may be produced over the distribution of the median nerve in a case of carpal tunnel syndrome (Fig. 18-9).

Finkelstein test. This test is used to rule out de Quervain's disease. The patient closes his fingers around his thumb and then ulnar deviates his wrist. Pain along the lateral wrist is a positive test.

Pathology of the Wrist and Hand
CARPAL TUNNEL SYNDROME
In carpal tunnel syndrome the median nerve is compressed in the tunnel by fibrous bands, scar tissue from chronic inflammation or microtrauma, arthritis, or myxedema due to hypothyroidism. The syndrome is characterized by pain or paresthesias such as tingling in the hand, particularly along the distribution of the median nerve. Numbness may be the presenting symptom. Weakness of the hand frequently occurs. On examination the thenar eminence may be atrophied. The flexor tendons might be slightly swollen. The Tinel sign and a positive Phalen test are valuable diagnostic clues.

Osteopathic treatment should be aimed at loosening tense fascia, freeing the area of edema fluid, and stretching fibrous bands. Any joint restrictions should be corrected.

DE QUERVAIN'S DISEASE
This condition is a stenosing tenosynovitis of the thumb. It is more common in women than in men and is related to repetitive movements of the thumb that cause inflammation within the tendon sheath. The main symptoms are pain and difficulty moving the thumb. Swelling around the anatomic snuffbox may be noted. There is pain on circumduction of the thumb. The specific test for this condition is the Finkelstein test. Injection with steroids may be necessary.

Osteopathic treatment is aimed at relieving edema and freeing motion of the joints and fascia. Counterstrain treatment of tender points may be helpful.

DUPUYTREN'S CONTRACTURE
This condition is characterized by contracture of the palmar fascia and nodule formation. There appears to be a genetic predisposition to the disease. It is frequently found in alcoholics. It can be triggered or aggravated by trauma. The nodules are tender. The palmar fascia contracts, flexing the fingers, particularly on the ulnar side. Finger and hand function can be severely limited.

Osteopathic treatment is aimed toward keeping the palmar fascia as free as possible: the metacar-

pophalangeal and proximal interphalangeal joints should be mobilized to prevent secondary joint immobilization and tethering of the flexor tendons. Surgical intervention may be required.

ARTHRITIS
Rheumatoid arthritis and osteoarthritis may involve the joints of the wrist and hand. Psoriatic arthritis and gouty arthritis may also affect this area. Many of the findings and specific deformities were mentioned earlier. In the arthritides, the small accessory motions of the joint are lost first. The osteopathic physician must articulate all joints once the acute inflammation has subsided. The patient should be encouraged to exercise the joints greatly to maintain mobility.

References
Arminio JA. 1982. DeQuervain's disease: The forgotten syndrome. Resident Staff Physician 28(6):84–88.

Bateman JE. 1978. The Shoulder and Neck. Philadelphia: W.B. Saunders.

Cailliet R. 1966. Shoulder Pain. Philadelphia: F.A. Davis.

———. 1976. Hand Pain and Impairment. 2nd ed. Philadelphia: F.A. Davis.

DiGiovanna E. 1981. Shoulder kinetics. Osteopath Ann 9(3):75–79.

Hoppenfeld S. 1995. Physical Examination of the Spine and Extremities. Norwalk, Conn: Appleton-Century-Crofts.

Janecki CJ, Field JH. 1984. Washerwoman's sprain, working woman's pain. Aches Pains 14:20.

Kapandji IA. 1972. The Physiology of the Joints. Vol 1. Upper Limb. Edinburgh: Churchill Livingstone.

Leddy JP, Hamilton JJ. 1984. Tennis elbow: Not just a case for the courts. Aches Pains 14:21.

Lipscomb PR. 1984. Carpal tunnel syndrome: Guide to office diagnosis. J Musculoskel Med 35:41.

Moseley HF. 1972. Shoulder Lesions. Edinburgh: Churchill Livingstone.

Nirschl RP. 1984. The prevention and management of tennis elbow. Pain Analg 6:10.

Paletta FX. 1981. Dupuytren's contracture. AFP 23:85–90.

Polley HF, Hunder GA. 1987. Physical Examination of the Joints. Philadelphia: W.B. Saunders.

Quiring DP. 1960. The Extremities. Philadelphia: Lea & Febiger.

Rasch PJ, Burke RK. 1978. Kinesiology and Applied Anatomy. Philadelphia: Lea & Febiger.

Roland AC, Cawley PW. 1984. Common elbow injuries. Family Practice Recertifications. MRA Publications, Inc., September 1984.

Weiss TE. 1984. Painful hands: Differential diagnosis by physical examination only. Consultant 24(12):51–65.

19

Diagnosis and Treatment of the Upper Extremity

THE SHOULDER GIRDLE
Eileen L. DiGiovanna

The two major goals of osteopathic manipulation of the shoulder girdle are to restore function and to prevent motion loss. This section describes several active, passive, and isometric techniques.

Spencer Techniques

The Spencer techniques are seven gentle stretching maneuvers used to treat shoulder restriction caused by hypertonic muscles, early adhesive capsulitis, healed fractures and dislocations, and any other traumatic or degenerative condition in which improved motion is needed. Motion testing is done passively or by using the Apley scratch test, described in Chapter 18. The general guidelines for performing all seven techniques are as follows:

1. **Patient position:** lateral recumbent position with the affected shoulder up. The patient's knees and hips are flexed, his back is straight and perpendicular to table, his lower arm is down and comfortable, and his head is supported by a pillow.
2. **Physician position:** standing at the side of the table, facing the patient.
3. **Technique:** The physician grasps the patient's forearm with one hand, flexing the patient's

elbow. The physician's other hand is placed on top of the patient's shoulder to lock the shoulder girdle, limiting scapular movement.

Each technique is repeated six to eight times; one should stop when it becomes painful to the patient or motion is restricted. With each movement, the physician tries to exceed the point reached in the previous excursion.

1. **To increase extension:** The physician moves the patient's arm in a horizontal plane, extending the shoulder and returning it to neutral position, gently increasing the excursion. The patient's elbow is kept in flexion (Fig. 19-1).
2. **To increase flexion:** The physician flexes the patient's shoulder, straightening the elbow, until the arm is over the patient's ear (Fig. 19-2). This maneuver is gently repeated in rhythmic motion, with the shoulder returned to neutral position each time. The physician may have to change the position of the hand locking the scapula to be comfortable during this maneuver.
3. **To increase circumduction:** The patient's elbow is flexed sharply and the shoulder is abducted to a 90-degree angle. The physician locks the patient's shoulder in this position and, using the patient's elbow as a pivot, gently ro-

An Osteopathic Approach to Diagnosis and Treatment, second edition
Eileen L. DiGiovanna and Stanley Schiowitz
Lippincott–Raven Publishers, Philadelphia © 1997.

295

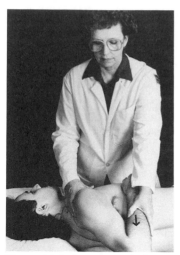

Figure 19-1. Spencer technique to increase shoulder extension.

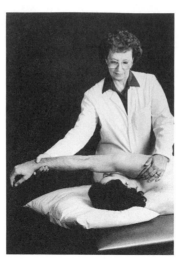

Figure 19-2. Spencer technique to increase shoulder flexion.

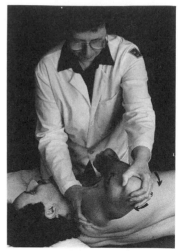

Figure 19-3. Spencer technique to increase shoulder circumduction.

tates the shoulder in gradually increasing circles, clockwise and then counterclockwise (Fig. 19-3).

4. **Circumduction with traction:** The physician extends the patient's elbow and abducts the arm to 90 degrees. The physician then locks the patient's scapula in this position and, using the patient's forearm as a pivot, gently rotates the humerus in gradually increasing circles, clockwise and then counterclockwise, maintaining a traction force at the patient's wrist (Fig. 19-4).

5. **To increase abduction:** The physician places her upper hand on the patient's shoulder. The patient's elbow is flexed and his hand rests on the physician's forearm below the elbow joint. The physician's lower arm gently exerts an upward pressure on the patient's flexed elbow, bringing the shoulder into abduction (Fig. 19-5).

6. **To increase adduction:** The physician places her upper hand on the patient's shoulder. The patient's elbow is flexed and the patient's hand may rest on the physician's forearm below the elbow joint. The physician's other hand gently exerts a downward pressure on the patient's flexed elbow bringing the patient's upper arm into adduction.

7. **To increase internal rotation:** The patient's hand, with the elbow flexed, is placed behind his lower ribs. The physician's upper hand locks the scapula; her lower hand gently draws the patient's elbow forward and down (Fig. 19-

6). The patient's elbow is released and the maneuver is repeated. An external rotation force may also be used in this position.

8. **Traction stretch:** The patient's hand is placed on the physician's shoulder with his elbow straight. The physician clasps her hands around the patient's shoulder over the humerus. The physician may then provide a gentle pull on the patient's shoulder. By leaning back, the physician uses her body weight rather than muscular force (Fig. 19-7).

Note: Patriquin reports that the original techniques designed by Spencer had step 5 carrying the shoulder into adduction by moving the elbow toward the table. This changed over time. Both abduction and adduction may be done as part of this step.

ISOMETRIC VARIATIONS
OF SPENCER TECHNIQUES
The positions used in the Spencer techniques may also be used to treat the shoulder with isometric therapy. The physician moves the arm to a barrier. The patient actively moves his arm against resistance in extension, flexion, abduction, adduction, and internal or external rotation.

For example, in the case of restricted motion in extension, the patient first assumes a position of maximum comfortable extension. The patient then tries to move his arm into flexion while the physician applies a mild isometric resistive force.

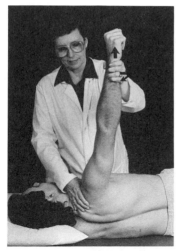

Figure 19-4. Spencer technique to improve circumduction, with traction.

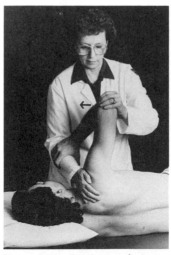

Figure 19-5. Spencer technique to increase shoulder abduction.

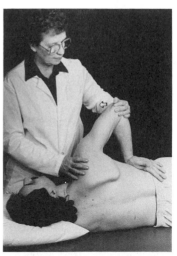

Figure 19-6. Spencer technique to increase internal rotation of the shoulder.

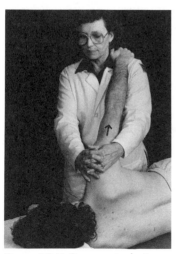

Figure 19-7. Spencer technique for traction stretch.

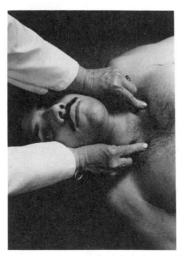

Figure 19-8. Test for abduction of the clavicle.

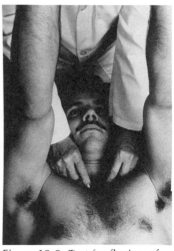

Figure 19-9. Test for flexion of the clavicle.

This position is held for 4 seconds; then the patient relaxes. The physician increases the patient's arm extension and the maneuver is repeated.

Muscle Energy Treatment of the Clavicle

TEST FOR CLAVICULAR MOTION

In **abduction,** the distal end of the clavicle moves superiorly and the proximal end moves inferiorly. The physician tests motion in abduction by placing her index finger on the clavicular head next to the sternum while the patient is supine; the physician then asks the patient to shrug (Fig. 19-8).

In **flexion,** the distal end of the clavicle moves anteriorly and the proximal end moves posteriorly on the sternum. The physician tests motion in flexion by placing her index finger on the clavicular head next to the sternum; the physician then asks the patient to flex his shoulder to 90 degrees and to reach up to the ceiling forcefully (Fig. 19-9).

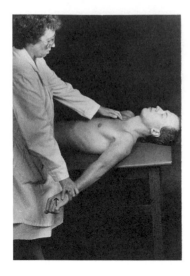
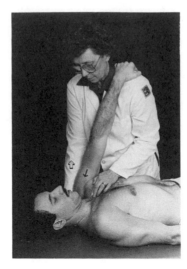

Figure 19-10. Muscle energy treatment for restricted abduction of the sternoclavicular joint.

Figure 19-11. Muscle energy treatment for restricted flexion of the sternoclavicular joint.

RESTRICTED ABDUCTION OF THE STERNOCLAVICULAR JOINT

1. **Patient position:** supine.
2. **Physician position:** standing at the side of the table, next to the affected shoulder.
3. **Technique:** The physician places one hand on the proximal clavicular head. With her other hand she grasps the patient's wrist and holds the arm extended and internally rotated (Fig. 19-10). The patient is instructed to raise his arm against the physician's hand, hold it in position, then relax. The technique is repeated twice more.

RESTRICTED FLEXION OF THE STERNOCLAVICULAR JOINT

1. **Patient position:** supine.
2. **Physician position:** standing at the side of the table, next to the affected shoulder.
3. **Technique:** The physician places one hand on the restricted clavicle and with the other reaches behind the axilla to cover the scapula. The patient holds the physician's shoulder with the hand of the affected side (Fig. 19-11). The physician flexes the clavicle toward the manubrium until movement is palpated in the sternoclavicular joint. This is done by straightening the body and pulling the scapula anteriorly. The patient is instructed to pull his shoulder down, hold this position for 2 to 3 seconds, and then relax. The maneuver is repeated twice more.

High-Velocity, Low-Amplitude Thrusting Techniques for the Shoulder Girdle

GLENOHUMERAL SOMATIC DYSFUNCTION

1. **Patient position:** prone.
2. **Physician position:** standing at the side of the table, on the side of the dysfunction.
3. **Technique:**
   a. The physician grasps the patient's glenohumeral joint by encircling the joint with both hands.
   b. The physician's thumbs rest in a crossed pattern on the posterior aspect of the patient's glenohumoral joint.
   c. The physician exerts a rapid downward and slightly lateral force through the patient's glenohumeral joint (Fig. 19-12).

SUPERIOR CLAVICULAR SOMATIC DYSFUNCTION

1. **Patient position:** supine.
2. **Physician position:** standing at the side of the table, on the same side as the dysfunction.
3. **Technique:**
   a. The physician grasps the superior surface of the restricted clavicle with the fingers of his monitoring hand.
   b. With his other hand, the physician flexes the patient's arm to 90 degrees (ipsilateral to the dysfunction).
   c. The physician exerts a simultaneous downward thrust on the clavicle and lateral trac-

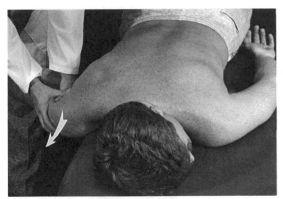

Figure 19-12. High-velocity, low-amplitude thrusting technique for somatic dysfunction of the glenohumeral joint.

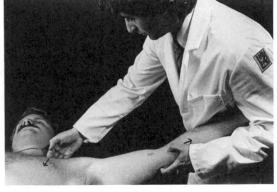

Figure 19-13. High-velocity, low-amplitude thrusting technique for somatic dysfunction of the superior clavicle.

tion on the patient's arm to produce the corrective force (Fig. 19-13).

STERNOCLAVICULAR SOMATIC
DYSFUNCTION
1. **Patient position:** supine.
2. **Physician position:** standing at the head of the table.
3. **Technique:**
   a. The physician rests the thenar eminence of his monitoring hand over the sternoclavicular joint that is restricted.
   b. The physician grasps the patient's arm on the side of the dysfunction and exerts a cephalad traction force on the arm.
   c. The physician achieves correction by exerting a downward thrust through the sternoclavicular joint while simultaneously inducing a rapid traction force through the patient's arm (Fig. 19-14).

ARTICULATORY TECHNIQUES FOR
CLAVICULAR RESTRICTIONS
The clavicle may be elevated or depressed at the sternal end. The techniques described are for an elevated clavicle.

Technique 1
1. **Patient position:** supine.
2. **Physician position:** seated at the head of the table.
3. **Technique:** The patient's neck, fully flexed, rests against the physician's chest. This posi-

tion locks out spinal motion. The physician places her thumb over the sternal end and exerts a downward and caudal pressure on the clavicle (Fig. 19-15). The patient is instructed to inhale and exhale fully. During exhalation the physician springs the clavicle to release the restriction.

Technique 2
1. **Patient position:** seated.
2. **Physician position:** standing close behind the patient.
3. **Technique:** The physician reaches under the affected arm and grasps the abducted humerus. With her other hand she reaches over the patient's shoulder and places the thumb or hypothenar eminence on the sternal end of the clavicle. The hand holding the humerus applies a lateral traction. The other hand provides a downward force on the clavicle (Fig. 19-16). This may be an articulatory or a high-velocity, low-amplitude force.

Counterstrain Techniques for the Shoulder
TENDER POINT LOCATIONS
The anterior tender points for the shoulder (Fig. 19-17) are the following:

1. Anterior acromioclavicular: anterior surface of distal clavicle
2. Long head of biceps: over the tendon

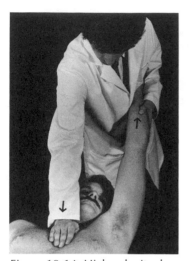

Figure 19-14. High-velocity, low-amplitude thrusting technique for somatic dysfunction of the sternoclavicular joint.

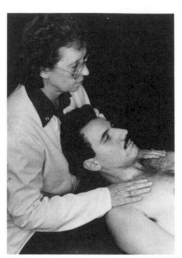

Figure 19-15. Articulatory technique for an elevated clavicle, patient supine.

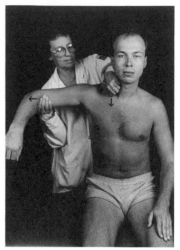

Figure 19-16. Articulatory technique for an elevated clavicle, patient seated.

3. Short head of biceps: inferolateral to the coracoid process

The posterior tender points (Fig. 19-18) are the following:

1. Posterior acromioclavicular: behind the lateral end of the clavicle
2. Supraspinatus: in the supraspinatus fossa

In the axilla lie the following:

1. Subscapularis tender point: on the anterior surface of the scapula
2. Latissimus dorsi tender point: deep in the axilla on the medial surface of the humerus

TREATMENT
Anterior Acromioclavicular Tender Point
1. **Patient position:** supine.
2. **Physician position:** at the side of the table opposite the tender point.
3. **Technique:** The tender point is monitored as the arm is adducted across the chest. The physician applies traction by pulling on the arm at the wrist (Fig. 19-19).

Long Head of Biceps Tender Point
1. **Patient position:** supine.
2. **Physician position:** at the side of the table, next

to the tender point and facing the head of the table.
3. **Technique:** The patient's arm is flexed to 90 degrees at the elbow and shoulder. The physician applies downward pressure at the elbow along the humerus to the monitoring finger (Fig. 19-20).

Short Head of Biceps Tender Point
1. The short head of biceps tender point is treated in the same manner as the long head, except that some fine-tuning into adduction is needed.

Posterior Acromioclavicular Tender Point
1. **Patient position:** prone.
2. **Physician position:** at the side of the table opposite the tender point.
3. **Technique:** The patient's arm is adducted across his back. The physician applies traction by pulling at the wrist (Fig. 19-21).

Supraspinatus Tender Point
1. **Patient position:** supine.
2. **Physician position:** at the side of the table next to the tender point.
3. **Technique:** The patient's arm is flexed and abducted to 120 degrees. The humerus is markedly externally rotated. The muscle should become very soft in this position (Fig. 19-22).

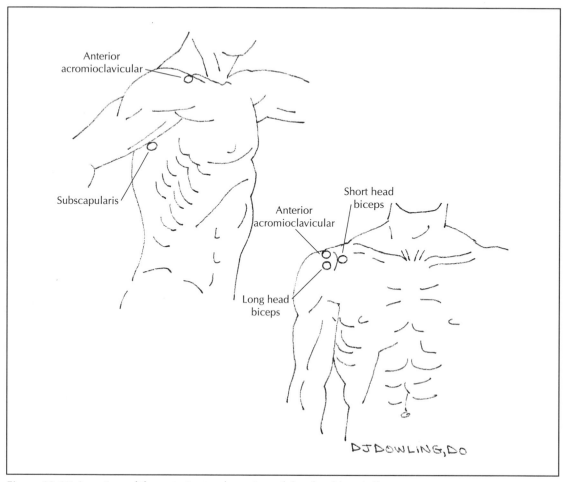

Figure 19-17. Location of the anterior tender points of the shoulder girdle.

Subscapularis Tender Point
1. **Patient position:** supine.
2. **Physician position:** at the side of the table next to the tender point.
3. **Technique:** The patient's arm is held posteriorly over the side of the table and toward his feet. His arm is internally rotated. No traction is applied.

Latissimus Dorsi Tender Point
1. The latissimus dorsi tender point is treated in the same manner as the subscapularis tender point except that traction is applied along the length of the arm.

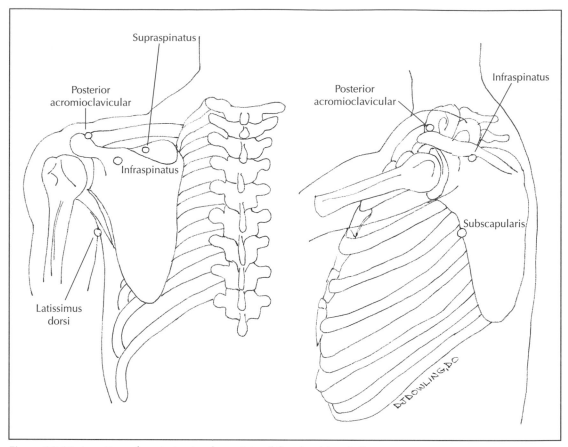

Figure 19-18. Location of posterior tender points of the shoulder girdle.

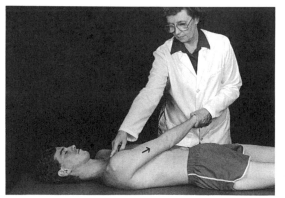

Figure 19-19. Counterstrain treatment for an anterior acromioclavicular tender point.

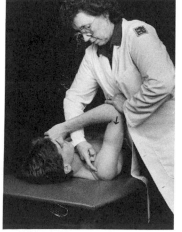

Figure 19-20. Counterstrain treatment for a tender point of the long head of the biceps.

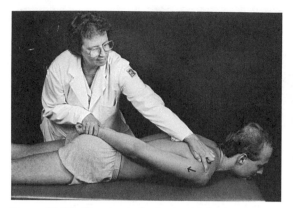

Figure 19-21. Counterstrain treatment for a posterior acromioclavicular tender point.

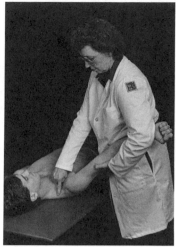

Figure 19-22. Counterstrain treatment for a supraspinatus tender point.

THE ELBOW
Eileen L. DiGiovanna

Adduction/Abduction

Adduction and abduction are accessory rocking motions of the upper part of the ulna on the trochlea of the humerus. Abduction is an accessory motion of pronation. Adduction is an accessory motion of supination.

MOTION TESTING

The patient's elbow is semiflexed about 45 degrees. The physician palpates the articulation by placing a finger on the dorsal aspect of the radial and ulnar sides of the olecranon, then tries to palpate into the trochlea. With his other hand the physician grasps the patient's forearm and, starting from a neutral position, fully supinates the forearm, inducing a rocking, adduction motion of the ulna. Reversing the forearm motion into full pronation induces a rocking abduction motion. The elbow is tested for restriction of either motion.

MUSCLE ENERGY TREATMENT
Adduction (Supination) Restriction
1. **Patient position:** supine.
2. **Physician position:** standing at the side of the table.

3. **Technique:**
   a. The physician places the patient's elbow into full supination.
   b. The patient gently tries to pronate his forearm against the physician's equal, restraining, isometric force.
   c. This position is held for 4 seconds, then the patient relaxes.
   d. The technique is repeated.

Abduction (Pronation) Restriction
1. To treat an abduction restriction, the position of the arm is reversed.

HIGH-VELOCITY, LOW-AMPLITUDE
THRUSTING TECHNIQUE FOR
ABDUCTION/ADDUCTION RESTRICTION
1. **Patient position:** seated.
2. **Physician position:** standing facing the patient.
3. **Technique:**
   a. The physician grasps the patient's elbow. The fingers of his monitoring hand are on either side of the olecranon. The other hand is used to hold and stabilize the patient's forearm, in supination/extension.

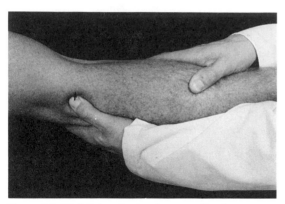

Figure 19-23. High-velocity, low-amplitude thrusting technique for adduction restriction of the elbow.

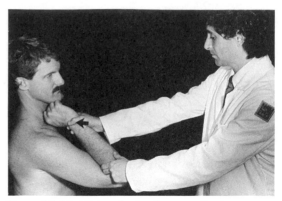

Figure 19-24. High-velocity, low-amplitude thrusting technique for anterior radial head.

b. The physician tests the motion of the radioulnar joint in adduction and abduction.

c. If restriction of motion is noted in abduction, the physician places the patient's elbow into abduction and exerts a hyperabduction corrective thrust. This is done with the elbow locked in extension.

d. If restriction of motion is noted in adduction, the physician places the patient's elbow into adduction and exerts a hyperadduction corrective thrust. This is done with the elbow locked in extension (Fig. 19-23).

Radial Head Dysfunctions

MOTION TESTING

1. **Patient position:** seated or supine.
2. **Physician position:** standing facing the patient. The radial head is palpated by flexing and extending the elbow.
3. **Technique:**
   a. The physician grasps the radial head between his thumb and index finger.
   b. The radial head is moved in a ventral and dorsal direction; any restriction of motion is noted.

   Note: The most common dysfunction of the radial head is a posterior radial head. This is diagnosed from the ability to move the radial head dorsally with restriction of motion ventrally. An anterior radial head is restricted in motion dorsally and has free motion ven-

trally. Posterior glide of the radius is coupled with pronation/extension, and anterior glide is coupled with supination/flexion.

HIGH-VELOCITY, LOW-AMPLITUDE THRUSTING TECHNIQUE FOR ANTERIOR RADIAL HEAD

1. **Patient position:** seated.
2. **Physician position:** standing facing the patient.
3. **Technique:**
   a. The physician grasps the patient's dysfunctioned oned arm, flexing it at the elbow and pronating it at the wrist.
   b. The physician places the second and third digits of his other hand into the crease of the patient's elbow, directly over the radial head.
   c. The physician exerts a rapid hyperflexion force on the elbow while simultaneously thrusting the radial head dorsally with the fingers of the other hand (Fig. 19-24).

POSTERIOR RADIAL HEAD SOMATIC DYSFUNCTION

1. **Patient position:** seated.
2. **Physician position:** standing facing the patient.
3. **Technique:**
   a. The physician encircles the patient's dysfunctioned elbow with both hands and extends it.
   b. The physician places his thumbs over the head of the radius anteriorly and the phalanx of his index finger over the radial head posteriorly.

c. The physician exerts a rapid hyperextension force on the patient's elbow while simultaneously inducing a ventral counterforce
through the radial head (Fig. 19-25).

Counterstrain Treatment of the Elbow
The tender points associated with the elbow are
shown in Figure 19-26. Radial head or lateral epicondyle tender points may be treated in the same
manner.

1. **Radial head/lateral epicondyle tender points**
   a. The elbow is held in full extension. This may
   be over a fulcrum of the table edge or the physician's knee.
   b. The arm is then supinated and abducted with
   varying amounts of force.
   c. The position is maintained for 90 seconds;
   then the arm is returned slowly to a neutral
   position (Fig. 19-27).

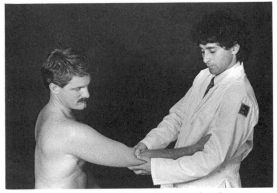

Figure 19-25. High-velocity, low-amplitude
thrusting technique for posterior radial head.

Figure 19-26. Tender points
associated with the elbow. *LE,*
lateral epicondyle; *ME,* medial
epicondyle.

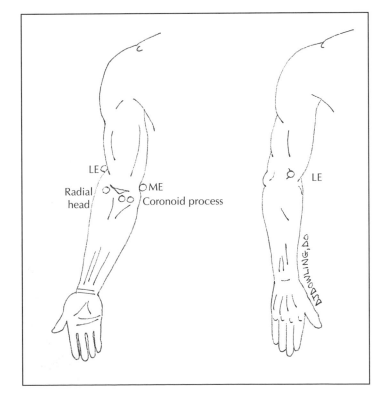

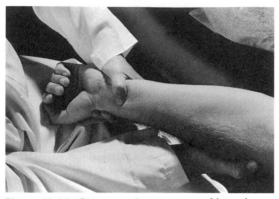

Figure 19-27. Counterstrain treatment of lateral epicondyle tender point.

2. **Coronoid tender points**
   a. The elbow is fully flexed.
   b. The forearm is pronated and abducted gently.
   c. The position is held for 90 seconds; then the arm is slowly returned to a neutral position.

THE WRIST AND HAND
Eileen L. DiGiovanna

The Wrist
TESTS FOR SOMATIC DYSFUNCTION
Somatic dysfunction of the wrist permits motion toward the dysfunction; motion away from the dysfunction will be restricted. The technique described below may be used to test motion of the radionavicular joint and each of the intercarpal joints. It may also be used to test the carpometacarpal and metacarpophalangeal joints.

1. **Physician position:** seated facing the patient.
2. **Technique:**
   a. The physician grasps the bones adjacent to the joint to be tested between his thumb and forefinger.
   b. The bones are moved through their range of motion and any restriction is noted.
   c. The motions tested are gliding in all directions and long-axis traction.

Gross motion is tested in flexion, extension, and radial and ulnar deviation. Both passive and active techniques may be used.

MUSCLE ENERGY (ISOMETRIC) TECHNIQUES
As in muscle energy techniques for treating dysfunction of any other joint, the wrist is moved to its barrier to motion and the patient is asked to push isometrically back toward the freedom of motion. The technique described below is used for wrist restriction in ulnar deviation.

1. **Technique:**
   a. The joint is moved into ulnar deviation to the barrier to motion.
   b. The patient is asked to push toward the radial aspect as the physician provides resistance.
   c. This position is held for 4 seconds, then released.
   d. The joint is moved to its new barrier.
   e. The maneuver is repeated three or four times.

Figure 19-28. High-velocity, low-amplitude thrusting technique for carpal dysfunction.

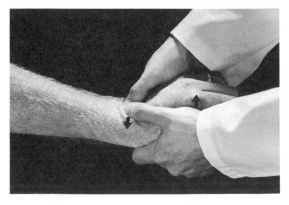

Figure 19-29. Dorsal tender points of the wrist and hand.

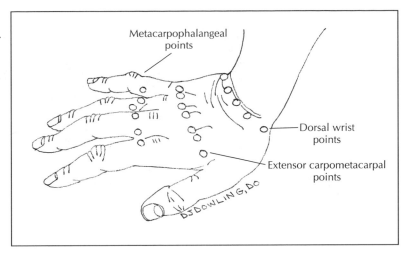

HIGH-VELOCITY, LOW-AMPLITUDE
THRUSTING TECHNIQUE FOR CARPAL
SOMATIC DYSFUNCTION
1. **Patient position:** seated on the table.
2. **Physician position:** standing facing the patient.
3. **Technique:**
   a. The physician grasps the patient's hand on the side of the dysfunction and localizes the dorsal radiocarpal joint with his thumbs.
   b. The physician exerts a whiplike thrust on the hand, moving it into rapid hyperflexion while simultaneously exerting a downward counterforce through the carpal somatic dysfunction (Fig. 19-28).

COUNTERSTRAIN TREATMENT
The locations of the tender points associated with the wrist are shown in Figures 19-29 and 19-30. All of these tender points respond to flexing or extending the wrist over the tender points (Figs. 19-31, 19-32).

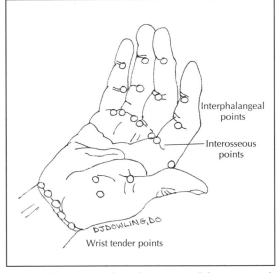

Figure 19-30. Ventral tender points of the wrist and hand.

The Hand
TESTS FOR SOMATIC DYSFUNCTION
1. **Physician position:** seated facing the patient.
2. **Technique:**
   a. The physician grasps the bones adjacent to the joint being tested between his thumb and index finger.
   b. The bones are moved through their range of motion as gentle traction is applied.

ARTICULATION TREATMENT
Intersegmental Articulations
1. **Physician position:** seated or standing, facing the patient.
2. **Technique:**
   a. The physician locks one metacarpal between the thumb and index finger of one hand.
   b. With the thumb and index finger of his other hand, the physician maneuvers the neighbor-

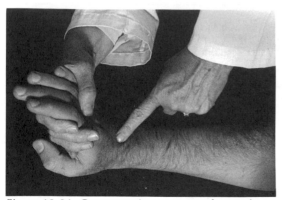

Figure 19-31. Counterstrain treatment of ventral tender point of the wrist by flexion of the wrist.

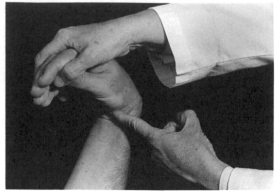

Figure 19-32. Counterstrain treatment of dorsal wrist tender points by extension of the wrist.

ing metacarpal into anterior or posterior glide or rotation, as desired.

Fingers
1. **Physician position:** seated or standing, facing the patient.
2. **Technique:**
   a. The physician locks the metacarpal, in this instance the second, between the thumb and index finger of one hand.
   b. The physician places the thumb of his other hand on the dorsum of the first phalanx and the index finger on the volar surface of the first phalanx.
   c. The physician applies long-axis extension (straight-line traction) or rotation or antero-posterior glide.

HIGH-VELOCITY, LOW-AMPLITUDE
THRUSTING TECHNIQUE FOR PHALANGEAL
DYSFUNCTION
1. **Patient position:** seated on the table.
2. **Physician position:** standing facing the patient.
3. **Technique:**
   a. With one hand, the physician holds and stabilizes the patient's wrist.
   b. The physician localizes the dysfunctional joint and exerts a simultaneous traction and hyperflexion thrust through the somatic dysfunction (Fig. 19-33).
   c. To treat the second or third phalanges, the physician holds the phalanx above the articulation being treated and maneuvers the distal phalanx through the desired motion.

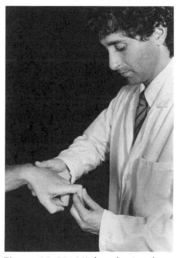

Figure 19-33. High-velocity, low-amplitude thrusting technique for phalangeal dysfunction.

COUNTERSTRAIN TREATMENT
The locations of the tender points associated with the hand are shown in Figures 19-29 and 19-30. A tender point of the first carpometacarpal joint that is associated with pain and weakness of the thumb is treated by markedly rotating the thumb toward the palm, with a slight amount of flexion. The interossei tender points are treated by flexing the joint and applying some traction. An extension carpometacarpal tender point is treated by extending the joint and applying traction.

EXERCISE THERAPY FOR THE UPPER EXTREMITY
Stanley Schiowitz
Albert R. DeRubertis

The Shoulder Girdle

The function and biomechanics of the shoulder girdle were reviewed in Chapter 18. The physician prescribing exercise therapy must take into account the three true articulations, the two pseudo-articulations, and the origins and insertions of all the muscles used in joint function.

GLENOHUMERAL JOINT

A. Pendulum exercise, acute phase—passive (Fig. 19-34)
  1. **Patient position:** bent forward, body supported by the good arm holding on to support, the back comfortable.
  2. **Instructions:**
    a. Allow your painful arm to hang down away from your body.
    b. Move your body forward and backward, then side to side. This creates shoulder joint motion without active participation of the shoulder muscles.
    c. Gradually increase body motion. Do not create pain. Start with 5 to 10 seconds of exercise.
    d. Slowly bring your body back to an upright position. Passively move the painful arm

back to your side, using your good arm to move it if necessary.
    e. Relax, rest, and repeat.
B. Pendulum exercise, after acute phase—active (Fig. 19-35)
  1. **Patient position:** bent forward, body supported by the good arm holding on to support, the back comfortable.
  2. **Instructions:**
    a. Allow your painful arm to hang down, away from your body.
    b. Swing your arm forward and backward, side to side, and in circles.
    c. Gradually increase the excursion of the arm motion. A weight may be held in your hand to increase the force used.
    d. Continue for 5 to 15 seconds; then slowly bring your body into the upright position.
    e. Relax, rest, and repeat.
      Note: Do not increase or create pain when performing this exercise.
C. Flexion stretch (Fig. 19-36)
  1. **Patient position:** standing facing a wall, an arm's length away.
  2. **Instructions:**
    a. Place the hand of the arm to be exercised

Figure 19-34. Pendulum exercise, acute phase—passive motion.

Figure 19-35. Pendulum exercise with active use of the shoulder.

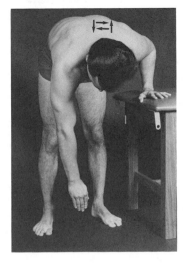

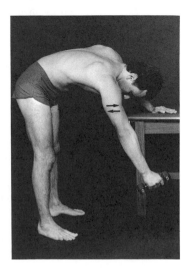

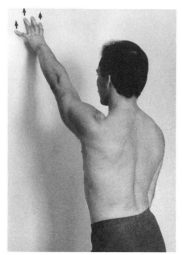

Figure 19-36. Flexion stretch.

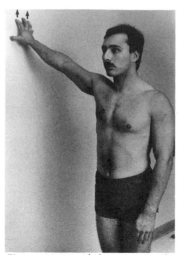

Figure 19-37. Abduction stretch.

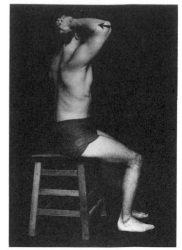

Figure 19-38. Abduction—external rotation stretch.

against the wall with the elbow fully extended.

b. Walk your fingers up the wall slowly, increasing flexion at the shoulder.

c. After reaching the limit of painless flexion, hold your arm in this position for 10 to 15 seconds. Then slowly walk your fingers higher on the wall, 1 inch at a time, to increase flexion. Hold your arm for 10 to 15 seconds at each new plateau of flexion; then walk the fingers higher.

d. At the end of 2 or 3 minutes, or if fatigued, slowly walk the arm down the wall.

e. Relax, rest, and repeat.

D. Abduction stretch (Fig. 19-37)

1. **Patient position:** standing with the side of the painful arm toward the wall.

2. **Instructions:** Repeat the technique described for flexion stretch, walking the arm up into abduction.

Note to physician: If the cause of the dysfunction is supraspinatus impingement, do not prescribe this exercise.

E. Abduction—external rotation stretch (Fig. 19-38).

1. **Patient position:** standing or sitting with both hands clasped behind the head and the elbows brought together in front of the body.

2. **Instructions:**

a. Slowly separate your elbows as far back as they can be painlessly stretched.

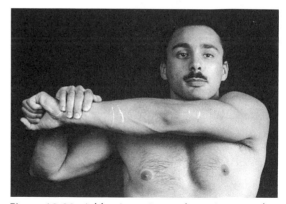

Figure 19-39. Adduction—internal rotation stretch (passive).

b. Hold this position for 5 to 15 seconds.

c. Return to the starting position.

d. Relax, rest, and repeat.

F. Adduction—internal rotation stretch (passive) (Fig. 19-39)

1. **Patient position:** standing with the arms at the sides.

2. **Instructions:**

a. Turn the hand of the arm to be treated inward (internal rotation).

b. Grasp that wrist with your other hand and pull it slowly across your chest to shoulder height.

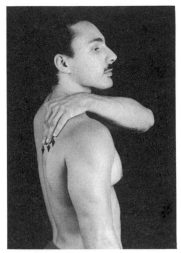

Figure 19-40. Adduction—internal rotation stretch (active).

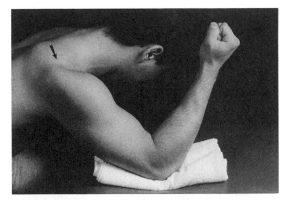

Figure 19-41. Forced flexion stretch.

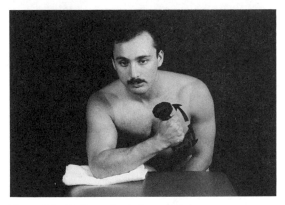

Figure 19-42. Forced rotation stretch.

c. Gradually increase your pull to maximum painless stretch. Hold for 5 to 15 seconds.
d. Return arm to the starting position.
e. Relax, rest, and repeat.
G. Adduction—internal rotation stretch (active) (Fig. 19-40)
1. **Patient position:** standing with both arms at the sides.
2. **Instructions:**
a. Bring the arm that is to be treated across your body and up over the opposite shoulder. Keep your palm pointing down.
b. Reach back over your shoulder and touch your scapula.
c. Walk your fingers down the scapula to achieve maximum painless stretch. Hold for 5 to 15 seconds.
d. Return your arm to the starting position.
e. Relax, rest, and repeat.

FROZEN SHOULDER FORCED STRETCH EXERCISES

These exercises are not performed during the acute phase of injury. Moderate wet heat should be applied as an aid to muscle relaxation before the patient begins exercising. If analgesics or non-steroidal anti-inflammatory drugs are prescribed, they should be taken 20 minutes before exercise. At the conclusion of these exercises, an ice pack should be applied for 20 minutes.

A. Forced flexion stretch (Fig. 19-41)
1. **Patient position:** seated facing a table, with the elbow on the side of the shoulder to be treated on the table.
2. **Instructions:**
a. Place the back of the elbow joint on the table, making a 90-degree angle between the forearm and the elbow.
b. Drop your body forward and downward, increasing shoulder flexion. Remain in this position for 15 seconds.
c. Allow your entire weight to rest on your elbow joint. With the increased flexion (stretch), you may feel mild pain.
d. Hold this position for 15 seconds. Raise your body up.
e. Relax, rest, and repeat.
f. Attempt to increase flexion motion with each repetition.
B. Forced rotation stretch (Fig. 19-42)

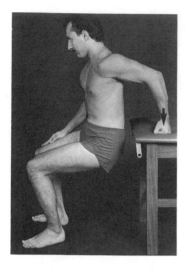
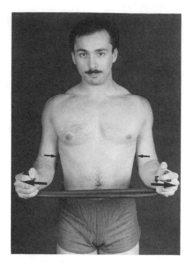

Figure 19-43. Forced extension stretch.

Figure 19-44. External rotator strengthening.

1. **Patient position:** seated facing a table, with the elbow on the side of the shoulder to be treated on the table. Hold a 3 to 5 pound weight in your hand.
2. **Instructions:**
   a. Allow your arm to pivot on the elbow inward, toward the table. The weight you are holding should slowly create forced internal rotation.
   b. Remain in this position for 10 seconds, then pivot the arm outward, creating external rotation.
   c. Return your arm to midline.
   d. Relax, rest, and repeat.
   e. Increase the weight held in your hand gradually, to force the rotation.
C. Forced extension stretch (Fig. 19-43)
   1. **Patient position:** stand with your back to a table. Bring your shoulder back with the elbow bent, until your fist rests upon the table.
   2. **Instructions:**
      a. Gently do a deep knee bend, resting your weight on your fist. This maneuver increases shoulder extension.
      b. Gradually increase the deep knee bend, resting all your weight on your fist.
      c. Hold this position of forced extension for 15 seconds.
      d. Return to the upright position.
      e. Relax, rest, and repeat.

STRENGTHENING EXERCISES WITH MECHANICAL AIDS
A. External rotators (Fig. 19-44)
   1. **Patient position:** standing, both arms at the sides, elbows bent to 90 degrees, holding a length of rubber tubing in both hands.
   2. **Instructions:**
      a. Pull the tubing horizontally between your hands as far as possible. Keep your elbows and arms against your body.
      b. Hold this position for 5 to 15 seconds.
      c. Return to the starting position.
      d. Relax, rest, and repeat.
B. Extensors (Fig. 19-45)
   1. **Patient position:** standing, both arms at the sides, holding a length of rubber tubing in both hands.

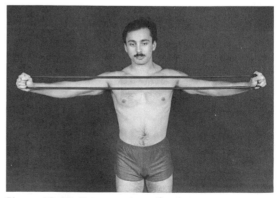

Figure 19-45. Extensor strengthening.

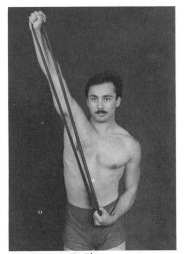

Figure 19-46. Flexor strengthening.

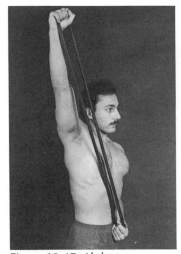

Figure 19-47. Abductor strengthening.

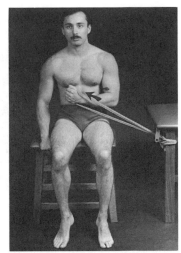

Figure 19-48. Internal rotator strengthening.

2. **Instructions:**
   a. Pull the rubber tubing horizontally as far as possible, while simultaneously raising both arms to shoulder height. Try to stretch out the arms fully.
   b. Hold this outstretched position for 5 to 15 seconds.
   c. Return to starting position.
   d. Relax, rest, and repeat.

C. Flexors (Fig. 19-46)
   1. **Patient position:** standing, one hand holding a length of rubber tubing firmly below the waist at the midbody line.
   2. **Instructions:**
      a. Grasp the other end of the rubber tubing with the arm to be treated.
      b. Pull on the tubing in a forward direction until your elbow is fully extended.
      c. Swing your fully extended arm over your head into full flexion.
      d. Hold this position for 15 seconds.
      e. Slowly return to the starting position.
      f. Relax, rest, and repeat.

D. Abductors (Fig. 19-47)
   1. **Patient position:** standing, one hand holding a length of rubber tubing firmly below the waist at the midbody line.
   2. **Instructions:**
      a. Grasp the other end of the rubber tubing with the arm to be treated.
      b. Pull sideways, stretching the tubing, until your elbow is fully extended.
      c. Swing your fully extended arm over your head into full abduction.
      d. Hold this position for 15 seconds.
      e. Slowly return to the starting position.
      f. Relax, rest, and repeat.

E. Internal rotators (Fig. 19-48)
   1. **Patient position:** seated next to a table with the side to be treated beside a leg of the table.
   2. **Instructions:**
      a. Place a length of rubber tubing around the table leg and grasp it with the hand next to the table leg.
      b. Keep that elbow flexed to 90 degrees and held firmly against your body.
      c. Pull and stretch the tubing by rotating your hand toward the midbody line. This creates internal rotation.
      d. Hold this position for 15 seconds.
      e. Slowly return to the starting position.
      f. Relax, rest, and repeat.

Elbow Joint

The exercises described in this section stretch the agonist muscles while strengthening the antagonist muscles. Each motion is performed slowly. The difficulty of the exercise is enhanced as the patient increases the weight used. To ensure maxi-

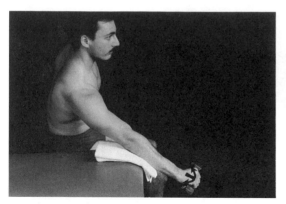

Figure 19-49. Flexion-extension pronation stretch.

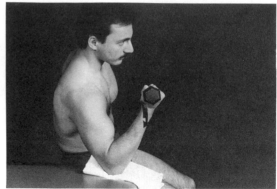

Figure 19-50. Flexion-extension supination stretch.

mum stretch, the patient uses his other arm to increase passively the motion after the extreme of voluntary stretch has been reached.

A. Flexion-extension pronation stretch (Fig. 19-49)
  1. **Patient position:** seated, with the side to be exercised next to a table. The elbow is placed near the edge of the table, with a towel or small pillow between it and the table.
  2. **Instructions:**
     a. Hold a 3- to 5-pound weight in your hand. Turn your hand so that the palm faces down (*pronation*).
     b. Allow the elbow to extend down to the table with the weight creating extension off the table. The elbow acts as a fulcrum. Use your other hand to gently push the elbow into forced extension. Hold this position for 5 seconds.
     c. Bring your arm up off the table into full elbow flexion. With your other hand, gently push the elbow into forced flexion. Hold for 5 seconds.
     d. Repeat the entire motion. Remember to keep your palm down in full wrist pronation at all times.
B. Flexion-extension supination stretch (Fig. 19-50)
  1. **Patient position:** seated, with the side to be exercised beside a table. The elbow is placed near the edge of the table, with a folded towel or small pillow between it and the table.
  2. **Instructions:**
     a. Hold a 3- to 5-pound weight in your hand.

Turn your hand so that the palm faces up (*supination*).
     b. Allow the elbow to extend down to the table with the weight creating extension off the table. The elbow acts as a fulcrum. With your other hand, gently push the elbow into forced extension. Hold this position for 5 seconds.
     c. Bring your arm up off the table into full elbow flexion. With your other hand, gently push the elbow into forced flexion. Hold for 5 seconds.
     d. Repeat the entire motion. Remember to keep your palm up in full wrist supination at all times.

Wrist
WRIST STRETCH
A. Extension—dorsiflexion stretch (Fig. 19-51)
  1. **Patient position:** standing, with the side to be treated next to a wall but far enough away to allow full elbow extension.
  2. **Instructions:**
     a. Place your palm, fingers pointing up, flat on the wall so that the elbow is fully extended.
     b. Lean on to the wall, causing extension stretch of the wrist. Hold for 5 seconds.
     c. Relax, rest, and repeat.
B. Extension—palmar flexion stretch (Fig. 19-52)
  1. **Patient position:** standing, with the side to be treated next to a wall but far enough away to allow full elbow extension.
  2. **Instructions:**
     a. Place your palm, fingers pointing down,

Figure 19-51. Wrist
extension—dorsiflexion stretch.

Figure 19-52. Wrist
extension—palmar flexion
stretch.

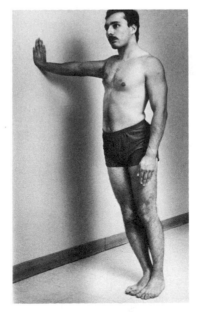

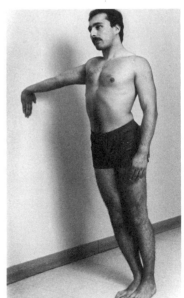

Figure 19-53. Wrist
flexion—palmar flexion stretch.

Figure 19-54. Wrist
flexion—dorsiflexion stretch.

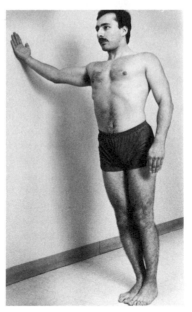

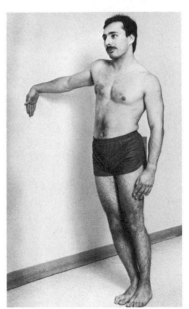

flat on wall so that the elbow is fully extended.
  b. Lean on to the wall, causing extension
     stretch of the wrist. Hold for 5 seconds.
  c. Relax, rest, and repeat.
C. Flexion—palmar flexion stretch (Fig. 19-53)
  1. **Patient position:** standing, with the side to
    be treated next to a wall but far enough away
    to allow full elbow extension.

2. **Instructions:**
  a. Place the back of your hand, fingers point-
    ing up, flat on the wall so that the elbow
    is fully extended.
  b. Lean on to the wall, causing flexion stretch
    of the wrist.
  c. Hold for 5 seconds.
  d. Relax, rest, and repeat.
D. Flexion—dorsiflexion stretch (Fig. 19-54)

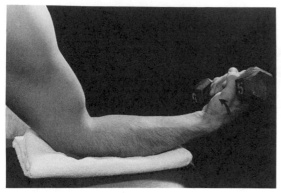

Figure 19-55. Wrist flexor strengthening.

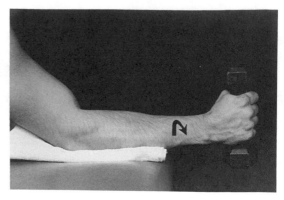

Figure 19-57. Wrist rotator strengthening.

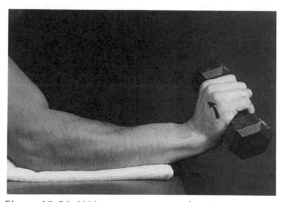

Figure 19-56. Wrist extensor strengthening.

2. **Instructions:**
   a. Hold a 3- to 5-pound weight in your hand. The palm faces up, putting the wrist in *supination*.
   b. Move the hand holding the weight up toward the ceiling (flex the wrist). Your forearm remains flat on the table.
   c. Hold for 5 to 15 seconds.
   d. Slowly lower the weight off the table, extending the wrist fully.
   e. Relax, rest, and repeat.
B. Wrist extensors (Fig. 19-56)
   1. **Patient position:** seated, with the side to be treated beside a table. The forearm rests on the table with the elbow at about 90 degrees of flexion. The wrist is off the table.
   2. **Instructions:**
      a. Hold a 3- to 5-pound weight in your hand. The palm faces down, placing the wrist in *pronation*.
      b. Bring the hand holding the weight up toward the ceiling (extend the wrist). The forearm remains on the table.
      c. Hold this position for 5 to 15 seconds.
      d. Slowly lower the weight off the table, flexing the wrist fully.
      e. Relax, rest, and repeat.
C. Wrist rotators (Fig. 19-57)
   1. **Patient position:** seated, with the side to be treated beside a table. The forearm rests on the table with the elbow at about 90 degrees of flexion. The wrist is off the table.
   2. **Instructions:**
      a. Hold a 3- to 5-pound weight in your hand. The palm faces down.

1. **Patient position:** standing, with the side to be treated next to a wall but far enough away to allow full elbow extension.
2. **Instructions:**
   a. Place the back of your hand, fingers pointing down, flat on the wall so that the elbow is fully extended.
   b. Lean on to the wall, causing flexion stretch of wrist.
   c. Hold for 5 seconds.
   d. Relax, rest, and repeat.

WRIST STRENGTHENING
A. Wrist flexors (Fig. 19-55)
   1. **Patient position:** seated, with the side to be treated beside a table. The forearm rests on the table with the elbow at about 90 degrees of flexion. The wrist is off the table.

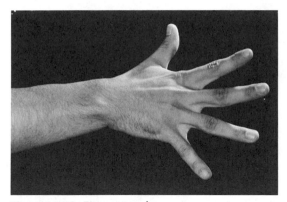

Figure 19-58. Finger stretch.

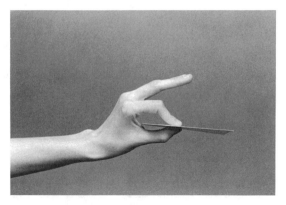

Figure 19-59. Finger coordination.

b. Slowly rotate your forearm, keeping the wrist stiff, until the palm faces up.

c. Hold this position for 5 seconds.

d. Slowly rotate your wrist back to the starting position.

e. Hold this position for 5 seconds.

f. Repeat the technique.

D. Ulnar-radial adduction

1. **Patient position:** seated, with the side to be treated beside a table. The forearm rests on the table with the elbow at about 90 degrees of flexion. The wrist is off the table.

2. **Instructions:**

a. Hold a 3- to 5-pound weight in your hand. The palm faces down. The wrist is held stiff.

b. Bend your wrist to the side, trying to touch your thumb to your arm.

c. Hold this position for 5 seconds.

d. Bend your wrist to the side in the opposite direction, trying to touch your small finger to your arm.

e. Hold this position for 5 seconds.

f. Repeat the technique.

The Hand

A. Finger stretch (Fig. 19-58)

1. **Patient position:** sitting or standing.

2. **Instructions:**

a. Make a tight fist and hold it for 5 seconds.

b. Open your fist and stretch your fingers as far out as possible.

c. Hold this position for 5 seconds.

d. Repeat the procedure.

B. Finger coordination (Fig. 19-59)

1. **Patient position:** sitting or standing.

2. **Instructions:**

a. Hold your hand with the palm down.

b. Hold a card firmly between the thumb and fingertips. Let go suddenly, so that the card falls to the floor.

c. Repeat, using the thumb and different fingers.

d. Repeat the entire process.

C. Finger coordination (Fig. 19-60)

1. **Patient position:** sitting or standing.

2. **Instructions:**

a. Hold your hand with the palm down.

b. Place a card between each of the fingers (four cards).

Figure 19-60. Finger coordination.

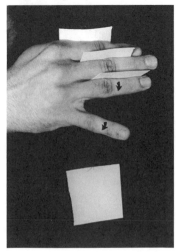

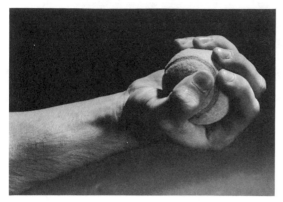

Figure 19-61. Finger-palm strengthening.

c. Release one card at a time by separating the fingers.
d. Repeat the technique, releasing the cards in different order:
D. Finger strengthening (Fig. 19-61)
   1. **Patient position:** sitting or standing.

2. **Instructions:**
   a. Hold a rubber ball in the hand to be treated.
   b. Alternately squeeze the ball between your thumb and little finger, thumb and ring finger, thumb and middle finger, thumb and index finger.
   c. Squeeze the ball with all your fingers.
   d. Hold each squeeze for 3 to 5 seconds.
   e. Repeat the sequence.

References

Jones L. 1981. Strain and Counterstrain. Colorado Springs: American Academy of Osteopathy.

Moran PS, Pruzzo NA, et al. 1973. An Evaluation and Treatment Manual of Osteopathic Manipulative Procedures, vol. I. Kansas City: Institute for Continuing Education in Osteopathic Principles.

Patriquin D. 1992. Evolution of osteopathic manipulative techniques: the Spencer technique. J Am Osteopath Assoc 92(9):1134–1136, 1139–1146.

20

The Lower

Extremity

THE HIP JOINT
Stanley Schiowitz

Functional Anatomy
The hip joint joins the pelvis to the lower extremity. It is a ball-and-socket articulation that allows motion in three planes and circumduction. Its bony components are the acetabulum, which is at the junction of the ilium, ischium, and pubic bones; and the head of the femur. The convex femoral head fits into the concave acetabulum. The articular surfaces are reciprocally curved but are not coextensive; nor are they fully congruent. The close-packed position of the hip joint is full extension, abduction, and medial rotation.

The hip joint is strongly maintained by its capsule and its ligaments—the iliofemoral ligament, the pubofemoral ligament, the ischiofemoral ligament, and, the ligament of the head of the femur. The ligaments slacken or tauten with motion, thereby stabilizing and limiting hip movement. In an upright human the femoral head and neck face medially, anteriorly, and cephalad. Any change in direction will influence pelvic tilt and gait.

The shaft of the femur descends medially, creating a mechanical genu valgus. The femoral shaft also undergoes torsional osseous changes so that the femoral condyles can articulate with the tibial condyles in a frontal plane. The genu valgus is exaggerated with increased pelvic width and contributes to the unstable gait patterns in elderly women.

A major bony landmark is the greater trochanter, easily palpated on the lateral superior aspect of the shaft. The lesser trochanter is on the medial aspect of the inferior end of the femoral neck. This trochanter, though not palpable, is very important, since it is the site of attachment of the iliopsoas tendon. At its distal end, the femoral condyles and epicondyles are easily palpable at the knee joint.

Gross Motion
The gross motions of the hip joint are flexion-extension, abduction-adduction, internal and external rotation, and circumduction. All hip joint motions should be measured with one hand stabilizing the pelvis. Average normal measurements are as follows:

1. Abduction-adduction, hip and knee flexed: 70 to 75 degrees.
2. Abduction, hip and knee extended: 40 to 45 degrees.
3. Adduction, crossing the anterior aspect of the opposite extended leg: 20 to 30 degrees.
4. Rotation, hip and knee extended or flexed,

An Osteopathic Approach to Diagnosis and Treatment, second edition
Eileen L. DiGiovanna and Stanley Schiowitz
Lippincott–Raven Publishers, Philadelphia © 1997.

should be similar: external rotation—about 45 degrees; internal rotation—about 35 degrees.

5. Flexion, knee flexed: 120 to 130 degrees.
6. Flexion, knee extended: usually less than 90 degrees, because it is limited by extensor muscle action.
7. Extension, subject prone: 20 to 30 degrees. If the opposite leg is placed in 90 degrees of flexion, hip extension is 90 to 120 degrees.

Major Muscles

1. **Iliopsoas.** The iliopsoas muscle is a major flexor of the hip upon the trunk. Its origins are very extensive, involving the vertebrae and their disks from the 12th thoracic vertebra to the sacrum, and the anterior ilium and sacrum. The iliopsoas muscle is affected by a wide variety of dysfunctions. Except in cases of nerve damage, it is always slightly hypertonic. The clinician should be aware of this when prescribing an exercise program and should avoid iliopsoas contracting and strengthening programs, especially for patients with low back pain. Athletes involved in major hip flexion sports, such as skating, soccer, and running, have overly developed iliopsoas muscles, creating an exaggerated lumbar-thoracic lordosis.

2. **Tensor fascia lata.** The tensor fascia lata originates in the anterior part of the external lip of the iliac crest and deep fascia lata and inserts on to the iliotibial tract of the fascia lata. This muscle flexes, medially rotates, and abducts the hip joint. Chronic dysfunction may manifest with a number of seemingly unrelated symptoms, including knee pain (especially at the fibular head), buttock pain, and a burning feeling in the lateral upper thigh.

3. **Gluteus medius.** The gluteus medius originates on the external surface of the ilium, below and between the iliac crest and the posterior gluteal line, and inserts on to the lateral surface of the greater trochanter. It is a major abductor of the hip joint and assists slightly in medial rotation and flexion. Hypotonic dysfunctions will affect stance and gait; hypertonic dysfunctions will usually be point-sensitive and mimic sciatic nerve symptoms.

4. **Gluteus maximus.** The gluteus maximus originates at the posterior gluteal line of the ilium, the posterior lower sacrum and coccyx, the aponeurosis of the erector spinae, the sacrotuberous ligament, and the gluteal aponeurosis. The major

actions of this muscle are to extend and laterally rotate the hip. Hypotonic dysfunctions will affect stance and gait. Hypertonic dysfunctions are usually greater in scope than those of the gluteus medius, involving sacral motion and ilial motion as well as hip joint motion.

The gluteus maximus follows the law of muscle detorsion. Therefore, to increase hip extension, as in ballet movement, the ilium must be rotated. Somatic dysfunction of the lumbar spine will limit lumbar regional motion, pelvic rotation, and hip extension.

5. **Hamstrings.** The hamstrings are three muscles, the semimembranosus, semitendinosus, and biceps femoris. All originate at the tuberosity of the ischium and insert on to various areas of the fibula and tibia. They are two-joint muscles that extend the hip and flex the knee. Both motions are interdependent and will affect each other's

Figure 20-1. Erichsen's test for sacroiliac dysfunction. Compression in a frontal plane.

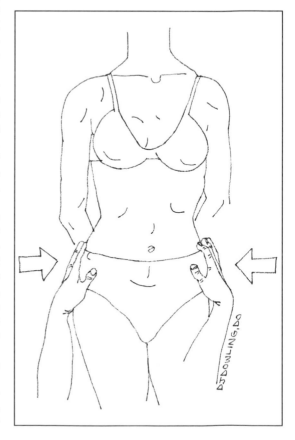

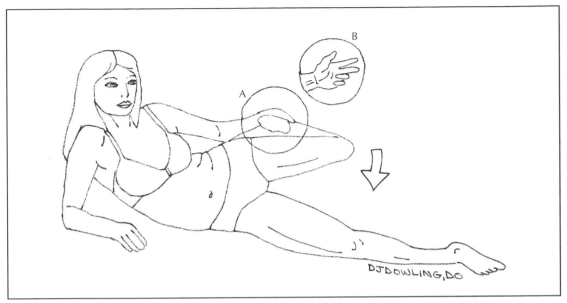

Figure 20-2. Ober's test for contracture of iliotibial fascia. (**A**) Patient holds leg in abducted position. (**B**) Patient lets go.

function. Dysfunctions are commonly found at the ischium, at the lateral aspect of the knee, and at the pes anserinus bursa.

6. **Piriformis.** The piriformis muscle originates on the pelvic surface of the sacrum, at the margin of the greater sciatic foramen, and at the sacrotuberous ligament. It inserts on to the superior border of the greater trochanter. The piriformis muscle is a lateral hip rotator, and its proximity to the sciatic nerve makes it a common site for dysfunction. When hypertonic, it is readily palpable in the lateral rectal mucosa. The piriformis symptom complex follows a sciatic neuritic pain distribution. Specific point tenderness can usually be evoked at a point in the buttocks halfway between the posterosuperior iliac spine and the superolateral aspect of the greater trochanter.

Tests for Evaluating Hip Dysfunction

This section describes several tests for evaluating specific dysfunctions of the hip. Most of the tests are done with the active assistance of the patient.

Erichsen's test. Erichsen's test is a test for sacroiliac disease and early spondylitic arthritis. The clinician grasps the iliac bones and presses them together (Fig. 20-1). A positive test result is indicated by pain.

Ludloff's sign. Ludloff's sign indicates traumatic separation of the epiphysis of the lesser trochanter. Ecchymosis is found at the base of the femoral triangle, and the subject cannot raise the thigh when seated.

Ober's test. Ober's test is a test for contracture of the iliotibial fascia. The patient lies on the good side with the knee and thigh flexed. The top leg is held by the patient in hip abduction, hip extension, and knee flexion (Fig. 20-2). The patient then drops the leg to the table. If the leg remains abducted, the test is positive.

Patrick's (FABERE) test. This test evaluates hip motion restriction in flexion, abduction, external rotation, and extension. The supine patient flexes the hip and knee of one leg and places its lateral malleous on the other leg just above the patella. The clinician gently presses the knee toward the table (Fig. 20-3). Pain or limitation of motion on extension usually indicates hip joint dysfunction (arthritis, synovitis). The hip motions are compared on the two sides.

Trendelenburg test. The Trendelenburg test evaluates gluteus medius weakness or congenital hip joint dislocation. The subject stands on the leg to be tested and raises the other leg (flex hip and knee) (Fig. 20-4). The clinician observes the gluteal crease lines. The test is positive (stance leg)

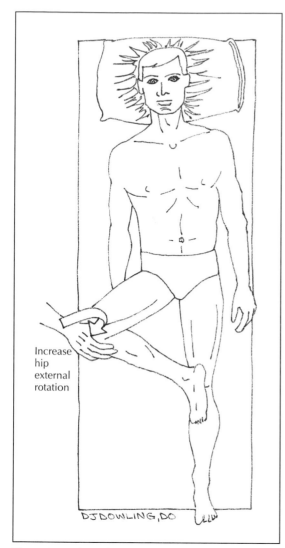

Increase
hip
external
rotation

DJDOWLING,DO

Figure 20-3. Patrick's (FABERE) test for hip joint motion restriction.

if the gluteal crease on the raised leg remains level or drops. Normally it should rise.

Thomas test. The Thomas test evaluates flexion contraction of the iliopsoas muscle. In a supine position, the patient flattens the lordotic curve by flexing both legs and knees to the abdomen, and then releases one leg to the table without creating lordosis (Fig. 20-5). The clinician measures the extension of the leg. The maneuver is repeated with the other leg, and the two sides are compared. Inability to fully extend the leg may indicate iliopsoas contracture.

Common Musculoskeletal Hip Joint Disorders

CONGENITAL DISLOCATION OF THE HIPS (NEWBORN)

Cardinal Diagnostic Findings

1. Asymmetry of gluteal skin folds.
2. Leg seems shorter.
3. Limitation of abduction present.
4. Positive Ortolani's sign; hip "clicks" with reduction as it is flexed, abducted, and externally rotated.
5. X-ray evidence.

TRANSIENT SYNOVITIS

Cardinal Diagnostic Findings

1. Child 3 to 12 years old.
2. Males predominate in 4:1 ratio.
3. No history of trauma, but limp is present.
4. Hip held in flexion, abduction, and external rotation.
5. Low-grade temperature is present.
6. Hip is tender to touch.
7. X-ray evidence.

LEGG-CALVÉ-PERTHES' DISEASE (OSTEOCHONDRITIS DEFORMANS JUVENILIS; ASEPTIC NECROSIS OF OSSIFICATION CENTER OF FEMORAL HEAD)

Cardinal Diagnostic Findings

1. Males predominate, ages 4 to 12, usually unilateral.
2. Antalgic gait present.
3. Pain is in groin, thigh, and may radiate to knee.
4. Sedimentation rate may be elevated. All other tests are normal.
5. Thomas test is positive: contracture of psoas and adductor muscles.
6. Limitation of hip abduction, extension, and internal rotation.
7. Disuse atrophy may develop in upper part of thigh.
8. X-ray evidence.

SLIPPED CAPITAL FEMORAL EPIPHYSIS

Cardinal Diagnostic Findings

1. Most common in adolescents, aged 10 to 15 years.
2. Males more commonly affected, in 3:1 or 4:1 ratio.
3. In a female, will occur at an earlier age because of advanced skeletal maturity.

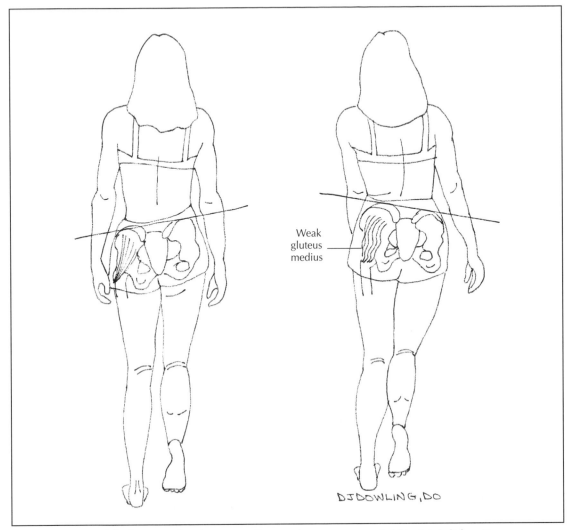

Weak
gluteus
medius

Figure 20-4. Trendelenburg test for gluteus medius weakness or congenital hip joint dislocation.

4. Bilateral involvement noted in 40% of patients.
5. Coxa vara will develop.
6. Antalgic gait present.
7. Limitation of hip motion.
8. Male may have female fat distribution with sexual underdevelopment.
9. X-ray evidence.

ISCHIOGLUTEAL BURSITIS
Common Diagnostic Findings
1. Adults with sedentary occupations.
2. Point tenderness over ischial tuberosity.
3. Pain relieved by local injection of anesthetic.

4. Pain relieved when patient takes weight off buttocks (stands up).
5. X-ray evidence usually not present.

TROCHANTERIC BURSITIS
Common Diagnostic Findings
1. Point tenderness on palpation of the greater trochanter.
2. Pain usually distributed down the lateral aspect of the leg; may mimic a neuritis.
3. Pain present with weight-bearing, walking.
4. X-ray evidence usually not present.

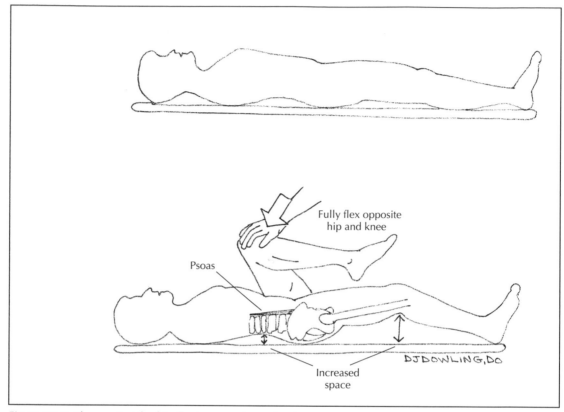

Figure 20-5. Thomas test for hip flexion muscle contracture.

MERALGIA PARESTHETICA
Common Diagnostic Findings
1. Usually caused by pressure on nerve, usually about anterior superior iliac spine. Good history necessary.
2. Persistent paresthesia, anesthesia, or hypesthesia at lateral buttock, down lateral thigh to the knee, for no apparent reason.
3. No point tenderness or muscle dysfunction.
4. Gait, weight-bearing normal.
5. Tinel sign may be present.
6. No x-ray evidence.

PSOATIC DYSFUNCTION
Common Causes
1. Trauma to lumbar spine, lesser trochanter, or pubes.
2. Psoatic myositis due to local inflammation or infection.
3. Psoatic bursitis.
4. Visceral dysfunction causing psoasitis, such as
   a. Appendicitis
   b. Renal or urethral dysfunction
   c. Fallopian tube infection
   d. Retroperitoneal lymphadenopathy
   e. Iliac or femoral phlebitis

Common Diagnostic Findings
1. Psoatic gait present.
2. On standing, hip and knee are flexed on pathologic side.
3. On standing, downward pelvic tilt on pathologic side.
4. In supine position, exaggerated lordosis.
5. Thomas sign present.
6. Point tenderness in femoral triangle.
7. Pelvis shifts to opposite side.
8. Occasionally no x-ray evidence.

THE KNEE JOINT
Stanley Schiowitz

Functional Anatomy

The knee joint is the largest and most complicated articulation in the body. It is a compound joint comprised of medial and lateral femoral-tibial articulations and a patella-femoral articulation, all within one joint capsule. Positioned midway in each supporting limb of the body, the knee is subjected to severe stresses as it performs its functions of weight-bearing and locomotion. The anatomic description of this articulation is simplified by considering it as two separate joints. The larger one, the femorotibial joint, consists of two condylar joints between corresponding femoral and tibial condyles. The second one, the femoropatellar joint, is between the patella and the femur.

THE FEMOROTIBIAL JOINT

The femoral condyles are convex in both planes and, viewed laterally, are spiral-shaped. The lateral condyle flattens more rapidly in the anteroposterior dimension than does the medial condyle, producing inequality in articular lengths. This is evident when the knee is placed in full extension. An automatic coupled rotation occurs to accommodate this inequality. Hoppenfeld describes a "screw home" motion in which the medial aspect of the tibia rotates laterally around the lateral femoral condyle, allowing the medial femoral condyle to complete its extension. This approximates a close-packed position, allowing prolonged periods of standing without relying on muscle function.

The tibial condyles are concave and end toward the midtibial line in intercondylar eminences. The condyles are separated by the intercondylar area.

The femorotibial joint is one of the few articulations with menisci. The medial meniscus is semicircular. Its anterior end is attached to the anterior intercondylar area in front of the anterior cruciate ligament. The lateral meniscus is almost a complete ring. Its anterior end is attached in front of the intercondylar eminence of the tibia, blending partially with the anterior cruciate ligament.

The femoral condyles roll and slide on the tibial condyles during flexion and extension, accompa-

nied by similar motions of the menisci. During extension the menisci are pulled anteriorly; with flexion they are moved posteriorly.

The femorotibial joint is stabilized by the capsule and its related ligaments and muscular attachments. Laterally, these attachments comprise the fibular collateral ligament, biceps tendon, popliteus tendon, and the iliotibial tract; medially, they comprise the pes anserinus, the medial head of the gastrocnemius, the tibial lateral ligament, and a portion of the quadriceps tendon. Posteriorly the joint is stabilized by both heads of the gastrocnemius, the semitendinous muscle, the biceps tendon, the oblique popliteal ligament, and the arcuate ligament. The anterior aspect is stabilized by the quadriceps muscles, the quadriceps tendon, the patella, the patellar tendon, and the medial and lateral retinacula.

The cruciate ligaments are intraarticular but extrasynovial. They stabilize the knee in the anteroposterior direction and allow the joint to function as a hinge while keeping the articular surfaces together. The *anterior cruciate ligament* arises from the tibia and runs backward, upward, and laterally to insert on to the lateral femoral condyle. During flexion, the anterior cruciate ligament slides the femoral condyle forward. The *posterior cruciate ligament* arises from the posterior aspect of the tibia and runs forward and upward obliquely to insert on to the lateral aspect of the medial femoral condyle. During extension the posterior cruciate ligament slides the femoral condyle posteriorly.

THE FEMOROPATELLAR JOINT

The femoropatellar joint is a sellar joint; the articulating surface of the patella is adapted to the patellar surface of the femur. This femoral articulation involves the anterior surface of both condyles. An oblique groove divides it into a large lateral and smaller medial area. The joint's stability is maintained by the quadriceps muscles, the quadriceps tendon, and the patellar tendon. Its major motions are vertical up-and-down movement on the femur, and movement in a sagittal plane with respect to the tibia. This allows a pulley function during flexion and extension of the knee.

Major Muscles

The quadriceps femoris is the extensor muscle of the knee. It consists of four muscles that have a common tendon of insertion on to the anterior tuberosity of the tibia. The rectus femoris arises from two tendinous heads, one from the anterior iliac spine and the second from a groove above the acetabulum and the hip joint capsule. It is directed downward along the anterior aspect of the thigh and ends in the common tendon. It functions as a two-joint muscle, producing both hip flexion and knee extension. The vastus lateralis is the largest part of the quadriceps. It arises from the upper intertrochanteric line and the anterior and inferior borders of the greater trochanter. The vastus medialis arises from the lower part of the intertrochanteric line, the spiral line, the medial lip of the linea aspera, the medial supracondylar line, and the tendons of the adductor longus and magnus. The vastus intermedius arises from the front and lateral surface of the upper shaft of the femur.

The flexor muscles of the knee are located in the posterior compartment of the thigh. They are the hamstrings, the gracilis, the sartorius, the popliteus, and the gastrocnemius muscles. All of these muscles are biarticular, with the exception of the popliteus and the short head of the biceps. Their action on knee flexion is related to the position of the hip. Rotation of the knee is also a function of these knee flexors.

Knee Movements

The active motions of the knee are classified as flexion-extension and medial-lateral rotation. Normally the knee flexes to 135 degrees; extension is a return from flexion to 0 degrees. Medial-lateral rotation, with the knee in flexion, is 10 degrees in each direction. With the foot on the ground, the last 30 degrees of extension is accompanied by a conjunct medial femoral rotation. With the foot off the ground, extension is accompanied by a conjunct lateral rotation of the tibia.

Accessory motions with the knee semiflexed are anteroposterior glide, abduction-adduction and long-axis extension.

Special Tests

VARUS-VALGUS STRESS TEST

This test evaluates the medial and lateral collateral structures. With the patient supine, the ankle joint is held between the examiner's side and arm, thus freeing both hands. The knee is tested in full extension by applying a valgus and then a varus force to the proximal tibia (abduction-adduction motion of leg) (Fig. 20-6). The examiner notes any instability or increased motion on application of force in either direction. Then the test is repeated with the knee slightly flexed. If the cruciate ligaments are intact, motion can be stable with the knee in full extension, even with collateral ligament rupture.

ROTARY INSTABILITY TESTING

Anterior Draw Test

The anterior draw test evaluates anterior cruciate ligament dysfunction. The patient is supine, with his knee flexed 90 degrees and his foot on the table. The examiner sits on the patient's foot or otherwise holds it firmly to stabilize it. The examiner then grasps the back of the proximal tibia with one or both hands and pulls it forward (Fig. 20-7). The patient's leg and foot are internally rotated 30 degrees, then externally rotated 15 degrees, and in a neutral position. On internal rotation, anterior shift of the lateral tibial plateau in conjunction with medial rotation implies injury to the anterior cruciate and lateral ligament. On external rotation, anterior shift of the medial tibial plateau in conjunction with lateral rotation implies injury to the anterior cruciate and medial collateral ligaments. With the foot in neutral position (anterior drawer sign) an anterior tibial shift indicates anterior cruciate ligament dysfunction, probably accompanied by medial and lateral ligamentous injury.

Posterior Draw Test

The posterior draw test evaluates posterior cruciate ligament dysfunction. The patient's foot is placed in neutral position, as for the anterior draw test. The examiner applies force on the anterior tibia in a posterior direction (Fig. 20-8). The femoral condyles become prominent anteriorly as the tibia subluxates posteriorly, indicating posterior cruciate ligament dysfunction.

EXTERNAL ROTATION—RECURVATUM TEST

With the patient supine, the examiner grasps one lower extremity under the heel. With his other hand he supports the calf. The knee is allowed to move from 10 degrees of flexion to full extension (Fig. 20-9). If the knee becomes hyperextended with external rotation of the tibia and tibial varus,

Figure 20-6. Varus-valgus stress for collateral structure dysfunction.

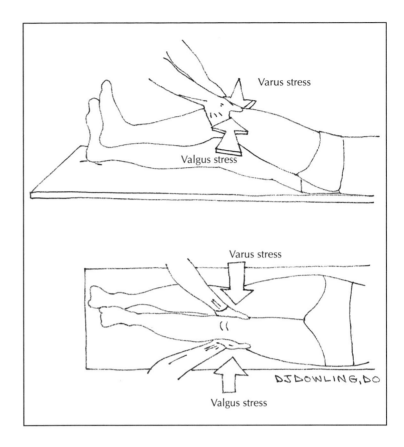

Figure 20-7. Anterior draw test for anterior cruciate ligament dysfunction.

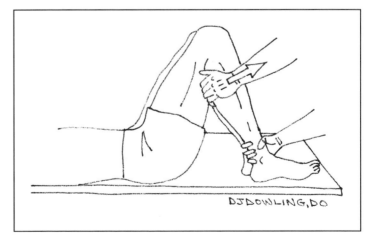

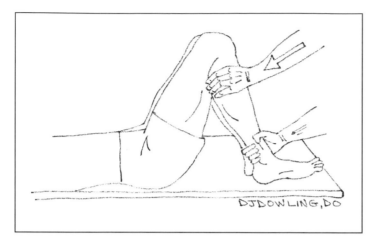

Figure 20-8. Posterior draw test for posterior cruciate ligament dysfunction.

the test is positive. This indicates injury to the arcuate ligament, popliteus, and fibular collateral ligament.

MCMURRAY TEST

The McMurray test evaluates for meniscal tears. With the patient supine, the examiner grasps the foot with one hand and palpates the knee joint line with the other hand. The examiner acutely flexes the knee and rotates the tibia into medial and lateral rotation. With the tibia held in lateral rotation the examiner applies a valgus stress and extends the knee (Fig. 20-10). The maneuver is repeated with the knee held in medial rotation and a varus stress applied while extending the knee. A palpable or audible click within the joint is considered a sign of a meniscal tear.

APLEY'S COMPRESSION TEST

With the patient prone, the knee is flexed to 90 degrees. The examiner stabilizes the patient's thigh and leans on the heel, compressing the menisci between the femur and tibia, then rotates the tibia medially while maintaining this compres-

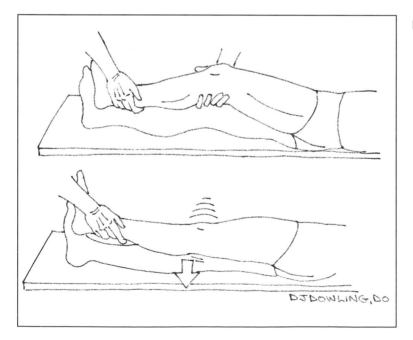

Figure 20-9. Recurvatum test.

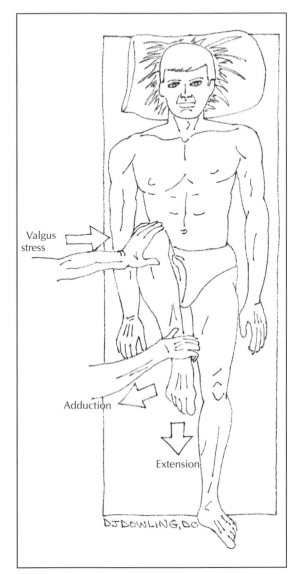

Figure 20-10. McMurray test for meniscal tears.

sion (Fig. 20-11). Medial joint pain produced by this maneuver suggests a medial meniscal tear, while lateral joint pain suggests a lateral meniscal tear.

APLEY'S DISTRACTION TEST

With the patient prone, the knee is flexed to 90 degrees. The examiner stabilizes the thigh by kneeling on it, then applies traction to the leg while rotating it medially and laterally (traction reduces meniscal pressure but increases ligamen-

tous strain) (Fig. 20-12). Any pain elicited by this maneuver indicates medial or lateral ligamentous dysfunction.

KNEE JOINT EFFUSION TEST

The knee joint effusion test is performed in the same manner as the test for external rotation. Failure of the knee to extend fully indicates increased joint fluid.

PATELLA FEMORAL GRINDING TEST

The patient is supine with the knee extended and relaxed. The examiner pushes the patella caudad in the trochlear groove, then holds it in this position. The patient is instructed to tighten the quadriceps muscle against the examiner's resistance. Palpable crepitation of patellar motion is an indication of roughness of the articulating surfaces, potentially due to chondromalacia of the patella.

Common Musculoskeletal Knee Joint Disorders

MENISCAL TEARS
Common Findings
1. History of trauma.
2. Pain, swelling, and complaint of knee locking.
3. McMurray's test and the Apley compression test positive.
4. Arthroscopy necessary for confirmation.

CHONDROMALACIA OF THE PATELLA
Common Findings
1. First attack occurred prior to bony fusion.
2. Pain on sitting, climbing stairs, or prolonged walking.
3. Minor joint effusion present.
4. Recurrence with squatting.
5. Stiffness after sitting.
6. Patella femoral grinding test positive.
7. X-ray findings may be present.

PATELLAR TENDON TENDINITIS
Common Findings
1. Repeated stress applied to the insertion of the quadriceps tendon on the patella, producing tendinitis (stress may be at proximal, or more often, distal pole of the patella).
2. Pain worse after exercise.
3. Severe localized point tenderness.
4. No joint effusion.
5. Bone scan showing increased activity, as in stress fracture.

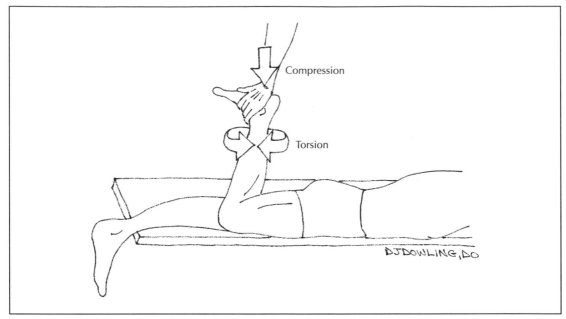

Figure 20-11. Apley's compression test for meniscal dysfunction.

Figure 20-12. Apley's distraction test for ligamentous dysfunction.

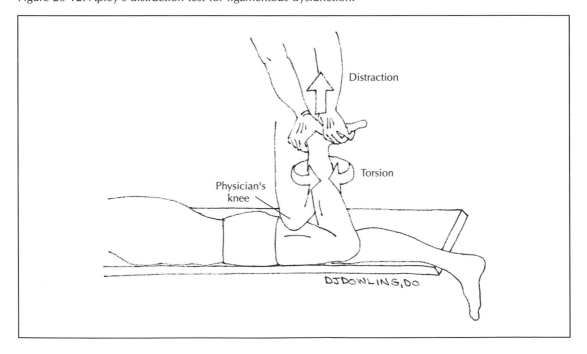

TRAUMATIC SYNOVITIS
Common Findings
1. Painful, swollen knee; difficulty with extension.
2. Suprapatellar pouch distended.
3. Patella is ballotable.
4. Knee only slightly warm.
5. History of trauma or chronic recurrence.

ANTERIOR FAT PAD LESION
Common Findings
1. Anterior knee pain of long duration.
2. Pain relieved by rest.
3. Pain relieved with knee in flexed position.
4. Tenderness anteriorly about the patellar tendon, usually of the fat pad itself on either side.
5. Joint line not involved.

OSGOOD-SCHLATTER DISEASE
Common Findings
1. Point tenderness and swelling of the tibial tubercle.
2. Relieved with rest.
3. Localized traction tendonitis.
4. Heals with bone fusion.

PES ANSERINUS BURSITIS
Common Findings
1. Located at insertion of pes anserinus.
2. At medial aspect of knee but below joint space.
3. Severe point tenderness.
4. Worsens with contraction of the sartorius, gracilis, and semitendinous muscles.

INFRAPATELLAR BURSITIS (HOUSEMAID'S KNEE)
Common Findings
1. Localized swelling of bursa.
2. Usually not painful.
3. Caused by local trauma, usually recurrent.
4. Outside of joint capsule, does not interfere with function.

BAKER'S CYST (POPLITEAL CYST)
Common Findings
1. Usually arises from semimembranous tendon bursa.
2. May communicate with the joint.
3. Benign posterior joint space effusion.
4. Not painful unless size hinders joint motion.
5. Frequently related to rheumatoid arthritis.

THE FOOT AND ANKLE JOINTS
Stanley Schiowitz

The foot and ankle joints make up a complex unit of 28 bones. This unit must perform the functions of weight-bearing and adapting to terrain during walking or running, yet still remain sufficiently elastic to accommodate to additional stress. Some 40% of the entire population have foot abnormalities, which makes the study of this region extremely important.

Functional Anatomy
The ankle articulation consists of the distal end of the tibia and the medial and lateral malleoli, which together form a concave surface, the crural arch, into which is fitted the body of the talus. These bones are connected by the joint capsule and by the deltoid, anterior and posterior talofibular, and calcaneofibular ligaments. The tibial malleolus extends about one third of the way down the medial surface of the talus and is anterior to the lateral malleolus. The fibular malleolus extends down the entire lateral aspect of the talus. When viewed from above, the entire articulation is laterally angled, thus creating a toeing-out of 15 degrees (Fig. 20-13).

The body of the talus is wedge-shaped and wider in its anterior portion. Dorsiflexion creates a close-packed position of the talus in the crural arch. Further dorsiflexion induces separation of the tibiofibular articulation, with lateral and caudal displacement of the distal fibula and medial rotation around the tibia. This motion of the fibula can be a major source of fibular head dysfunction.

The major joint motions of the ankle are plantar flexion (to 50 degrees) and dorsiflexion (to 20 degrees) (Fig. 20-14). Accessory motions of side-to-

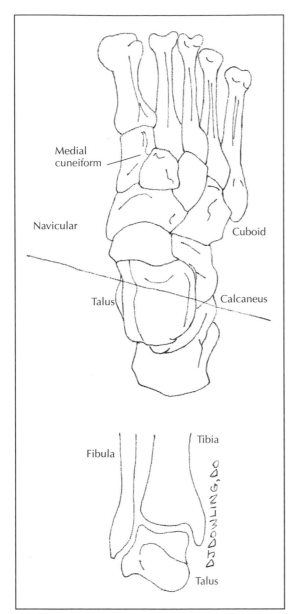

Figure 20-13. Regional functional anatomy of the ankle joint.

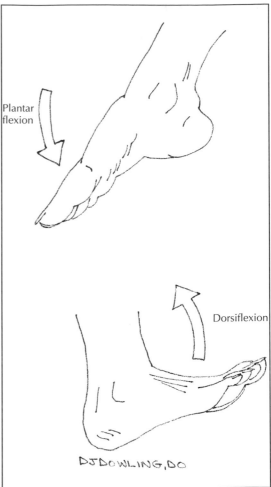

Figure 20-14. Major motions of the ankle joint.

side glide, rotation, abduction, and adduction are present if the joint is in plantar flexion.

The triangular deltoid ligament is located medially and is attached above to the medial malleolus and below to the tuberosity of the navicular, the sustentaculum tali of the calcaneus, and the me-

dial tubercle of the talus. The deltoid ligament is so strong that trauma often causes fractures of its bony attachments rather than rupture of the ligament itself.

The anterior talofibular ligament goes from the anterior margin of the lateral malleolus forward and medially to attach to the lateral aspect of the neck and the lateral articular facet of the talus. The posterior talofibular ligament runs from the lower part of the lateral malleolus to the lateral tubercle of the posterior process of the talus. The calcaneofibular ligament runs from the apex of the lateral malleolus downward and backward to the tubercle on the lateral surface of the calcaneus (Fig. 20-15).

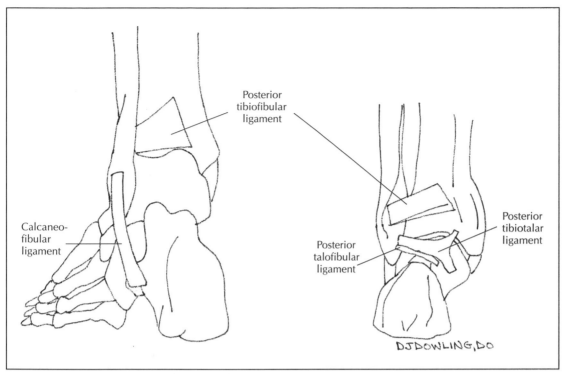

Figure 20-15. Ligamentous attachments at the ankle, posterior view.

The shape of the crural concavity, the extent of the lateral malleolus on the talus, and the strong ligamentous attachments deter joint dislocations unless accompanied by fracture of the malleoli.

The most common sprain represents an inversion and is usually caused by a combination of plantar flexion, internal rotation, and inversion. The lateral ankle ligaments sustain the initial impact. The type of ligamentous tear or fracture-dislocation will depend on the severity of the force.

The major muscle of ankle dorsiflexion is the tibialis anterior, assisted by the extensor digitorum longus, the extensor hallucis longus, and the peroneus tertius. The major muscles of ankle plantar flexion are the gastrocnemius and soleus, assisted by the plantaris, tibialis posterior, flexor hallucis longus, and flexor digitorum longus.

The subtalar articulation consists of the talus on the calcaneus. These bones have two separate concave-convex articulations. The major motions are calcaneal abduction (valgus) and calcaneal adduction (varus), in relationship to the fixed talus.

The talus articulates with the navicular and the calcaneus articulates with the cuboid.

The combined motions of these joints create foot inversion and eversion (Fig. 20-16). Inversion is created by calcaneal adduction, navicular rotation, and glide on the talus. These motions raise the navicular and the medial border and depress the lateral border of the foot. Eversion is produced by an opposite series of motions. The muscles involved in the motion of inversion are the tibialis anterior and posterior. The muscles involved in the motion of eversion are the peroneus longus and brevis.

The cuboid motions on the calcaneus are glide with conjunct rotation. This usually accompanies the inversion-eversion motions of the combined articulations.

The forefoot consists of the metatarsals and phalanges. These bones have a combined motion of forefoot abduction and adduction (Fig. 20-17).

Pronation and supination of the foot are commonly described as a combination of various mo-

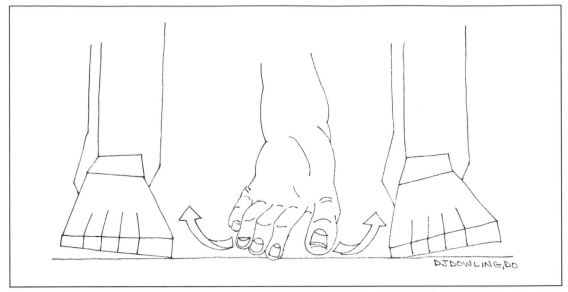

Figure 20-16. **(A)** Eversion of the ankle. **(B)** Inversion of the ankle.

tions. Pronation consists of calcaneal abduction, subtalar-cuboid-navicular eversion, forefoot abduction, and ankle dorsiflexion. Supination consists of calcaneal adduction, subtalar-cuboid-navicular inversion, forefoot adduction, and ankle plantar flexion.

ARCHES OF THE FOOT

The longitudinal curve of the foot can be divided into medial and lateral longitudinal arches. The lateral arch is composed of the calcaneus, cuboid, and fourth and fifth metatarsal bones. This arch is low, with limited mobility: it is designed to

Figure 20-17. **(A)** Abduction of the forefoot. **(B)** Adduction of the forefoot.

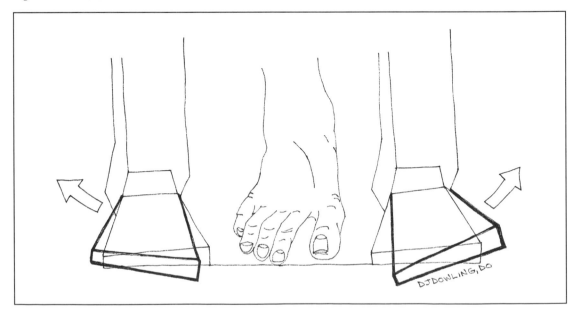

transmit weight and thrust to the ground. Its major articulation is the calcaneocuboid, which has a limited range of motion. Stress through this arch can create a typical cuboid somatic dysfunction. Torsion through the anterior aspect of this arch will readily cause fracture of the fifth metatarsal.

The medial longitudinal arch is composed of the calcaneus, the talus, the navicular, the cuneiforms, and the first three metatarsal bones. This arch is considerably higher and more mobile than its lateral counterpart. The plantar ligaments, plantar fascia, and the tibialis posterior, flexor digitorum longus, flexor hallucis longus, and intrinsic muscles of the foot assist in controlling the medial arch.

Evidently muscles contribute little to the main-tenance of the arch, which instead is supported passively by the skeletal structure and ligaments. Muscles do play an active role in balance and gait.

Many authors describe a number of transverse arches (Fig. 20-18). With the exception of the metatarsal heads, these arches do not transmit forces to the ground. The anterior metatarsal transverse arch consists of the five metatarsal heads, with the second metatarsal as its highest point. With weight-bearing this arch is flattened. Depression of the anterior metatarsal transverse arch increases the weight-bearing burden of the metatarsal heads, creating dysfunction. A second, posterior metatarsal arch consists of the bases of the five metatarsals. A third, tarsal arch has been described, consisting of the navicular, cuneiform, and cuboid

Figure 20-18. Transverse arches of the foot.

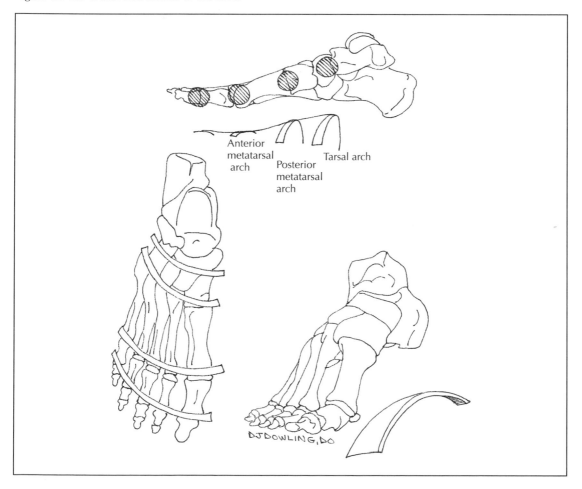

bones. This arch assists in flexibility and the rotation motions of the foot. Diminution or absence of the tarsal arch is evident in pes planus (flat feet).

Common Musculoskeletal Disorders
PEDIATRIC CONGENITAL DEFORMITIES:
ANATOMIC DEFINITIONS
Pes planus: Flattened longitudinal arches.
Equinus: Toes pointed down, foot in plantar flexion (Fig. 20-19A).
Calcaneus: Toes pointed up, foot in dorsiflexion (Fig. 20-19B).

Figure 20-19. Pediatric congenital deformities. **(A)** Equinus. **(B)** Calcaneus.

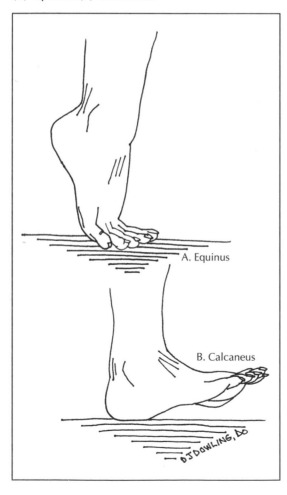

A. Equinus

B. Calcaneus

Valgus: Toes pointed out, foot in abduction.
Varus: Toes pointed in, foot in adduction.
Eversion: Foot rotated externally on its longitudinal arch; sole faces laterally.
Inversion: Foot rotated internally on its longitudinal arch; sole faces medially.

COMMON CONGENITAL
PEDIATRIC CONDITIONS
1. **Pes planus (dropped longitudinal arches).** Pes planus may be a normal finding in a child; however, it may also represent a congenital condition, either flexible calcaneal valgus or rigid vertical talus.
2. **Talipes equinovarus (clubfoot).** The foot is in the position of inversion, adduction of the forefoot, calcaneal varus, and equinus. The calf muscles are contracted.
3. **Metatarsus varus.** This condition is characterized by calcaneal valgus, the forefoot in adduction, and a convex lateral foot border.
4. **Tibial torsion.** In tibial torsion the tibia is twisted on its longitudinal axis and the relationship between the patella and the foot is abnormal. The condition can be secondary to femoral torsion. Bilateral torsion can create "pigeon toeing" or a Charlie Chaplin type of gait.

COMMON ADULT CONDITIONS
1. **Foot strains.** Foot strains are of several types, including (a) plantar fascia involvement of the medial longitudinal arch or at the calcaneal insertions, (b) medial and lateral ligament involvement secondary to chronic or acute strains, and (c) metatarsalgia secondary to abnormal weight-bearing by the metatarsal heads.
2. **Morton's syndrome.** Morton's syndrome is a metatarsalgia caused by a short first metatarsal bone.
3. **Morton's neuroma.** Morton's neuroma is a fibroneuromatous reaction between the heads of the third and fourth metatarsals.
4. **March fracture.** March fracture is a stress fracture, usually involving the shaft of the second or third metatarsal.
5. **Hallux valgus.** Hallux valgus is a lateral deviation of the proximal phalanx of the first toe associated with soft tissue changes, pain, swelling, and inflammation at the medial as-

pect of the head of the first metatarsal, which is angled medially. This condition is also called a bunion.

6. **Hallux rigidus.** Hallux rigidus is an osteoarthrosis of the first metatarsophalangeal articulation. Joint motion is severely limited: there is no first toe push-off, and localized pain is present at that joint.

7. **Claw toe.** Claw toe is a fixed flexion deformity of the proximal interphalangeal joints associated with hyperextension of the metatarsophalangeal articulations.

8. **Hammer toe.** Hammer toe is similar to claw toe, but the distal interphalangeal articulation is in hyperextension. Usually only one toe is involved.

9. **Callus.** A callus is a hyperkeratotic response of the skin to excessive pressure.

10. **Corns.** Soft corns are hyperkeratotic lesions found between the toes, usually the fourth and fifth toes. They are extremely painful. Hard corns are usually found when hammer or claw toes cause abnormal shoe pressure on the hyperflexed or hyperextended joint.

The treatment and prevention of many of these adult dysfunctions require the proper fit of shoes and orthotic devices, as well as knowledge of osteopathic diagnostic and manipulative procedures.

References

Basmajian JV. 1978. Muscles Alive. Baltimore: Williams & Wilkins.

Cailliet R. 1968. Foot and Ankle Pain. Philadelphia: F.A. Davis.

D'Ambrosia RD. 1977. Musculoskeletal Disorders. Philadelphia: J.B. Lippincott.

Hoppenfeld S. 1986. Physical Examination of the Spine and Extremities. Norwalk, Conn: Appleton-Century-Crofts.

Jones L. 1955. The Postural Complex. St. Louis: Charles C Thomas.

Kapandji IA. 1970. The Physiology of the Joints. Vol II. Edinburgh: Churchill Livingstone.

MacConaill MA, Basmajian JV. 1977. Muscles and Movements. New York: Robert E. Krieger.

O'Donoghue DH. 1970. Treatment of Injuries to Athletes. Philadelphia: W.B. Saunders.

Rasch PJ, Burke RK. 1978. Kinesiology and Applied Anatomy. Baltimore: Lea & Febiger.

Warwick RB, Williams PL. 1973. Gray's Anatomy, 35th British Ed. Philadelphia: W.B. Saunders.

Wells KF, Luttgens K. 1976. Kinesiology. Philadelphia: W.B. Saunders.

Wilson FC. 1983. The Musculoskeletal System, 2nd ed. Philadelphia: J.B. Lippincott.

21

Diagnosis and
Treatment of the
Lower Extremity

THE HIP
Stanley Schiowitz

This section describes the diagnosis and treatment of soft tissue dysfunctions of the hip joint. In most instances, these dysfunctions are evaluated by testing the range of anatomic or physiologic joint motion. The diagnosis of restrictive movements in the extremities can usually be simplified by comparing both sides. However, arthritic involvement of the hip joint can confuse the diagnosis, and it may be difficult to ascertain how much of the restriction is due to myofascial dysfunction and how much to joint lining disease. The techniques described here can be utilized when both conditions are present. After a few treatments the soft tissue components will improve, and any remaining restriction can be attributed to degenerative joint changes.

Most physicians treating musculoskeletal problems use the anatomic barriers to passive motion as their guide. The following discussion is presented with that in mind.

Screening Tests for Somatic Dysfunctions of the Hip
The following screening tests are performed to evaluate gross motions of the hip joint. Individual joint motions should be tested if any of the screen-

ing procedures are positive. Individual joint motions include abduction and adduction, internal and external rotation, flexion, and extension. Extending these procedures to their anatomic barriers of motion will result in full anatomic barrier motion measurements.

FABERE test. The FABERE test evaluates flexion, abduction, external rotation, and extension of one hip joint as compared with the other. The test is described in Chapter 20.

Squatting. The patient attempts to squat while holding on to support. Hip joint restriction will prevent this movement, as will knee joint dysfunction (Fig. 21-1).

Straight leg raising. The patient is supine with the legs together and extended. The physician stands on the side of the leg to be tested and grasps the patient's ankle with one hand while placing the other hand on the patient's opposite anterior superior iliac spine (Fig. 21-2). With the patient's knee extended, the physician lifts the patient's leg, flexing the hip, until motion is felt at the opposite anterior superior iliac spine. The angle of flexion from the table top is measured. The physician returns the leg to the table and repeats the maneuver from the other side of the table with the other leg. Any limitation of flexion

An Osteopathic Approach to Diagnosis and Treatment, second edition
Eileen L. DiGiovanna and Stanley Schiowitz
Lippincott–Raven Publishers, Philadelphia © 1997

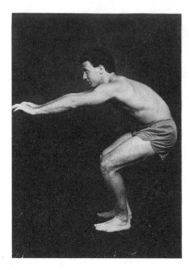

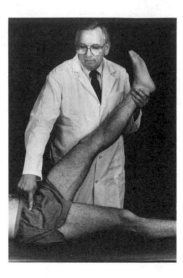

Figure 21-1. Squatting test for hip joint restriction.

Figure 21-2. Straight leg raising test for limitation in flexion of the hip joint.

is interpreted as being caused by contracted hamstring muscles.

Thomas test for psoas contraction. In a supine position, the patient flattens the lumbar lordotic curve by flexing both hips and knees to the abdomen, then releases one leg to the table without creating lordosis. The clinician measures the extension of the leg. The maneuver is repeated with the other leg, and the two sides are compared. Inability to fully extend the leg may indicate iliopsoas contracture.

Treatment

MYOFASCIAL STRETCH—PASSIVE AND ACTIVE

1. **Patient position:** supine.
2. **Physician position:** standing on the side of dysfunction, facing the table.
3. **Technique:**
   a. The patient's hip and knee are flexed.
   b. The physician places his hands on the posterior aspect of the patient's thigh, near the popliteal region.
   c. The physician passively applies increasing force to the patient's thigh in the direction of limitation of motion, to the point of creating pain. This position is held for 3 seconds.
   d. The patient pushes his thigh against the physician's resisting hands, creating an isometric contraction in the direction opposite to the

passive motion. This position is held for 3 seconds (Fig. 21-3).
   e. The physician relaxes all force and returns the hip to the starting position.
   f. The patient rests for 3 seconds; then the procedure is repeated.

This maneuver should be performed three times, with each repetition allowing greater freedom of motion. The technique can be repeated in another direction of limitation of motion.

PASSIVE MYOFASCIAL RELEASE—COMBINED HIP AND KNEE

1. **Patient position:** supine.
2. **Physician position:** standing on the side of the dysfunction, facing the table.
3. **Technique:**
   a. The patient's hip and knee are flexed to 90 degrees, if possible.
   b. The patient's hip is placed into abduction and external rotation up to full pain-free motion.
   c. The physician places one hand on the medial aspect of the patient's knee, firmly holding that limb in its abduction—external rotation position.
   d. With his other hand, the physician grasps the patient's foot or shin and externally rotates

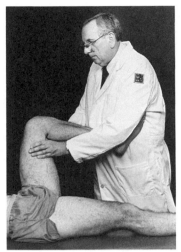

Figure 21-3. Passive-active myofascial stretch of the hip.

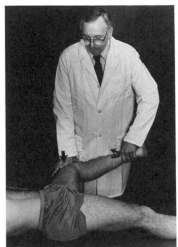

A

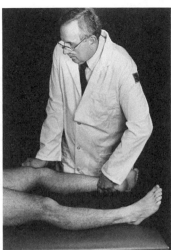

B

Figure 21-4. **(A)** Passive myofascial release of the hip and knee, abduction–external rotation. **(B)** The hip and knee are returned to full extension.

the tibia to its maximum pain-free position (Fig. 21-4A).

e. The physician holds this position for 3 seconds, increasing the motion pressure of both hands until the muscles relax.

f. Maintaining pressure with both hands, the physician slowly returns the patient's hip and knee to full extension on the table, releasing the pressure of both hands only at the last 5 degrees of full extension (Fig. 21-4B).

g. The patient rests; then the treatment is repeated.

This procedure can be performed with the patient's hip in adduction and internal rotation. The physician places one hand on the lateral aspect of the patient's knee and moves the tibia into internal rotation (Fig. 21-5).

PSOAS ADDUCTOR STRETCH—PASSIVE AND ACTIVE

1. **Patient position:** supine.
2. **Physician position:** standing beside the table, on the side to be treated.
3. **Technique:**
   a. The patient flexes the dysfunctional hip and

knee and places that foot on table beside the other knee, which is in full extension.

b. The patient then abducts and externally rotates the flexed hip, so that the plantar aspect of the foot lies beside the medial aspect of the extended knee.

c. The physician places one hand on the anterior superior iliac spine of the nondysfunctional side and the other hand on the medial aspect of the patient's flexed knee, holding it in its position of flexion, hip abduction–external rotation.

d. The physician adds a gentle passive stretching force toward the table. This position is held for 3 seconds.

e. The patient exerts a gentle force upward into adduction, internal rotation–flexion, against the physician's isometrically resisting right hand (Fig. 21-6). This position is held for 3 seconds.

f. The patient relaxes. After 3 seconds the procedure is repeated.

MYOFASCIAL RELEASE WITH TRACTION OF THE HIP JOINT

1. **Patient position:** supine.
2. **Physician position:** sitting beside the table on

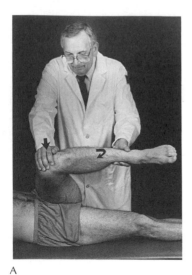
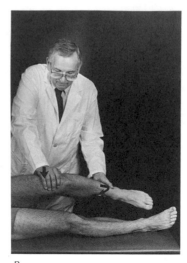

Figure 21-5. **(A)** Active myofascial release of the hip and knee, adduction–internal rotation. **(B)** The hip and knee are returned to full extension.

A

B

the side of the dysfunction, facing toward the patient's head.

3. **Technique:**
   a. The patient's ankle and shin are placed in the physician's axilla and maintained in position by firm adduction of the arm.
   b. The physician grasps the patient's extended leg above the knee and rotates the hip internally and externally, testing for ease of motion.

   c. The hip is placed into its freedom of motion and firmly held there.
   d. The physician then applies traction to the entire leg by leaning back, creating a pull of the leg that is snugged in his axilla and gradually increasing rotation into the freedom of motion (Fig. 21-7). This position is held for 3 seconds; then the physician quickly rotates the hip fully in the opposite direction. This position is held for 3 seconds.

Figure 21-6. Myofascial release with traction of the hip joint.

Figure 21-7. Passive-active psoas adductor stretch.

Figure 21-8. Passive-active hamstring stretch.

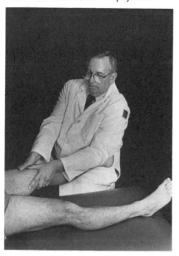
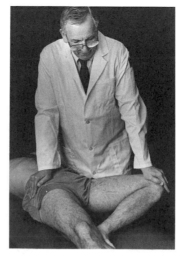
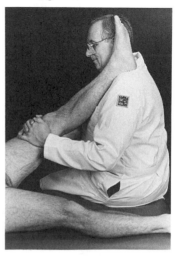

e. The physician releases the leg and relaxes the position.

f. The patient rests for 3 seconds; then the technique is repeated.

HAMSTRING STRETCH—PASSIVE AND ACTIVE

1. **Patient position:** supine.
2. **Physician position:** sitting on the table on the side of the dysfunction, facing the patient.
3. **Technique:**
   a. The patient's ankle is placed on the physician's shoulder. The physician places both his hands on the anterior aspect of the patient's knee to maintain the leg in full extension.
   b. The physician stands up, raising the straightened leg higher into hip flexion. The hip is stretched to the point of onset of pain and held at maximum painless stretch for 3 seconds.
   c. The patient presses that leg down on to the physician's shoulder for 3 seconds (Fig. 21-8).
   d. The leg is released, the patient relaxes for 3 seconds, and the technique is repeated.

Counterstrain Treatment

Three significant tender points are associated with the hip joint (Fig. 21-9). One might also consider the piriformis tender point when treating hip pain: the piriformis tender point is most closely associated with sacral dysfunctions and was discussed in Chapter 14.

POSTEROLATERAL TROCHANTERIC TENDER POINT

1. **Tender point:** on the posterolateral surface of the greater trochanter.
2. **Patient position:** prone.
3. **Physician position:** standing or seated beside the table.
4. **Technique:**
   a. The hip is extended and abducted (Fig. 21-10).
   b. External rotation may be needed.

LATERAL TROCHANTERIC TENDER POINT

1. **Tender point:** 5 to 6 inches below the trochanter on the lateral thigh.

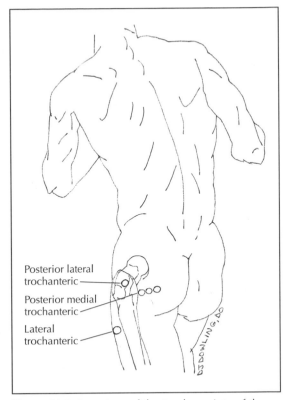

Posterior lateral trochanteric

Posterior medial trochanteric

Lateral trochanteric

Figure 21-9. Locations of the tender points of the hips.

2. **Patient position:** prone.
3. **Physician position:** standing or seated beside the table.
4. **Technique:**
   a. The leg is abducted (Fig. 21-11).
   b. Some flexion may be introduced.

POSTEROMEDIAL TROCHANTERIC TENDER POINTS

1. **Tender point:** 2 to 3 inches below the trochanter along posterior shaft of femur over to the ischial tuberosity.
2. **Patient position:** prone.
3. **Physician position:** standing beside the table, opposite the tender point.
4. **Technique:**
   The thigh is extended, adducted and externally rotated (Fig. 21-12).

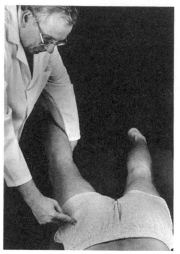

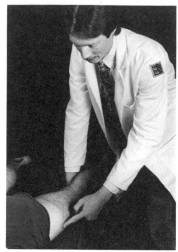

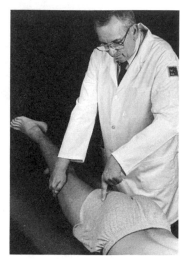

Figure 21-10. Counterstrain treatment of posterolateral trochanteric tender point.

Figure 21-11. Counterstrain treatment of lateral trochanteric tender point.

Figure 21-12. Counterstrain treatment of posteromedial trochanteric tender point.

THE KNEE
Stanley Schiowitz

The knee joint is subject to numerous stresses in normal daily activities. Simply standing up from a sitting position can be difficult or painful if the knee joint is not fully functional. In addition, the resurgence of health consciousness has created a number of enthusiastic walkers, joggers, runners, and tennis players. Each of these activities can add greatly to knee joint dysfunction.

Before treating specific osteopathic articular somatic dysfunctions, the physician must evaluate and treat any soft tissue dysfunctions. The localized osteopathic joint motion dysfunctions discussed in this chapter involve minor or accessory motions.

Diagnosis of Somatic Dysfunctions of the Knee Joint

ABDUCTION—TIBIA ON FEMUR
This is a condition of varus stress of the tibia on the femur. It can be created by a blow to the medial knee joint or by a twisting motion that produces lateral ligamentous sprain. The lateral joint structures are lax, the medial knee joint approximates, and tibial motion on the femur is restricted in medial translatory slide.

1. **Patient position:** supine, with the knee fully extended.
2. **Physician position:** standing on the side of the somatic dysfunction, facing the table.
3. **Technique:**
   a. The physician's cephalic hand grasps the patient's distal femur, holding it firmly and restricting its movement.
   b. With his other hand the physician grasps the patient's lower ankle and creates valgus-varus stress of the tibia on the femur. The varus motion should be greater than the valgus motion.
   c. The physician moves his hand up to the proximal tibia, then induces a straight medial-lateral translatory slide of the tibia upon the femur (Fig. 21-13). The lateral translatory motion should be greater than the medial translatory motion.

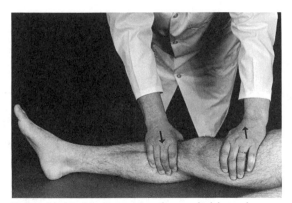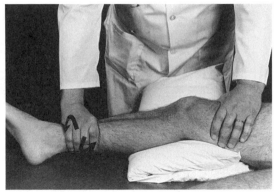

Figure 21-13. Motion testing for medial-lateral translatory slide dysfunctions.

Figure 21-14. Motion testing for internal and external rotation of the tibia on the femur.

ADDUCTION—TIBIA ON FEMUR

This is a condition of valgus stress of the tibia on the femur. It can be created by a blow to the lateral knee joint or by a twisting motion that produces medial ligamentous sprain. The medial joint structures are lax, the lateral knee joint approximates, and tibial motion on the femur is restricted in lateral translatory slide.

1. **Patient position:** supine, with the knee fully extended.
2. **Physician position:** standing on the side of the dysfunction, facing the patient.
3. **Technique:**
   All positions are as described above for abduction; however, the findings are reversed: valgus motion is greater than varus, and medial translatory motion is greater than lateral.

INTERNAL AND EXTERNAL ROTATION—TIBIA ON FEMUR

1. **Patient position:** supine. A pillow is placed under the knee to be examined to maintain slight flexion.
2. **Physician position:** standing on the side of the dysfunction, facing the table.
3. **Technique:**
   a. The physician's cephalic (with respect to the patient) hand grasps the patient's distal femur, holding it firmly and restricting its movement.
   b. With his other hand the physician grasps the patient's lower ankle and induces internal

and external rotary motion of the tibia on the femur (Fig. 21-14).
4. **Interpretation:**
   Increased internal rotation with restricted external rotation signifies internal rotation dysfunction; increased external rotation with restricted internal rotation signifies external rotation dysfunction.

ANTEROPOSTERIOR SLIDE DYSFUNCTION—TIBIA ON FEMUR

In this condition the tibia is restricted in anterior or posterior slide. This motion is coupled to knee flexion-extension. Movement of the tibia on the femur into extension is coupled with anterior slide. Movement of the tibia on the femur into flexion is coupled with posterior slide. The initial complaints or findings are restrictions of flexion or extension movements. The physician must look for these dysfunctions.

The technique described below is a modified drawer test.

1. **Patient position:** supine, with the dysfunctional knee flexed and the foot flat on the table.
2. **Physician position:** sitting on the patient's foot, anchoring it to the table.
3. **Technique:**
   a. The physician wraps both hands around the proximal tibia with his thumbs in front of the medial and lateral condyles and pressing on them. The physician's hand encircles the leg and grasps it firmly below the popliteal space.

b. The physician creates a direct anteroposterior translatory slide of the tibia on the femur by first pulling the tibia forward with both hands and then pushing it backward with both thumbs (Fig. 21-15).

   Note: In performing this test, the physician is not evaluating for cruciate ligamentous tears. The anteroposterior force used must be greatly reduced.

4. **Interpretation:**

   a. Increased anterior slide with decreased posterior slide signifies anterior slide dysfunction; increased posterior slide with decreased anterior slide signifies posterior slide dysfunction.

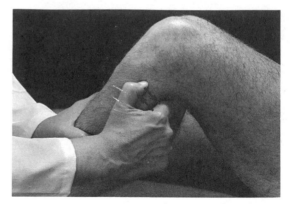

Figure 21-16. Motion testing for proximal fibular head dysfunctions.

PROXIMAL FIBULAR HEAD
DYSFUNCTION—FIBULA ON TIBIA

These dysfunctions are not anatomically part of the knee joint. However, the proximity of the fibular head to the knee joint and the overlapping symptom complexes warrant inclusion of these dysfunctions here. When evaluating or treating a fibular head dysfunction, the physician should completely examine the distal articulation as well as the ankle joint.

1. **Patient position:** supine, with the dysfunctional knee flexed and the foot flat on the table.

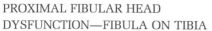

Figure 21-15. Motion testing for anteroposterior slide dysfunctions of the tibia on the femur.

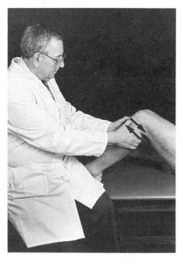

2. **Physician position:** sitting on the patient's foot.
3. **Technique:**

   a. The initial steps are as in the modified drawer test (see anteroposterior slide dysfunction).

   b. The physician grasps the head of the fibula with his thumb and index finger (Fig. 21-16).

   c. A firm anteroposterior slide motion of the fibular head on the tibia is created.

4. **Interpretation:**

   a. Increased anterior slide with decreased posterior slide signifies anterior fibular head dysfunction; increased posterior slide with decreased anterior slide signifies posterior fibular head dysfunction.

Treatment

Treatment of somatic dysfunctions of the knee begins with myofascial ligament-release techniques that encourage motion. The hip and ankle joints are included in the treatment. The somatic dysfunctions described in this chapter usually occur in combination. The techniques described below involve more than one joint or more than one dysfunction.

PASSIVE MYOFASCIAL
RELEASE—COMBINED HIP AND KNEE

This treatment combines myofascial release of the hip joint with increasing internal and external rotation of the tibia on the femur (previously described under hip joint).

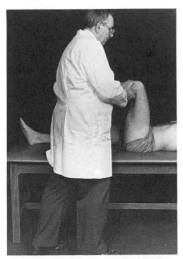

Figure 21-17. Treatment of the knee using flexion-extension with anteroposterior translatory slide.

FLEXION-EXTENSION WITH ANTEROPOSTERIOR TRANSLATORY SLIDE

1. **Patient position:** supine, the hip and knee on the side of the dysfunction flexed to 110 to 120 degrees.
2. **Physician position:** standing on the side of the dysfunction, facing the patient.
3. **Technique:**
   a. The patient's ankle is placed in the physician's axilla. The axillary grip must be firm enough that flexion-extension of the knee can be created by the to-and-fro rocking of the physician's body.
   b. The physician grasps the proximal end of the tibia with his thumbs on the anterior tibia and his fingers clasped behind the leg, below the popliteal space.
   c. The physician rocks forward, increasing knee flexion 5 to 10 degrees, and simultaneously pushes the tibia into posterior slide by the pressure of his thumbs (Fig. 21-17).
   d. The physician rocks backward, decreasing the flexion, and simultaneously pulls the tibia into anterior slide with his fingers.
   e. The to-and-fro rocking motion is repeated 3 to 4 times, increasing the anterior and posterior slide motions each time.

MYOFASCIAL RELEASE WITH TRACTION OF THE KNEE JOINT—INTERNAL AND EXTERNAL ROTATION

1. **Patient position:** supine. A pillow is placed under the knee to be treated, creating 10 to 15 degrees of flexion.
2. **Physician position:** sitting beside the table on the side of the dysfunction, facing the patient.
3. **Technique:**
   a. The patient's ankle and shin are placed in the physician's axilla and maintained in position by firm adduction of the physician's arm.
   b. The physician grasps that tibia at its proximal end, then translates the tibia on the femur anteriorly and applies traction by leaning back.
   c. The physician translates the tibia on the femur posteriorly and applies traction by leaning back.
   d. The physician rotates the tibia on the femur internally and applies traction by leaning back.
   e. The physician rotates the tibia on the femur externally and applies traction by leaning back (Fig. 21-18).
   f. The physician rests briefly, then repeats the set of maneuvers, increasing the rotation and slide motions but not the traction pull with each repetition.

KNEE AND ANKLE JOINT— LONG-AXIS EXTENSION

1. **Patient position:** supine, with the hip and knee on the side of the dysfunction in 90 degrees of flexion.
2. **Physician position:** standing beside the table on the side of the dysfunction, facing the foot of the table.
3. **Technique:**
   a. The physician places his flexed elbow (closer to the table) in the patient's popliteal space and grasps the calcaneus with that hand.
   b. With his other hand the physician grasps the anterior aspect of the patient's ankle at the talus. A small towel or pillow can be inserted between the physician's elbow and patient's popliteal space for comfort, or if the patient's leg is longer than the physician's forearm.
   c. As the physician rocks backward, his elbow should separate the femur from the tibia,

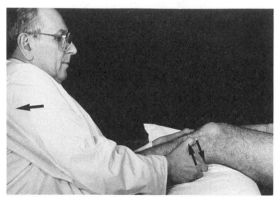

Figure 21-18. Myofascial release with traction of the knee joint used for internal and external rotation, anterior and posterior translatory slide.

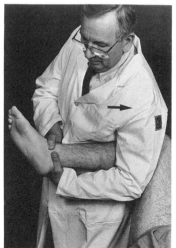

Figure 21-19. Treatment of the knee and ankle joints using long-axis extension.

while his hands on the calcaneus and talus should separate the talus from the crural arch (Fig. 21-19).

d. This position is held for 3 seconds; then the physician rocks forward to relax the traction force.

e. Rest and repeat.

Any of these techniques can be modified by introducing isometric resistance to create myofascial relaxation: for abduction, adduction, and internal or external rotation dysfunctions. The principle is the same in all cases. The joint is placed into its barrier to motion; then the patient actively attempts to reverse that motion against the isometric resistive force supplied by the physician.

Counterstrain Treatment

The locations of the tender points around the knee are shown in Figure 21-20.

ANTERIOR TENDER POINTS

The major anterior tender point is the patellar tender point, located just below the patella.

1. **Patient position:** supine.
2. **Physician position:** standing beside the table.
3. **Technique:**

a. A rolled pillow is placed beneath the patient's calf.
b. The knee is hyperextended by the physician pressing down on the anterior thigh just above the patella with a fair amount of force.
c. The foot is internally rotated (Fig. 21-21).

POSTERIOR TENDER POINTS

A. Anterior cruciate tender point
   1. **Patient position:** supine.
   2. **Physician position:** standing beside the table.
   3. **Technique:**
      a. A rolled pillow is placed under the thigh of the involved leg.
      b. The physician presses down on the lower leg just below the joint with a large amount of force (Fig. 21-22).
      c. This technique shortens the anterior cruciate ligaments.
B. Posterior cruciate tender point
   1. **Patient position:** supine.
   2. **Physician position:** standing beside the table.
   3. **Technique:**
      a. A rolled pillow is placed behind the knee below the joint.
      b. The physician presses down on the dorsum of the ankle with a large amount of force.
      c. The foot is internally rotated (Fig. 21-23).
      d. This maneuver shortens the posterior cruciate ligament.

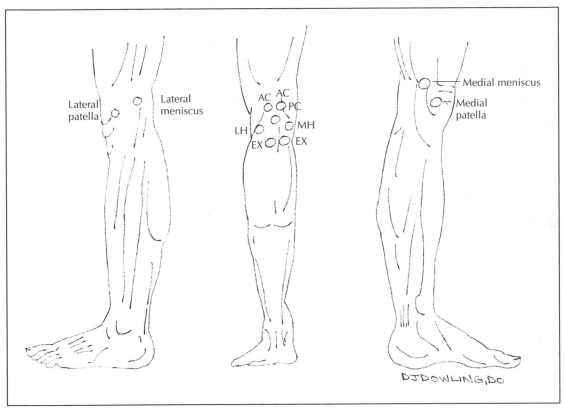

Figure 21-20. Location of the tender points around the knee. *PAT*, patellar; *LM*, lateral meniscus; *LH*, lateral hamstring; *MM*, medial meniscus; *MH*, medial hamstring; *EX*, gastrocnemius; *AC*, anterior cruciate; *PC*, posterior cruciate.

Figure 21-21. Counterstrain treatment of patellar tender point.

Figure 21-22. Counterstrain treatment for anterior cruciate tender point.

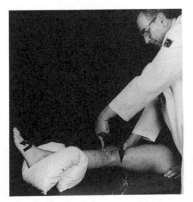

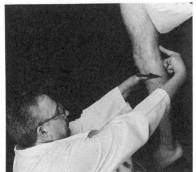

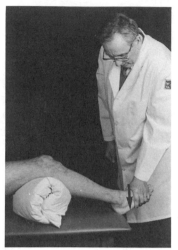

Figure 21-23. Counterstrain treatment for posterior cruciate tender point.

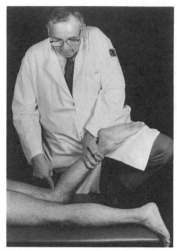

Figure 21-24. Counterstrain treatment for gastrocnemius tender point.

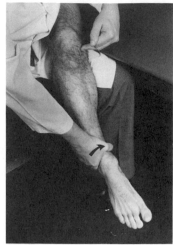

Figure 21-25. Counterstrain treatment for medial meniscus tender point.

C. Gastrocnemius tender points
   1. **Patient position:** prone.
   2. **Physician position:** standing beside the table with his foot on the table.
   3. **Technique:**
      a. The foot is hyperextended over the physician's knee by a downward force on the posterior ankle (Fig. 21-24).
      b. This maneuver shortens the gastrocnemius muscle.

MEDIAL TENDER POINTS
A. Medial meniscus tender point
   1. **Patient position:** supine, involved leg off the table.
   2. **Physician position:** seated beside the table.
   3. **Technique:**
      a. The physician grasps the patient's foot and internally rotates the lower leg, keeping the knee slightly flexed.
      b. The knee is adducted slightly against the edge of the table (Fig. 21-25).
B. Medial hamstring tender point
   1. **Patient position:** supine.
   2. **Physician position:** standing beside the table.
   3. **Technique:**
      a. The knee is flexed to about 60 degrees.
      b. The leg is externally rotated with a slight amount of adduction. This may be accomplished by grasping the patient's foot or ankle to use it as a lever.

LATERAL TENDER POINTS
A. Lateral meniscus tender point
   1. **Patient position:** supine, with the leg off the table.
   2. **Physician position:** seated beside the table.
   3. **Technique:**
      a. The leg is off the table with the knee slightly flexed.
      b. The physician grasps the patient's foot and internally rotates it (Fig. 21-26).
      c. The lower leg is slightly abducted.
      d. Occasionally external rotation may be needed.

Figure 21-26. Counterstrain treatment for lateral meniscus tender point.

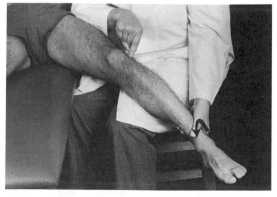

Figure 21-27. Counterstrain treatment for lateral hamstring tender point.

Figure 21-28. High-velocity, low-amplitude thrusting technique for an anterior fibular head somatic dysfunction.

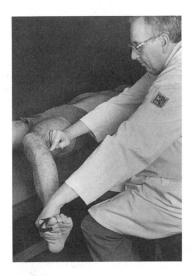

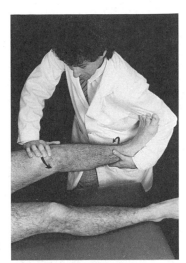

B. Lateral hamstring tender point
   1. **Patient position:** supine, with the leg off the table.
   2. **Physician position:** seated next to the table.
   3. **Technique:**
      a. The physician grasps the patient's foot and externally rotates it.
      b. The knee is flexed about 30 degrees and an abduction force is applied to the leg (Fig. 21-27).

High-Velocity, Low-Amplitude Thrusting Techniques

A. Anterior fibular head somatic dysfunction
   1. **Patient position:** supine.
   2. **Physician position:** standing beside the table, on the same side as the dysfunction.
   3. **Technique:**
      a. The physician grasps the patient's foot on the side of the somatic dysfunction with his nonthrusting hand.
      b. The physician places the thenar eminence of his thrusting hand over the superolateral aspect of the fibular head.
      c. The patient's knee is placed in the close-packed position, then mildly flexed.
      d. The physician exerts a rapid knee extension while simultaneously introducing a downward and medial thrust through the fibular head (Fig. 21-28).

   e. Slight internal rotation of the tibia facilitates the motion.
B. Posterior fibular head somatic dysfunction
   1. **Patient position:** supine.
   2. **Physician position:** standing beside the table, opposite the dysfunction.
   3. **Technique:**
      a. The physician grasps the patient's foot and ankle on the side of the dysfunction with his nonthrusting hand.
      b. The physician flexes the patient's hip and knee to 90 degrees.

Figure 21-29. High-velocity, low-amplitude thrusting technique for a posterior fibular head somatic dysfunction.

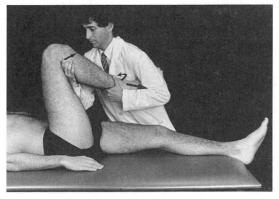

c. The physician places the index finger of his thrusting hand into the patient's popliteal crease, monitoring the dysfunctional fibular head.

d. The physician locks the patient's foot on the side of the dysfunction in his armpit.

e. The physician exerts a rapid downward thrust on the distal tibia and fibula while simultaneously pulling the fibular head anteriorly with his index finger (Fig. 21-29).

f. Slight external rotation of the tibia facilitates the motion.

THE FOOT AND ANKLE
Stanley Schiowitz

The walking foot is constantly adapting to terrain. Beyond the calcaneus, the tarsal, metatarsal, and phalanges act as stabilizers, rising, falling, twisting, and turning to accommodate to every change in the road or our style of movement. These motions in turn are transmitted through the calcaneus, talus, and ankle mortice. This articulation is a secondary balancing mechanism, allowing dorsiflexion and plantar flexion, rotation, abduction, and adduction at the ankle.

Unexpected or uncompensated stresses or strains of the foot will create dysfunctions. These can occur at the articulations of the foot or at the ankle joint. A diagnosis is based on loss of joint mobility and tissue changes. Because the foot and ankle are attached to the body, the physician must always search out secondary dysfunctions.

Diagnosis of Somatic Dysfunctions of the Foot and Ankle Joint

The ankle joint is commonly involved in eversion and inversion strains or sprains, as well as in malleolar fractures. A thorough history, physical examination, and ancillary studies should be done before treatment is instituted. Dysfunction often follows immobilization treatment procedures. People with healed fractures may still have unresolved somatic dysfunctions.

The clinician should first examine a healthy extremity and test its motions. The findings in a healthy extremity provide a standard for comparison with a dysfunctional extremity.

MOTION TESTING

A. Dorsiflexion and plantar flexion
   1. **Patient position:** supine, with the knee slightly flexed and supported by a pillow.
   2. **Physician position:** standing at the foot of the table, facing the patient.
   3. **Technique:**
      a. With one hand the physician grasps the anterior ankle, locking both malleoli.
      b. With the other hand he grasps the forefoot, close to but not on the talus.
      c. The physician inverts the forefoot and, maintaining this position, places the foot into dorsiflexion and then plantar flexion (Fig. 21-30).
      d. Note degrees and freedom of motions as compared with the other foot.

B. Abduction-adduction (subtalar)
   1. **Patient position:** supine, with the knee slightly flexed and supported by a pillow.
   2. **Physician position:** standing at the foot of the table, facing the patient.
   3. **Technique:**
      a. The physician grasps the forefoot and places it into abduction and adduction (Fig. 21-31).
      b. Note degrees and freedom of motions as compared to the other foot.

C. Calcaneal inversion-eversion
   1. **Patient position:** supine, with the knee slightly flexed and supported by a pillow.
   2. **Physician position:** standing at the foot of the table, facing the patient.

Figure 21-30. Motion testing for dorsiflexion and plantar flexion.

Figure 21-31. Motion testing for subtalar abduction-adduction.

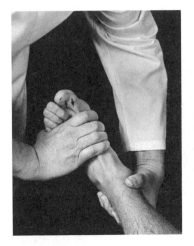
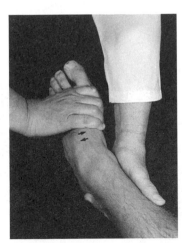

Figure 21-32. Motion testing for calcaneal inversion-eversion.

Figure 21-33. Motion testing for a cuboid dysfunction.

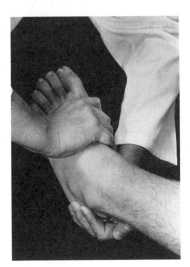
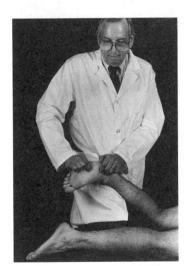

3. **Technique:**
  a. The physician grasps the calcaneus in one hand. His other hand is on the forefoot, locking the talus.
  b. The physician inverts and everts the calcaneus on the talus (Fig. 21-32).
  c. Note degrees and freedom of motions as compared to the other foot.
D. Cuboid dysfunction
  1. **Patient position:** prone.
  2. **Physician position:** standing beside the table, with one knee on the table.

3. **Technique:**
  a. The patient's knee is flexed, with the foot resting on the physician's knee.
  b. The physician grasps the calcaneus with one hand, locking it.
  c. With the thumb and index finger of the other hand, the physician grasps the cuboid and moves it dorsally and ventrally (Fig. 21-33).
  d. Note degrees and freedom of motion as compared to the other foot.
E. Fifth metatarsal dysfunction

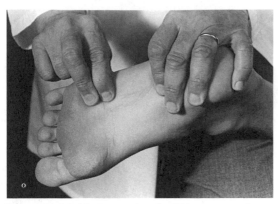

Figure 21-34. Motion testing for fifth metatarsal dysfunction.

1. **Patient position:** prone.
2. **Physician position:** standing beside the table, with one knee on the table.
3. **Technique:**
   a. The physician grasps the cuboid with one hand, locking it.
   b. With his other hand he grasps the fifth metatarsal and moves it dorsally and ventrally (Fig. 21-34).
   c. To examine rotary motion of the metatarsal, the physician locks the fourth metatarsal and examines motion of the fifth. To examine motion of the fourth metatarsal, he locks the third metatarsal.
   d. Note degrees and freedom of motions as compared to the other foot.
F. Navicular dysfunction
   1. **Patient position:** supine.
   2. **Physician position:** seated at the foot of the table with his back to the patient. The foot to be examined lies on a pillow on his lap.
   3. **Technique:**
      a. The physician grasps the foot, including and locking the talus with one hand.
      b. With his other hand he grasps the navicular and moves it dorsally and ventrally (Fig. 21-35).
      c. Note degrees and freedom of motions as compared to the other foot.
G. Cuneiform dysfunction
   1. **Patient position:** supine.
   2. **Physician position:** seated at the foot of the table with his back to the patient. The foot to be examined lies on a pillow on his lap.

3. **Technique:**
   a. The physician grasps and locks the navicular.
   b. The physician moves the cuneiform on the navicular.
H. First metatarsal dysfunction
   1. **Patient position:** supine.
   2. **Physician position:** seated at the foot of the table with his back to the patient. The foot to be examined lies on a pillow on his lap.
   3. **Technique:**
      a. The physician grasps and locks the first cuneiform.
      b. He grasps the first metatarsal and moves it dorsally and ventrally.
      c. To examine for rotary motion of the metatarsals, the physician locks the second metatarsal to evaluate the first, and locks the third to evaluate the second.
      d. Note degrees and freedom of motions as compared to the other foot.
I. Phalangeal dysfunction
   1. **Patient position:** supine.
   2. **Physician position:** seated at the foot of the table with his back to the patient. The foot to be examined lies on a pillow on his lap.
   3. **Technique:**
      a. The physician grasps the metatarsal and locks it with one hand.
      b. With his other hand he grasps the first phalanx articulating with that metatarsal.
      c. After applying slight traction, the physician evaluates dorsal, ventral, abduction, adduction, and rotary motions (Fig. 21-36).
      d. Note degrees and freedom of motions as compared to the other foot.

TREATMENT
A. Knee and ankle joint, long-axis extension
   1. **Patient position:** supine.
   2. **Physician position:** standing with his back to the patient.
   3. **Technique:**
      a. With the caudal (relative to the patient) hand the physician firmly grasps the forefoot and talus. With his other hand he holds the calcaneus.
      b. The physician's elbow maintains long-axis extension, with pressure at the popliteal region.

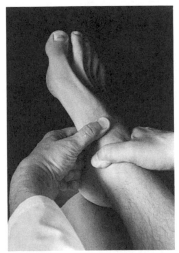

Figure 21-35. Motion testing for navicular dysfunction.

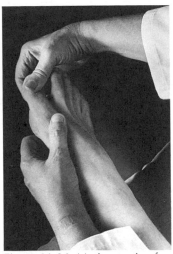

Figure 21-36. Motion testing for phalangeal dysfunction.

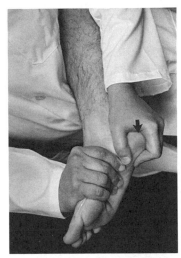

Figure 21-37. Modified hand position for knee and ankle joint long-axis extension, used for treatment.

c. The physician places the foot into corrective flexion-extension and abduction-adduction motions (Fig. 21-37).

d. Maintaining the above position, the physician uses his cephalic hand to create calcaneal inversion and eversion.

B. Myofascial and joint motion—passive release

1. **Patient position:** supine.

2. **Physician position:** standing at the foot of the table.

3. **Technique:** The physician applies mild traction force, then places the joint into the corrective motion direction.

   Note: This technique is applicable to all the joints examined as described in the first section of this chapter.

Counterstrain Treatment

The locations of the tender points on the lateral and medial aspects of the ankle and the dorsum of the foot are shown in Figure 21-38. There is also a tender point on the sole of the foot at the anterior end of the calcaneus.

A. Calcaneal tender point

1. **Patient position:** prone.

2. **Physician position:** standing, with one foot on the table.

3. **Technique:**

   a. The patient's foot rests on the physician's knee.

   b. The foot is plantar-flexed against the physician's knee (Fig. 21-39).

   c. The physician grasps behind the heel and pushes toward the toes.

B. Dorsal metatarsal tender points

1. **Patient position:** prone, with the knee flexed to 90 degrees.

2. **Physician position:** standing beside the table.

3. **Technique:**

   a. The physician strongly dorsiflexes the foot by placing a downward pressure on it (Fig. 21-40).

C. Medial ankle tender point

1. **Patient position:** lying on his side, with the involved leg up.

2. **Physician position:** seated beside the table.

3. **Technique:**

   a. The patient's foot is brought off the table.

   b. A rolled towel is placed under the anterior ankle.

   c. The physician inverts the foot by pressing forcefully on the lateral side of the foot (Fig. 21-41).

Figure 21-38. Locations of
foot and ankle tender points.
DM, dorsal metatarsal; *MA*,
medial ankle; *LA*, lateral
ankle; *TAL*, talus; *DC*, dorsal
cuboid; *NA*, navicular; *LC*,
lateral calcaneal.

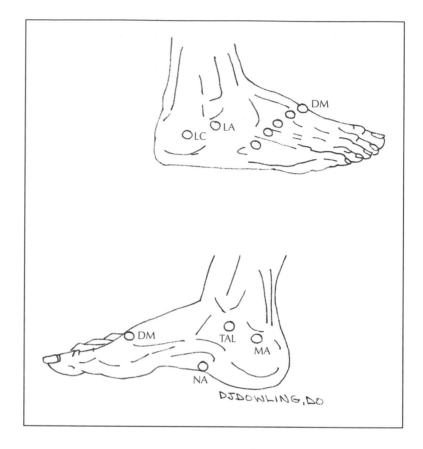

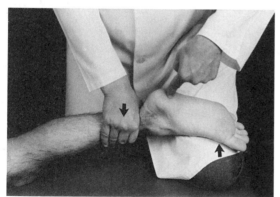

Figure 21-39. Counterstrain treatment of calcaneal
tender point.

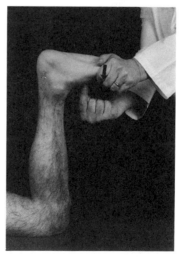

Figure 21-40. Counterstrain treatment for dorsal
metatarsal tender point.

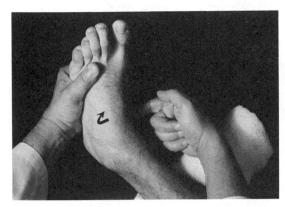

Figure 21-41. Counterstrain treatment for medial ankle tender point.

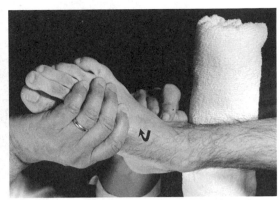

Figure 21-42. Counterstrain treatment for lateral ankle tender point.

D. Lateral ankle tender point

This technique is the same as for the medial ankle tender point except that the ankle is forcefully everted (Fig. 21-42).

E. Talar tender point

This tender point is on the anteromedial ankle deep to the talus.

1. **Patient position:** prone, with the foot up.
2. **Physician position:** seated at the foot of the table.
3. **Technique:**
   a. The foot is dorsiflexed, inverted, and internally rotated (Fig. 21-43).

F. Dorsal cuboid tender point

1. **Patient position:** prone.

2. **Physician position:** standing beside the table.
3. **Technique:**
   a. The physician grasps the patient's foot and inverts it by applying pressure on the lateral side (Fig. 21-44).

G. Navicular tender point

1. **Patient position:** prone.
2. **Physician position:** seated or standing beside the table.
3. **Technique:**
   a. The physician places his thumb or two fingers over the navicular bone to cause an inversion of the navicular.
   b. A slight amount of flexion is added (Fig. 21-45).

Figure 21-43. Counterstrain treatment for talus tender point.

Figure 21-44. Counterstrain treatment of dorsal cuboid tender point.

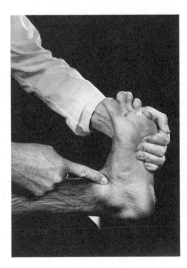

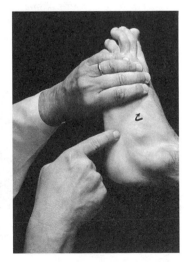

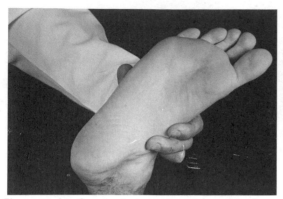

Figure 21-45. Counterstrain treatment for navicular tender point.

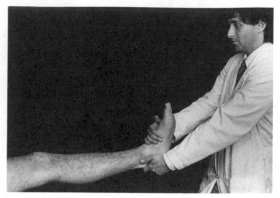

Figure 21-46. High-velocity, low-amplitude thrusting technique for an eversion-inversion somatic dysfunction.

High-Velocity, Low-Amplitude Thrusting Techniques

A. Eversion-inversion somatic dysfunction of the ankle
   1. **Patient position:** supine.
   2. **Physician position:** standing at the foot of the table.
   3. **Technique:**
      a. The physician grasps the patient's foot on the side of the dysfunction, placing one hand on the dorsal midtarsal region and using the other to grasp the calcaneus.
      b. The physician applies traction to the patient's leg (Fig. 21-46).
      c. If an inversion somatic dysfunction (i.e., eversion restriction) is present, the physician exerts rapid traction caudad through the calcaneus with simultaneous hyper-eversion of the ankle.
      d. If an eversion somatic dysfunction (i.e., inversion restriction) is present, the physician exerts traction through the calcaneus while simultaneously hyperinverting the ankle.
B. Tibiocalcaneal somatic dysfunction
   1. **Patient position:** supine.
   2. **Physician position:** standing beside the table on the side of the somatic dysfunction.
   3. **Technique:**
      a. The physician cups the patient's tibia and fibula with one hand and places the thenar

eminence of the other hand over the dorsum of the patient's forefoot.
      b. The physician applies traction cephalad on the patient's leg, through the tibia/fibula.
      c. The physician exerts traction and a rapid posterior thrust through the hand on the patient's forefoot. The physician's other hand stabilizes the ankle joint (Fig. 21-47).
C. Metatarsal somatic dysfunction
   1. **Patient position:** supine.
   2. **Physician position:** standing beside the table on the side of the somatic dysfunction.
   3. **Technique:**
      a. The physician grasps the patient's involved foot and places the pads of his thumbs, facing one another, over the junction of the metatarsal somatic dysfunction.
      b. The physician exerts a downward thrust through the thumbs, separating the joint articulation (Fig. 21-48).
D. Transtarsal somatic dysfunction
   1. **Patient position:** supine.
   2. **Physician position:** standing beside the table on the side of the somatic dysfunction.
   3. **Technique:**
      a. The physician places the patient's knee in flexion, abduction, and external rotation.
      b. The physician places the thenar eminence of one hand over the calcaneus; the other hand is placed over the first metatarsal and talus.

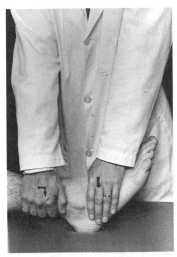

Figure 21-47. High-velocity, low-amplitude thrusting technique for tibiocalcaneal somatic dysfunction.

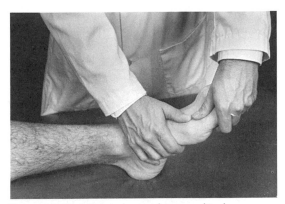

Figure 21-48. High-velocity, low-amplitude thrusting technique for metatarsal somatic dysfunction.

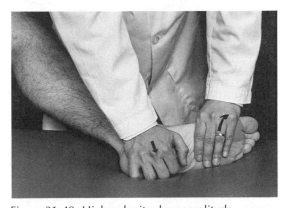

Figure 21-49. High-velocity, low-amplitude thrusting technique for transtarsal somatic dysfunction.

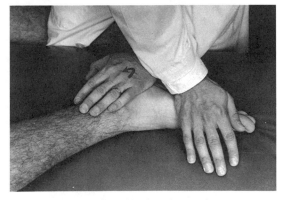

Figure 21-50. Modified high-velocity, low-amplitude thrusting technique for transtarsal somatic dysfunction.

      c. The physician exerts a counterclockwise rotary thrust with the hand holding the talus while simultaneously exerting a downward thrust through the calcaneus with the other hand (Fig. 21-49).

E. Modified technique for transtarsal somatic dysfunction
  1. **Patient position:** supine and in FABERE position.
  2. **Physician position:** standing beside the table.
  3. **Technique:**
    a. The physician exerts a simultaneous downward, lateral, and rotary thrust with the hand over the calcaneus. His other hand stabilizes the foot (Fig. 21-50).

F. Cuboid-navicular somatic dysfunction
  1. **Patient position:** prone.
  2. **Physician position:** standing beside the table on the side of the dysfunction.
  3. **Technique:**
    a. The physician flexes the patient's hip and knee on the dysfunctional side, then drops the leg off the side of the table.
    b. The physician grasps the patient's foot with both hands and places his thumbs in a V shape over the plantar surface of the cuboid or navicular.

c. The physician exerts a downward thrust through his thumbs while simultaneously inducing a whiplike action at the patient's ankle and knee (Fig. 21-51).

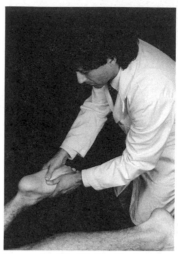

Figure 21-51. High-velocity, low-amplitude thrusting technique for a cuboid-navicular somatic dysfunction.

EXERCISE THERAPY FOR THE LOWER EXTREMITY
Stanley Schiowitz
Albert R. DeRubertis

The Hip

Related exercises are described in Chapter 11 (Treatment of the Lumbar Spine—Exercise Therapy). The clinician should review these exercises when prescribing exercise therapy for the hip.

MUSCLE STRETCH
A. Groin muscle stretch (Fig. 21-52)
  1. **Patient position:** standing, facing a firm support such as a table.
  2. **Instructions:**
    a. Place the sole of the foot of the leg to be treated on the edge of the table (the left foot is used as an example). The other foot remains on the floor, fully extended, with the toes pointing toward the table.
    b. Flex your left hip and knee as you lean your body toward the table. Continue leaning until you have achieved maximum painless stretch of the left groin muscles.
    c. Hold this position for 5 to 15 seconds.
    d. Straighten out the left leg. Relax, rest, and repeat.

    e. The stretch should affect the muscles of the medial, anterior, and posterior groin. To stretch the right groin, repeat the exercise with your right foot on the table.
B. Groin muscle stretch (Fig. 21-53)
  1. **Patient position:** standing, facing a firm support such as a table.
  2. **Instructions:**
    a. Place the sole of the foot of the nondysfunctional leg on the edge of the table (the left leg is used as an example). The right leg is fully extended with the foot on the floor and parallel to the table.
    b. Flex your left hip and knee as you lean your body toward the table. Continue leaning until you have achieved maximum painless stretch of the right medial groin muscles.
    c. Hold this position for 5 to 15 seconds.
    d. Straighten out the left leg. Relax, rest, and repeat.
    e. To stretch the left groin, repeat the exercise with your right foot on the table.

Figure 21-52. Groin muscle stretch.

Figure 21-53. Groin muscle stretch.

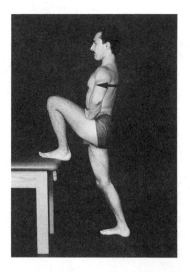 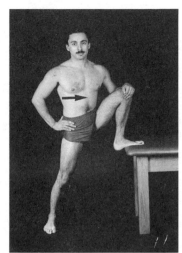

C. Bilateral groin muscle stretch (Fig. 21-54)
   1. **Patient position:** seated on the floor, with the hips and knees flexed and the soles of the feet resting against each other. The hands hold the toes or ankles.
   2. **Instructions:**
      a. Pull your body forward, bending from the hips, while keeping your back flat to avoid strain. Create a groin stretch.
      b. Place your elbows forward and resting on your legs. Lean on your elbows to push your thighs toward the floor.
      c. Hold a position of maximum painless stretch for 5 to 15 seconds.
      d. Relax, rest, and repeat.

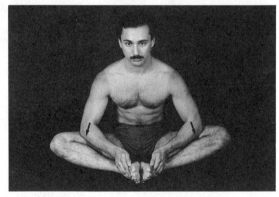

Figure 21-54. Bilateral groin muscle stretch.

MUSCLE STRENGTHENING
A. Hip flexors (Fig. 21-55)
   1. **Patient position:** standing, holding on to a firm support that is behind the patient; or seated with the legs dangling off a high table. A 3- to 5-pound weight is attached to the ankle of the leg to be exercised.
   2. **Instructions:**
      a. Slowly flex your knee and hip to 90 degrees.
      b. Hold this position for 5 to 15 seconds.
      c. Lower foot slowly to the floor.
      d. Relax, rest, and repeat.
B. Hip extensors (Fig. 21-56)
   1. **Patient position:** standing, holding on to a firm support with the hand opposite the leg

to be exercised; or prone. A 3- to 5-pound weight is attached to the ankle.
   2. **Instructions:**
      a. Move your fully extended leg backward, keeping your low back flat.
      b. Hold this position for 5 to 15 seconds.
      c. Slowly return to the starting position.
      d. Relax, rest, and repeat.
C. Hip abductors (Fig. 21-57)
   1. **Patient position:** standing, holding on to a firm support with hand opposite the leg to be exercised; or lying on the side. A 3- to 5-pound weight is attached to the ankle.
   2. **Instructions:**
      a. Move the leg to be exercised directly sideways, fully extended, away from the midline of the body.

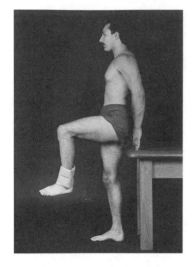

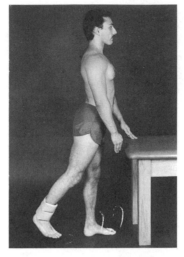

Figure 21-55. Hip flexor strengthening.

Figure 21-56. Hip extensor strengthening.

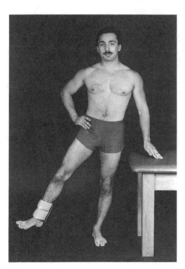

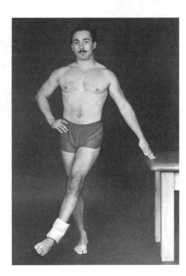

Figure 21-57. Hip abductor strengthening.

Figure 21-58. Hip adductor strengthening.

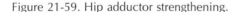

Figure 21-59. Hip adductor strengthening.

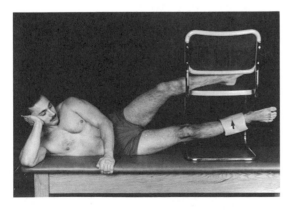

b. Hold this position for 5 to 15 seconds.
c. Slowly return to the starting position.
d. Relax, rest, and repeat.

D. Hip abductors (Fig. 21-58)
   1. **Patient position:** standing, holding on to a firm support with the hand on the same side as the leg to be exercised. A 3- to 5-pound weight is attached to the ankle.
   2. **Instructions:**
      a. Extend the leg to be exercised and move it in front of the other leg and across the midline of the body.
      b. Hold this position for 5 to 15 seconds.

Figure 21-60. Quadriceps stretch.

Figure 21-61. Knee flexor strengthening.

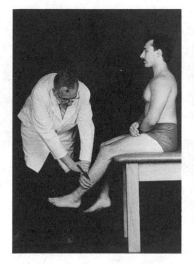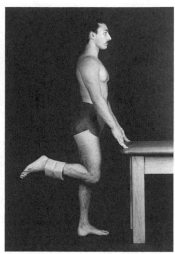

c. Slowly return to the starting position.
d. Relax, rest, and repeat.

E. Hip abductors (Fig. 21-59)

1. **Patient position:** lying on the side to be exercised. The upper leg rests on a box or a chair, 8 to 10 inches above the floor. A 3- to 5-pound weight is attached to the ankle.

2. **Instructions:**
   a. Raise the leg to be exercised off the floor toward the other leg. Keep the leg fully extended.
   b. Hold for 5 to 15 seconds.
   c. Slowly return to the starting position.
   d. Relax, rest, and repeat.

The Knee

MUSCLE STRETCH

A. Quadriceps (Fig. 21-60)

1. **Patient position:** seated on a table with the hips and knees bent. The knee with contracted quadriceps will not fully flex to 90 degrees.

2. **Instructions:**
   a. Place increasingly heavier weights on the ankle, forcing the knee into flexion and quadriceps stretch. Or,
   b. Have someone push down on your leg slowly, creating quadriceps stretch.
   c. Hold for 5 to 15 seconds. Return to the starting position.
   d. Relax, rest, and repeat.

MUSCLE STRENGTHENING

A. Knee flexors (Fig. 21-61)

1. **Patient position:** standing, holding on to a support in front of the body. A 3- to 5-pound weight is attached to the ankle.

2. **Instructions:**
   a. Flex your knee as far as it will go. Keep your back straight.
   b. Lower your leg, slowly straightening out your knee. Count slowly to ten as you lower the foot to the floor.
   c. Relax, rest and repeat.

B. Knee flexors—prone position (Fig. 21-62)

1. **Patient position:** prone, with a 3- to 5-pound weight attached to the ankle.

2. **Instructions:**

Figure 21-62. Knee flexor strengthening.

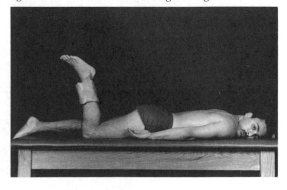

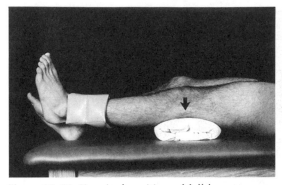

Figure 21-63. Terminal position of full knee extension.

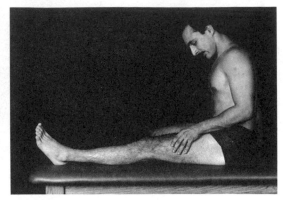

Figure 21-64. Isometric quadriceps contraction.

a. Bend your knee to 90 degrees.
b. Very slowly lower that leg down into full extension.
c. Relax, rest and repeat.

C. Terminal position of full knee extension (Fig. 21-63)
1. **Patient position:** seated on the floor or a table. A rolled towel or pillow is placed under the knee to be exercised (about 6 inches high). A 3- to 5-pound weight is attached to the ankle.
2. **Instructions:**
a. Push your knee down against the pillow, toward the floor, so that the weighted ankle comes off the table as the knee straightens out. Concentrate on pushing

the knee down; do not try to extend the knee.
b. Hold this position for 5 to 15 seconds.
c. Slowly lower the weight to the table.
d. Relax, rest, and repeat.

D. Isometric quadriceps contraction (Fig. 21-64)
1. **Patient position:** seated, with one hand on the quadriceps muscle on the side to be treated.
2. **Instructions:**
a. Without moving your leg, try to contract the muscle you are touching so that the kneecap moves upward toward your hand.
b. If the exercise is performed correctly, you will see the kneecap move and feel the muscle tighten.

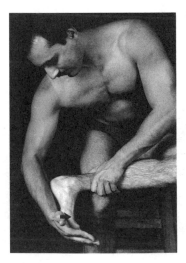

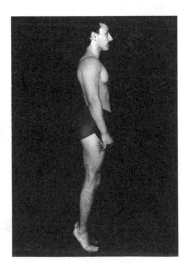

Figure 21-65. Passive foot and ankle stretch.

Figure 21-66. Heel raising to strengthen the gastrocnemius and stretch dorsiflexors.

Figure 21-67. Toe raising to strengthen dorsiflexors and stretch the gastrocnemius.

Figure 21-68. Toe stretch to stretch the arch and strengthen the peroneus longus.

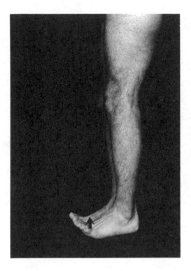
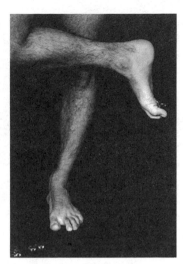

The Foot and Ankle

STRETCH

A. Passive foot and ankle stretch (Fig. 21-65)
   1. **Patient position:** sitting, holding the foot to be stretched with one hand above the ankle and the other hand on the forefoot.
   2. **Instructions:**
      a. Push your forefoot down. Hold for 3 seconds. Relax.
      b. Push your forefoot up. Hold for 3 seconds. Relax.
      c. Push your forefoot in. Hold for 3 seconds. Relax.
      d. Push your forefoot out. Hold for 3 seconds. Relax.
      e. Rotate your forefoot in a clockwise and then counterclockwise direction, four times each way. Relax.
      f. Rest and repeat the entire exercise.

STRETCH–STRENGTHENING

A. Heel raising (Fig. 21-66)
   1. **Patient position:** standing with both feet flat on floor, 6 to 8 inches apart.
   2. **Instructions:**
      a. Rise up on your toes. Hold on to something for balance, if necessary.
      b. Maintain this position for 5 to 15 seconds.
      c. Return to the starting position.
      d. Relax, rest, and repeat.
B. Toe walking
   1. Toe walking is performed in the same posi-

tion as the heel-raising exercise. Walk forward on the toes for ten steps.
C. Toe raising (Fig. 21-67)
   1. **Patient position:** standing, with both feet flat on floor and 6 to 8 inches apart.
   2. **Instructions:**
      a. Lean back on your heels.
      b. Maintain this position for 5 to 15 seconds.
      c. Return to the starting position.
      d. Relax, rest, and repeat.
D. Heel walking
   1. With the weight on the heels and the toes off the ground, walk backward on your heels for ten steps.
E. Picking up marbles (Fig. 21-68)
   1. **Patient position:** standing near support. Marbles are placed on the floor within reach of the foot to be exercised.
   2. **Instructions:**
      a. Pick up one marble with your toes.
      b. Lift this foot off the floor, cross it in front of the other leg, and release the marble into a container placed 6 to 8 inches off the floor to the side of your stationary leg.
      c. In this manner pick up all the marbles on the floor, one at a time.
F. Toe stretch (Fig. 21-69)
   1. **Patient position:** seated, with both feet resting flat on a book resting firmly on the floor.
   2. **Instructions:**
      a. Lift up your toes only. Hold for 3 seconds. Relax.

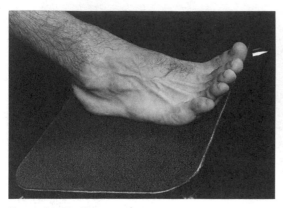

Figure 21-69. Toe stretch.

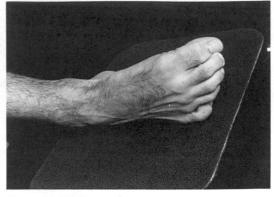

Figure 21-70. Toe curl.

b. Put your toes over the edge of the platform and push them down. Hold for 3 seconds. Relax.

c. Spread the toes far apart. Hold for 3 seconds. Bring them firmly together.

d. Curl your toes down as you bring your foot facing inward. Place your weight on the outer surface of your feet (Fig. 21-70). Hold for 3 seconds. Relax.

e. Place one foot forward and resting on its heel, with the foot and toes pointing up. Press down on that heel as you turn your foot in clockwise and counterclockwise circles. Your big toe should make complete circles. Repeat three times.

f. Relax, rest, and repeat the entire exercise.

22

The Temporo-mandibular Joint

ANATOMY AND BIOMECHANICS
Donald E. Phykitt

The temporomandibular joint (TMJ) is a synovial joint formed by the articulation of the condyle of the mandible with the mandibular (glenoid) fossa and the articular tubercle of the temporal bone. The joint is divided into superior and inferior compartments by a fibrocartilaginous disk. The major motions of the TMJ are depression of the mandible (opening the mouth) and elevation of the mandible (closing the mouth). These motions are achieved by rotation of the condyle in the mandibular fossa, accompanied by anterior or posterior glide on the articular tubercle, respectively. Furthermore, the joint allows protraction, retraction, and side-to-side glide of the mandible.

Anatomy
The mandibular fossa is an oval depression in the temporal bone just anterior to the external auditory meatus. It is bounded anteriorly by the articular tubercle, laterally by the zygomatic process, and posteriorly by the tympanic plate. The close proximity of the mandibular fossa to the external auditory meatus allows fingers placed in the meatus of each ear to palpate condylar motion as it rotates and glides in the fossa. Occasionally, a small ridge of bone (the postglenoid tubercle)

forms a prominence at the posterior border of the fossa.

The shape of the mandibular fossa does not exactly conform to the mandibular condyle. The articular disk molds the two surfaces together.

The mandibular condyle varies considerably in size and shape. The anteroposterior dimension of the condyle is approximately half the transverse dimension. The long axis of the condyle faces slightly posteriorly to the frontal plane and slightly medially.

The articular surfaces of the condyle are at its anterior and superior surfaces. These surfaces are convex. The posterior surface is broad and flat.

The articular disk is fibrous and is molded to the bony surfaces. It is variable in thickness, being thinnest centrally. Its margins merge with the joint capsule. The disk is more firmly attached to the mandible than to the temporal bone. Therefore, when the head of the mandible glides anteriorly on the articular tubercle (as when opening the mouth), the articular disk slides anteriorly against the tubercle.

The fibrous capsule of the TMJ is loose. It is attached to the margins of the articular area on the temporal bone and to the neck of the mandible. It is thickened laterally to form the temporomandib-

An Osteopathic Approach to Diagnosis and Treatment, second edition
Eileen L. DiGiovanna and Stanley Schiowitz
Lippincott–Raven Publishers, Philadelphia © 1997.

ular ligament. This is a triangular ligament whose base attaches to the zygomatic process and the articular tubercle. Its apex is fixed to the lateral aspect of the neck of the mandible. The accessory ligaments of the TMJ are the stylomandibular, sphenomandibular, and pterygomandibular ligaments; none has any significant effect on joint movement.

The innervation of the joint is mainly supplied by the auriculotemporal branch of the mandibular division of the trigeminal nerve. Additional fibers are supplied by the masseteric branch of the mandibular nerve. The vascular supply is derived from the superficial artery and the deep auricular branch of the maxillary artery.

Movements of the TMJ result chiefly from the actions of the muscles of mastication—the temporalis, masseter, medial pterygoid, and lateral pterygoid muscles. The various movements of the TMJ result from the cooperative activity of several muscles, either bilaterally or unilaterally.

1. **Temporalis:** Extensive fan-shaped muscle covering the temporal region.
   Origin: Temporal fossa and temporal fascia.
   Insertion: Coronoid process and anterior border of the ramus of the mandible.
   Actions: Elevates the mandible (closes the mouth) and retracts the mandible after closure.
2. **Masseter:** A quadrangular muscle that covers the coronoid process and ramus of the mandible. It is easily palpated at the cheek when the teeth are clenched.
   Origin: Inferior margin and deep surface of the zygomatic arch.
   Insertion: Lateral surface of the ramus and corocoid process of the mandible.
   Actions: Elevates the mandible, clenches the teeth, and aids in protraction of the mandible.
3. **Lateral pterygoid:** A short, thick muscle with two heads of origin.
   Origin: Superior head—infratemporal surface of the greater wing of the sphenoid; inferior head—lateral surface of the lateral pterygoid plate.
   Insertion: Neck of mandible and the articular disk.
   Actions: When contracted bilaterally, the lateral pterygoid muscles protract and depress the mandible. When contracted unilaterally they

produce contralateral lateral glide of the mandible.
4. **Medial pterygoid:** A thick quadralateral muscle located deep to the ramus of the mandible: it embraces the inferior head of the lateral pterygoid muscle.
   Origin: Deep head—medial surface of lateral pterygoid plate; superficial head—tuberosity of the maxilla.
   Insertion: Medial surface of mandible, near its angle.
   Actions: Contracting bilaterally, it assists in elevating and protracting the mandible; contracting unilaterally, it produces contralateral lateral glide of the mandible.

Biomechanics

Mandibular movements may be classified as bilaterally symmetric or bilaterally asymmetric. Because the mandible is a single bone with two joints, movement through one joint cannot occur without a similar coordinating or dissimilar reactive movement in the other joint. Depression, elevation, protraction, and retraction of the mandible are bilaterally symmetric motions since they require similar motions in both joints. Lateral excursions (side-to-side movements) are bilaterally asymmetric, since there are dissimilar movements of the joints.

Depression. Hingelike rotation of the mandibular condyle is accompanied by simultaneous anterior glide of the condyles and articular disks on the articular tubercles. This is mainly produced by the lateral pterygoid muscles. Some assistance is gained from the suprahyoid and infrahyoid muscles. The axis of rotation is through the head of the mandible; the axis of glide is through the mandibular foramen.

Elevation. Elevation is the opposite of depression. The motion is achieved mainly through the actions of the temporalis and medial pterygoid muscles, with assistance from the anterior fibers of the masseter.

Protraction (protrusion). This motion involves anterior glide of both condyles and articular disks along the articular tubercles. It is achieved through bilateral contraction of the medial and lateral pterygoid muscles.

Retraction. This movement is opposite to that of protraction. It is produced by bilateral contraction of the horizontal fibers of the masseter muscles.

Lateral excursion. This movement involves lateral glide of the ipsilateral mandibular condyle, accompanied by slight medial rotation of the contralateral condyle about the medial, shifting axis. It is achieved by unilateral contraction of the contralateral medial and lateral pterygoid muscles.

EVALUATION AND TREATMENT OF TMJ DYSFUNCTION
Mary-Theresa Ferris
Eileen L. DiGiovanna

Temporomandibular joint (TMJ) dysfunction affects approximately 20% of the American population, with a 3:1 female-male preponderance. Pain associated with the temporomandibular joint was first described in the 1830s. The first treatment was an ostectomy.

The etiology of TMJ dysfunction appears to be a combination of various factors, including malocclusion, trauma, psychological or emotional status, the neuromuscular apparatus, and the general health of a patient. Internal derangement is another etiologic factor, described as an abnormal relationship of the articular disk to the mandibular condyle, fossa, and articular eminence. Included in this category are perforation, fragmentation, and displacement of the disk.

Dental procedures such as forceful extractions can be considered traumatic, and bruxism (teeth grinding) is seen as repeated microtrauma to the TMJ. Muscular imbalance is another etiologic factor that may be a cause of or may be caused by malocclusion. Malocclusion may occur with the loss of a single tooth or several teeth, improper alignment of dentures, and other factors.

Signs and Symptoms
The most common signs of TMJ dysfunction are clicking or popping sounds in the joint, preauricular pain, limited jaw movements, and tenderness on palpation. Additional frequently encountered symptoms include jaw, ear, and facial pain, headache, masticatory muscle pain, fatigue, and tightness. Although not as common, the following symptoms have also been reported: swallowing difficulties, tinnitus, backache, mouth dryness, nervousness, sleep disorders, snoring, loss of balance, and mental disorders.

Evaluation
HISTORY
A thorough history is extremely important and must include trauma (not just to the head and neck), dental work, gum chewing, clenching or grinding of teeth, stress, psychological makeup, and postural habits. The TMJ stressor may be present for a long time before it manifests itself as a symptom.

PHYSICAL EXAMINATION
The entire person must be taken into consideration when approaching the physical examination. A complete physical must be performed and any possible organic causes ruled out. Muscle spasms, scoliosis, leg length discrepancies, arches of the feet, craniosacral motion, and somatic dysfunctions must be evaluated.

Examination of the TMJ should include the following:

1. Observation of facial symmetry or asymmetry.
2. Observation of a midline deviation of the mandible and palpation of the TMJ during opening and closing of the mouth.
3. Measurement of the jaw opening. The average adult opening is 40 mm.
4. Assessment of joint noises—when a click occurs with mandibular opening.
5. Palpation of the joint and surrounding areas for bony abnormalities and tenderness.

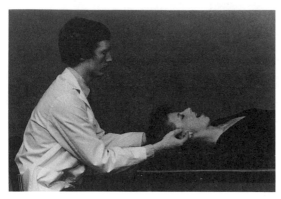

Figure 22-1. Evaluating TMJ function by observing tracking while palpating the joint through the auditory meatus.

6. Assessment of musculature—spasms, imbalance, etc.
7. Evaluation of craniosacral motion, especially the temporal bones.
8. Palpation of the TMJ through the external auditory meatus, noting tenderness or deviation with motion.

A dental examination is also essential for a complete evaluation of a TMJ dysfunction.

To evaluate joint motion, the examiner places one finger in the meatus of each ear and palpates the joint as the patient opens and closes the mouth. The physician observes the quality of motion, any asymmetry, and the presence of clicking or grinding of the joint (palpable or audible) (Fig. 22-1).

The cervical spine needs to be evaluated because it is fairly common to find dysfunctions of the occipitoatlantal joint, C2, and C3.

TMJ IMAGING
TMJ imaging may also be employed in the diagnostic evaluation.

1. **X-ray or tomograph.** This provides information on symmetry, bony positioning, and degenerative changes.
2. **Magnetic resonance imaging.** This is the procedure of choice for internal derangements. It will demonstrate bony detail as well as soft tissues in both anatomic and semifunctional relationships in all planes.

Treatment

The treatment of TMJ dysfunction has three components:

1. Identifying and eliminating any treatable cause
2. Osteopathic manipulative treatment
3. Prescribing an exercise regimen for the patient to use at home

Conservative treatment following the above guidelines should be used before any consideration of surgical intervention.

Interocclusal stabilization devices, also known as splints or appliances, may be helpful. There are two types of these devices, the first of which attempts to reposition the malocclusion. Repositioning is accomplished over several months and involves frequent readjustments as the muscles relax and the mandible shifts. The second type of occlusal device does not change the natural occlusion. This type is fitted to allow the muscles of mastication to function at their proper length and to decrease the spasticity of these muscles, which in turn will help decrease myofascial pain.

OSTEOPATHIC MANIPULATIVE TECHNIQUES
Persons with TMJ dysfunction may benefit greatly from one or more of the manipulative techniques described below.

Muscle Energy Techniques
Muscle energy techniques are designed to treat and relax the various muscles of mastication—those that open and close the jaw, and those that move it from side to side.

1. **Patient position:** supine.
2. **Physician position:** seated at the head of the table.
3. **Technique:**
    a. To treat the muscles that close the jaw, ask the patient to open her mouth. Place two fingers on the patient's chin. Ask her to attempt to close her mouth against your resistance (Fig. 22-2). Repeat three times.
    b. To treat the muscles that open the jaw, ask the patient to close her mouth. Place two fingers on the patient's chin. Ask her to attempt to open her mouth against your resistance (Fig. 22-3). Repeat three times.
    c. To treat the muscles that move the jaw laterally, ask the patient to move her jaw away

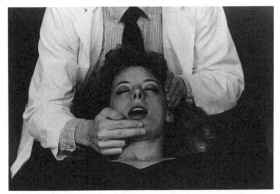

Figure 22-2. Muscle energy treatment for muscles that close the jaw.

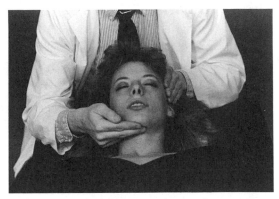

Figure 22-3. Muscle energy treatment for muscles that open the jaw.

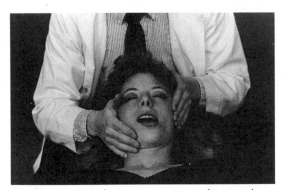

Figure 22-4. Muscle energy treatment for muscles that move the jaw laterally.

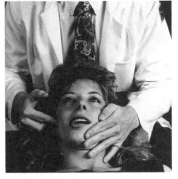

Figure 22-5. Counterstrain treatment for tender point in the right masseter muscle.

from the affected side. Place two fingers on the side of her jaw, and ask her to move her jaw back against your fingers as you provide a resistance (Fig. 22-4). Repeat three times, attempting to move the jaw through its restriction.

Counterstrain Technique
1. **Patient position:** supine.
2. **Physician position:** seated at the head of the table.
3. **Technique:**
   a. One finger monitors the tender point in the muscle.
   b. The patient is asked to relax her jaw. With the other hand the physician moves the jaw toward the affected side until the point is no longer tender (Fig. 22-5).
   c. This position is held for 90 seconds. The jaw is then returned to the neutral position.

Stretching the Pterygoid Muscles
In some cases of TMJ dysfunction the pterygoid muscles are hypertonic. These muscles can be passively stretched by applying pressure with a gloved finger inside the mouth. The finger is gently slid along the muscle, massaging and stretching it. Inhibition of tender points in these muscles may also be used.

Cranial Concepts
Because the temporal bone is intimately involved in most TMJ cases, it must be evaluated and treated for any motion restriction found (see Chapter 25, Cranial Concepts). Evaluation and treatment of the sacrum may provide important help as well.

References

Berkowitz BKB, Moxham BJ. 1988. A Textbook of Head and Neck Anatomy. Chicago: Year Book Medical Publishers.

Blood SD. 1986. The craniosacral mechanism and the temporomandibular joint. JAOA 86:512–519.

Clemente CD. 1987. Anatomy: A Regional Atlas of the Human Body, 3rd ed. Baltimore: Urban and Schwarzenberg.

DiGiovanna EL, Schiowitz S. 1991. An Osteopathic Approach to Diagnosis and Treatment. New York: J.B. Lippincott.

Downs JR. 1976. Treating TMJ dysfunction. Osteopath Phys 106–113.

Gelb H. 1985. Clinical management of head, neck, and TMJ pain and dysfunction. Philadelphia: W.B. Saunders.

Goulet JP, Clark GT. 1990. Clinical TMJ examination methods. CDA Journal 25–33.

Greenberg SA, Jacobs JS, Bessette RW. 1989. Temporomandibular joint dysfunction: evaluation and treatment. Clin Plast Surg 16:707–24.

Hasso AH, Christiansen EL, Alder ME. 1989. The temporomandibular joint. Radiol Clin North Am 27:301–314.

Jones LH. 1981. Strain and Counterstrain. Colorado Springs, Colorado: American Academy of Osteopathy.

Levitt SR, McKinney MW, Willis WA. 1993. Measuring the impact of a dental practice on TM disorder symptoms. J Craniomand Prac 11:211–216.

Mohl ND, Ohrbach R. 1992. Clinical decision making for temporomandibular disorders. J Dent Educ 56:823–833.

Moore KL. 1985. Clinically Oriented Anatomy, 2nd ed. Baltimore: Williams & Wilkins.

Royder JO. 1981. Structural influences in temporomandibular joint pain and dysfunction. JAOA 80:60–67.

Smith SD. 1980. Head pain and stress from jaw-joint problems: Diagnosis and treatment in temporomandibular orthopedics. Osteopath Med 35–51.

Woodburne RT. 1973. Essentials of Human Anatomy. New York: Oxford University Press.

23

Sinus Drainage Techniques

EILEEN L. DiGIOVANNA

Functional Anatomy

The nasal sinuses are a significant site of infection and a possible origin of headache. They include four pairs of aerated cells in the bones of the skull, named after the bones in which they are located: frontal, sphenoid, ethmoid, and maxillary.

Normally, secretions of the nasal sinuses drain into the nasal passages. The frontal sinuses drain primarily by gravity; the ethmoid, sphenoid, and maxillary sinuses rely heavily on the ciliated cells that line them to move mucus toward the nasal passages. The lining of the sinuses is similar to that of the upper respiratory tract and is affected by the same infectious processes and allergic responses.

Edema or tenacious mucus as well as slowing of ciliary movement may affect the discharge of secretions out of the sinuses. Secretory fluids build up, the passage of air is blocked, and unequal pressures result, leading to pain. This pain may be located over the sinuses or in the forehead, the orbits, or the cheeks, and may be referred via reflexes to the occiput and neck, the teeth, the temples, or the ears.

Sympathetic innervation to the sinuses arises in the upper thoracic area and passes through the cervical ganglia. The upper thoracic and cervical areas should be evaluated for the presence of somatic dysfunction, and any dysfunction found should be treated. Probably the most consistent mechanical finding associated with sinusitis is oc-

cipitoatlantal dysfunction, which requires treatment for relief.

The osteopathic treatment of sinusitis has several goals: to relieve obstruction and pain; to improve venous and lymphatic flow from the area; to effect reflex changes; and to improve mucociliary clearance. Several manual techniques have been designed to aid in achieving these goals. Although only one set of sinuses may produce pain, the entire series of techniques should be performed, to assist drainage of all the sinus areas.

Treatment Techniques

The positions of patient and operator, described below, are identical for all the techniques:

1. **Patient position:** supine on the table, with her eyes closed, and relaxed.
2. **Physician position:** seated comfortably at the head of the table.

DIRECT PRESSURE AND "MILKING"

Pressure may be applied directly with the thumbs over the frontal sinuses. The pressure is gradually increased and released in a gentle, rhythmic motion, never hard enough to cause severe pain. The cycle is repeated several times (Fig. 23-1).

The thumbs are then placed side by side in the center of the forehead and, with gentle pressure downward, are moved laterally toward the temples. At the edge of the temporal fossae the thumbs

An Osteopathic Approach to Diagnosis and Treatment, second edition
Eileen L. DiGiovanna and Stanley Schiowitz
Lippincott–Raven Publishers, Philadelphia © 1997.

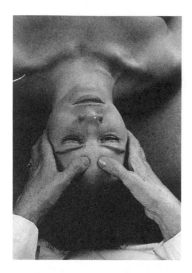

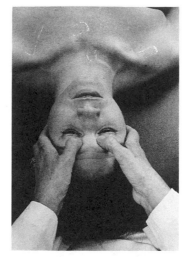

Figure 23-1. Direct pressure applied over the frontal sinuses.

Figure 23-2. Gentle pressure applied over the supraorbital notch.

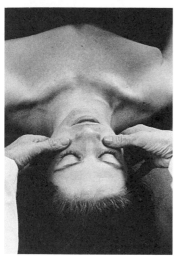

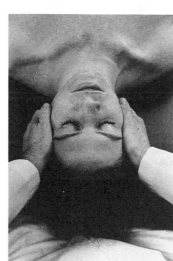

Figure 23-3. Pressure applied over the maxillary sinuses.

Figure 23-4. Direct pressure applied over the temporal areas.

are directed caudad to the zygoma. This cycle is repeated six or eight times.

Supraorbital notch. Gentle pressure may be applied over the supraorbital notch; then the thumbs are swept along the eyebrow ridge bilaterally (Fig. 23-2).

Maxillary sinuses. The same technique can be applied to the maxillary sinuses. Pressure is applied over the sinuses with the thumbs. The nasal passages are "milked" by beginning with the thumb on each side of the nose and pressing down while sweeping the thumbs laterally along the maxilla (Fig. 23-3).

Temporal areas. Direct pressure may be applied over the temporal areas by gently placing the thenar eminences in the temporal fossae bilaterally and compressing these areas between the hands. Pressure is applied and released in gentle, rhythmic motions (Fig. 23-4).

INDIRECT PRESSURE

The fingers of the operator's hands are interlaced and laid palm up on the table under the patient's head. The thenar eminence of each hand is placed against the patient's head laterally on the occiput. Gentle, rhythmic pressure is applied to the head

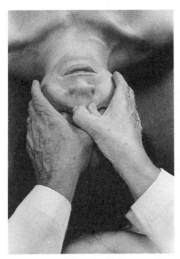

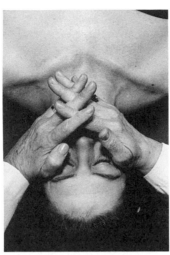

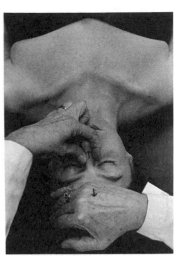

Figure 23-5. Sinus drainage technique for nasal congestion.

Figure 23-6. Counterstrain technique for the maxillary sinuses.

Figure 23-7. Counterstrain technique for supraorbital tender points.

by pressing the hands together and releasing them. A counterstrain technique is applied in the same manner. The pressure is maintained for 90 seconds, then released very slowly. A similar technique involves cupping the occiput in one hand and placing the heel of the other hand in the center of the patient's forehead, compressing the head between the two hands in a gentle, rhythmic motion.

NASAL DECONGESTION

The nasal passages are milked by the examiner, who places the thumb of the right hand on the left side of the patient's nose and the left thumb on the right side of the nose, the thumbs crossing above the bridge of the nose. Pressure is applied alternately by each thumb, moving down the length of the nose (Fig. 23-5). This is done several times; then the thumbs are reversed and a sweeping motion is made bilaterally down the sides of the nose and out over the maxillae.

COUNTERSTRAIN TECHNIQUES

Maxillary sinuses. The tender points are over the infraorbital nerves. An effective counterstrain technique for the maxillary sinuses is to interlace the fingers above the bridge of the nose with the thenar eminences resting on the lateral curve of the zygoma. Pressure through the thenar eminences, in a compressing and lifting motion, is maintained for 90 seconds, then released (Fig. 23-6).

Supraorbital tender points. The supraorbital tender points are located near the site of the supraorbital nerves. One arm rests on the patient's forehead, lightly pulling it superiorly, and, with fingers of the other hand pinching the bridge of the nose, the examiner distracts the nose caudad (Fig. 23-7).

24 Myofascial Release Concepts

PAULA SCARIATI
DENNIS J. DOWLING

Fascia is a sheet or band of fibrous tissue that lies deep to the skin and invests all structures of the body. Every nerve, bone, muscle, and organ is covered with some form of fascia. The term, which is Latin for band or bandage, is descriptive of the pervading presence of the material. If all of the other structures, visceral and somatic, were somehow dissolved, a ghostly fascial image would persist and retain recognizable form.

Function

Some authors (Kuchera and Kuchera) have described the functions of fascia as the 4 Ps: packaging, protection, posture, and passageways. There is a rich nervous supply to the fascia, and all nerves perforate or are encompassed by fascia. Muscles—smooth, cardiac, and skeletal—are enveloped by it. Contraction and motion of the muscles are guided by fascia, and the balance of structures is maintained by stresses distributed throughout. As an encasement and as a tether, fascia protects underlying structures. Usually this means that forces are absorbed or redistributed. Because of its reactivity to forces, its configuration may change and precede changes in other structures, such as the muscles. The processes of circulation, both vascular and lymphatic, are maintained and regulated through fascial influence. When change does occur in the structure of fascia, with reorganization, directionality, and thicken-

ing, all of the functions may be altered and/or reduced. Sudden stretching of fascia may be accompanied by a sensation of burning pain and irritation of membranous components and may result in sharp or stabbing sensations. Regional muscles may contract in reflex to these stimuli.

Organization

Much of the regional and localized named fascia is artificially divided. Fascia forms a continuity and is a form of connective tissue. The cellular components include fibroblasts, osteoblasts, chondroblasts, osteocytes, chondrocytes, reticular cells, mast cells, and formed elements of blood.

There are two types of general connective tissue: loose and dense. Dense tissue may be regular or irregular. *Dense regular connective tissue* has either long or overlapping layers. Tendons and ligaments are formed of dense connective tissue. The dermis, organ capsules, periosteum, and perichondrium are forms of *dense irregular connective tissue*. The fibers are meshlike, lack a distinct pattern, and are oriented in many different directions.

Loose connective tissue is found in subcutaneous fascia, in the lamina propria beneath epithelium, and in the mesenteries. There is a rich assortment of nonfibrous material such as fibroblasts, mast cells, and macrophages contained throughout. Any formed blood element, with the exception of erythrocytes and platelets, may exist in this tissue.

An Osteopathic Approach to Diagnosis and Treatment, second edition
Eileen L. DiGiovanna and Stanley Schiowitz
Lippincott–Raven Publishers, Philadelphia © 1997.

Components

Fibroblasts prepare and secrete collagen, elastin, and other proteoglycans. When there is increased need for repair, they can proliferate to accommodate the increased demand. In conjuction with macrophages known as histiocytes, they comprise the reconstructive component of reconstruction. The macrophages phagocytose absorbed debris and are developed from monocyte precursors.

Collagens are composed of many smaller fibers and are the most abundant and widely distributed proteins in the body. Although they are typically soft and flexible, they contribute high tensile strength to many structures. Four classes exist as determined by location and type: I is found in dermis, tendon, and bone; II forms cartilage; III is located in the cardiovascular tract, gastrointestinal tract, and integument; and IV is in the basement membranes of epithelium.

The protein *elastin* is the major component of elastic fibers. They have a distinct ability to be stretched and then return to their original disposition without being permanently deformed. Abundant in regions subjected to cyclical expansion and relaxation, they appear in cardiac, pulmonary, and skin structures. Stressors such as cigarette smoke and sunlight break down the elastic fibers of elastin.

All connective tissues have a spacial fill-in material of varying amounts known as *amorphous ground substance*, which is a mixture of macromolecules known as proteoglycans and glycoproteins. Both contain carbohydrates and proteinaceous material. Glycosaminoglycans are of several types, with some regional specificity. Along with proteoglycans, they give a large net negative charge to the amalgam and can bind to large amounts of water. This allows for free diffusion of smaller molecules throughout; it also gives the amorphous ground substance a gel-like consistency.

Both nutrients and waste products diffuse through the liquid material. Approximately 70% of connective tissue is composed of water, of which the ground substance is primarily responsible. Hyaluronic acid, a component of ground substance, is very hydrophilic. This aspect gives the fascia a colloid-like capacity. Intermittent or low-force impulses can create wavelike fluid mechanics. *Drag* is the amount of resistance to motion as determined by internal molecular resistance. Sudden focal force evokes a more rigid reaction. Injury or constant tension may reduce the water component, leaving the remaining components drier and relatively stiffer. Adhesions, which are abnormal cross-linkages between collagen fibers, are then more likely to occur.

As a connective tissue, *adipose* is both subcutaneous and found around some internal organs. An energy storage site, it also serves as an insulator against temperature extremes and as support for some structures. A rich blood supply and reticular mesh are found, and the relative size of each of the cells varies, depending on the activity and nutritional status of the individual.

Types

Fascia is also described as superficial, deep, and subserous. A continuous layer of *superficial fascia* lies beneath and is continuous with the skin's dermis layer. Two layers exist, with a potential space between capable of accommodating fluid accumulation. Superficial fascia invests the outer components of skeletal muscle and helps to give form to the skin. In concept, it is a sac which helps to insulate and separate the body from the external environment. Small fibrils act as anchors from the skin to the deeper fascia. Forces directed through palpation perpendicular to these tethers but parallel to the deep fasciae allow the examiner to appreciate a sense of resistance ("*drag*" or "bind") or freedom ("*ease*") to movement.

The *deep fascia* serves more of a compartmentalization role. Woven in a tighter, more compact fashion, it encapsulates and separates muscles and visceral organs. Variously named regions of fascia are the locations of thicker, deep fascia. The fibrous pericardium, parietal pleura, perineurium, and perimysium are some forms. The septa of the muscles are also examples. These coverings give some form and guidance to the structures they envelop. A condition such as "shin splints" results from ischemia due to muscular enlargement within a confining space.

Subserous fascia is a loose, fibroelastic connective tissue. The pleura, pericardium, peritoneum, and other capsular coverings of the visceral organs are representative examples. The tissue is also subject to inflammatory and infectious processes such as pleuritis or peritonitis. Pericarditis can severely tamponade the function of the heart.

Interconnection

Rather than exist in a segregated fashion, the various fasciae show continuous communication. Suspensory ligaments of the heart and other organs represent continuities. The recently discovered connection between the dura and the rectus capitis posterior minor is an example of the continuity and interrelatedness of bodily structures. The inguinal ligament is a reflection of the inrolled lower edge of the external oblique muscle aponeurosis.

As connective tissue, other elements such as the blood and osseous structures of the body act to maintain communication among the various areas of the body. Blood is a connective tissue in its ability to remove, replace, nourish, and deliver to all regions of the body. The musculoskeletal system allows interaction of various parts of the body and helps in the process of fluid flow. The replacement and maintenance of elemental substances such as calcium are dependent on the storage sites in the bone, and the process of hematopoiesis occurs in the marrow.

Bones must be thought of as more like plastic than like stone. They have a good deal of flexibility and can accommodate and distribute stresses within a certain capacity of tolerance. The amount, interval, and impulse of the force as well as the vector, direction, and individual structure, age, and nutritional status of the bone help to determine the result. Sudden forces may create bending, as in a green-stick fracture in children, or rupture of the components and related structures. Sometimes the force is transmitted to surrounding or underlying structures of other types. Head trauma may avoid frank skull fracture but result in disruption of blood vessels or contusion of the brain. Constant or intermittent forces of relatively less intensity may result in deformation and/or reformation of bone.

According to Wolff's law, alteration of function results in a change in the structure of bone. The mastoid processes are barely existent in a newborn infant but become larger, knoblike projections from the temporal bone by adulthood. Asymmetric or even symmetric stressors on bone or other bodily components bring about long-term changes in structure.

The principle of Wolff's law also applies to the fascial tissue. When subjected to stress, previously ambiguous tissue develops directionality. The ability to return to a more elastic state is hampered or eliminated. The longer the force and the responsive reaction continue, the less likely the tissue is to reformulate itself. Fiber adhesions develop from both the approximation of tissue and inflammatory processes. As an acute process, the compression the material undergoes is protective. Contraction and reformation restrict and resist further destruction. With removal of the irritating event, the body's self-healing mechanisms help restore the tissue's capacity. However, inappropriate persistence of the reaction or further injury results in more chronic changes, and perhaps even scarring. Fasciae retain a memory of the forces which have been inflicted through the reorganization of tissue. These histochemical changes may occur parallel to the vector force when there is shearing of the fascia or perpendicular when there is focal impact. Conditions such as fibromyalgia may represent chronic inflammatory changes at multiple sites. In other words, the connective tissues easily exhibit a structure-function interrelationship. The corollary of abnormal function promoting development of abnormal structure is apparent.

Reconstruction

The repair and proliferation of the type and amount of tissue have multiple determinants. Tobacco, sun exposure, and age reduce the facility to produce elastin. Piezoelectric currents develop due to ionic charges following irritation or injury. Fibroblasts align along the electric fields and determine the direction of repair and proliferation. Certain specialized fasciae such as the thoracolumbar fascia and the falx cerebri show lines of force based on chronic normal stresses.

Patterns of Fascial Strain

As a compensatory organ, the fascia absorbs and distributes forces. When examining patients for somatic dysfunction, one often sees patterns to the findings. Most frequently areas of restriction are found at transitional zones, with an apparent preference for alteration from side to side from one region to the next successive one. These were called *compensatory patterns* by J. Gordon Zink. He found that 80% of the people he examined who described themselves as "well" exhibited this pattern. The remaining group of "well" people also showed an alternating sequence but in the exact opposite directions. He termed these *common* and *uncommon compensatory patterns*, respectively. They are as follows:

	Common (CCP)	Uncommon (UCCP)
Occipitoatlantoid	L	R
Cervicothoracic	R	L
Thoracolumbar	L	R
Lumbosacral	R	L

Some subjects may not show a preference to one side or other and have tissue that is equally responsive bilaterally. These are fairly healthy and adaptive tissues.

The reason for the compensatory patterns may be handedness, eye dominance, or foot preference. Postural imbalance such as leg length discrepancies and eye-level imbalance may also play a role. The tendency to move in one direction results in attempts to maintain a center of gravity and a balance of all forces to attain equilibrium. Some authors have even suggested a genetic basis in the natural formation of helical patterns, even as small as DNA.

Individuals who did not fit either of these compensatory patterns were noted to have *uncompensated patterns*, in which there may be no alternation or the alteration is incomplete. Dr. Zink reasoned that the compensated patterns were more adaptive and that these individuals responded more favorably to any stress or illness. Injuries tend to exaggerate already existent patterns. People with uncompensated patterns were more likely to have suffered trauma, were slower to recover from illness, and required more chronic treatment.

Therapeutic Considerations

All manipulative medical interventions rely upon the physical interaction of the physician or therapist with the somatic elements of the patient. The process is guided by various considerations. All of the soft tissues have a tolerance for stretch based on their condition, within certain limits. Some of the structures, such as muscle, have the ability to contract. They may do so under voluntary control or reflexively. Injury, chronicity, nutritional sta-

tus, and position all affect responsiveness. The origins and insertions of the tendons and ligaments determine available motion. The fascia shows decreased elasticity with age and relatively undiminished contractility. The nature of the surrounded structures, regional force and tension requirements, and nutritional status further modify the stretch or contract reactivity. The bones act as levers, both in their function and when used by the physician therapeutically.

Connective tissue release modalities have been called "myofascial release" techniques historically. In truth, they are "myo-fascial-tendon-ligament-osseous-viscera" techniques. Most of the proponents of these techniques have used the responsiveness of the tissue as a guideline for further movement.

Practically all of the modalities are passive in that the patient is to make no conscious effort at moving a region. When active involvement is requested, it is usually to facilitate relaxation, either through a contract/relax response or reflexively through reciprocal inhibition. In both of these situations, the patient's involvement is in short pulses.

The modalities can be described as either direct or indirect. *Direct* techniques bring the region in question into one or more of the relative barriers to motion, with the intent that the tissue relaxes and stretches toward the physiologic limits. A response called *creep* has been used to describe the relaxation of myofascial tissue to a gentle force load and the decreased resistance to subsequent applications. Varieties of *indirect* techniques all position the region into the various freedoms. Some are static in that the position is held. Others are dynamic and use either continuous motion in response to feedback experienced by the physician or the application of facilitating forces or motions. After treatment, reassessment or mobilization into the barriers is engaged. Some of these modalities and specific techniques are also described in other sections of this book.

Myofascial Release Techniques

Counterstrain is a myofascial release technique originally described as "spontaneous release by positioning." A tender point is noted on palpation and the region or entire body is positioned into freedoms for the purpose of shortening muscles. The positions are held for 90 to 120 seconds. Subsequent tissue softening and/or reduced tenderness is noted.

Facilitated positional release involves positioning a region or joint into neutral, unloading the joint, adding a facilitating force (compression and/or torsion), adding motion in all three planes of freedom, and monitoring for release. The time interval is a few seconds.

Functional techniques appear to have started with Dr. Still. Palpation of specific joint and tissue compliance determines positioning in three cardinal planes, translation in two planes (transverse and anterior or posterior), and compression or traction. An additional element is reaction to a respiratory component (inhalation or exhalation).

Torque unwinding is an unpublished modality which has been taught at seminars. It has a theoretical construct of bodily cubes with regions of restriction being reflected on opposing surfaces due to vectors of force resulting from injury. Treatment involves bringing the two ends into alignment, mimicking the position of the original injury, and waiting for release and/or adding slight oscillatory torsional forces into both locations at the same time. These techniques are attempts to balance the stress load by adding limited forces in the direction opposite to the original vector of injury.

Balanced ligamentous release (articular ligamentous release) uses the palpating hands as both monitors and fulcrums. The regions of the joints and ligaments are balanced to create relaxation and gapping. Release occurs as the tissue further relaxes and more normal motion is established.

Unwinding is a dynamic technique. The patient gives constant feedback to the examiner while moving a portion of the body in response to sensations of movement. The technique can be localized using impulses of drag and ease over wider regions. The neck or extremities can be treated regionally or used as levers to manipulate the trunk. The physician facilitates the process by resisting influences such as gravity while following small muscular motions or fascial ease.

Direct fascial release requires that a torsion, compression, and/or traction force be maintained into the barrier while one waits for a release (fascial creep). After this occurs, the region can be moved in all planes more easily.

Cranial osteopathy is a form of fascial release that attempts to balance forces of the five components, as proposed by William Garner Sutherland.

Visceral manipulation uses manual techniques (the physician's contact with the somatic system) to balance forces which create stresses on the visceral organs.

The Still technique is a recently "rediscovered" application of manipulative techniques believed to be used by Dr. Still. Richard VanBuskirk has developed this modality after discerning written descriptions by Dr. Still and Dr. Hazard, an early student. It combines indirect technique with a subsequent quick articulatory procedure. A journal article reviewing this modality is awaiting publication.

Even though these modalities are mentioned as distinct units, they may occur as a continuity. The physician may switch from one to another to adapt to tissue response.

Examples of Indirect Techniques
CERVICAL SPINE FUNCTIONAL TECHNIQUE
1. **Patient position:** supine.
2. **Physician position:** seated at the head of the table.
3. **Technique:**
   a. The physician places the index finger of either hand on the transverse process of the vertebra to be released.
   b. Range of motion of the vertebral unit is assessed in all three planes—flexion-extension, side-bending, and rotation.
   c. Response to translation laterally in the coronal plane and anteriorly/posteriorly along the sagittal plane is assessed.
   d. Tissue responsiveness at the monitoring site is assessed for compression or traction.
   e. The vertebra is positioned in all three cardinal planes of freedom.
   f. The two directions of translation are added.
   g. Respiration is used to determine tissue relaxation. If the tissue feels more relaxed during inhalation, then the patient is instructed to take a deep breath and hold it. If exhalation is the freer modifier, then the patient takes a breath and exhales fully and maintains full exhalation for several seconds.
   h. The physician follows the vertebra into the direction of ease at each release.
   i. The region is reassessed.

THORACIC SPINE/UPPER EXTREMITY UNWINDING

1. **Patient position:** supine.
2. **Physician position:** standing or seated at the side of the table along the side to be treated.
3. **Technique:**
   a. The physician grasps the patient's forearm with both hands.
   b. The patient's arm is brought to approximately 90° of shoulder flexion.
   c. Slight tension is introduced by traction and the whole arm is subjected to a mild amount of torsion by internally and then externally rotating the arm.
   d. The tension is reduced and effort is directed toward supporting the arm against gravity.
   e. Tissue responsiveness at the monitoring site is assessed.
   f. The physician allows the arm to drift in any or all directions. If the extremity hits a barrier, there will be a tendency for the muscles to tighten. The physician should attempt to use the least amount of interaction necessary.
   g. As the movement becomes more active, the physician can give less and less support.
   h. If a pattern of movement is repeated three times or more, the physician should hold the arm at one or another extreme of the movement and hold it in place. Any tugging motion which leads to the same repetitive motion should be resisted by maintaining the extremity in place.
   i. Elimination of the resistance should occur when the extremity begins to move in a direction which does not fit the previous pattern.
   j. The endpoint occurs when the arm comes to rest alongside or across the patient's abdomen. Palpated impulses to movement should be absent.
   k. The region is reassessed.
   l. Large movements of the shoulder involve the thoracic spine, whereas smaller conical types of movement may support only regional extremity movement.

SCAPULA RELEASE

1. **Patient position:** lying on his side, with the side to be treated facing upward.
2. **Physician position:** standing, facing the patient.
3. **Technique:**
   a. The physician abducts the patient's arm and

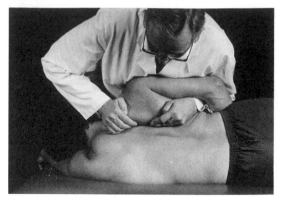

Figure 24-1. Fascial release of the scapula.

places his caudad arm (relative to the patient) between the patient's arm and his chest wall.
   b. The physician grasps the patient's scapula at the medial edge and inferior angle with his caudad hand and the medial edge and superior medial angle with his cephalad hand (Fig. 24-1).
   c. With a slight amount of traction, the scapula is tested in the following directions:
      i. Cephalad (elevation) and caudad (depression)
      ii. Lateral (distraction) and medial (retraction)
      iii. Rotation clockwise and counterclockwise
   d. The scapula is placed into all three directions of freedom successively and held in place.
   e. The physician waits for a further loosening into one or more directions of freedom, indicating a release.
   f. The region is reassessed.

SACRAL BALANCING

1. **Patient position:** supine.
2. **Physician position:** seated to one side of the patient facing toward the patient's head.
3. **Technique:**
   a. Depending on the patient's comfort, one of the following two positions can be used:
      i. Both knees bent, feet flat on the table, separated and adducted.
      ii. Legs extended.
   b. The physician places the hand of the arm which is closer to the patient beneath the patient's sacrum. The physician's fingertips extend to the patient's sacral base and the apex

of the sacrum rests between the physician's thenar and hypothenar eminences. The hand contours to the sacrum. The physician rests his forearm on the table.

c. The physician places the forearm of his other arm across the ASISs of the patient's pelvis. The physician's arm, which is now close to the patient's head, rests on the ipsilateral ASIS while the hand holds the outer edge of the opposite iliac crest.

d. A medial force is engaged across these two contact points with this arm.

e. The physician monitors the motion of the sacrum during inhalation and exhalation. The sacral base moves posteriorly in inhalation and anteriorly in exhalation.

f. The physician evaluates the motion for symmetry and quality.

g. The physician attempts to balance the sacrum in all directions of ease.

h. When symmetry is established, the physician assesses the efficacy of the treatment.

KNEE TORQUE UNWINDING

1. **Patient position:** supine.
2. **Physician position:** seated or standing to one side of the patient facing toward the patient's head.
3. **Technique:**
   a. The physician finds a point tenderness, motion restriction, or tissue tension at any given location about the knee.
   b. The physician should imagine that the knee is encased in a cube.
   c. Drawing an imaginary line diagonally across from the location of the original point, the physician must realize that this point is a reflection of the original point. The second point may also be found by palpating the original point, tapping it, and feeling for a resonance of the impulse. If the point is two fingerbreadths below the upper edge of the cube, the resonance point will be two fingerbreadths above the lower edge of the opposite face of the cube. The same relationship is maintained for the point relative to the lateral edges of the cube.
   d. One or two fingers of each hand cover each point.
   e. A rotary motion is introduced at both locations at the same time. The preferred manner

is to rotate one side clockwise while the other moves counterclockwise, and then reverse directions. The angle of the rotary motion is narrow, and the oscillation of motion is a few cycles per second for up to a minute.

f. Alternating points found on opposite faces of imaginary cubes can be located throughout the lower extremity.

g. The region is reassessed.

LARGE INTESTINE/VISCERAL MANIPULATION

1. **Patient position:** supine, hips and knees flexed, feet on the table and spread apart.
2. **Physician position:** standing or seated to the patient's right side.
3. **Technique:**
   a. The physician uses the hypothenar eminence of his right hand and places it medial to the patient's left ASIS. A mild pressure is directed inward toward the pelvis and upward toward the umbilicus. This position is held until there is a softening. This is directed at relaxing the fascial components of the sigmoid colon.
   b. Keeping the fingers curved, the physician then uses the fingertip pads of both hands and reaches across the patient and grasps the abdomen between the left iliac crest and the costal cartilage along the anterior axillary line. A gentle tug is directed medially. A softening or release of the subcutaneous structures, specifically the descending colon, is desired.
   c. The edge of the left hand is placed across the epigastric region and a caudad mild force is directed toward the umbilicus for releasing the transverse colon.
   d. The physician can remain on the patient's right and use the heels of both hands to direct the abdomen between the right crest and rib margin in the anterior axillary line medially. Otherwise, the physician can move to the patient's left side and treat the ascending colon much in the same way as the descending colon was treated in b.
   e. If standing on the patient's right side, the physician uses the hypothenar eminence of his right hand and places it medial to the patient's right ASIS. A mild pressure is directed inward toward the pelvis and upward toward

the umbilicus. This position is held until there is a softening. This is directed at relaxing the fascial components of the cecum.

f. Other visceral techniques directed toward improving gastrointestinal function can be added.

THE STILL TECHNIQUE FOR THE THORACIC SPINE

1. **Patient position:** seated
2. **Physician position:** standing facing the patient
3. **Technique:**
   a. The physician place his forearms across the patient's shoulders.
   b. The physician palpates the transverse process of the diagnosed thoracic somatic dysfunction.
   c. A downward force is placed by the physician's forearms onto the patient's shoulders until it is noted by the physician's palpating fingers.
   d. If the somatic dysfunction is sidebent and rotated to one side, the physician mimics this by introducing side-bending and rotation down to the involved level while maintaining the downward force through the shoulders.
   e. This position is maintained for a few seconds.
   f. The physician then reverses the process while maintaining the downward force through the shoulders. The patient is sidebent and rotated opposite to the original manuever and therefore opposite to the somatic dysfunction.
   g. Articulation of the joint may be noted.
   h. The region is reassessed.

References

Barral JP, Mercier P. 1988. Visceral Manipulation. Seattle: Eastland Press.

Bowles CH. 1992. Functional technique: a modern perspective. In: Beal MC, ed. The Principles of Palpatory Diagnosis and Manipulative Technique. Newark, Ohio: American Academy of Osteopathy, 174–178.

Greenman PE. 1989. Principles of Manual Medicine. Baltimore: Williams & Wilkins.

Jones LH. 1992. Spontaneous release by positioning. In: Beal MC, ed. The Principles of Palpatory Diagnosis and Manipulative Technique. Newark, Ohio: American Academy of Osteopathy, 179–185.

Kuchera WA, Kuchera ML. 1994. Osteopathic Principles in Practice, 2nd ed. Columbus, Ohio: Greyden Press.

Van Buskirk R. 1996. The Still Technique. Personal communication.

Wallace EM. 1995. Torque Unwind. Presented at the Convocation of the American Academy of Osteopathy, Nashville.

25 Cranial Concepts

HUGH ETTLINGER
BONNIE GINTIS

The cranial concept was originally conceived and developed by William Garner Sutherland from 1899 until his death in 1954. Sutherland's teachings are a direct extension of the principles of osteopathy as taught by Andrew Taylor Still at the American School of Osteopathy.

Dr. Sutherland's study began after careful examination of a disarticulated skull. He first identified a design for motion in the structure of the sutures. After lengthy study he concluded that motion occurred between the cranial bones. Dr. Sutherland realized that there were no muscles that could account for the motion he palpated between the bones of the cranium. He concluded that the motion must be the response to an involuntary mechanism. He named this mechanism the *primary respiratory mechanism* (PRM).

This section introduces the basic principles of the cranial concept and the primary respiratory mechanism. It should be used as a stepping-stone to a more in-depth study of this field. In addition to didactic study, individualized palpatory training is a mandatory adjunct to the study of this aspect of osteopathy.

The Primary Respiratory Mechanism

The primary respiratory mechanism is palpable in the cranium and throughout the body. Its action is part of the normal physiology of the living human body. It has two alternating phases, referred to as the *inhalation* and *exhalation* phases. The primary respiratory mechanism is not a wave that travels from head to foot.

Five phenomena function together as the primary respiratory mechanism:

1. The fluctuation of the cerebrospinal fluid (CSF), and the potency of the tide
2. The mobility of the intracranial and intraspinal membranes and the function of the reciprocal tension membrane
3. The inherent motility of the central nervous system
4. The articular mobility of the cranial bones
5. The involuntary mobility of the sacrum between the ilia

Together, these five phenomena form a structure-function relationship between the central nervous system and its container.

Phases of the Primary Respiratory Mechanism

As mentioned, the two phases of the primary respiratory mechanism are referred to as inhalation and exhalation phases. These phases are palpable simultaneously throughout the five phenomena and the entire body. During the inhalation phase, midline bones flex and paired bones externally rotate, moving the basicranium superiorly. The resultant increased transverse diameter of the cranium is accompanied by a simultaneous decrease

An Osteopathic Approach to Diagnosis and Treatment, second edition
Eileen L. DiGiovanna and Stanley Schiowitz
Lippincott–Raven Publishers, Philadelphia © 1997.

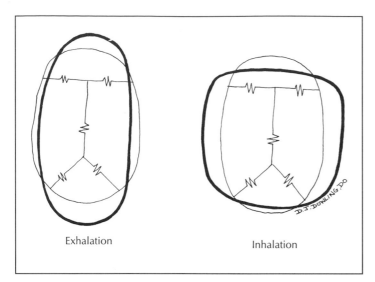

Figure 25-1. Inhalation and exhalation phases of the primary respiratory mechanism.

Exhalation   Inhalation

in anteroposterior diameter and a decrease in vertical dimension (Fig. 25-1). The foramen magnum moves superiorly, drawing the sacral base posteriorly by means of its dural attachment at the second sacral segment. The space that contains the CSF and the fluid itself are affected by the alternating phases of the primary respiratory mechanism. The dural membranes change shape around a suspended, automatically shifting fulcrum, maintaining balance and constant tension during the phases of the primary respiratory mechanism. There is a rhythmic expansion and contraction of the brain and spinal cord during the phases of the primary respiratory mechanism.

In the exhalation phase these motions are reversed.

The study of the primary respiratory mechanism begins with a detailed examination of each of its five phenomena.

The Fluctuation of the Cerebrospinal Fluid and the Potency of the Tide

The fluctuation of the CSF is considered the first principle in the primary respiratory mechanism. Within the fluid is a potency or force that manifests as a fluctuant movement. Dr. Sutherland referred to this force as the "breath of life."

Within that cerebrospinal fluid there is an invisible element that I refer to as the "Breath of Life." I want you to visualize this Breath of Life as a fluid

within this fluid, something that does not mix, something that has potency as the thing that makes it move. Is it really necessary to know what makes the fluid move?

Although Dr. Sutherland did not theorize on the origin of the breath of life and its fluctuation, he did clearly distinguish it from the actions created by arterial pulse and respiration.

Movement of CSF involves both circulation and fluctuation. Circulation of the CSF, which occurs via hydrostatic forces at choroid plexuses and arachnoid granulations, has been well documented. Seventy percent of CSF is formed at the choroid plexus in the ventricles. These plexuses are formed by the pia and intracranial capillary beds, and are part of the blood-brain barrier. The other 30% is formed as CNS extracellular fluid moves into the subarachnoid space, providing a drainage pathway for the brain (Fig. 25-2). The intraventricular and subarachnoid distribution of CSF is connected by two small foramina in the fourth ventricle, the foramen of Magendie and the foramen of Luschka. CSF is drained via arachnoid granulations, formed by arachnoid and the inner layer of the dura. Arachnoid granulations are found in the superior sagittal sinus and near the dorsal root ganglia in the spinal cord.

Forces generated by hydrostatic gradients are not sufficient to account for the exchange of CSF with the circulation of the body. Fluctuation, a

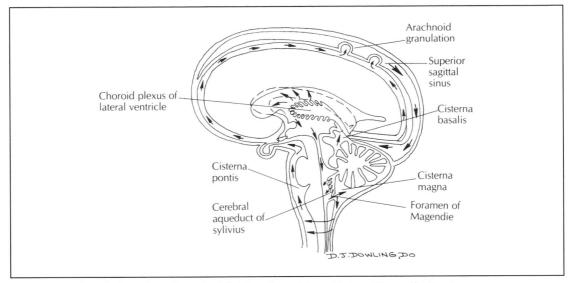

Figure 25-2. Circulation of cerebrospinal fluid. (Adapted from Netter, Ciba collection.)

back-and-forth movement of the fluid, contributes to this process.

Fluctuation of CSF has been documented recently by MRI studies. These studies demonstrate fluctuant movement of CSF in response to arterial pulse and respiration. The primary respiratory mechanism also fluctuates the CSF. CSF fluctuation provides a continuous mixing which, combined with the small circulatory forces, allows for adequate exchange of the CSF with the circulation of the body. Circulatory forces alone are inadequate to account for this process.

Dr. Sutherland likened the fluctuation of the CSF to the tide in the ocean. In her book, *The Sea Around Us*, Rachel Carson describes the difference between waves, currents, and the tide. Her analogy illustrates concepts that also apply to circulation and fluctuation in the human body.

There is no drop of water in the ocean, not even the deepest parts of the abyss that does not know and respond to the mysterious forces that create the Tide. No other force that affects the sea is so strong. Compared with the tide, the wind created waves are surface movements. So, despite their impressive sweep, are the planetary currents, which seldom involve more than the upper several hundred fathoms.

Currents are similar to a circulation, carrying fluid from one place to another at relatively rapid speed. The tide is a fluctuation, which creates a mixing by to-and-fro movement of the fluid. Dr. Carson continues:

The influence of the tide over the affairs of sea creatures as well as men may be seen all over the world. The billions upon billions of sessile animals like oysters, mussels, and barnacles owe their very existence to the sweep of the tides which brings them the food which they are unable to go in search of.

The sessile cells of the central nervous system (CNS) also depend on a constant mix of their fluid surroundings to maintain concentration gradients adequate for nutrition and waste disposal. The fluctuation of the CSF helps maintain these gradients.

Dr. Sutherland referred to the effect of the fluctuation of the CSF on the physiological function in the body. "Through the functions of the Primary Respiratory Mechanism, the physiologic centers in the medulla relate to the secondary physiology of the living human body." The discovery of the circumventricular organs in the walls of the third and fourth ventricles thirty to forty years after Dr. Sutherland's statement sheds light on a possible mechanism for this relationship. These organs are sensory apparatuses designed to monitor the CSF for the operation of various feedback mechanisms of the CNS. The circumventricular organs have been shown to be involved in the regulation of temperature, electrolyte balance, hypothalamic-pituitary function, and cardiovascular and respiratory function. Adequate exchange of the CSF is necessary for these organs to receive accurate information and appropriately regulate body function.

The Mobility of the Intracranial and Intraspinal Membranes and the Function of the Reciprocal Tension Membrane

The Reciprocal Tension Membrane (RTM) is a function of the mobility of the intracranial and intraspinal membranes; the pia, arachnoid, and dura. Understanding the development and the anatomy of the membranes helps illustrate their function.

Membranous structures in the body are all composed of connective tissue derived from embryonic mesenchyme. All membranes are continuous with all other mesenchymally derived connective tissues of the body. The intracranial membranes are intimately related to the rest of the body through fascial connections from the cranial base throughout the entire spine, the diaphragm, extremities, and viscera.

The newborn skull has no interlocking sutures. The only joint in the cranium is that between the condyles of the occiput and the atlas. A newborn's cranial bones are suspended in dura, and the shape of the skull is maintained by dura, by fluid, and by the central nervous system's motion within. Developmentally prior to bone formation, membranes provide shape and protection and also guide and limit motion.

THE PIA, ARACHNOID, AND DURA

The pia mater is a thin membrane that is adherent to the brain and spinal cord. It is highly vascular. A cranial portion sheathes nerve roots, extending down into fissures and sulci. Its vessels form the choroid plexus of the ventricles. The spinal portion sheathes spinal nerves. Lateral extensions form the denticulate ligaments and blend with the filum terminale internale.

The arachnoid is a gauzy membrane that contains CSF in the space between the pia and arachnoid, the subarachnoid space. Subarachnoid cis-

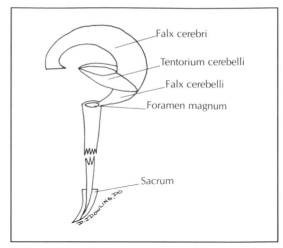

Figure 25-3. Dural membranes, lateral view.

terns are enlargements of the arachnoid space containing CSF. Cisterns function as "waterbeds," cushioning the brain. Arachnoid granulations, also called Pacchionian bodies, lie along the longitudinal fissure and function to resorb CSF. There are also spinal arachnoid granulations along the arachnoid layer in the spinal canal.

The dura mater is described as having cranial and spinal portions. In actuality there is one continuous membrane. These two parts are named only for anatomical convenience (Fig. 25-3).

There are two layers of cranial dura. This membrane is tough and inelastic. In the adult, the layers are tightly adherent to each other except where they form the venous sinuses.

The external layer of dura is the internal periosteum of cranial bones, the pericranium. Pericranium is continuous with periosteum of sutures and foramina, and with the external periosteum of the cranial bones. Compressive and tensile forces generated on the dura by the growing brain stimulate this membranous connective tissue to form bone between these layers of dura. Therefore, the bones of the cranium "float" within layers of dural membrane.

The periosteum of all cranial bones is continuous with all the dura. All adjacent membranous or fascial structures are continuous with each other. The dura and bone of the skull are examples of this continuity of connective tissues of differing densities.

Figure 25-4. Reciprocal tension membrane system.

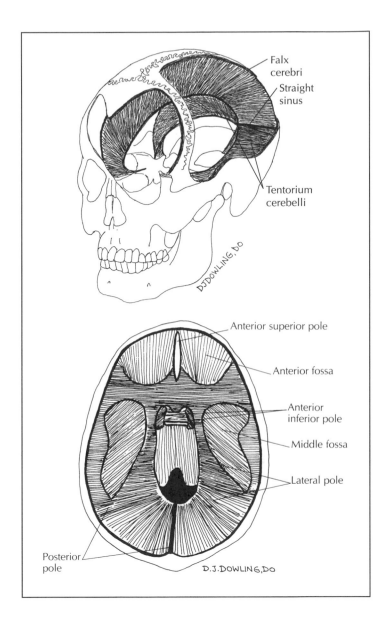

CRANIAL STRUCTURES FORMED BY DURA

The internal layer of dura is called the *meningeal layer*. This layer surrounds the brain and comes together in two layers to form the falx cerebri, the tentorium cerebelli, and the falx cerebelli.

The falx cerebri is a sickle-shaped arc between the two hemispheres of the brain that has three poles of attachment (Fig. 25-4). The anterior inferior pole attaches to the crista galli of the ethmoid. The superior pole attaches to the surface of the skull along the metopic and sagittal sutures. The posterior pole attaches to the superior surface of the tentorium in the area of the straight sinus and the internal occipital protuberance.

The tentorium cerebelli is a double sickle-shaped membrane in the posterior fossa. It is transversely oriented and concave anteriorly. The occipital lobes are above, and the cerebellum is below it. It has poles of attachment that relate to the free and attached borders.

The free or inner concave border forms the tentorial notch, which surrounds the midbrain and attaches to the anterior clinoid processes of the sphenoid. The attached or outer convex border attaches to five areas: the transverse ridge of the sulcus of the transverse sinus of the occiput, the posteroinferior angle of the parietal bone at the asterion, the mastoid portion of the temporal bone, the petrous ridge of the temporal bone, and the posterior clinoid process of the sphenoid.

The falx cerebelli is a small sickle of dura that extends between the two hemispheres of the cerebellum. Its superior attachment is to the inferior surface of the tentorium cerebelli in the area of the straight sinus. Its inferior attachment is to the vertical crest on the inner surface of the occiput. The inferior aspect of the attachment extends posteriorly, where it has a strong attachment to the foramen magnum. It is continuous with the dura of the spinal canal.

Dural membranes fold or form a sac to form three important structures. The diaphragma sellae is a small fold of dura that covers the hypophyseal fossa of the sella turcica of the sphenoid, encasing the pituitary. Meckel's cave is formed from a fold of dura and sits on the anterior surface of the petrous portion of the temporal bone. It encases the semilunar ganglion, which is composed of three sensory branches of the fifth cranial nerve, the trigeminal nerve. The endolymphatic sac is part of the membranous labyrinth system of the inner ear. It is composed of dura and is suspended from the inferior aspect of the petrous portion of the temporal bone.

The spinal portion of the dura is continuous with the inner layer of the cranial dura. Only one layer extends into the spinal canal. The other layer remains as the periosteum of the outside of the cranium. The spinal dura surrounds the spinal cord within the spinal canal. There are many attachments within the spinal canal. Firm attachments of spinal dura include the foramen magnum, the posterior aspect of the dens, the posterior aspect of the body of C3, the posterior aspect of the body of S2, the posterior aspect of the coccyx via the filum terminale, and fibrous slips to the posterior longitudinal ligament along the entire spine.

The arterial supply to the dura is derived from terminal branches of the external and internal carotid arteries. Arteries passing through the dura are not just supplying the brain. The dura has its own rich blood supply.

The nerve supply to the dura is derived from all three branches of the trigeminal nerve, from sympathetic nerves from the carotid plexus and the superior cervical ganglion, and from cervical sensory nerves from C1 and C2.

DURAL VENOUS SINUSES

The venous sinuses are spaces within dural layers that convey venous blood from veins within the cranium to the systemic venous circulation (Fig. 25-5). Venous sinuses are devoid of the elastic and muscle tissue found in all other veins, and so have no elasticity and muscular contraction to enhance drainage. Circulation is dependent on motion. During the flexion phase, the sinuses change from V-shaped to ovoid, with a resultant increase in capacity. During this phase the tributary veins increase drainage into the sinuses.

Venous sinuses drain 95% of blood from the cranium via the internal jugular vein. It is of crucial importance that there is proper functional motion of the occipital and temporal bones, which comprise the jugular foramen, to have unimpeded venous drainage. The remaining 5% of venous blood drains via facial veins and the external jugular vein.

The superior sagittal sinus lies in the attached margin of the falx cerebri and drains primarily to the right transverse sinus, the sigmoid sinus, and then to the internal jugular vein.

The inferior sagittal sinus lies in the posterior two thirds of the free margin of the falx cerebri. It drains to the great vein of Galen, the straight sinus, the left transverse sinus, the sigmoid sinus, and then to the internal jugular vein.

The straight sinus is at the junction of the falx cerebri and the tentorium cerebelli. It is also the point of union of the great vein of Galen and the inferior sagittal sinus. These sinuses drain primarily to the left transverse sinus, the sigmoid sinus, and then to the internal jugular vein.

The occipital sinus lies in the attached margin of the falx cerebelli, extending from the foramen magnum to the internal occipital protuberance. It drains primarily to the left transverse sinus, the sigmoid sinus, and then to the internal jugular vein.

The bilaterally paired cavernous sinuses are found lateral to the sella turcica and extend from the sphenoidal fissure to the apex of the petrous portion of the temporal bone. Cranial nerves III,

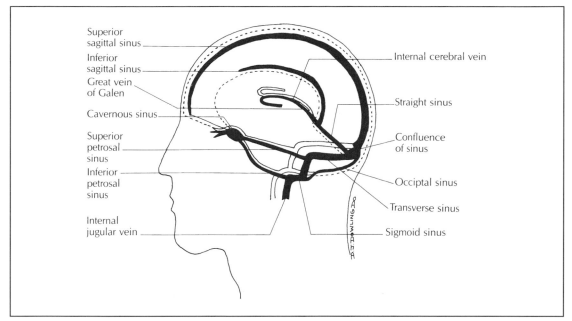

Figure 25-5. Venous sinus system.

IV, VI, the ophthalmic division of V, and the internal carotid artery are all found in relation to the cavernous sinuses. These sinuses are fed by ophthalmic veins, and drain to the superior and inferior petrosal sinuses, the sigmoid sinus, and then to the internal jugular vein.

The circular sinus or intercavernous sinus surrounds the pituitary and connects the cavernous sinuses via two transverse vessels. The circular sinus drains to the superior and inferior petrosal sinuses, the sigmoid sinus, and then to the internal jugular vein.

The superior petrosal sinuses lie in the attached margin of the tentorium cerebelli along the superior border of the petrous portion of the temporal bone. They drain into the sigmoid sinus, and then to the internal jugular vein.

The inferior petrosal sinuses lie at the junction of the posterior border of the petrous portion of the temporal bone with the basilar process of the occiput. They drain into the internal jugular vein.

The transverse sinuses lie in the attached margin of the tentorium cerebelli and extend from the area of the confluence of sinuses (internal occipital protuberance) to the jugular fossae. They lie in grooves in the occipital squama and mastoid angles of the parietals. The transverse sinuses become the sigmoid sinuses along the mastoid portion of the temporal bones and the jugular process of the occiput and drain into the internal jugular vein.

The basilar sinus or basilar plexus overlies the basisphenoid and basiocciput, connecting the inferior petrosal sinuses. This plexus consists of several interfacing veins between the layers of the dura, connecting the circular sinus with the internal vertebral venous plexus.

RECIPROCAL TENSION MEMBRANE (RTM)

The RTM is a single unit of structure and function. All membranes change shape during the phases of the primary respiratory mechanism. Membranes balance and maintain a constant level of tension during the rhythmic, simultaneous, alternating shape change of the phases of the primary respiratory mechanism. Just as ligaments allow joints to move through a range of motion, the intracranial and intraspinal membranes allow a range of motion of the bones that are suspended within them. This reciprocal action functions around a fulcrum in a dynamic relationship, guiding and limiting motion in the cranium and responding to motion throughout the body.

The RTM functions in the phases of flexion and extension around a suspended, automatically shifting fulcrum. Dr. Magoun named this fulcrum the *Sutherland fulcrum* in honor of its discoverer. This fulcrum shifts and adjusts to maintain balanced tension in response to normal motion or trauma. The Sutherland fulcrum normally functions at the junction of the falx and the tentorium, along the straight sinus. It is not located at a fixed anatomical point. It is automatically shifting and suspended to be able to adapt to changing forces.

Dr. Sutherland stressed the importance of learning to observe the functioning of this fulcrum. If the membranes can be brought to a state of balanced membranous tension, the inherent forces within the body have an opportunity to resolve dysfunctions.

The Inherent Motility
of the Central Nervous System

There is a rhythmic expansion and contraction of the brain and spinal cord during the phases of the primary respiratory mechanism. This change of shape occurs simultaneously with movements in membrane, bone, and fluid during the phases of the primary respiratory mechanism. This coiling and uncoiling motion of the nervous system occurs about a fulcrum located at the lamina terminalis, the most anterior point of the primitive neural tube.

The Articular Mobility
of the Cranial Bones

The study of cadaveric bone specimens has enabled anatomists to obtain extensive information regarding the form of bone, but has led to inaccurate information regarding its function. According to *Gray's Anatomy*, "Bones from preserved cadavers yield misleading values, especially in regards to plastic deformation, but also in elasticity, hardness, and compressive and tensile properties."

Living bone is approximately 70 percent water. Its properties are closer to other connective tissues than cadaveric study would lead one to believe. The limited mobility allowed by sutures makes the plasticity of bone a relatively important source of motion for the cranium. The thin, flat bones of the cranium are well suited to plastic deformity.

Study of the embryological development of cranial bone provides important information regarding their form and function. Compressive forces early in development create a cartilaginous matrix in the area that becomes the cranial base. Tensile forces create membrane in the area that develops into the cranial vault. Dr. Sutherland considered the motion in the cranial base primary, the motion in the vault being accommodative to the base.

The primary respiratory mechanism is palpable in the newborn, whose cranium is predominantly cartilage and membrane and lacks sutures between the bones. As the skull ossifies, sutures form to accommodate this motion, which is already present. The shape of the suture therefore reflects its motion. The basic suture types and their respective motions are shown in Figure 25-6 and are listed below:

Serrate: Sawtoothed (e.g., the sagittal suture). Allows a rocking motion.
Squamous: Scalelike, or overlapping, such as the temporoparietal (squamoparietal) suture. Allows a gliding motion, determined by the bevel and groove direction of the two surfaces.
Harmonic: Edge to edge (e.g., The lacrimoethmoidal suture). Allows shearing.
Squamoserrate: A combination, found in the lambdoidal and coronal sutures.

The motion of a bone may be deduced from the shape of its sutures (Fig. 25-7). When an axis of motion crosses a suture line, the suture changes shape and develops a bevel, since motions on opposite sides of an axis are different. These points are called pivots (Fig. 25-8).

This section examines the bones of the cranial base and vault, their sutures, the pivots within them, and their motions. The facial bones are not considered, although they are affected by cranial mechanics.

THE SPHENOID

The sphenoid articulates with 12 bones (Fig. 25-9). It is influential in the motion of the frontal and facial bones.

Parts
Structurally, the sphenoid consists of the body, the greater and lesser wings laterally, and the pterygoid plates inferiorly.

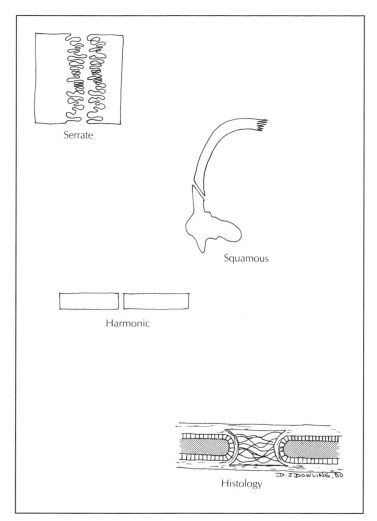

Serrate

Squamous

Harmonic

D. J DOWLING, DO

Histology

Figure 25-6. Types of sutures found in the skull.

Articulations

1. **Occiput:** The sphenoid articulates with the basilar portion of the occiput (the sphenobasilar joint), a synchrondrosis that is cartilaginous until age 20 to 25 years, then converts to cancellous bone. It exhibits flexibility, not articular mobility.

2. **Temporals:** The sphenoid articulates with the temporal in three areas. The articulation of the squamosal border of the greater wing of the sphenoid with the inferior border of the temporal squama is important. Within this articulation is a change in bevel called the sphenosquamous pivot (S.S. pivot; Fig. 25-10). A line connecting the S.S. pivot on either side of the bone reflects the axis of motion of the sphenoid. It is found directly behind the zygomatic arch. Above the sphenosquamous pivot, the articulation is mostly squamous and the sphenoid is externally beveled (the suture is on the external surface). The temporal bone is internally beveled (the suture is on the internal surface). More simply, the temporal bone overlaps the sphenoid here, and a primarily gliding motion exists. Below the sphenosquamous pivot, the articulation is more serrate, less vertical, and more evenly beveled. The motion is more of a rocking motion.

3. **Parietals:** A small articulation exists at the pterion between the posterosuperior surface of the

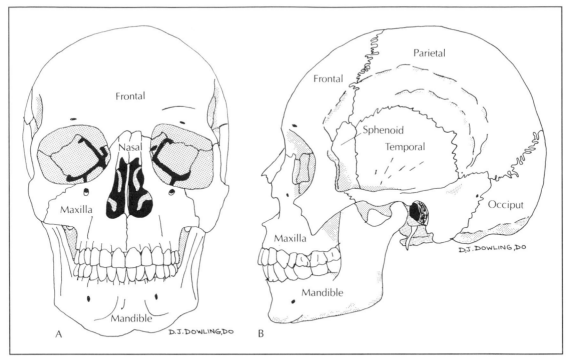

Figure 25-7. The skull **(A)** frontal view. **(B)** Lateral view.

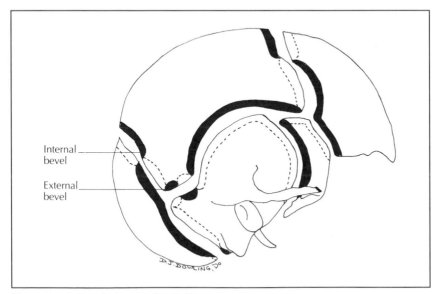

Figure 25-8. Bevel changes in skull sutures.

Figure 25-9. Sphenoid.

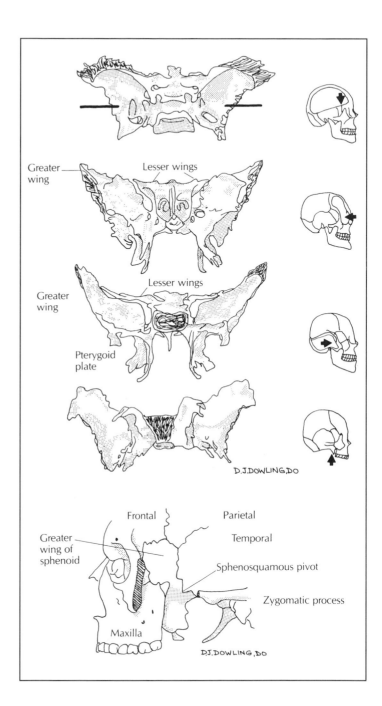

Figure 25-10. Sphenosquamous pivot.

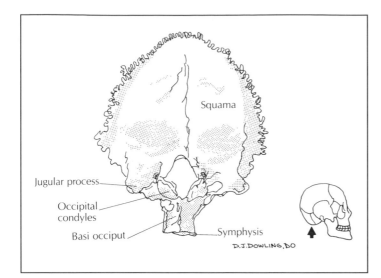

Figure 25-11. Occiput.

greater wing and the anterior inferior angle of the parietal bone. It is a squamous suture, allowing gliding motion. The sphenoid overlaps the parietal bone.

4. **Frontal bone:**
   a. An L-shaped articulation exists between the anterosuperior surface of the greater wings and the lateral inferior surfaces of the frontal bone. It is a serrate suture.
   b. Two other articulations, also serrate, exist between the anterior border of the lesser wings laterally and the orbital surface of the frontal bone, and between the anterosuperior surface of the body medially and the orbital surface of the frontal bone. Together, these two articulations allow the sphenoid to influence the lateral surfaces of the frontal bone laterally, anteriorly, and slightly superiorly as the sphenoid flexes.

5. **Ethmoid:**
   a. The anterior body of the sphenoid (ethmoid spine) articulates with the posterior border of the cribriform plate. This articulation is a gomphosis or peg-in-socket joint.
   b. Two other articulations, both harmonic, allow flexibility of motion in these areas of contact (laterally in the horizontal plane and midline in a vertical plane).

6. **Palatines** (2)
7. **Vomer**
8. **Zygomae** (2)

The palatines, vomer, and zygomae are intermediaries between the sphenoid and maxillae.

Motion
In flexion, the sphenoid rotates anteriorly about a transverse axis through its body at the level of the zygomatic arch. This motion is discussed in detail later.

THE OCCIPUT
The occiput is influential in the motion of the posterior part of the cranium.

Parts
The structures of the occiput are shown in Figures 25-11 and 25-12.

1. **Basilar occiput (basiocciput):** anterior to and forming the anterior border of the foramen magnum.
2. **Condyles:** adjacent to and forming the lateral borders of the foramen magnum.
3. **Squama:** body of the occiput, forming the posterior border of the foramen magnum.

Ossification of all parts is not complete until approximately 5 years.

Articulations
Articulating with six bones, the occiput is influential in the movement of the temporals and parietals (Fig. 25-13).

Figure 25-12. Base of
skull—occiput.

Figure 25-13. Superior view of skull
with calvaria removed, showing
articulations of the occiput.

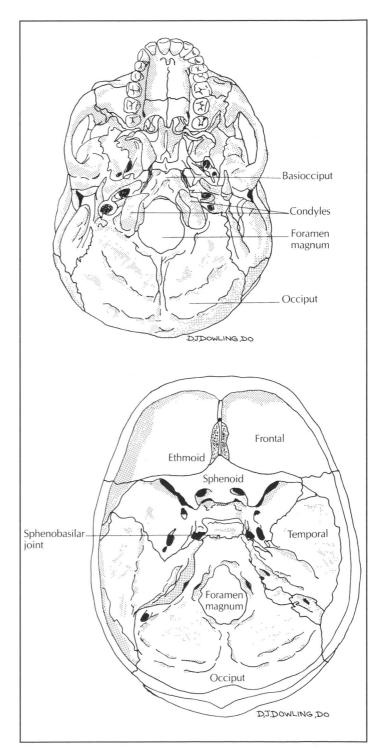

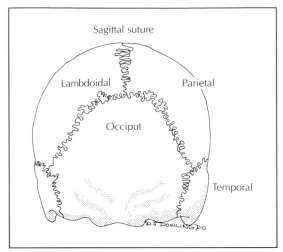

Figure 25-14. Posterior view of skull articulations of the occiput.

1. **Sphenoid:** The articulation of the occiput with the sphenoid was discussed under the sphenoid bone.
2. **Parietals:** The lambdoidal suture between the superior surface of the occiput and the postero-inferior surface of the parietal bone is the site of articulation. The change in bevel along this articulation can be found by extending the superior temporal line from the parietal bone posteriorly to this suture (Fig. 25-14). The change in bevel occurs at the point at which the orienta-

tion of both bones changes from primarily the coronal plane (superior) to primarily the horizontal plane (inferior). From the midline to this point, the occiput is internally beveled (overlapping the parietal) and the suture is more serrate, although squamoserrate. Lateral to this point, the occiput is externally beveled (overlapped by the parietal bone) and the suture is less serrate, although still squamoserrate (see Fig. 25-14). The motion is primarily rocking, but there is some slide as the occiput slides anteriorly into flexion. The parietal motion is almost entirely lateral.

3. **Temporals:** There are three distinct areas of contact of the occiput with the temporal bones (Fig. 25-15).

a. The lateral posterior surface of the occiput articulates with the mastoid portion of temporal bone. The joint is convex on the temporal bone and concave on the occiput, almost describing an L shape. The point at which the legs meet is a point of bevel change, called the condylosquamomastoid pivot. Superior and posterior to this point, the occiput is externally beveled (overlapped by the temporal bone); anterior to this point it is internally beveled (or flat). The joint is serrate, accommodating a rocking motion.

b. The jugular process of the occiput articulates with the jugular surface of the temporal bone.

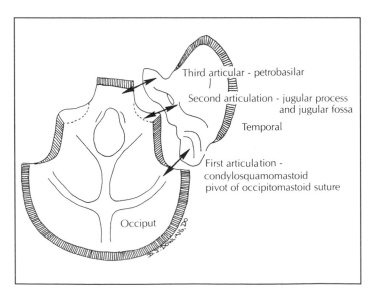

Figure 25-15. Articulation between the occiput and the temporal bone, superior aspect.

There are two parts to this articulation:

i. The jugular notch of the occiput articulates with the jugular fossa of the temporal bone, forming a smooth, quadrangular articulation in the coronal plane.

ii. An irregular, flat, rough surface posterior to the notch articulates with a surface on the temporal bone. It is in the horizontal plane. This is an extremely important articulation because it is the fulcrum around which the occiput and temporal bones move in relation to each other. The temporal bone moves anteriorly and superiorly posterior to this point, anteriorly and inferiorly anterior to the point, laterally above this point, and medially below it.

iii. The upper edge of the lateral border of the basiocciput articulates with the petrous portion of the temporal bone (inferior border). This is a tongue-and-groove articulation, allowing a hinge and glide motion.

4. **Atlas:** The occipitoatlantal articulation is a synovial joint. The articular surfaces converge anteriorly and inferiorly, predisposing the articulation to compression when hyperextended, such as in whiplash or the birth process. Birth trauma involving the craniocervical junction can have serious clinical consequences, since the condylar parts of the occiput are still separate and can be forced medially, changing the size and shape of the foramen magnum. The atlas is less often affected by birth trauma because the transverse ligament of the atlas prevents widening of the atlas facets.

Motions
The primary motion of the occiput on the atlas is flexion-extension, with the occipital condyles convex and the superior articular facets of the atlas concave.

THE TEMPORAL BONE
Parts
The structure of the temporal bone is shown in Figure 25-16.

1. **Squama:** smooth body of the temporal bone.
2. **Mastoid portion:** posterior, including the mastoid process.
3. **Zygomatic arch:** anterior and lateral.

4. **Petrous portion:** medial, containing the auditory and vestibular apparatus. It is the surface for the attachment of the tentorium cerebelli.

Articulations
The temporal bone articulates with seven other bones.

1. **Sphenoid:** The articulation of the temporal bone with the sphenoid was discussed under the sphenoid bone.
2. **Occiput:** The articulation of the temporal bone with the occiput was discussed under the occiput. This is the major influence on temporal motion.
3. **Zygoma:** The temporozygoma articulation forms the zygomatic arch, a serrate suture that allows rocking.
4. **Parietal:** The temporoparietal articulation can be considered as two separate articulations, or as one articulation with a change in bevel where the mastoid and squamous portions of the temporal bone meet. For present purposes it is considered as two separate articulations.

   a. The superior surface of the temporal bone, broadly beveled internally, articulates with the inferior anterior surface of the parietal bone, broadly beveled externally (the temporal bone overlaps the parietal bone). This suture is squamous, allowing medial and lateral glide of both bones as they rotate internally and externally.

   b. The superior surface of the mastoid portion of the temporal bone articulates with the posteroinferior surface of the parietal bone, forming an irregular, cobblestone articulation. There is a change in bevel at the center. This suture accommodates the rotary motion of the petrous portion of the temporal bone.

5. **Mandible:** The temporomandibular articulation is a synovial joint, found underneath the most posterior portion of the zygomatic arch.

THE PARIETAL BONES
Parts
The parietal bone has only one part (Fig. 25-17).

Articulations
The parietal bones articulate with five bones (Fig. 25-18).

1. **Parietal:** The interparietal (sagittal) suture is serrate, allowing a rocking motion as the pari-

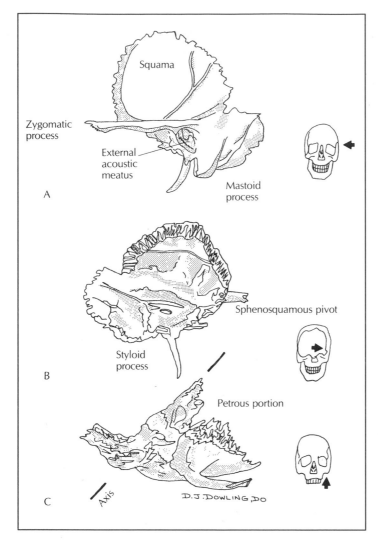

Figure 25-16. Structure of the temporal bone. **(A)** External view; **(B)** Internal view; **(C)** Inferior view.

etal bones rotate internally and externally. It has fewer but wider serrations posteriorly to accommodate greater motion there.
2. **Frontal:** The coronal suture is squamoserrate with an external bevel medially and an internal bevel laterally on the parietal.
3. **Sphenoid**
4. **Occiput**
5. **Temporal**

FRONTAL BONE
Parts
1. **Nasal part:** inferior and midline, articulates with the ethmoid.

2. **Orbital parts:** lateral and inferior, forming the roof of the orbit.
3. **Squama:** forehead area, with frontal eminences laterally. A metopic suture exists in the midline in 10% of adults.

Articulations
The frontal bone articulates with 11 bones (Fig. 25-19).

1. **Parietal bones**
2. **Sphenoid**
3. **Ethmoid:** three sutures, two lateral, one in the midline anteriorly, all harmonic to accommodate gliding (Fig. 25-20).

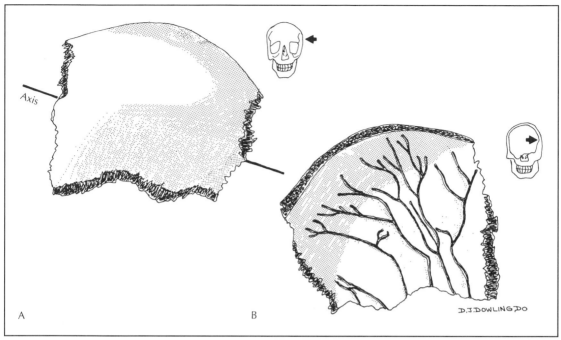

Figure 25-17. Structure of the parietal bone. **(A)** External view; **(B)** Internal view.

Figure 25-18. Sutures and articulations of the parietal bones of the skull, superior view.

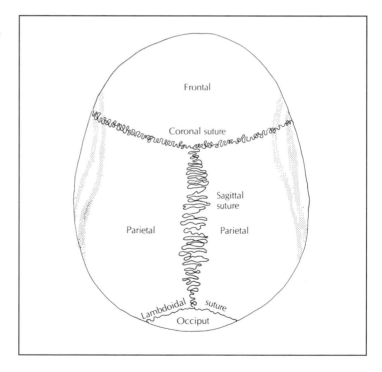

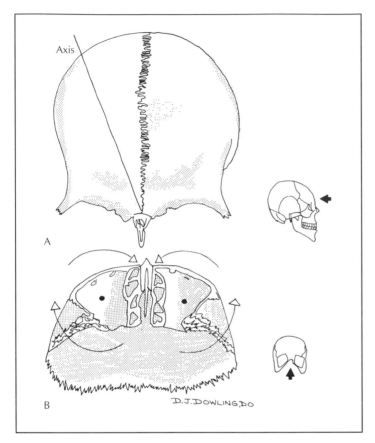

Figure 25-19. Frontal bone.
(**A**) Anterior view; (**B**) Inferior view.

4. **Lacrimals**
5. **Maxillae**
6. **Nasal bones**
7. **Zygomae**

ETHMOID
Parts
1. **Horizontal cribriform plate:** where the falx cerebri attaches.
2. **Lateral masses** (2)
3. **Perpendicular plate**

Articulations
The ethmoid articulates with 12 bones.

1. **Frontal bone**
2. **Sphenoid**
3. **Palatines** (2)
4. **Nasals** (2)
5. **Vomer**
6. **Inferior conchae**

7. **Maxillae** (2)
8. **Lacrimals** (2)

Involuntary Mobility of the Sacrum Between the Ilia
The sacrum rocks on a transverse axis through the articular pillar of the second sacral segment, posterior to the sacral canal (Fig. 25-21). This motion must be differentiated from respiratory sacral motion, which is caused by spinal motion and contraction of the pelvic diaphragm. The axis of involuntary sacral motion lies anterior to the sacral canal and passes through the body of S2 at the junction of the short and long arms of the L-shaped sacral articulation.

Patterns of Motion in the Cranium
No cranial bone moves independently. Restriction originating in any part of the cranium will cause

Figure 25-20. Structure and articulations of the ethmoid. (A) Superior view; (B) Lateral view; (C) Inferior view.

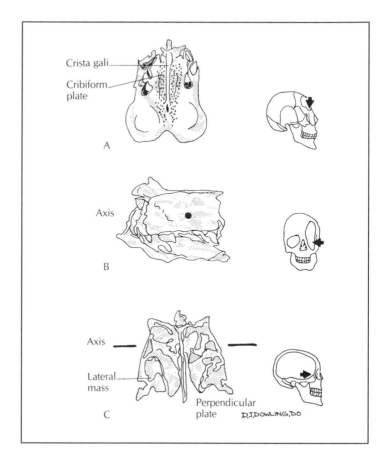

changes in the motion patterns of the entire cranium.

Magoun has identified three factors essential for cranial articular motion.

1. **Plastic resiliency.** Every bone must be sufficiently resilient in itself and mobile in its sutures to move through its normal range without strain.
2. **Resiliency of contiguous bones.** The contiguous bones must be similarly resilient and mobile to accompany movement or compensate for it without strain.
3. **Unrestricted movement of dural membranes.** The dural membranes must be unrestricted in their arcs of reciprocal tension to allow such movement to occur within normal limits.

To this list one may add the influence of cervical fascia and muscles attaching to the cranial base, as well as sacral articular mobility.

Magoun emphasizes one further point referring to palpation of the cranium. "Do not look for movement as in the other joints of the body. This is merely a resiliency—a combination of slight yielding or suppleness in the articulation plus the flexibility of live and pliant bone."

The sphenobasilar junction is the reference point for discussion of physiologic and nonphysiologic cranial motion patterns.

FLEXION AND EXTENSION

Flexion of the sphenobasilar junction results in slight elevation of that articulation. The midline bones all rotate about a transverse axis into flexion (Fig. 25-22). Paired lateral bones move into external rotation. During extension, opposite motions occur (Fig. 25-23). All motions are subtle.

Occiput. In flexion, the occiput rotates about a transverse axis directly above the foramen magnum at the level of the confluence of sinuses. As it rotates, the basilar part and the condyles move anteriorly and superiorly, directly influencing the

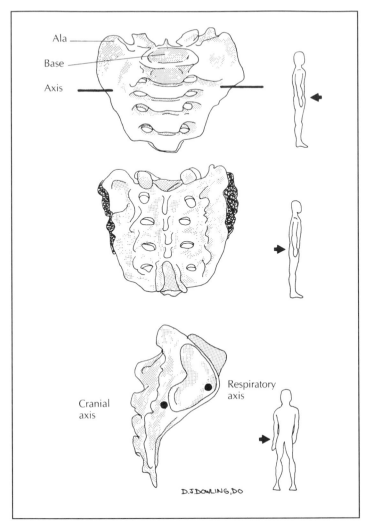

Ala

Base

Axis

Cranial
axis

Respiratory
axis

D.J.DOWLING, DO

Figure 25-21. Axes of sacral motion.

temporal bones, and the squama moves posteriorly and slightly laterally. The greatest lateral deviation occurs at the lateral angles.

Sphenoid. The sphenoid rotates on a transverse axis through the center of its body at the level of the floor of the sella turcica. The greater wings move forward, slightly laterally, and inferiorly, influencing the lateral edges of the frontal bone anteriorly and laterally. The pterygoid processes move posteriorly and slightly laterally.

Temporal bone. The temporal bone externally rotates around an axis running from the jugular surface to the petrous apex. This approximates a line running through the petrous portion along its long axis. The squamous portion and zygomatic arch move anteriorly, laterally, and inferiorly; the mastoid moves medially, superiorly, and slightly posteriorly; and the top of the petrous portion rotates laterally and slightly superiorly. The motion of the temporals has been likened to a wobbly wheel.

Parietal bones. The inferior surface of the parietal bone moves laterally around an axis connecting the anterior and posterior bevel changes (on the coronal and lambdoidal sutures). The posterior surface moves more laterally than the anterior surface.

Ethmoid. Influenced by the sphenoid and falx cerebri, the ethmoid rotates about a transverse axis through the middle of the bone, in the same direc-

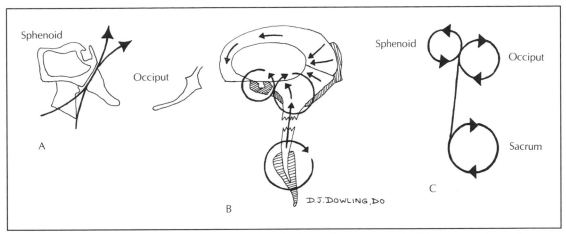

Figure 25-22. PRM, flexion phase. (A) Relationship of sphenoid to occiput. (B) Effects on reciprocal tension membrane system. (C) Direction of force in flexion.

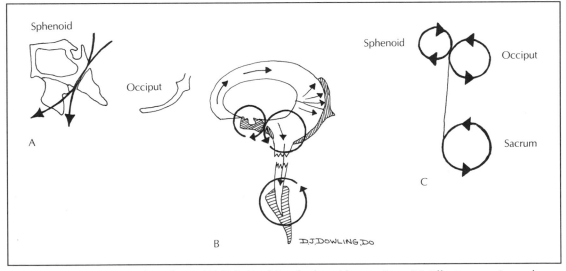

Figure 25-23. PRM, extension phase. (A) Relationship of sphenoid to occiput. (B) Effects on reciprocal tension membrane system. (C) Direction of force in extension.

tion as the occiput. The lateral masses move as paired bones into external rotation.

Frontal bone. The frontal bone acts as paired bones do, rotating externally under the influence of the sphenoid. The axis of rotation runs from the frontal eminence through the center of the orbital plate. The inferior lateral angles move laterally and anteriorly. The glabella recedes slightly under the influence of the falx.

Sacrum. Pulled by dura, the sacral base moves posteriorly and the apex moves anteriorly about a transverse axis through the second sacral segment.

TORSION
Cranial torsion is a rotation of the sphenobasilar symphysis along an anteroposterior axis (Fig. 25-24). The sphenoid and occiput rotate in opposite directions. The axis runs from nasion to opisthion.

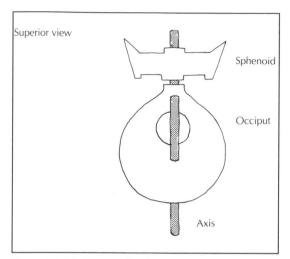

Figure 25-24. Torsional axis.

The torsion is named for the side of the high wing of the sphenoid (Figs. 25-25, 25-26).

The following changes take place in the other bones and the membranes.

Figure 25-25. Right torsion.

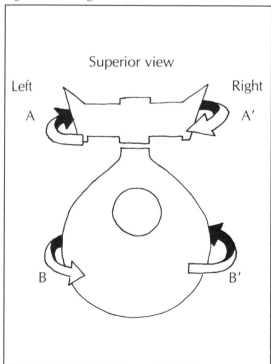

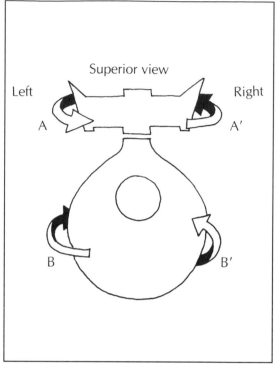

Figure 25-26. Left torsion.

1. **Temporal bone:** relative external rotation on the side of the torsion.
2. **Parietal bone:** relative external rotation on the side of the torsion.
3. **Mandible:** shifted toward the side of the torsion.
4. **Orbit:** smaller on the side of the torsion.
5. **Membranes:**
   a. Falx cerebri: also torsioned, with the anterior end twisting in the same direction the sphenoid rotates, and the posterior end twisting in the same direction the occiput rotates.
   b. Tentorium cerebelli: The tentorium is side-bent in the same direction as the occiput rotates.
   c. Spinal dura: relaxed on the side of the low occiput, allowing the sacral base on that side to move inferiorly.

Side-Bending and Rotation
Side-bending and rotation are two separate motions of the sphenobasilar symphysis that occur simultaneously (Fig. 25-27). Side-bending occurs by rotation around two vertical axes, one through the center of the body of the sphenoid and the

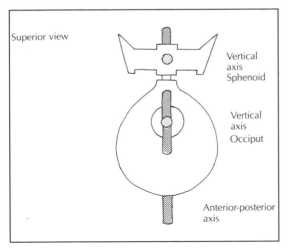

Figure 25-27. Side-bending and rotation axes.

other through the center of the foramen magnum (Figs. 25-28, 25-29). The sphenoid and occiput rotate in opposite directions on these axes, causing the side-bending.

Rotation occurs on the same axis as torsion; however, the sphenoid and occiput rotate in the same direction. Rotation occurs toward the side of the convexity (convexity is lowered).

The following motions occur in the other bones and membranes:

1. **Temporal bones:** externally rotated on the convex side.
2. **Parietal bones:** externally rotated on the convex side.
3. **Mandible:** shifted to the convex side.
4. **Frontal bone:** anterior on convex side.
5. **Orbit:** anterior on convex side.
6. **Membranes:**
   a. Falx cerebri: side-bent, following the convexity of the side-bending of the sphenobasilar symphysis.
   b. Tentorium: follows occipital motion.
   c. Spinal dura: inferior on the side of the convexity (low occiput), dropping the sacral base on that side.

Strains

Strains are nonphysiologic dysfunctions and are usually induced traumatically. There are vertical

Figure 25-28. Right side-bending and rotation.

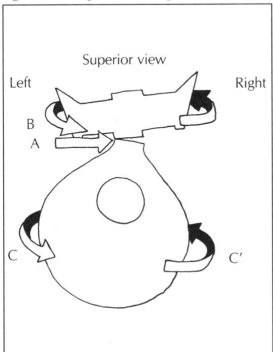

Figure 25-29. Left side-bending and rotation.

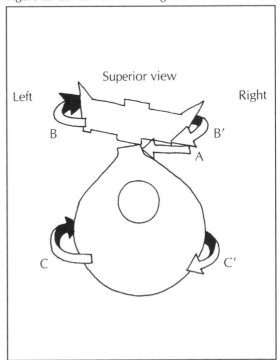

and lateral strains. They are discussed in the section on diagnosis and treatment.

DIAGNOSIS AND TREATMENT

The diagnosis and treatment of the primary respiratory mechanism involves more than simply reducing cranial strains. Dysfunction may exist in any of the five phenomena. Diagnostic skill must be developed to distinguish whether the dysfunction is in fluid, membrane, bone, and/or the nervous system. Dysfunctions in different aspects of the primary respiratory mechanism may create similar-appearing motion changes in the cranium but require significantly different treatment.

In diagnosis and in treatment a light touch and gentle handling are essential. Magoun states, "To employ other than skillful and delicate sense perception is to lose the shades of physiological reaction so necessary for success. Living cells prefer persuasion to force, consideration to trauma, intelligence to ill-expended energy. *One must work with the tissues, not against them.*"

Diagnosis

History and observation are primary tools used in diagnosis. A history of trauma is important. The direction and amount of force of the trauma should be noted. Observation will disclose general tendencies as well as asymmetries. Photographs of the individual taken before the traumatic incident are helpful for comparison. Asymmetry may represent a functionally normal anatomic variant. Functional and dysfunctional asymmetries should be distinguished.

Palpation and perception are the most important tools for osteopathic diagnosis. Before starting, the patient should be warm, relaxed, and comfortable. The operator must also be comfortable, with forearms supported. The motions being palpated are small, and operator tension may block or confuse signals coming from the palpating fingers.

Diagnosis can be made by passive observation or by motion testing. Observation can reveal any dysfunctional patterns that may be present during the phases of the primary respiratory mechanism. This diagnostic information may also be obtained by testing for motion. Whenever possible, motion should be initiated when the primary respiratory mechanism begins the phase closest to the motion being tested. Motion is initiated slowly and gently. When a response is observed, the practitioner sim-

ply follows the motion as the inherent forces carry it to its limit.

Treatment

Three common principles used to treat dysfunctions are indirect, direct, and disengagement. Molding and opposite physiologic motion are other approaches to treatment that will not be described in this chapter.

1. **Indirect (exaggeration):** The dysfunction is moved in the direction opposite the restriction, toward the freedom of motion. It is the direction in which the point of balanced membranous tension is usually found.
2. **Direct:** The dysfunction is moved in the direction of the restriction to the motion barrier. Gentle encouragement is maintained against the restrictive barrier until release occurs.
3. **Disengagement:** The articulation is separated. Traction or compression may be necessary for disengagement, according to the anatomy of the articulation involved.

Two additional forces may be used to enhance the treatment:

1. **Directing the tide:** The practitioner places a finger at a spot on the skull at the greatest contralateral diameter from the restriction. This will be described in the next section.
2. **Respiratory assist:** Inhalation accentuates flexion and external rotation, and exhalation accentuates extension and internal rotation. If treatment requires positioning in flexion, deep inhalation may aid in release. Treatment may use a series of deep breaths, or the practitioner may ask the patient to hold his or her breath in inhalation. Exhalation may be used for positioning in extension in the same manner.

Techniques to Alter the Pattern of Fluid Fluctuation

COMPRESSION OF THE FOURTH VENTRICLE (CV-4)

This technique is commonly called the CV-4 technique because its effects are postulated to be due to compression of the fourth ventricle, which lies anterior to the occipital squama. It is one of the most useful of all cranial techniques.

The technique has been used successfully to relieve headaches, reduce fever, assist in difficult labor, relieve congested sinuses and lungs, and reduce edema. It can also be used to reduce trauma, such as a whiplash injury, or even the trauma of noncranial manipulative treatment.

One way to perform the CV-4 is for the practitioner to place her thenar eminences on the occipital squama, below the superior nuchal line. The hands must not be on the temporal bone or the occipitomastoid (O-M) suture, since this will create dysfunctions. The O-M suture should be palpated before the hands are placed. Then the practitioner interlocks her fingers or overlaps her hands underneath.

The practitioner begins by monitoring the primary respiratory mechanism through several cycles. The mechanism is then followed into the exhalation phase, with the practitioner gently resisting its motion toward the inhalation phase.

After a time the fluid flux will slow to a still point, during which no flux will be palpable. At this point the practitioner may notice warmth in her palms or sweat on the patient's forehead, and the patient's breathing may change. To finish, the practitioner maintains her hand position, applying no pressure, until she feels the primary respiratory mechanism return, slowly, to full force. This may take from 15 seconds to several minutes. This signifies the end of the treatment. In cases of acute head trauma or tenderness, this technique may be applied to the sacrum, with extension encouraged by directing the base anteriorly, resisting flexion.

VENOUS SINUS DRAINAGE

This nontraumatic technique may increase venous drainage. Before treatment is initiated, the thoracic outlet, cervical, and O-A dysfunctions must be mobilized to allow drainage into the thoracic cavity.

Step 1. The physician places four fingers across the superior nuchal line, pointed directly anteriorly toward the patient's face. This position is maintained with slight pressure (usually the weight of the head will suffice) until release or an apparent softening of the bone is felt beneath the fingers. This release is followed, to maintain balance of tension, until both sides release (this may take several minutes). This step promotes drainage of the transverse sinus.

Step 2. To promote drainage of the confluence of sinuses, one finger is placed on the inion with the hands cradling the back of the head. The same procedure is followed until a "softening" response is felt.

Step 3. To promote drainage of the superior sagittal sinus, the sagittal suture may be spread by moving superiorly and anteriorly from the lambda with two crossed thumbs on either side of the suture, disengaging the suture. Wait for release, then work up the suture, one thumb at a time, toward the bregma.

Continue anteriorly on the frontal bone with fingers lined up along both sides of the midline until a response is felt.

V-SPREAD

V-spread is a combination of disengagement and directing the tide. The physician places two fingers of one hand on either side of the suture to be released and exerts gentle traction to disengage the suture. Simultaneously, she places one or two fingers on the point of greatest distance from the suture on the contralateral side. Gentle pressure with these fingers will send a fluid wave toward that suture. This wave should be palpated by the V-spread fingers within a few seconds and will continue between the two hands. The physician adjusts the directing fingers until the pulse is palpated between the two V-spread fingers. Release or an apparent softening of the tissues will occur.

LATERAL FLUCTUATION

Lateral fluctuation is a general palliative technique. It is useful in calming patients after traumatic or other stressful situations. A lateral fluctuation may be initiated with a bilateral temporal hold, the thumbs over the anterior aspects of the mastoid processes and the fingers cupping the occipital squama. Motion is initiated by directing one temporal bone toward external rotation and the other toward internal rotation, shifting fluid toward the side of external rotation. Attention is placed on the shifting fluid, not the rotation of bone. Motion should be followed gently to its endpoint, then initiated in the opposite direction, again focusing on the shift of the fluid. Repeat this process until the fluid shifts persist without assistance. At this point, allow the fluctuation to continue, resisting each phase gently until a still point is reached. The treatment is complete when the primary respiratory mechanism has resumed.

Somatic Dysfunction Diagnosis and Treatment

Dysfunctions of the sphenobasilar junction and the temporal, frontal, and parietal bones will be discussed. Dysfunctions of the facial bones, although relevant to complete cranial diagnosis and treatment, are beyond the scope of this chapter.

SPHENOBASILAR JUNCTION

The sphenobasilar junction is the point around which diagnostic motion patterns are described. These general patterns represent the adaptation of the cranium to strain. The strain may be the result of dysfunction anywhere in the body. Cranial treatment is most effective when it is part of a complete osteopathic treatment plan.

Sphenobasilar diagnosis may be accomplished by either observation of motion patterns or by the perceived response to initiation of motion. To observe or motion-test for sphenobasilar patterns, the clinician may use either the vault hold or the fronto-occipital hold; both holds are described for each pattern. Always palpate gently for cranial motion as described earlier for general finding before undertaking specific motion testing.

1. **Vault hold.** The physician places his hands on either side of the head with the thumbs touching each other just behind the sagittal suture (they should not be touching the patient's head). The index fingers contact the greater wings of the sphenoid, the little fingers contact the occiput, and the middle two fingers contact the temporal and parietal bones (one on each side of the ear). The finger pads, not the tips are used. The entire finger and palm of the hand should contact the head.
2. **Fronto-occipital hold.** The physician places one hand under the patient's head, cupping the occipital squama. The other hand is placed across the forehead so that the thumb and index or middle finger of that hand contact the greater wings laterally. The entire hand, not just the finger pads, should contact the patient's head.

FLEXION AND EXTENSION

Although flexion and extension are the normal physiologic motion present, they may be restricted in one direction. This dysfunction may occur without other associated nonphysiologic dysfunctions.

Table 25-1. Findings in a Flexion or Extension Dysfunction of the Sphenobasilar Symphysis

Parameter Evaluated	Flexion Dysfunction	Extension Dysfunction
Restricted motion	Extension	Flexion
Head diameter	Increased in transverse dimension	Increased in longitudinal dimension
Forehead	Wide and sloping	Vertical
Eyes	Prominent	Receded
Paired bones	Externally rotated	Internally rotated
Ears	Protruding	Close to head

General Findings and Observations
The general findings of a flexion or extension dysfunction are listed in Table 25-1.

Palpation for Motion
Do not encourage motion out of phase with the primary respiratory mechanism.

1. **Vault hold.** The physician places his hands in the vault hold. Flexion is initiated by directing both the greater wing of the sphenoid and the occipital squama inferiorly. Both hands move symmetrically caudad and expand laterally. Motion is initiated at the beginning of physiologic flexion and followed until resistance is met. This is the limit of flexion. Extension involves an opposite set of maneuvers: the hands (index finger and fifth finger) move cephalad and medially until resistance is met.
2. **Fronto-occipital hold.** The physician positions his hands in the fronto-occipital hold. To test flexion, he rotates the greater wings anteriorly and inferiorly and simultaneously rotates the occipital squama inferiorly and anteriorly. These motions are reversed to evaluate extension.

Dysfunction Correction
Indirect or exaggeration techniques may be used to correct cranial dysfunction patterns. The same holds and motions are used as were described for motion testing. Flexion is encouraged for a flexion dysfunction (extension restriction); extension is encouraged for an extension dysfunction (flexion

Table 25-2. Findings in Torsion Dysfunction of the Sphenobasilar Symphysis

Parameter Evaluated	Side of High Sphenoid Wing	Side of Low Sphenoid Wing
Frontal lateral angle	Anterior	Posterior
Orbit	Wide	Narrow
Frontozygomatic angle	Increased	Lessened
Eyeball	Protruded	Retruded
Zygomatic orbital rim	Everted and externally rotated	Inverted and internally rotated
Symphysis menti	To this side	Away from this side
Mastoid tip	Posteromedial	Anterolateral
Ear	Protruding	Close to head

restriction). However, instead of moving the joint to its limit of motion, the movement is stopped at the point of balanced membranous tension. The correction is then made by the inherent forces. If this alone does not correct the dysfunction, two assistive forces may be used:

1. **Directing the tide.** This force is called on by the physician placing a finger directly on the vertex. The technique is easiest with the vault hold, where the thumbs are over the point of contact. With the fronto-occipital hold, the index finger on the frontal side may be stretched to this point. Fluid is directed to the sphenobasilar symphysis.
2. **Respiratory assist.** For a flexion dysfunction, the patient is asked to inhale and hold the breath for as long as possible. For an extension dysfunction, the patient is asked to exhale and hold for as long as possible.

TORSION

The reader should review the motion pattern described earlier. On one side the sphenoid wing is high and the occiput low, as rotation occurs about an anteroposterior axis.

General Findings and Observation

The side of the high sphenoid wing (and low occiput) is in relative external rotation. The side of the

low sphenoid wing and high occiput is in relative internal rotation. Table 25-2 lists the important findings.

Palpation for Motion

1. **Vault hold.** Test motion by symmetrically rotating each hand in opposite directions around a horizontal axis.
2. **Fronto-occipital hold.** The frontal hand elevates one greater wing. The occipital hand lowers the occipital squama on the same side.

Dysfunction Correction

The sphenobasilar symphysis is moved into free motion until the point of balanced membranous tension is reached. This position is held until release occurs. Directing fluid from the vertex to the symphysis may help. Having the patient inhale fully and holding for as long as possible may also encourage release. The range of motion is then rechecked.

SIDE-BENDING AND ROTATION

Side-bending and rotation dysfunctions are named for the convexity of the side-bending motion. The dysfunction was described previously.

General Findings and Observation

In side-bending and rotation dysfunctions, one side of the head is relatively convex, the other relatively flat. Table 25-3 lists the important findings.

Table 25-3. Findings in Side-Bending and Rotation Dysfunctions of the Sphenobasilar Symphysis

Landmark	Convexity	Concavity
Lateral frontal angle	Posterior	Anterior
Orbit	Narrow	Wide
Frontozygomatic angle	Lessened	Increased
Eyeball	Retruded	Protruded
Zygomatic orbital rim	Prominent	Flat
Symphysis menti	To this side	Away from this side
Mastoid tip	Posteromedial	Anterolateral
Mastoid portion	Anterolateral	Posteromedial
Ear	Protruding	Close to head

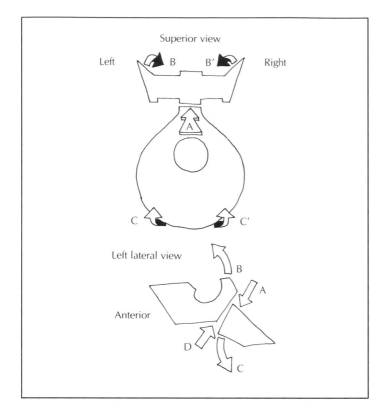

Figure 25-30. Superior strain.

Palpation for Motion
1. **Vault hold**. The physician approximates the fingers of one hand while simultaneously lifting cephalad. The fingers on the opposite hand are spread and moved caudad.
2. **Fronto-occipital hold.** Side-bending is initiated first by approximating the fingers of both hands. Then rotation, which occurs automatically, can be assisted by rotating the hands about a vertical axis.

Dysfunction Correction
The motion is brought to its freest position, the point of balanced membrane tension. Directing fluid from vertex will assist, as will the patient's respiratory assistance.

STRAINS
Strains are serious dysfunctions and are almost always traumatically induced. There are two types of strains, vertical strains and lateral strains. Each is discussed separately.

Vertical Strains
Vertical strains are named according to the position of the basisphenoid. It can move superiorly or inferiorly, creating superior and inferior vertical strains.

General findings and observation. A vertical strain is flexion of the sphenoid accompanied by extension of the occiput, or extension of the sphenoid with flexion of the occiput. Side-to-side findings are symmetrical. Evidence of the anterior quadrants in external rotation would indicate a superior vertical strain (Fig. 25-30); if they are in internal rotation, there is inferior strain (Fig. 25-31).

Palpation for motion
1. **Vault hold.** To test for superior vertical strain, the physician rotates both hands forward, carrying the greater wings into flexion and the occiput into extension. These motions are reversed to test for inferior vertical strain.
2. **Fronto-occipital hold.** To test for superior vertical strain, the physician moves the frontal hand caudad, influencing the sphenoid toward flexion, and simultaneously moves the occipital hand cephalad, influencing the occiput toward

Figure 25-31. Inferior strain.

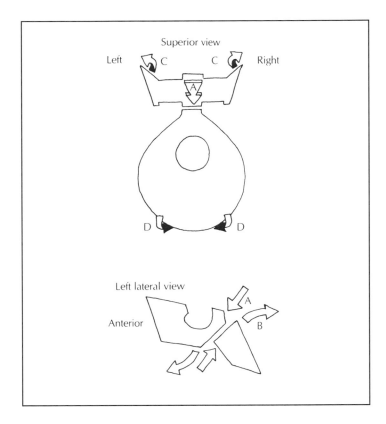

extension. The directions of each hand are reversed to test for inferior vertical strain.

Dysfunction correction. This dysfunction is corrected in the same manner as other dysfunctions of the sphenobasilar symphysis. The physician finds the point of balanced membrane tension and holds it, directing fluid from the vertex.

Lateral Strain

A lateral strain is a side-to-side shearing of the sphenobasilar symphysis (Fig. 25-32). It is usually caused by trauma lateral to one side of the anterior cranium or the opposite posterior cranium (anterior or posterior to the sphenobasilar symphysis) (Figs. 25-33, 25-34).

General findings and observation. Both bones rotate on a vertical axis in the same direction. The head may take on the appearance of a parallelogram (especially noticeable in infants). Regardless of age, side-to-side findings will not be symmetric.

Palpation for motion

1. **Vault hold.** To test for lateral strain, the physician directs the sphenoid laterally in one direction with his index fingers while directing the occiput in the opposite direction with the fifth fingers.

2. **Fronto-occipital hold.** The physician directs the sphenoid laterally in one direction with the frontal hand and directs the occiput in the opposite direction with the occipital hand.

Figure 25-32. Lateral strain axes.

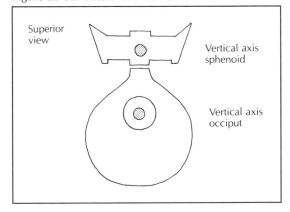

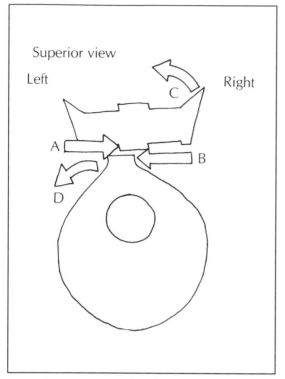

Figure 25-33. Left lateral strain.

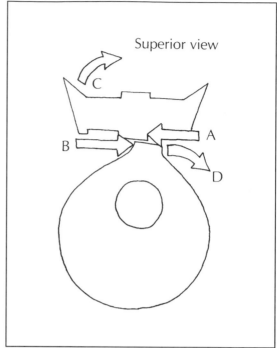

Figure 25-34. Right lateral strain.

Dysfunction correction. The physician finds the point of balanced membrane tension (toward the freedom of motion), then assists by directing fluid from the vertex or by using the patient's respiratory assistance.

COMPRESSION OF THE SPHENOBASILAR SYMPHYSIS
This dysfunction occurs as a result of pressure or trauma to the front of the head or face, to the back of the head, or to the entire periphery (i.e., compression of the infant cranium during a difficult birth) (Fig. 25-35).

General Findings and Observation
This dysfunction manifests as a restriction (mild, moderate, or severe) of all motions at the sphenobasilar symphysis. With severe compression, the cranium feels rigid.

Motion Testing
Any hold may be used. The dysfunction is recognized as the practitioner tests for all motion pat-terns and becomes aware of limited or absent motion in the sphenobasilar symphysis.

Dysfunction Correction
Correction of this dysfunction is difficult, often requiring more than one practitioner. The technique will not be described here.

Conclusion
This chapter has been an introduction to osteopathic cranial concepts. This overview of the anatomy and the basic principles of the primary respiratory mechanism should be used as a steppingstone to further studies of this subject matter. In addition, individualized palpatory training is a central aspect of the study of osteopathy.

The student is encouraged to study *Teachings in the Science of Osteopathy* by William G. Sutherland and *Osteopathy in the Cranial Field* by Harold I. Magoun.

Dr. Sutherland considered the cranial concept a direct extension of the osteopathic concept of

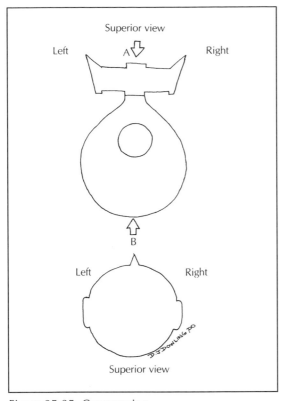

Figure 25-35. Compression.

Dr. Still. It is not a separate field of study, nor is it a technique. The cranium and the primary respiratory mechanism should be evaluated and treated as part of a total osteopathic plan for any patient. The application of the cranial concept is as broad as the scope of osteopathy.

26

Osteopathic Manipulative Treatment: Contraindications, Precautions, and Side Effects

EILEEN L. DiGIOVANNA

Although osteopathic manipulation is a highly effective treatment for many conditions and a useful adjunct in the treatment of others, certain precautions, contraindications, and side effects must be taken into consideration when formulating a treatment plan. Because of the wide variety of techniques available to osteopathic physicians, there is no absolute contraindication to at least some form of manipulation in any given patient or condition as long as the patient's condition is stable and motion is permitted.

Before any form of manipulation is begun, a careful medical history and physical examination of the patient should be done and a differential diagnosis considered with a working diagnosis established. After this evaluation is completed, a treatment plan should be devised consistent with the patient's needs. Just as medication should not be prescribed without a thorough knowledge of the patient's history and physical status, neither should manipulation be done solely on the basis of the chief complaint.

Manipulation has proven to be not only effective, but quite safe. Since manipulation is practiced not only by D.O.'s but also by many M.D.'s, chiropractors, physical therapists, and others involved in manual medicine, it is obvious that millions of such treatments are given annually to patients with but few complications reported in the literature.

Thrusting Techniques

Most of the severe iatrogenic complications reported as a result of manipulation are related to thrusting techniques. According to reports in the literature, most have resulted from chiropractic manipulation and have involved the upper cervical spine. Complications include neurovascular accidents, aggravation of disk syndromes, and fractures. Missed diagnoses contributed significantly to complications, emphasizing the need for careful patient evaluation.

Physician-related problems include lack of skill, diagnostic error, and the use of inappropriate force. Patient-related problems include abnormal bony structure, pathologic entities, intolerance of head motion leading to vertigo, and psychological intolerance of manipulation.

Perhaps the most significant complication reported is vertebrobasilar accident with rotary cervical manipulation, such as reported by Gittinger. In some persons, rotation and extension of the cer-

An Osteopathic Approach to Diagnosis and Treatment, second edition
Eileen L. DiGiovanna and Stanley Schiowitz
Lippincott Raven Publishers, Philadelphia © 1997.

vical spine cause narrowing of the vertebral artery on the side opposite the rotation. Pre-existent compromise of cranial collaterals, such as the carotids, must be considered. Occipital infarction may result, with various neurologic sequelae. Some considerations when using cervical high-velocity, low-amplitude techniques include preventing extreme extension, carrying the head out of the midline, using minimal to no rotation, and testing the patient's tolerance by rotating the patient's head for 30 seconds while watching for nystagmus, nausea, or dizziness.

One of the more common side effects of cervical HVLA appears to be vertigo. Although this may indicate impending vascular problems, in most cases it is of positional origin. Contraindications to thrusting techniques likely include the acute phase of rheumatoid arthritis, osteoporosis, bone cancers, fractures, atherosclerotic plaques, and cervical spondylosis with vertebral artery ischemia. Care should be exercised in treating patients with radicular pain from herniated disks, pregnant women, or patients with acute whiplash, Scheuermann's disease, and postsurgical conditions. Patients on anticoagulant therapy should be treated with great caution.

Muscle Energy Treatment

Muscle energy treatment is quite safe. Occasionally some muscle stiffness and soreness occur after the treatment. If the area being treated is not localized well or if too much contractive force is used, pain may be increased.

Sometimes the patient is in too much pain to contract a muscle, or for some reason is unable to cooperate with the physician's instructions or positioning. In such instances muscle energy treatment may be difficult to apply.

Some complications reported as a result of muscle energy treatment include aggravation of herniated disk syndrome, increased pain, costochondral separation, neurovascular accident, and fractures.

Counterstrain Techniques

Counterstrain is one of the safest of the techniques because it is purely positional and no force is generated by the patient or physician. Patients do need to be warned that they may feel sore after a treatment, because this is a common side effect.

Muscle spasm, aggravation of herniated disk syndrome, dizziness, and fracture have all been reported as resulting from counterstrain.

Facilitated Positional Release (FPR)

Although FPR is a positional technique, some facilitating force is used. FPR with a compressive force should not be used in radiculopathy of the cervical spine. Aggravation of herniated disk syndrome and fractures have been reported with this technique.

Myofascial Release

Perhaps the gentlest of all the techniques when done in an indirect manner, this still has some complications and side effects to be aware of. Aggravation of disk symptoms and muscle spasm are perhaps the most common. Headaches, increased pain, and costochondral separation have been reported.

Cranial Treatment

These techniques are generally nontraumatic; however, they may have the farthest-reaching effects when complications and side effects do occur.

Fatigue and lethargy are the most common side effects. Nausea, vomiting, headache, dizziness, and loss of appetite are seen. The most serious complication the author has heard of is hypopituitarism following an intraoral technique that was a reversible problem. Emotional release, which may occur with any type of manipulation, most commonly occurs with cranial treatment, and the physician needs to be prepared to deal with this situation.

Eclectic Manipulation

Mastery of the multiple techniques of manipulative treatment will help the clinician determine and apply the most appropriate treatment in each patient. An analogy can be drawn with prescribing drugs: the more one knows about medications, their interactions, and their effects, the better one can tailor treatment to the individual case. Similarly, the more manipulative techniques the clinician knows, the more safely and effectively he or she can use them. Each patient and each physician are different. The manipulative procedures used should reflect these differences.

References

Bourdillon JF. 1982. Spinal Manipulation, 3rd ed. Norwalk, Conn: Appleton-Century-Crofts.

Brownson RJ, et al. 1986. Sudden sensorineural hearing loss following manipulation of the cervical spine. Laryngoscope 96:166–170.

DiGiovanna EL, Banihashem M, et al. 1996. Survey of American Academy of Osteopathy. unpublished.

Gittinger JW. 1986. Occipital infarction following chiropractic cervical manipulation. J Clin Neuroophthalmol 6:11–13.

Grayson MF. 1987. Horner's syndrome after manipulation of the neck. Br Med J 295:6610:1381–1382.

Hoag JM, Cole WV, Bradford SG. 1969. Osteopathic Medicine. New York: McGraw-Hill.

Laughlin TM. 1987. Complications of spinal manipulation: a literature review 1975–1984. Osteopath Ann 14 (1):21–23.

Maitland GD. 1977. Vertebral Manipulation, 4th ed. Stoneham, Mass: Butterworths.

27

Practical Applications of Osteopathic Manipulative Treatment

WHIPLASH INJURIES
Donald E. Phykitt

"Whiplash" is commonly used to describe an injury caused by acute hyperextension-hyperflexion of the cervical spine. Motor vehicle accidents account for a significant proportion of such injuries. The victims commonly are passengers in a stationary or slowly moving vehicle that is struck from behind, or passengers in a moving vehicle that strikes an immovable object (deceleration injury). Tissue damage and injury can occur when the offending vehicle is moving as slowly as 7 miles per hour.

Whiplash injuries are more accurately described as inertial injuries, since they result from a discrepancy between the inertia (resistance to movement) of the head and the momentum (tendency to keep moving) of the trunk. Inertia and momentum meet in the highly mobile cervical spine; for this reason, considerable research has focused on cervical injury.

Osteopathic medicine, however, regards whiplash as an insult to the entire body, including the pelvis, spine, and cranium and their connecting soft tissues (fascia, tendons, ligaments, muscles). This insult results in both local and distant reflexes that affect every organ system in the body. Heilig in 1963 aptly summarized the situation:

"Whiplash" describes the mechanism of a whole series of vertebral and paravertebral injuries. It is not a typical syndrome, nor any particular injury. It is characterized only by the fact that damage has occurred to tissues as a result of forces of inertia and their effect on contiguous or connecting tissues and not because of external contact of the injured area.

Evaluation of the whiplash patient includes a complete history and physical examination. Special attention should be given to neurologic deficits, structural deviations, primary and compensatory somatic dysfunctions (cervical, thoracic, lumbar, sacral, cranial), and areas of sympathetic hyperactivity. The clinician should attempt to reconstruct the events of the accident and to uncover any predisposing structural or medical conditions.

Treatment is individualized for each patient. It will include osteopathic manipulative treatment, exercise, thermal and physical modalities, pharmacologic therapy, and emotional support.

Mechanism of Injury
Three theories are commonly proposed to explain the mechanism of injury in whiplash. All three

An Osteopathic Approach to Diagnosis and Treatment, second edition
Eileen L. DiGiovanna and Stanley Schiowitz
Lippincott–Raven Publishers, Philadelphia © 1997.

recognize that the impact producing whiplash propels the body in a linear horizontal direction. Because of inertia, the head momentarily remains in its original position. It then abruptly moves in the direction opposite the impact force vector. Cessation of the impact, along with an acute stretch reflex of the neck muscles, causes the head to recoil in the same direction as the initial impact force vector.

For example, if a stopped car is struck from behind, the driver's body is propelled forward. After a brief pause the head moves backward into hyperextension, damaging the soft tissues on the anterior aspect of the neck. The head then recoils forward into hyperflexion, damaging the soft tissues in the posterior cervical region. Both motions can cause vertebral injuries as well.

The three theories on causation differ, however, with respect to the exact paths followed by the head and neck during the hyperextension and hyperflexion, and with respect to the forces that result in vertebral injury. According to the most widely held theory, the head follows an arc above the shoulders, and damage results from rapid tissue stretch secondary to traction, hyperflexion, and hyperextension.

A second theory, proposed by McKeever, contends that the injurious force results from horizontal translation of the body with respect to the head. McKeever postulates that the head remains at the same horizontal level throughout the injury (i.e., it does not follow an arc). Thus there is shortening of the neck with resultant severe compression when the head is directly above the shoulders. These compressive forces result in avulsion injuries of vertebral structures.

A third theory agrees that the cervical vertebrae are compressed. However, it postulates the concomitant presence of torques at the level of C1 and C7. It proposes that horizontal translation of the body is accompanied by an extension torque of the head at C1 and a flexion torque of the trunk at C7. Accordingly, the most severe injury is thought to occur in the midcervical region.

It is most likely that the actual mechanism of injury combines elements of all three theories. Most investigators believe that hyperextension causes greater injury than hyperflexion, for the following reasons:

1. The original force (usually directed from behind) most often comes as a surprise, giving the

victim less chance to prepare by tightening his muscles.
2. Flexion is restricted by the impact of the chin on the chest. This motion is within the physiologic and anatomic limits of cervical motion.
3. However, nothing restricts extension until the occiput strikes the back of the seat. This motion is well beyond the anatomic barriers to motion and soft tissue and osseous injury can occur.

Pathophysiology

Regardless of the mechanism of injury in whiplash, the damage caused to the cervical tissues remains the same. Tissue and structural injury in the cervical spine will be discussed in reference to the superficial soft tissues, the vertebral complex (vertebrae, ligaments, tendons), the peripheral and sympathetic nervous systems, the vascular system, and the cerebrum.

SUPERFICIAL SOFT TISSUE
Hyperextension
Abrupt elongation of relaxed, unprepared muscles initiates an acute stretch reflex. Rear-end acceleration accidents result in hyperextension of the cervical spine with concomitant stretching of the neck flexors. Similarly, hyperflexion during deceleration accidents is accompanied by stretching of the extensor muscles.

When a muscle is stretched acutely, most of the stretch is sustained by the intrafusal muscle fibers of the muscle spindles, which normally monitor muscle length. Abrupt, forceful elongation of the muscle initiates a neural reflex and results in a proportionately stronger contraction of that muscle. The reflex does not cause the subsequent spasm directly but contributes strongly to the recoil of the neck after the initial hyperflexion or hyperextension.

If the degree of stretch is sufficient, the fibrils of the extrafusal fibers (contractile elements of the muscle) will tear. The gross muscle is not injured, so there is usually no gross hemorrhage or edema. And because major nerves are not initially involved, there may be no immediate pain, paresthesia, or paresis. Severe injury, however, can cause nerve damage and gross bleeding.

Edema and microhemorrhage can serve as foci of muscle irritability, resulting in painful muscle spasm. Sustained contraction inhibits motion and impedes circulation, resulting in the buildup of metabolites, notably lactic acid. This compounds the muscle hyperirritability. The final result is fibrous contracture, trigger point formation, and chronic pain and immobility.

Hyperextension results in damage to the anterior cervical muscles. Minor injury may only traumatize the sternocleidomastoid muscle. However, this can lead to pain and trigger point formation along the whole muscle, especially at the origin, and can result in the head tilt and painful torticollis experienced by many patients.

More severe hyperextension damages the deeper neck flexors, notably the scalenes and longissimus colli. Severe hyperextension is often accompanied by stretching and subsequent edema of the pharynx and esophagus. Retropharyngeal hematoma can develop, causing dysphagia and pain on swallowing soon after an accident.

The prevertebral fascia of the anterior neck is continuous with the fascia of the mediastinum, which in turn is continuous with the crura of the diaphragm and the fascia surrounding the psoas major muscles. Thus, hyperextension can set up fascial strain patterns that can contribute to dysfunction in the thorax, abdomen, pelvis, and even the lower extremities.

Hyperflexion

Hyperflexion injuries cause less severe damage than hyperextension injuries but still contribute greatly to a patient's symptoms and incapacitation, for the following reasons:

1. The musculature of the posterior neck is both intricate and widespread. It includes the intrinsic muscles (e.g., the multifid and rotator muscles) as well as the extensive paravertebral muscles and the muscles of the shoulder girdle (the levator scapulae, rhomboid, and trapezius muscles). Moreover, numerous muscles attach to the occipital and suboccipital joints. These joints are highly mobile and consequently highly susceptible to injury. From these anatomic relationships, it can be understood why patients often complain of cervical pain radiating up to the occiput and down to both shoulders and the midthoracic region.

2. The posterior neck is richly innervated by afferent fibers. Not only do these fibers travel to the muscles, but they also pierce the muscles on their way to innervating the skin of the posterior neck and scalp. Muscle spasm and waste buildup irritate the nerves. Such irritation of the occipital nerves (sensory for the scalp) causes much of the cephalgia reported.

VERTEBRAL COMPLEX

When muscles are elongated beyond their physiologic limits, tendons, ligaments, and articular capsules are stretched or torn. Vertebral subluxations or fractures can result.

Hyperextension is accompanied by posterior translation of a vertebra on the one below it. It may also involve traction on the anterior portion of the vertebral body and compression of the posterior articulation, with these consequences:

1. Anterior traction can result in strain or even tearing of the anterior longitudinal ligament and annulus fibrosis, with hemorrhage and edema.
2. Posterior compression can lead to fractures of the vertebral body or the spinous process.
3. Posterior glide causes facet encroachment onto the intervertebral foramen, with possible impingement on the nerve root.
4. Posterior translation accompanied by posterior compression can lead to acute facet impingement.

Hyperflexion is accompanied by anterior translation of a vertebra on the one below it. It may also include anterior compression and posterior traction, with the following consequences:

1. Anterior compression can cause fracture of the vertebral body.
2. Posterior traction can result in sprain or tearing of the supraspinal ligaments, interspinal ligaments, or posterior longitudinal ligaments.
3. Anterior glide can cause capsular tears of the articulation with or without facet subluxation or dislocation. This translation is also associated with foraminal narrowing and possible nerve root impingement.
4. Rarely, hyperflexion can cause posterior disk herniation. This injury is most often associated with rotational forces or horizontal shear forces at the time of impact.

Strains, sprains, and tears of the muscles, ligaments, tendons, and capsules can all contribute to myofascial pain reflexes. They cause alterations in the function of bony articulations. They also lead to gross, usually palpable restrictions of vertebral motion.

After the acute injury, scar tissue forms in the overstretched tissues. Chronic pain and joint disability ensue as a result of osteophyte formation, traumatic arthritis, bony overgrowth, and synovitis at intervertebral joints. Delayed disk degeneration is often observed.

PERIPHERAL NERVES

Peripheral nerves can be injured anywhere along their course. Impingement on the nerve roots as they exit the vertebral foramina occurs during subluxation, dislocation, and facet synovitis. Other nerve injuries can occur:

1. Acutely, when the nerve is irritated as it pierces contracted or inflamed musculature or fascia
2. Chronically, as perineural scar tissue forms
3. As part of a neurovascular compression syndrome (usually scalenius anticus, hyperabduction, or costoclavicular)

A significant example of peripheral nerve irritation is seen in the occipital region. The intricate musculature in the suboccipital region and the torque forces sustained during impact make this area especially vulnerable to extensive muscle strain. The greater and lesser occipital nerves as well as the suboccipital nerve (C1-C2) pierce these tissues. Irritation of these nerves causes much of the cephalgia and neck pain experienced by whiplash victims.

Conversely, injury to the deep anterior structures of the neck is likely to cause brachial plexus damage. The plexus passes laterally between the anterior and middle scalene muscles. Plexus injury can result from stretching (extension, contralateral lateral flexion) during impact or from hypertonicity and inflammation of the scalenes.

SYMPATHETIC NERVOUS SYSTEM

Sympathetic nervous system symptoms are common after whiplash injuries. No sympathetic fibers are found in the intermediolateral cell column of the cervical spine. The cervical nerves are connected to the sympathetic nervous system via preganglionic fibers that arise in the lateral horn cells from T1 to T6. These fibers proceed up the sympathetic chain to enter the cervical ganglia and synapse with postganglionic fibers.

The inferior cervical ganglion is usually fused with the superior thoracic ganglion, in which case it is referred to as the cervicothoracic or stellate ganglion. It lies at the level of the superior border of the first rib, just anterior to C7. Some postganglionic fibers join the seventh and eighth cervical nerves to supply the blood vessels, sweat glands, and piloerector muscles of the upper extremity. The inferior cervical ganglion also sends branches to the heart.

The middle cervical ganglion lies anterior to the vertebral artery at about the level of the transverse process of C6. Postganglionic fibers pass to the fifth and sixth cervical nerves. Some fibers are also sent to the heart and thyroid gland.

The superior cervical ganglion lies at the level of the atlantoaxial joint. Some postganglionic fibers accompany the internal carotid and ophthalmic arteries into the orbit, where they supply the dilator muscles and smooth muscles of the upper lid. Other fibers accompany the external carotid artery to supply glands of the head and face. The superior cervical ganglion also contributes fibers to the first four cervical nerves.

A final path the sympathetic fibers in the cervical region can take is in the form of the vertebral nerve. Postganglionic fibers accompany the vertebral arteries and enter the skull to supply the vestibular portion of the ear, certain cranial nerves, and the pharynx.

Sympathetic symptoms can occur as a result of stimulation of peripheral nerves (containing sympathetic nerves) as they pierce inflamed soft tissue, stimulation of sensory elements of C1 and C2, simultaneous sympathetic irritation during nerve root compression in its foraminal passage, and compression of the vertebral artery. Sympathetic symptoms can be aural (tinnitus, deafness, postural dizziness), ocular (blurred vision, retrobulbar pain, and a pupil that dilates when the head is turned and returns to normal in the neutral position), vestibular (vertigo), and others, such as miosis, rhinorrhea, sweating, lacrimation, photophobia.

VASCULAR SYSTEM

Vascular compromise often occurs as a result of vertebral artery compression or spasm. The vertebral artery can be compressed anywhere along its course as it passes through the foramina in the transverse processes of the cervical spine. However, compression most often occurs at the levels of C1 and C2. The prevalence of compression here is due to the susceptibility of the region to injury and to the acute turn the artery makes as it enters the skull. Vertigo, syncope, near syncope, or nystagmus on rotation of the head are highly suggestive of vertebral artery compromise.

CEREBRUM

Patients with inertial injuries may also sustain cerebral concussion. This is most likely the result of the impact of the brain against the vault during rapid flexion and extension of the neck. Although head trauma is not necessary for concussion to occur, its presence makes the diagnosis more likely. The patient usually describes a "blinding" or "exploding" sensation in the head at the time of impact, followed immediately by headache, restlessness, insomnia, or mood change.

Factors Affecting Degree of Injury

Individuals subjected to identical forces may sustain different injuries or have different courses of recovery. A number of variables, including both the mechanics of the impact and the individual's condition at the time of the accident, determine the type and degree of injury sustained. Among these factors are the following.

1. **Force of impact:** The severity of injury is directly related to the force of impact. The force of impact is determined by the size of the offending vehicle and the speed at the time of impact.
2. **Position of the head:** Quite often, at the time of impact the victim has his head turned, to speak to someone or to look in the mirror. Head rotation at the time of impact increases the severity of the injury sustained and predisposes to greater injury on the side of the neck toward which the head is turned, for the following reasons:
   a. Rotation of the spine results in narrowing of the intervertebral foramen on the side to which the head is turned. This increases the likelihood of unilateral nerve root compression on that side.
   b. Rotation of the head greatly reduces the physiologic range of extension in the cervical spine. This increases the chance that the physiologic range of extension will be exceeded at impact, producing tissue damage.

   c. Many authorities believe that vertebral fracture and intervertebral disk herniation are more likely to occur when rotation accompanies flexion and extension at the time of impact.
3. **Position of the hands:** Bracing the hands against the steering wheel reduces anterior translation of the body, thereby reducing cervical injury but increasing the probability of injury to the shoulders, ribs, and thoracic region.
4. **Awareness of impending accident:** When the victim is aware that impact is about to occur, he may tense his muscles, in this manner reducing the pendular action of the head and the subsequent tissue damage.
5. **Head rests:** Properly adjusted head rests at the level of the occiput reduce hyperextension and the recoil into flexion by reducing the stretch reflex. This greatly decreases the severity of injury.
6. **Preexisting conditions:** Preexisting medical conditions (e.g., degenerative joint disease, osteoporosis) and previous trauma increase the likelihood of injuries such as fractures or nerve root impingement.

The Scope of Whiplash Injury

From an osteopathic viewpoint, the body is a unit mechanism, and all parts are deranged in a whiplash injury. This discussion considers the widespread effects of whiplash injury.

SACRAL INJURY

Injury to the sacrum occurs simultaneously with injury to the cervical and thoracic regions. These sacral dysfunctions apparently serve to maintain disability in cases that fail to respond to therapy (Becker, 1961).

The anterior longitudinal ligament fastens to the basiocciput, runs anterior to the bodies of the cervical vertebrae, and then attaches to the anterior vertebral bodies from T2 to the second sacral segment. The posterior longitudinal ligament extends from the occiput to the coccyx. Posteriorly, the supraspinal and interspinal ligaments and the ligamentum nuchae connect the spinous process. The dura is firmly attached at the basiocciput and the first two cervical vertebrae, then continues down the spinal canal without attachments until it reaches the anterior aspect of the second sacral segment, where it is again attached.

During cervical hyperflexion and hyperextension, the continuity of the various muscular, ligamentous, and dural attachments causes the sacrum to be forcibly lifted and dislodged from its floating position between the ilia. On rebound the sacrum lodges at varying degrees between the ilia. Locking invariably results in restriction of the involuntary flexion-extension movements of the sacrum in relation to the craniosacral mechanism. Craniosacral restriction may be accompanied by gross lumbosacral and sacroiliac dysfunctions (e.g., unilateral sacral flexion, sacral torsion).

The diagnostic and therapeutic consequences are several:

1. Freedom of voluntary sacral motion depends on freedom of craniosacral motion. Thus, the unilateral sacral flexion or sacral torsion cannot be successfully treated until the craniosacral mechanism has been restored.
2. Restriction of sacral motion locks the entire craniosacral mechanism, preventing it from carrying out its healing and life-sustaining functions. Restriction of craniosacral function can result in pain, fatigue, and disability of the whole body.
3. Loss of sacral motion places greater stress on the already injured tissues of the cervical and thoracic regions, hindering the self-reparative process. In essence, sacral dysfunction disturbs the body's balance and homeostatic mechanism, which hinders the healing process.

PELVIC INJURY

Iliosacral lesions are common after motor vehicle accidents. They are most frequently associated with having one foot planted, as when the driver sharply depresses the brake pedal at the time of impact. Both ilial rotations and superior pubic shears are observed. The paravertebral muscles of the spine and the latissimus dorsi attach to the iliac crests. Therefore, movements of the spine and shoulder girdle operate against the resistance of the locked ilium.

THORACIC AND LUMBAR INJURY

Many anatomic factors promote thoracic and lumbar dysfunction after whiplash injury. First, the continuity of the cervical, thoracic, and lumbar spine that is provided by the ligamentous attachments and paravertebral musculature transmits the acute strain to the thoracic and lumbar region.

Second, lateral and rotary forces are experienced in the thoracic and lumbar region, which results in alteration of the normal anteroposterior and lateral curves, narrowing of the intervertebral foramina, and establishment of somatic dysfunctions. Third, the thoracic spine's proximity to the cervical spine and its intimate relationship with the muscles of the shoulder girdle make it especially susceptible to dysfunction. Special attention should be given to the upper thoracic region and the upper ribs.

CRANIAL INJURY

Dysfunctions of the cranium are almost invariably present after whiplash injuries. As a rule, the occiput and sacrum exhibit the same restriction (e.g., flexion or extension, to the right or left). The same forces that act on the cervical spine act on the cranium. Asymmetric traction by muscles that attach to the cranium can result in torsions and side-bending or rotary dysfunctions. The temporal bones are especially vulnerable to these forces. Strain patterns are usually present if the victim's head has struck any object.

UPPER EXTREMITY INJURY

Injury to the upper extremity usually results from having the hand braced against an immovable object, such as the steering wheel or dashboard. Injuries usually involve the soft tissues of the shoulder—the glenohumeral capsule, the acromioclavicular and coracoclavicular ligaments, the rotator cuff muscles, and the trapezius. Tender points and fascial strains are common in the supraspinatus, trapezius, and latissimus dorsi muscles.

Pain radiating down the arm, with or without weakness or parethesias, does not necessarily indicate foraminal nerve root compression. It can be secondary to peripheral nerve irritation, neurovascular compression of the brachial plexus, or sympathetic nervous system irritation (referred pain). A careful neurologic and structural examination should be performed to uncover the cause.

Localized dysfunctions of the hands, wrists, and elbows may also occur.

LOWER EXTREMITY INJURY

The lower extremity can be involved in whiplash injury, exhibiting pain and decreased range of motion of various articulations secondary to sacral and ilial dysfunction, iliopsoas strains, and strain or sprain of the hip, knee, foot, and ankle. Hip and pelvic fractures are quite common if the victim's foot was firmly planted at the time of impact.

THORACIC, ABDOMINAL, AND PELVIC CAVITY INJURY

Fascial connections with the deep cervical fascia make the mediastinum and abdominal diaphragm susceptible to fascial strain. Fascial strain can limit thoracic visceral function and weaken the structures supporting the abdominal viscera. Sacral and ilial restrictions can weaken the support of the pelvic viscera and cause strains in the pelvic diaphragm. Contractures of the abdominal and pelvic diaphragms impede lymphatic and venous return, creating visceral congestion.

Symptoms

The whiplash patient often has no immediate pain and refuses medical treatment at the scene of the accident. A few hours later she may experience minor pain and stiffness in the neck and back. By the following day, sufficient edema and inflammation have accumulated to increase the severity of the pain and stiffness. Pain may be felt in the anterior or posterior aspect of the neck and radiating to the occiput, one or both shoulders, and the midthoracic region. The pain may radiate down either or both arms and may or may not be accompanied by numbness, weakness, and paresthesias.

Headaches are usually occipital but may radiate to the frontal region. Occasionally they are frontal or retrobulbar; rarely, they are bitemporal.

Other symptoms may not be evident for a few days to two or three weeks. These may include symptoms caused by involvement of the sympathetic nervous system, vascular impairment, dysphagia, nausea, vomiting, fatigue, low back pain, temporomandibular joint dysfunction, and severe emotional and psychological symptoms.

The multiple areas of body involvement, the potential severity, and the variety of symptom complexes that may develop mandate a comprehensive history and physical examination in the patient with whiplash injury, even if the original complaints seem minor.

Treatment

Treatment of whiplash injuries is individualized for each patient, by stage of recovery and with con-

sideration for the patient's total health needs. Common pitfalls in treatment are treating only the cervical and upper thoracic regions, and overtreating injured tissues. It must be remembered that the body has sustained tissue injury and the physician only aids the body's own reparative mechanisms. Extensive therapy may exceed the point of restoration of health and add to the injury.

This section presents guidelines and suggestions for a treatment regimen based on the severity and time of the patient's injury. The stages are not well demarcated, and the time frames are only guidelines. A patient's course of recovery will vary according to the severity of the injury, preexisting conditions, and the individual patient's physiology. Furthermore, many patients are first seen long after the onset of the injury. Delay before initiation of treatment greatly alters recovery time. The most accurate way to assess the patient's condition is with a comprehensive history and physical examination.

The treatments described below fit into the following three classifications: (1) osteopathic manipulative treatment, (2) adjunctive therapy (thermal, physical, and pharmacologic modalities), and (3) physical activities. Each category is reviewed separately for acute, early chronic, and late chronic stages of injury.

ACUTE STAGE (3 TO 5 DAYS)

The acute phase of whiplash injury is characterized by acute muscle contraction and moderate to severe limitation of motion. Tissues often are warm and edematous. Occasionally ecchymosis is present. Pain is usually confined to the neck and upper thoracic area, with or without radiation to the skull, shoulders, and upper extremities. Low back pain, dysphagia, and sympathetic nervous system symptoms may be present.

A patient seen immediately after injury may exhibit no signs or symptoms. This is not a reason to withhold therapy. On the contrary, proper treatment initiated early may greatly reduce the edema and resultant incapacitation.

Osteopathic Manipulative Treatment
Osteopathic manipulation should be instituted as soon as possible after the patient has been stabilized. The goals are to minimize edema and tissue reaction. The treatment is gentle, indirect, and perilesional; that is, it addresses areas adjacent to the injured tissues.

A useful approach is to restore respiratory motion in both the cranium and the sacrum, followed by treatment of the pelvis and voluntary sacral motion. Myofascial release or muscle energy therapy is commonly employed. If the patient cannot cooperate or cannot be positioned for muscle energy therapy, the pelvis can be treated positionally either with fascial release (using the lower extremities) or with counterstrain techniques. Sacral motion in the incapacitated patient may be induced by sacral rocking, similar to the method described for the obstetric patient later in this chapter. This is followed by treatment of the lumbar and thoracic regions. Treatment should be restricted to soft tissue techniques. If the patient is bedridden, the physician may treat the spinal areas by placing her hands under the patient and applying steady pressure with her fingertips against the paravertebral muscles. Specific techniques are described in Chapters 9, 11, 14, and 17.

A major purpose of manipulation is to restore circulation. Many experienced clinicians avoid vigorous manipulation of acutely inflamed areas, believing that the increased blood flow may increase hemorrhage and fluid leak, thus causing more damage. Perilesional treatment may divert blood flow from the injured tissues to those in adjacent areas. This, combined with gentle lymphatic drainage of injured areas, may reduce the edema.

Manipulation of acutely injured areas should be both gentle and brief. It entails (1) indirect treatment of soft tissues in the cervical and upper thoracic region, (2) passive range of motion exercises, and (3) lymphatic drainage. Gentle occipital traction is useful and well tolerated. Tender points in the occipital region, sternocleidomastoid, levator scapulae, and rhomboids should be sought and treated.

The anterior neck is best treated by counterstrain techniques applied to the anterior tender points and by fascial release of the hyoid bone. Passive range of motion therapy should be instituted without creating pain.

Adjunctive Therapy

1. **Thermal.** Ice packs or ice massage (7 minutes each hour) should be instituted for the first 18 hours after injury, followed by heat therapy, dry or moist. Moist heat may be used at home. Ultra-

sound or diathermy have also been recommended any time after the initial 48 hours of injury.
2. **Immobilization.** The whiplash injury is a sprain/strain injury. For this reason, many clinicians recommend using a cervical collar, with the following stipulations:
   a. It is used only when acute inflammation is evident.
   b. It must be properly applied, usually with the spine in slight flexion.
   c. Its use should be limited to the acute period. Prolonged use results in muscle atrophy and disability. As the patient improves, the hours of wear should be reduced. First the patient wears the collar only while sleeping and driving, then only while sleeping.
3. **Traction.** Mechanical or manual traction should be used only if the patient obtains relief with its use. Mechanical traction is begun with a light weight (6 to 8 lb) that is slowly increased as the patient improves.
4. **Pharmacologic therapy.** Nonsteroidal anti-inflammatory drugs may be useful during the acute inflammatory stage. A lower analgesic dose can be prescribed once the inflammation has been controlled.

Physical Activity

Severely injured patients should be placed on bed rest for at least 2 to 3 days. If they feel better after this period, they may begin limited activity. If they have not improved, they should stay in bed for the remainder of the week. Passive exercises may be started in bed to avoid tissue atrophy.

Patients not confined to bed should be encouraged to begin limited activities immediately as tolerated. Passive range of motion exercises can be performed daily. Patients should also be instructed in which activities to avoid (e.g., rapid turning of the head).

EARLY CHRONIC PHASE (1 WEEK
TO 1 MONTH)

Acute inflammation has subsided but increased tissue tension remains. Range of motion has improved. Pain is usually still present but is not as acute. Radiation of pain may still be present. Sympathetic nervous system symptoms may have begun or persist.

Osteopathic Manipulative Treatment

More aggressive treatment may now be employed. It is useful to treat in the same order as during the acute phase, but direct techniques may be added. Muscle energy techniques as well as high-velocity, low-amplitude thrusting techniques directed toward the lumbar and thoracic region may be tolerated. The cervical spine should be treated with muscle energy techniques and more vigorous lymphatic drainage techniques, in addition to occipital release, counterstrain therapy, and fascial release. Direct thrusting techniques to the cervical region should be avoided. Careful attention is paid to the cranium, sacrum, and anterior neck. Active myofascial treatment for range of motion may be instituted.

Adjunctive Therapy

1. **Thermal.** Moist heat, ultrasound, and diathermy may be continued.
2. **Immobilization.** A cervical collar should be minimal if at all.
3. **Pharmacologic therapy.** Nonsteroidal anti-inflammatory agents may be continued in analgesic dosage if necessary.
4. **Physical modalities.** Electrical muscle stimulation is often useful to induce muscle relaxation.

Physical Activity

The patient should be walking and at close to or full activity. The patient should be encouraged to increase his cervical range of motion exercises. Both active and passive isometric resistance can be added if tolerated. He should also begin range of motion exercises as needed for other spinal regions. Weight lifting is to be avoided.

LATE CHRONIC PHASE (1 TO 3 MONTHS OR LONGER)

Mild pain with or without radiation is all that remains. There may be residual limitation in range of motion, especially in the neck or upper extremities. Tissue changes are usually chronic in nature.

Osteopathic Manipulative Treatment

Treatment includes the whole body. High-velocity, low-amplitude thrusting techniques may now be employed in the cervical region. A good practice is to begin with soft tissue techniques, then position the neck and spring it a few times. If this does not cause pain, the thrust may be performed. If springing causes pain, thrusting should not be performed. Vigorous, active range of motion therapy should be employed.

Adjunctive Therapy

Adjunctive therapy is similar to that in the early chronic phase, with the following differences:

1. Electrical stimulation should be adjusted to stimulate the muscle and thus decrease atrophy.
2. Trigger point therapy may be employed, using either vapocoolant sprays, deep pressure, or injection of a local anesthetic.
3. Physical therapy is begun to strengthen the extremities and improve aerobic capacity.

Physical Activity

The patient should be encouraged to work toward full activity. He participates in physical therapy, as previously described.

Emotional Support

Throughout the recovery process, the patient should be given strong emotional support. The following are guidelines for the physician.

1. Explain the injury and describe the plan of treatment.
2. Empathize with the patient's incapacity.
3. Encourage the patient and point out progress.
4. Describe the prognosis fully, in language that the patient understands. Do not guarantee results.
5. Set goals that are realistic. Review these goals with the patient as the treatment progresses.

HEADACHES
Donald Hankinson

Headache is commonly seen by physicians in general practice. According to the Cecil's *Textbook of Medicine*, headache is the ninth most common reason for visiting a physician. In a New York Hospital study, 46% of patients in the hospital complained of headache.

The causes of headache are many and varied and include muscle tension, migraine, sinus congestion, trauma, hypertension, premenstrual syndrome, tumors, and meningitis. The vast majority of headaches are due to muscle tension or migraine. A 28-year study at the Headache Unit of Montefiore Hospital found that 90% of patients had either migraine, tension headaches, or a combination of the two. Even head pain usually attributed to other causes, most notably sinus congestion and mild hypertension, are thought by some clinicians to be misdiagnosed tension or migraine headaches. Although standard textbooks of medicine agree on a musculoskeletal pathologic basis for cephalgia, this factor is rarely considered in the diagnosis or treatment of headache.

This section explores the role of the musculoskeletal system in the pathogenesis, diagnosis, and treatment of migraine and tension headaches.

Pathogenesis

The brain itself is almost totally insensitive to pain. Extracranially, the pain-sensitive structures are the scalp, arteries, muscles, mucous membranes of the sinuses, external and middle ear, and the teeth. The musculoskeletal pathogenesis of tension headaches is fairly straightforward. According to Cecil's *Textbook of Medicine*, "The contracting muscles or nerves supplying them may release vasoactive substances such as lactate, serotonin, bradykinin and prostaglandins which lower the pain threshold." The crucial area here is the suboccipital and upper cervical area. In the upper two cervical segments the sensory fibers of the first three cervical segments are joined by the descending tracts of cranial nerves V, IX, and X. These three cranial nerves, along with the second cervical nerve, mediate the referral of excessive connective tissue tension in the cervical area as pain in the cranial vault, or cephalgia.

Intracranially, only the dura and large arteries at the base of the skull, the dural arteries, and the venous sinuses are sensitive to pain. Guyton states that the pain of migraines is secondary either to stretching of the dura at the cranial base, tugging on the venous sinuses, or damage to the tentorium. This prolonged tension causes a reflex vasospasm. The ischemia that develops results in loss of vascular tone for as long as 48 hours. The subsequent excessive stretching of the arteries causes the actual pain of a migraine. Biochemical substances, specifically norepinephrine (increased) and serotonin (decreased), are postulated to mediate the vasodilatory and vasoconstrictive phases, but their role remains speculative. What is known is that connective tissue stresses that cause tension or drag on dural structures create an environment for the development of migraines. Thus, headache is part of an evolving process, not an isolated event. In both migraine and tension headache, excessive tonus of connective tissue structures is a primary etiologic factor.

Evaluation

How should the osteopathic physician approach the patient with headache? A complete history is essential to determine whether a tension or migraine headache is present or whether further diagnostic workup is necessary to evaluate the possibility of a less common, potentially more ominous etiology. These two types of headaches have rather characteristic presentations, which, in allopathic medical practice, form the basis of diagnosis.

Tension headaches are bilateral, are usually preceded by emotionally stressful situations, and worsen as the day progresses. The pain is described as a constant tight pressure encircling the head like a hat band. The pain may last for weeks, months, or years. It remits with alcohol ingestion but is often unchanged with rest. Migraine is often preceded by an aura consisting of sensory, motor, and mood changes. The pain is usually unilateral, although the site can vary. Migraine headaches can be precipitated by flashing lights, foods with high concentrations of tyramine, certain vasodilatory drugs, alcohol, and especially red wine. Sleeping or lying down in a dark room often affords relief. Migraines tend to be familial.

The physical examination is where the osteopathic physician first departs from allopathic medical management of headaches. A complete physical examination with vital signs and thorough neurologic evaluation is essential. In the vast majority of cases, the only positive findings will be on the musculoskeletal examination, which, unfortunately, is often neglected.

Palpation is used to uncover the fascial stresses involved in the pathogenesis of the patients' complaints. Several areas are particularly common trouble spots in the patient with cephalgia. The cervical spine, especially C1, C2, and C3, is involved in most headaches. The second and third cervical nerves via the greater and lesser occipital nerves respectively provide sensory innervation for the cranial vault posterior to the ear, the mastoids, and the suboccipital area. The first cervical nerve provides motor innervation to the muscles of the suboccipital triangle. This area is also significant because it refers pain to the cranial nerves V, IX, and X.

Lawrence Jones in *Strain and Counterstrain* identifies tender points that commonly occur with different types of headaches. Frontal and orbital headaches usually are associated with C1 and occipitomastoid tender points. Periorbital headaches are associated with C2, occipitomastoid, squamosal, infraorbital, and nasal tender points. Occipital headaches are associated with C4 tender points. Generalized, vague headaches are associated with C5 tender points.

The cervical evaluation, therefore, includes any restrictions of vertebral motion, paravertebral muscle contractures, tender points, or other types of fascial stress.

The suboccipital area, evaluated next, is of crucial importance. In this area the muscles of the trunk attach to the cranium, the body compensates for motion or restrictions of motion in the rest of the cervical spine, and many of the neuromuscular elements implicated in the pathogenesis of cephalgia are found. Restrictions of motion of the occiput on the atlas and the quality of the soft tissues in the occipitoatlantal sulcus must be evaluated. Some clinicians have detected a series of tender points along the inferoposterior borders of the occiput between the inion and the mastoid process. Pressure on one of these tender points will often elicit the patient's pain.

The third area evaluated is the cranium. Cranial somatic dysfunction produces fascial stress on the dura, just as vertebral somatic dysfunction results in fascial stress of the connective tissue structures attached to the vertebrae. In addition, many of the main venous sinuses and cranial arteries run along the inner table of the cranial bones and may be affected directly by restrictions in cranial motion. The middle meningeal artery (the largest intracranial artery) along the sagittal sinus and the confluence of sinuses on the occiput are examples.

In *Osteopathy in the Cranial Field*, Harold Magoun offers some of Sutherland's observations. "The sphenoid is usually found rotated around its antero-posterior axis with the greater wing more prominent (lower) on the side of the pain." Magoun also emphasizes the importance of evaluating the temporals and the occipitomastoid.

The temporal bone is important to the body's effort to maintain homeostasis. The tentorium attaches to its petrous ridges; it contains the primary relay station for sensory impulses of the 5th to the 12th cranial nerves as well as the motor nuclei of all cranial nerves. Nearly a dozen muscles attach to its aspects. Finally, the superior petrosal sinus and middle meningeal artery run along its inner border.

The occipitomastoid is important, among other things, for its association with the jugular foramen, which conducts the vagus nerve. In *Craniosacral Therapy*, John Upledger observes that headaches are often more severe in patients with an overall extension pattern. He adds that this pattern, as well as temporal dysfunction, is very common in patients with migraine headaches.

The sacrum must also be carefully evaluated. A common area affected by fascial stress is the dura at the base of the cranium. This dura is continuous with its attachment to the second sacral segment, with only connections to C2 and C3 in between. Therefore, sacral somatic dysfunction can exert a fascial drag on the dura at the cranial base. The sacral range of motion with pulmonary respiration, sacroiliac and lumbosacral somatic dysfunctions, the quality of the surrounding soft tissue structures, and tender points (both anterior and posterior) must all be evaluated.

Management

It is only common sense that osteopathic manipulative treatment be added to the traditional allopathic management of migraine and tension headaches. Most internal medicine texts recommend the following for this fundamentally musculoskeletal disorder: rest, exercise, diet, anti-inflammatory drugs, analgesics, and ergot preparations. Treatment of the musculoskeletal system is conspicuously absent. However, as Magoun states, "Structure is not the only cause, but corrections of structural imbalances permit the total organism to return to the level of adaptation below the threshold for cephalgia."

In treating the dysfunctions, any form of osteopathic manipulative treatment with which the clinician is comfortable is appropriate if the patient can tolerate it. Myofascial techniques, muscle energy techniques, thrusting techniques, fascial release, and counterstrain treatment will address problems not only in the areas mentioned but wherever they occur. For clinicians who do not practice cranial osteopathy, treatment of the rest of the mechanisms, with emphasis on the cervical, suboccipital, and sacral areas, will help or cure many patients.

Direct action techniques should be preceded by soft tissue techniques. In fact, many somatic dysfunctions relate to the soft tissues.

In cranial treatment, freeing of the temporal bones is very difficult in patients with recurrent headaches and should be attempted between attacks. All borders of the temporal bones must be freed, including the occipitomastoid. Fluid congestion resulting from dilation of venous and arterial structures and from dural stresses is an important factor in the pathogenesis of headaches. Venous drainage techniques may lessen this congestion. Otherwise, any of the standard cranial techniques can be employed to relieve any restrictions that are found.

The osteopathic physician, with special training in musculoskeletal diagnosis and treatment, can offer an invaluable service to the patient with tension or migraine headaches. The relief of fascial stresses at very least affords a decrease in the severity and frequency of cephalgic episodes. Proper diagnosis and treatment of specific somatic components will help relieve debilitating headaches, with only periodic treatments to maintain normal physiologic function.

SCOLIOSIS
Sandra D. Yale

Structural scoliosis is a pathologic spinal condition that produces lateral curvature of the spine and is accompanied by rotation of the vertebrae and ribs in a horizontal plane. The Greeks used the word *skoliosis*, which means crookedness, to describe this condition.

Scoliosis is an ancient disease. Cave drawings and woodcuts made at the time of Hippocrates attest to the significance of this disease to patients and physicians alike. In modern times, it is still the most common deforming orthopedic problem in children.

The disease most often affects adolescents at the time of their pubertal growth spurt and slows at the end of skeletal growth. The effects of scoliosis are both physiologic and cosmetic. The more significant physical side effects are pain and cardiopulmonary complications.

Prevalence and Etiology

The prevalence of scoliosis varies in different areas of the world because of factors both medical and socioeconomic. The prevalence of scoliosis in the United States is variably reported as 0.3% to 15.3%, depending on the school-age screening study used. It is present in approximately 2% of all adults. In children its frequency is 1.4/1,000, with four times more girls affected than boys. Possibly one sixth of all scolioses may have a familial background.

There are many theories on the etiology of scoliosis. Steindler contends that it is due to inability of the spine to resist ordinary functional stresses: he suggests that the root cause is some inherent muscular weakness or skeletal or musculoskeletal deficiency. Others contend that scoliosis occurs secondary to central and peripheral postural mechanisms. One study in animals found an increase in type I oxidative fibers on the convex side of scoliotic curves. However, it is unclear whether this finding is part of the neuromuscular dysfunction or a secondary development. The results of many other studies in animals and humans indicate that the etiology is probably multifactorial, and the condition is partially hereditary.

Denslow and Korr state that "[t]he osteopathic lesion represents a hyperexcitable segment of the spinal cord through which impulses are channelled into muscles receiving innervation from that segment." If these segments persist, proprioceptive nerve endings in the peripheral muscles and joints could be maintained under continuous bombardment. This continuous stimulation could lead to increased muscle tension, and the segment would eventually be less able to withstand the stresses of daily living. Such persistent lesions could be a factor in the etiology of scoliosis.

Clinical Findings

Scoliosis can be divided into *structural* and *functional* groups; some curves have features of both. A structural curve does not correct on lateral bending of the trunk. This type of curve is relatively fixed and inflexible. There are changes in bone symmetry, with shortened ligaments and muscles on the concave side of the curve. Structural curves can occur due to fracture of the vertebrae, congenital anomalies, or soft tissue trauma such as burns or irradiation.

Functional curves can be partially or completely straightened by lateral bending in the opposite direction. Functional curves may be either *postural* or *compensatory*. Postural curves are slight deviations in a normal spine that correct voluntarily and disappear with movement. Compensatory curves are a manifestation of an underlying dysfunction that produces a lateral curve. A short leg produces a compensatory spinal curve. Uncorrected functional curves eventually develop a structural component.

Some 80% of all structural scoliotic curves are idiopathic. This condition is thought to be inherited in autosomal dominant fashion with incomplete penetrance. Idiopathic scoliosis is commonly divided into infantile, juvenile, and adolescent kinds. *Infantile idiopathic scoliosis* occurs from birth to 3 years of age. It is more common in boys and in Europeans. Potential causes include

molding in utero, injury to the skull during birth, or cranial asymmetry caused by laying babies in cribs on their sides. However, none of these causes has been demonstrated experimentally. Infantile idiopathic scoliosis usually resolves spontaneously.

Juvenile scoliosis occurs from 4 to 10 years of age. It may represent a late infantile form of scoliosis that resolves or a more serious form that persists into adolescence.

Adolescent idiopathic scoliosis occurs from age 10 until skeletal maturity. It is often present at an earlier age but remains unnoticed until the adolescent growth spurt occurs. This form of idiopathic scoliosis is the most significant and prevalent form and can become progressively worse during the growth spurt.

Idiopathic curves can occur at any area in the spine. Five of the most common curves are listed below:

1. Right thoracic curve
2. Right thoracolumbar curve
3. Double major curve—usually right thoracic, left lumbar
4. Lumbar curve
5. Cervicothoracic curve

The right thoracic curve is usually highly structural and the ribs can have increased angles on the convex side. This curve can develop quickly and requires early intervention to achieve a functional and cosmetic outcome. When a thoracic curve reaches 70 degrees, there can be significant cardiopulmonary dysfunction. The right thoracolumbar curve is usually less disruptive and cosmetically deforming but can cause severe rib and flank distortion due to rotation. The lumbar major curve can be very rigid, causing severe pain and dysfunction during childbirth and leading to arthritic changes later in life.

The remaining 20% of structural scolioses (nonidiopathic) occur secondary to congenital anomalies, neuromuscular diseases, tumors, trauma, infections, and iatrogenic causes. Congenital scoliosis occurs due to malformation of spinal elements or the development of bony bridges over growth areas. There are open and closed vertebral forms. Meningomyelocoele and spina bifida are two examples of the open form in which closed parts of vertebrae are unfused or missing altogether. The closed vertebral forms are various, some bizarre. There can be failure of vertebral formation, in which hemivertebrae form, or failure of segmentation, in which unilateral and bilateral bars form. Hemivertebrae cause severe curves because they tend to grow. Unilateral bars and hemivertebrae are the worst combination; they progress rapidly until spinal fusion is needed.

Neuromuscular scoliosis occurs secondary to muscle weakness and imbalance caused by central or peripheral nervous system disease. These scolioses can be divided into neuropathic and myopathic forms. The neuropathic form is due to central nervous system dysfunction and damage. Some examples are poliomyelitis, cerebral palsy, and syringomyelia. The myopathic form includes muscular dystrophy, amyotonia congenita, and Friedreich's ataxia.

The neuromuscular scolioses are generally relentlessly progressive. Victims have decreased respiratory function due to the scoliosis and respiratory muscle weakness. Their scolioses are difficult to manage because of multiple anomalies and medical problems.

Traumatic scoliosis can occur secondary to fracture in which the epiphyseal growth plate is injured, causing asymmetric growth of the vertebrae. Irradiation of the thorax or abdomen can cause similar damage to the growth plate. Wedge fractures in older persons can also cause slight curve formation.

Scoliosis capitis is probably caused by persistent malfunction of the occiput secondary to the stress of labor and delivery. The occipital dysfunction causes cranial obliquity with flattening on one side of the face and increased roundness on the opposite side. The sacrum and pelvis assume the same obliquity and increase the scoliotic tendency.

OSTEOPATHIC NOTES
The body always tries to keep the eyes level. If for whatever reason there is a curve in the spine, the compensatory curves will form to keep the body balanced.

Scoliosis is not just pure lateral flexion; there is also a significant rotational component. The vertebrae involved follow Fryette's first law of vertebral motion. That is, in the neutral position, adjacent vertebrae rotate and side-bend in opposite directions. The ribs follow the vertebral motion. The ribs on the convex side separate and move poste-

riorly, producing the rib hump noted in scoliosis. The ribs on the concave side move closer together and anterior. Rotational stresses in scoliosis occur with enough force to deform the vertebral body. Disk spaces are narrowed on the concave side of the curve. The vertebral body tends to be wedged and thickened on the concave side of the curve. The vertebral canal may also be narrowed on the convex side of the curve.

The body changes follow Wolf's law, according to which the bony shapes and internal structures reflect the habitual stresses that have acted on the plastic osseous tissue. The changes that occur in a scoliotic patient with growth follow the Hueter-Volkman principle. The three basic parts of this principle are:

1. Increased pressure on a vertebral growth plate retards growth.
2. The less pressured side of the plate grows more.
3. This unequal growth influences the endochondral ossification and causes wedging.

The change from a functional to a structural scoliosis also follows this principle. There are progressive soft tissue shortening, body changes, and disk degeneration. The ligaments and fascia become more fibrotic, and there is decreased active and passive range of motion.

Diagnosis and Evaluation
Certain clues in the history may help establish the diagnosis. Although back pain is a rare symptom in children, 40% to 80% of adults with scoliosis may present with back pain. The pain is usually mild to moderate and worse at the end of the work day or after strenuous activity. The area of pain is variable but is often at the apex or junction of a curve. In a child, the parents may have noticed a round back or shoulders, or prominence of one hip. The patient may complain of difficulty in fitting a hem or sleeve lengths.

The physical examination begins with observation of the patient's gait. Observe for patterns indicating asymmetric pelvic rotation or drop which may indicate a short leg. Examine the patient from the back, sides, and front. Any asymmetry of the neck musculature or unequal scapular angle level is noted. Decide if the trunk seems to be balanced over the pelvis. If a plumb line dropped from the inion does not divide the body in half, the scoliosis is probably more severe. Look for a rib hump, unilateral muscle prominence, an asymmetric waist crease, or an unequal distance between the arms and trunk.

Ask the patient to bend forward from the hips with the knees extended. Observe the patient's back at eye level from in back and in front. A rib hump will become more prominent in this position. The rib hump represents posterior rotation of the spine and ribs on the side of the convexity of the curve. A curve with 10 degrees of angulation can be detected visually.

Assess the flexibility of the curve by having the patient side-bend without flexing forward. Mark how far down the lateral leg the patient can reach. Functional curves are more flexible, but it is not uncommon for a structural curve to have a functional component.

The degree of chest wall flexibility should also be examined. Place both hands over the ribs and note any asymmetry of inspiration or expiration. A cardiopulmonary assessment should be considered in severe scoliosis or in any patient with signs of cor pulmonale, dyspnea on exertion, or repeated bouts of respiratory illness. This should include an electrocardiogram to look for right ventricular hypertrophy, and baseline pulmonary function studies.

Radiographic studies are used to determine the type and magnitude of the spinal curve. Scoliosis patients tend to receive a large amount of radiation in the course of a lifetime, so each study should yield maximum information with minimum radiation. Standing PA films on 30 × 90 cm cassettes have been suggested. The initial study can also include a lateral radiograph to determine the degree of kyphosis and lordosis of the spine.

The magnitude of the curve is generally measured by the Cobb method:

1. Locate the vertebral bodies at the extreme ends of the curve. The top of the superior vertebrae and the bottom of the inferior vertebrae tilt toward each other more than the other vertebrae.
2. Draw horizontal lines from the top of the superior vertebrae and the bottom of the inferior vertebrae into the concavity of the curve.
3. Drop intersecting perpendicular lines from the horizontal lines and measure the acute angles.

There is a great deal of controversy as to how often a curve should be reassessed. Curves of less than 10 degrees should be reevaluated in 6 months to a year. Curves of more than 10 degrees should be reexamined in 4 to 6 months. Curves of more than 20 degrees should be examined at 4-month intervals.

Progression of 5 degrees or more is an indication for treatment. Curves of more than 30 degrees should be treated. A curve of less than 20 degrees in a skeletally mature adult usually will not progress, but the patient should be followed if she is symptomatic because she is at greater risk for degenerative disk disease and back strain. Skeletally mature adults with curves of 20 degrees or more should ideally be followed up at 1- to 2-year intervals.

Progression of a scoliotic curve is defined as an increase of greater than 5 degrees of curve magnitude between two visits. Bracing with either the Milwaukee brace or the Boston brace (molded orthosis) effectively prevents progression in about 90% of cases.

Treatment

Transcutaneous electrical nerve stimulation is used at night to involuntarily contract the paraspinal musculature on the convex side. The effectiveness of this treatment is inconclusive: some studies show improvement and some failure.

Nonoperative treatment consists of braces, active and passive stimulation, and exercise. There is a great deal of controversy as to whether exercise is beneficial in conjunction with other treatment modalities such as bracing to preserve muscle tone and keep the correction. The exercises should stress pelvic tilt, trunk shifting, and flexibility. Noncontact sports such as swimming are also beneficial.

Surgery is considered if bracing does not prevent progression or if the curve is greater than 50 degrees on initial evaluation. The most common reason for surgical correction is to prevent the cardiopulmonary complications of severe scoliosis. The most commonly used device is the Harrington rod.

Osteopathic manipulation should be aimed at increasing the intrinsic sustaining forces of the musculoskeletal system. This can be done by using active and passive techniques to increase muscle balance on both sides of the curve. The technique used depends on the physician's expertise and experience. Muscle energy and fascial release will increase muscle balance and relieve stress caused by muscle spasm and contracture. High-velocity, low-amplitude techniques can be used to correct specific acute somatic dysfunctions that occur in the curve. Craniosacral techniques can be used to alleviate strain patterns that occur in the cranium and sacrum secondary to the scoliosis or primary patterns that may have precipitated formation of the scoliosis.

The prognosis of untreated scolioses depends on many factors, such as age, sex, skeletal maturity, and curve magnitude. About 75% of all scolioses progress, so the likelihood of spontaneous remission is low. Girls generally progress more often than boys. The larger the curve at initial diagnosis,

the more progression is to be expected. Curves may also progress after skeletal maturity is achieved. Certain patients who have had a compensated scoliosis throughout life may start to progress as they grow older.

The goals of the primary care physician in treating scoliosis are twofold. The first goal is to prevent severe scoliosis, which causes deformity and cardiopulmonary crowding, through early screening of children for scoliosis, with periodic rechecks. The second goal is to coordinate the treatment of the patient with scoliosis by making sure the patient gets thorough and adequate follow-up with timely referral to a specialist in the treatment of scoliosis where needed.

THORACIC OUTLET SYNDROME
Eileen L. DiGiovanna

Thoracic outlet syndrome is an umbrella term for a complex of signs and symptoms of various causes. The common denominator is compression of nerves or vascular structures as they pass through the thoracic inlet, traverse the shoulder girdle and axilla, and begin their descent into the arm. The axillary artery or components of the brachial plexus may be compressed.

Symptoms of nerve compression are pain or dysesthesia of the upper extremity. Arterial compression results in typical ischemic signs and symptoms whose severity depends on the degree of compression. These manifestations may include coldness, pallor, cyanosis, and occasionally Raynaud's phenomena. The anatomic location of the veins in this area protects them from the forces acting on the nerves and arteries, so venous compression is rarely a problem.

Etiology
The anatomy of the area may contribute to the development of thoracic outlet syndrome. The neurovascular structures must pass through several narrow passageways. Three passageways are of particular concern. One is the triangle formed by the anterior and medial scalene muscles and the first rib, which provides a passageway for the subclavian artery and nerve plexus. The second is

where the neurovascular bundle passes between the clavicle and the first rib. The third is along the border of the pectoralis minor near its attachment to the coracoid process as the neurovascular bundle passes between it and the rib cage. As the arm is hyperabducted, the pectoralis minor is pulled taut and may compress the neurovascular bundle against the rib cage.

There are numerous causes for narrowing of these areas. Some require orthopedic or neurosurgical treatment, such as cervical ribs (which may be asymptomatic), improperly healed clavicle or first rib fractures, aberrant muscle slips, and the like. However, many other causes of thoracic outlet syndrome are amenable to osteopathic manipulation. Tension in muscles and fascia may compromise the free passage of nerves and arteries. Restricted motion of joints in the area, particularly at the junction of the clavicle and first rib, may be a source of chronic pressure on these structures. Edema as a result of somatic dysfunction is another source of pressure. All of these causes respond to osteopathic manipulation.

Evaluation
Before treatment is initiated, a thorough assessment is necessary. The clinician must identify conditions that should be referred for specialist

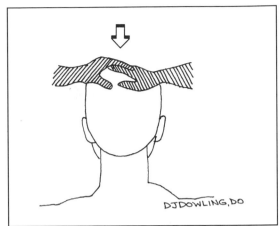

Figure 27-2. Spurling maneuver.

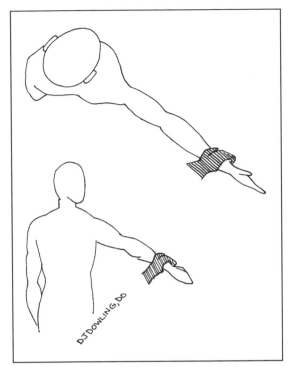

Figure 27-1. Adson test.

care and rule out conditions that produce referred pain, numbness, or paresthesia of the arm and hand. A differential diagnosis would include cervical root compression or radiculitis, Pancoast tumor, Sudek's dystrophy or shoulder-hand syndrome, and carpal tunnel syndrome. The patient should be examined for joint motion of the upper ribs, clavicles, and cervical and thoracic spine. Tissue tension should be assessed in the area of the thoracic inlet.

Depending on which structures are involved, impingement may occur in any of several patient positions. Several special tests have been designed to better localize the area of impingement.

1. Adson test. The patient's affected arm is abducted and the physician palpates the radial pulse. The patient is instructed to turn her head toward the affected side and extend the neck, then take a deep breath (Fig. 27-1). The test is positive if the pulse disappears or diminishes or if the patient's symptoms are elicited. If nothing happens with this maneuver, the patient is asked to turn her head away from the affected arm.

2. Spurling maneuver. The Spurling maneuver is done with the patient seated. The physician applies a compressive force to the top of the patient's head (Fig. 27-2). Pain down the arm indicates that the problem is probably not thoracic outlet syndrome but rather a nerve root compression.

3. Hyperabduction test. As in the Adson test, the radial pulse is monitored. The patient's arm is elevated 180 degrees (Fig. 27-3). The test is positive if the pulse diminishes or if symptoms are elicited.

4. Costoclavicular test. The patient is asked to assume a "military" posture—chest out, shoulders back and down (Fig. 27-4). Again, the radial pulse is monitored. The test is positive if the pulse diminishes or if symptoms are elicited.

If the Adson is positive but cervical rib radiographs are normal, the area of the scalenes should be examined. The osteopathic physician may be able to relieve the symptoms by gentle stretching and relaxation of the scalenes if they exhibit increased tension or fibrosis. Fibrous bands may also be stretched sufficiently to relieve some of the symptoms. The patient should be placed on an exercise program for use at home. Stretching exercises rather than isometric exercises should be used if there is any evidence of muscle hypertrophy.

If hyperabduction of the arm is the problem, any abnormal tensions of the pectoralis muscles should be addressed. However, the patient will likely have to avoid holding the arm in this posi-

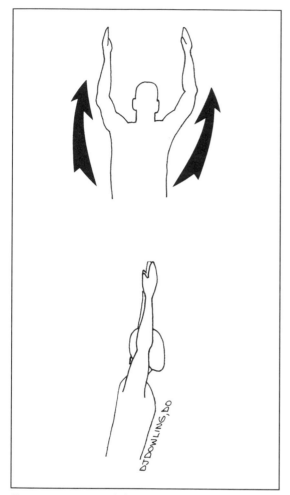

Figure 27-3. Hyperabduction test.

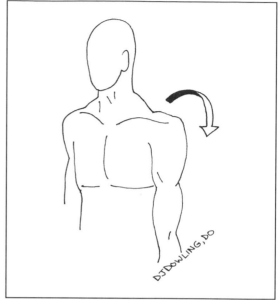

Figure 27-4. Costoclavicular test.

tion for extended periods of time, as in painting ceilings or trimming trees.

If the patient sleeps with her arm over her head, awareness of the problem is usually sufficient to correct it. Some patients find it helpful to tie their wrist with a piece of gauze or nylon stocking that is long enough to allow motion but not long enough for the arm to be placed over the head.

Restrictions of the clavicle and first rib are commonly seen and quite responsive to manipulation. Any somatic dysfunction involving the clavicle, the first rib, the seventh cervical, vertebra, or the first thoracic vertebrae seems capable of producing thoracic outlet syndrome symptoms. Frequently such dysfunctions occur in combinations. Structural motion in addition to tissue changes

in the area should be assessed. The second thoracic vertebra and the second rib are commonly involved. Somatic dysfunctions must be diagnosed and corrected if the problem is to be solved.

Three motions should be restored to the clavicle: motion in abduction-adduction, flexion-extension, and longitudinal rotation. Both sternoclavicular joints should be examined. Articulation of these joints may be sufficient, or muscle energy techniques may be used.

The first rib may be examined by the clinician sitting at the head of the supine patient and placing his thumbs on the flat posterosuperior portion of the rib, then springing it gently. It may also be assessed by following its motion during inhalation and exhalation. Motion may be improved using muscle energy techniques or high-velocity, low-amplitude thrusting techniques.

Any somatic dysfunctions involving the upper thoracic area should be treated. The cervical spine should be assessed and treated to restore motion to all vertebrae.

After motion is restored to all ribs and vertebrae, it may be helpful to reevaluate the area for any fascial tensions or tender points which remain. These should be treated with myofascial release or counterstrain. The removal of tender points seems to decrease proprioceptive overactivity, which may recreate the former dysfunctions. Stretching of any tight muscles or fibrous bands is helpful. The patient should be placed on an exercise program at home to continue stretching the muscles of the cervical and upper thoracic spine, pectorals, and shoulder girdle.

The patient's posture needs to be evaluated and corrected, since drooping shoulders, forward carriage of the head, and rounded thoracic spine may contribute to the problem.

LUMBAR RADICULOPATHIES
Barbara Polstein

The term *radiculopathy* refers to a disease process involving one or more spinal nerve roots. There are three common causes of lumbar radicular syndromes: herniated nucleus pulposus, central spinal stenosis, and lateral spinal stenosis. In addition, three pseudoradicular syndromes are frequently responsible for low back pain radiating to the buttock and lower extremity: posterior facet joint syndrome, sacroiliac joint syndrome, and piriformis and other myofascial syndromes. These pseudoradicular syndromes do not compress the spinal nerves. Their manifestations are often similar to those of true radiculopathies, they may occur alone or in combination with disk herniation or spinal stenosis, and they respond favorably to manipulative treatment.

Functional Anatomy

The basic functional unit of the spine is a three-joint complex—an intervertebral disk set between two vertebral bodies anteriorly, and two posterior facet joints. In the absence of pathology, this three-joint complex serves to house and protect the spinal cord, offers unhindered passage of the spinal nerve roots to the periphery, helps to disperse external forces during normal weight-bearing and more vigorous activity, and facilitates spinal motion. When the balance in this complex is lost, as it may be in degenerative diseases, its functions are compromised, often resulting in compression of one or more spinal nerve roots.

INTERVERTEBRAL DISKS

The intervertebral disks act as hydrolic shock absorbers. Each is composed of strong, concentrically arranged fibers, the annuli fibrosi, that enclose a gelatinous, mucopolysaccharide nucleus pulposus. Forces exerted on the disk are evenly distributed within the containment of the disk. The functions of the intervertebral disk are twofold: constant intradiskal pressure maintains separation of the two adjacent vertebrae, and mobility of the nucleus pulposus facilitates vertebral motion. For example, during flexion the nucleus pulposus moves posteriorly and during extension it moves anteriorly.

The loss of blood supply to the disk normally occurs between the ages of 20 and 30 years. In adults, the disk receives its nutrition by diffusion of solutes through the vertebral endplates and by the imbibing properties of the nucleus pulposus. The annulus fibrosus attaches to the edges of hyaline cartilage of adjacent vertebral endplates by the insertion of annular fibers. The disk is ensheathed by periosteum, which has two thickenings, the anterior and posterior longitudinal ligaments.

The annulus fibrosus is innervated by twigs of the recurrent sinovertebral nerve and by skeletal branches of the primary central rami. It contains both free (nocioceptive) nerve endings and complex surface receptors, that may be used for proprioception.

Intervertebral disk degeneration is often initiated simply by wear and tear. Repeated microtrauma, especially when induced by rotational forces, further predisposes the disk to damage. Typically, circumferential tears appear in the outer portion of the annulus. The weakened annulus, no longer able to contain the nucleus pulposus under pressure, may bulge. After severe or repeated stress, circumferential tears may coalesce, forming a radial tear through which nuclear material can herniate. The loss of disk height with herniation disrupts normal joint function, initiating a cycle of progressive degeneration and joint instability.

POSTERIOR FACET JOINTS

Posterior facet joints are typical synovial joints formed by the inferior and superior facets. The articular capsule is richly innervated by twigs from the recurrent sinovertebral nerve and branches of the primary dorsal ramus of the mixed spinal nerve, each supplying at least two facet joints.

Kirkaldy-Willis often describes degenerative changes in the three-joint complex as occurring in three phases. Central to this model is the recognition that the posterior facet joints and intervertebral disk are intimately related. Instability of one, whether due to degenerative processes or trauma, will always affect the other. During the first phase, repeated microtrauma leads to synovitis and hypomobility of the posterior facet joints. Progression of this process produces instability and capsular laxity, with possible subluxation of the posterior joints. Stage three is heralded by an attempt at stability of the involved joints, accomplished by fibrosis and the formation of osteophytes. Osteophyte formation on the superior facets produces lateral stenosis, whereas osteophyte formation on the inferior facets limits the central canal.

Similar changes occur at the disk. These include annular tears with possible herniation, advanced disk degeneration, and osteophyte formation. The final result is spondylosis at one or more levels.

SPINAL NERVES

There are 31 pairs of spinal nerves; 5 are in the lumbar area. Each pair exits the spine through the intervertebral canal just below the vertebral body it is named for. Hence, a herniated L4-L5 disk compresses the L5 nerve root. The lumbar spinal nerve roots arise from a series of filaments that blend together to form distinct ventral and dorsal roots. These travel through the subarachnoid space until they exit at the intervertebral canal.

As the nerve roots traverse the subarachnoid space they acquire meningeal coverings—the pia mater, arachnoid, and finally dura mater. Just lateral to the dorsal root ganglion, the dural investments of the two nerve roots combine to form a common sheath around the mixed spinal nerve,

and the dura mater becomes continuous with the epineurium. Proximal to the dorsal root ganglion, each of the mixed spinal nerves divides into a primary ventral ramus and a primary dorsal ramus. The primary ventral rami proceed to the lumbar or sacral plexus. They also send skeletal branches to the posterolateral and lateral aspects of the intervertebral disk, anterior longitudinal ligament, and periosteum.

The smaller primary dorsal rami have medial, intermediate, and lateral branches. The medial branch passes under the mammiloaccessory ligament on its way to the lumbar intrinsic muscles. Deep to the multifidus muscle a branch arises to supply sensory innervation to the interspinous ligament and posterior facet joints both above and below each branch. The intermediate branches supply the lumbar fibers of the longissimus muscles. The first through fourth lumbar primary dorsal rami innervate the iliocostalis muscles by their lateral branches. The first through third lateral branches continue past the iliac crest to provide sensation to the skin of the lateral buttock as far as the greater trochanter.

The recurrent sinovertebral nerve is formed by twigs from the anterior primary rami (somatic input) and the gray ramus communicantes (autonomic innervation). It reenters the intervertebral canal to innervate the posterior longitudinal ligament, posterior and posterolateral disk, anterior meninges, the nerve root sleeve as far as the intervertebral foramen, the ligamentum flavum, and the posterior facet joints.

Four large mixed nerves innervate the entire lower extremity. The second through fourth lumbar primary ventral rami, after exiting the intervertebral foramen, travel within the body of the psoas muscle and form the lumbar plexus with its two divisions. The obturator nerve (anterior division) innervates the hip adductors and the gracilis muscle; the femoral nerve (posterior division) innervates the hip flexors and knee extensors.

The lumbosacral plexus is formed by the primary ventral rami of the fourth and fifth lumbar nerves and the first through third sacral nerves. It also forms two large mixed nerves that are initially bound by a common sheath. The sciatic nerve exits the pelvis through the greater sciatic foramen. It travels beneath the piriformis muscle into the posterior thigh. Just proximal to the popliteal fossa, the common peroneal (posterior division) and tibial (anterior division) components of the sciatic nerve separate. The tibial nerve innervates the foot, ankle, and knee flexors; the common peroneal nerve supplies the toe and ankle extensors as well as ankle evertors by way of its superficial and deep branches.

Any of these nerves may become inflamed. The resulting peripheral neuritis is a potential source of confusion with the lower extremity pain, numbness, or paresthesias associated with a lumbar radiculopathy. Sciatic neuritis will be discussed in greater detail in the section on the piriformis syndrome.

Physical Examination

The diagnosis of lumbar radiculopathy is based on a thorough history and physical examination. Sciatica is not difficult to diagnose. However, accurate delineation of the etiology of the symptoms is not only challenging but is essential for an effective treatment plan. The physical examination outlined below is performed in conjunction with a routine physical examination, with special emphasis on the musculoskeletal and nervous systems.

GAIT

Observe the patient during the swing and stance phases of gait, looking for ease of motion. Note antalgia, ataxia, "simian gait," and signs of neurologic deficit such as foot drop. Have the patient walk on his toes and heels and squat to assess the S1, L5, and L4 nerve roots, respectively.

STANDING

Observe static symmetry. Examine the lordotic and kyphotic curves. Is scoliosis present? Evaluate the gross range of motion in flexion, extension, side-bending, and rotation. Perform a standing flexion test. Note any guarding or overdramatization of pain.

SEATED

Examiner in Front of the Patient

Test the deep tendon reflexes at L4 (patellar tendon) and S1 (Achilles tendon). Asymmetry may indicate neural compromise. With the patient seated, perform the 90-degree straight leg raising test. This is less obvious to the patient and should be compared with results on a supine straight leg raising test.

Generally assess the muscle strength of all lower extremity muscle groups. Note any asymmetry. The myotomes are L2—hip flexion, L3—knee extension, L4—ankle dorsiflexion and inversion, L5—great toe extension, S1—plantar flexion, ankle eversion, and hip extension, and S2—knee flexion.

Check sensation in response to both dull and sharp stimuli. Check joint position sense; it can be altered peripherally in diabetes mellitus or centrally with posterior column damage (i.e., subacute combined degeneration). Note any muscle atrophy or fasciculations.

Examiner in Back of the Patient

Note skin temperature, drag, and consistency of the paravertebral muscles (ropy v. boggy). Test gross range of motion and lumbar intersegmental vertebral motion. Perform the seated flexion test.

SUPINE

The straight leg raising test with and without dorsiflexion helps to delineate sciatic nerve irritation (positive with dorsiflexion) from hamstring muscle contracture. Note the performance of the nondysfunctional leg on the straight leg raising test. The Thomas test for psoas muscle contracture and the FABERE test for hip joint pathology are performed. Palpate the greater trochanteric area for trochanteric bursitis. Palpate for tender points at the tensor fascia lata and iliotibial bands, and perform the Ober test. Check for anterior tender points (Jones test). Roll your fingers over the skin of the iliac crests. Point tenderness may indicate Maigne's syndrome. The Hoover test may be used when malingering is suspected.

PRONE

Palpate for paravertebral muscle consistency (ropy vs. boggy) and for changes in tissue texture. Evaluate for sacral motion restriction. Note accentuation or flattening of the normal lumbar lordosis, and perform a spring test. Palpate for tender points at the intervertebral disk spaces, the transverse and spinous processes, the lumbosacral junction, the lumbar and sacral tender areas (Jones tender points), and over the piriformis, gluteal, and quadratus lumborum muscles. Perianal or saddle paresthesia may indicate a cauda equina syndrome.

OTHER TESTS

A rectal examination may be performed to evaluate sphincter tone, prostate enlargement, occult blood masses, and piriformis tenderness. Check for testicular masses.

Adjunctive tests should include blood and urine chemistries; supine or standing (postural) anteroposterior, lateral, and indicated oblique radiography of the lumbar spine and pelvis; and computed tomography (CT), magnetic resonance imaging (MRI), or myelography. Chest radiography, skeletal scintigraphy, angiography, and diskography are performed as needed, as are tests of the erythrocyte sedimentation rate, C-reactive protein assays, rheumatoid factor assays, serum protein electrophoresis, serum immunoelectrophoresis, acid phosphatase or prostate-specific antigen assays, lumbar puncture, and HLA typing.

Herniated Nucleus Pulposus

Intervertebral disk herniation can occur in three directions: posterolaterally, purely laterally, and centrally. Posterolateral disk herniation is most common. It often presents as sharp pain of sudden or gradual onset. Increased intraabdominal pressure accompanying a cough, sneeze, lifting, or a Valsalva maneuver will accentuate symptoms. The L5-S1 and L4-L5 disks account for 95% of disk herniation in the lumbar region. The lower lumbar segments bear more weight and act as a fulcrum for forward and backward bending; therefore, they are subjected to greater mechanical stress.

Because of this distribution, radicular symptoms typically present as sciatica or low back pain that radiates to the hip, buttock, posterior thigh, and sometimes the leg and foot. Persistent radiculopathy without back pain may occur once the nuclear material has passed the posterior longitudinal ligament. Atypical pain patterns, such as anterior thigh and groin pain, may be associated with disk herniation at a higher level or with a massive midline herniation.

PHYSICAL FINDINGS

The patient may stand with the affected leg slightly flexed and may walk with an antalgic gait, which reduces tension on the sciatic nerve and its connective tissue wrappings. Protrusion of the disk lateral to the nerve root causes side-bending away from the involved side. Disk protrusion medial to the nerve root causes side-bending toward the lesion. Protective paravertebral muscle spasm with flattening of the normal lumbar lordosis and decreased range of motion is common. A compensatory scoliosis and pelvic side shift with forward flexion are usually present.

The straight leg raising test is most specific for disk herniation affecting the L4, L5, S1, and S2 nerve roots. The straight leg raising test produces tension along the sciatic nerve, the lumbosacral nerve roots, and the dura mater. Unilateral straight leg raising between 0 and 35 degrees places some tension on the sciatic nerve; between 35 and 70 degrees it maximally involves the sciatic nerve, its nerve roots, and the dura. Pain associated with unilateral straight leg raising beyond 70 degrees is most likely joint pain.

A positive straight leg raising test is one that produces pain radiating along the distribution of the sciatic nerve. However, a positive test result is not coequivalent with disk herniation, just as a negative test result does not exclude the possibility of disk herniation. One study found a 64% correlation of results on the straight leg raising test with herniation demonstrated by CT. On the other hand, 97% of patients with positive results on a straight leg raising test of an apparently normal leg had herniated disks demonstrated on CT. Kosteljanetz et al. reported that 43 (88%) of 49 patients with positive results on the straight leg raising test and 19 (95%) of 20 patients with a positive test of the apparently normal leg had disk herniation confirmed surgically.

Neurologic deficit is an important physical finding that helps differentiate radicular from referred pain. Motor weakness, sensory deficit, or reflex changes depend on the level of the involved nerve roots and the extent of the herniation.

The clinical diagnosis can be confirmed with CT, myelography, or MRI. Asymptomatic disk defects have been shown by CT and myelography to occur in up to 25% of the general population. Thus, none of these imaging studies is diagnostic, and clinical correlation is mandatory. CT and MRI arc of equal value in demonstrating herniated intervertebral disks. MRI offers more detail on the degree of disk degeneration and is more accurate in demonstrating small, nonherniated disk protrusions.

Myelography has not been completely replaced by CT or MRI and remains an important diagnostic modality. Since the substitution of water-based for oil-based dye, the incidence of arachnoiditis secondary to myelography has decreased.

Most patients with disk herniation can be treated conservatively. Conservative treatment includes bedrest (less than 1 week), moist heat or ice, nonsteroidal anti-inflammatory agents, and dose pack corticosteroids or muscle relaxants in the acute phase, followed by osteopathic manipulation and an exercise program. Prolonged bedrest, traction, corsets, most centrally acting muscle relaxants, and ultrasound treatment are of debated therapeutic efficacy.

The results of manipulative treatment, osteopathic or nonosteopathic, are mixed. Siehl and Bradford treated over 700 patients between 1950 and 1960 with manipulation under anesthesia. Of these, 185 were diagnosed as having a herniated disk, 171 with myelography. Most of the patients were followed for at least 2 years. Twenty-six percent of the 186 responded with good results (i.e., they were able to resume normal activities relatively symptom free), and 44% of the patients had fair results (they resumed a relatively normal activity level but with some residual symptoms). The remaining 30% responded poorly. These patients showed little to no improvement, reported exacerbation, or had early recurrence of symptoms.

Similarly, Chrisman et al. treated 39 patients with rotatory manipulation under anesthesia, one treatment each. The diagnosis of herniated disk was made in 27 patients both clinically and with myelography. The remaining 12 patients had normal myelograms and were diagnosed from clinical findings alone. Approximately one third of the patients with an abnormal myelogram responded favorably. Ten of the 12 with a normal myelogram also had good to excellent results. In general, those with normal myelograms consistently did better.

Myelography was performed both before and after rotatory manipulation. No reduction of herniation was noted. However, in several operations rotatory manipulation was performed and was noted to cause the two adjacent laminae, on either side of the herniated disk, to move apart at least 5 mm. The authors proposed that stretching of the lower fibers of the ligamentum flavum and the superolateral position of the posterior joint capsule, rather than an actual reduction in herniation, was a possible mechanism for symptom relief. They also discussed the possibility of adhesions over the spinal nerve roots as a cause for radicular symptoms that are freed by rotatory manipulation.

Steiner has stressed the distinction between a reducible versus a nonreducible herniated disk, or a protruding versus a degenerated or sequestered disk. As long as the annulus has retained its inherent elasticity and the disk herniation is not fragmented or massive, it should be reducible with manipulation. However, only clinical or subjective improvement has been reported; the disk lesion has not demonstrably resolved on CT or myelography.

Surgery is indicated when there is progressive neurologic deficit or moderate to severe neurologic deficit (e.g., bowel or bladder dysfunction, foot drop, paralysis), or persistent, intolerable radicular symptoms despite an adequate trial of manipulation.

It has been reported that surgery offers more of a short-term than long-term solution. On 4- to 10-year follow-ups of patients in a randomized study who had been treated surgically, the same functional capacity and complaints existed as in patients treated nonoperatively. By contrast, careful patient selection, accurate preoperative diagnosis, and the absence of psychosocial impairment greatly increased the likelihood of surgical success. The risk of a poor surgical outcome is associated with lack of clinical correlation, abnormal pain drawing, a pending Workmen's Compensation case, and a psychological profile indicating hysteria, hypochondriasis, or somatization.

Osteopathic manipulation is directed toward eliminating or reducing muscle spasm and restoring normal joint motion. These goals can be achieved through a combination of specifically applied soft tissue techniques. Once muscle spasm has been sufficiently relieved, high-velocity, low-amplitude thrusting techniques are often necessary to normalize joint motion. Trigger points can be treated with a vapocoolant spray and injection of a local anesthetic.

CENTRAL DISK HERNIATION

When large enough, central disk herniation produces a compressive lesion of the cauda equina at one or more levels. The cauda equina syndrome is characterized by bilateral or unilateral sciatica, "saddle" anesthesia, and lower extremity weakness that may progress to paraplegia with bowel and bladder incontinence. Physical examination may reveal unilateral or bilateral weakness and decreased sensation in the lower extremities, decreased anal sphincter tone, urinary retention, saddle paresthesia, a positive straight leg raising test on the dysfunctional or nondysfunctional side, and bilaterally depressed deep tendon reflexes. Definitive diagnosis requires CT or MRI.

Reported cases of cauda equina syndrome secondary to central disk herniation range from 1% to 16% of all herniated lumbar disks. There is no indication for conservative treatment. Prompt and accurate diagnosis is essential to ensure quick surgical decompression. Irreparable damage to bladder function is likely unless surgical decompression is performed within 12 hours of the initial loss of bladder control.

Spinal Stenosis

LATERAL SPINAL STENOSIS

Lateral spinal stenosis can involve any one of the three segments of the lateral spinal canal: the entrance zone (spinal canal), the midzone (nerve root canal), or the exit zone (intervertebral foramen). As with a herniated disk, lateral stenosis most commonly occurs at the L4-L5 or L5-S1 levels. The patient usually complains of unilateral or bilateral sciatica without concurrent low back pain. The symptoms are exacerbated by extension and rotation of the lumbar spine and are often intermittent. Neurologic deficit, if present, is usually mild. However, progressive degeneration can result in fixed stenosis with constant resting pain and dysesthesia.

Lateral radiographs may show decreased intervertebral disk height and/or enlarged superior articular processes or spondylolisthesis. Oblique x-ray is best to demonstrate spondylolysis. CT or MRI will usually demonstrate stenosis of any one of the three portions of the lateral spinal canal.

Conservative treatment includes an exercise program with the avoidance of rotational exercises, instruction in back care, and an abdominal support. Manipulative treatment was shown by Kirkaldy-Willis and Cassidy to offer significant relief of symptoms in 50% of patients diagnosed with lateral spinal stenosis. If the condition is severe enough, laminectomy is indicated.

CENTRAL SPINAL STENOSIS

Central spinal stenosis is also called pseudoclaudication or neurogenic claudication. The symptoms are similar to those of intermittent claudication due to occlusive aortoiliac disease. However, there are differentiating features between the two. The pain of neurogenic claudication is usually described as a burning or numbness in the low back and buttock which is exacerbated by walking up an incline and by extending of the lumbar spine. Relief is reported after 20 to 30 minutes of rest and by sitting with the hips and trunk flexed. The patient may walk in a "simian" posture with his trunk flexed at the hips.

Vascular intermittent claudication, on the other hand, typically manifests as an aching or cramp-like pain in the hips, thighs, and buttocks with radiation into the calves. The pain is usually initiated by walking and is relieved within a few minutes of resting. Spinal motion (e.g., extension) does not exacerbate symptoms.

Physical examination in a patient with vascular disease may demonstrate femoral bruits, decreased peripheral pulses, and cool, pale lower extremities, with one leg usually worse than the other. Neurologic deficit is absent. In contrast, neurogenic claudication is often significant for unilateral or bilateral radicular symptoms. Deep tendon reflexes may be depressed at more than one spinal level. If the deep tendon reflexes are initially normal, an abnormality may be revealed when tested immediately after exercise. A neurogenic bladder also frequently accompanies neurogenic claudication. Although subtle, a history of frequency, urgency, or incomplete bladder emptying is an indication. Perianal anesthesia and hypotonicity of the anal sphincter may also be present.

Some authors have suggested that degenerative changes of the spine are accompanied by hypertension of the vertebral venous plexuses. The pain experienced in central stenosis may be the result of edema with subsequent compression of the small nerves innervating vertebrae, the annulus fibrosus, and ligaments, as well as compression of the vertebral arterial supply, producing ischemia of the cauda equida.

Conservative therapy includes an exercise program emphasizing lumbar flexion, and abdominal support. Kirkaldy-Willis and Cassidy found that high-velocity, low-amplitude thrusting techniques offered significant symptom relief in 5 of 11 patients with central spinal stenosis. Soft tissue and articular techniques and occasionally thrusting techniques are used to treat palpable findings such as muscle spasm, decreased joint mobility, and tender points. Flexion should be encouraged and extension avoided, since either may exacerbate symptoms. Surgery is generally indicated in cases of pain refractory to conservative measures, marked exercise intolerance, significant muscle weakness, numbness or paresthesia, and bladder or bowel dysfunction.

The resolution of symptoms in some patients treated by high-velocity, low-amplitude thrusting techniques for documented spinal stenosis raises two important questions. The manipulation itself does not reduce bony stenosis. Therefore, what is the actual source of symptoms in these patients, and are the symptoms relieved? Only speculative answers are available. Are radicular symptoms due to abnormal fascial and dural strains or to adhesions that compress the arterial, venous, and nerve supply to the vertebrae, spinal cord, disks, and posterior joints? Do radicular symptoms represent an abnormal sympathetic reflex mediated by the sinovertebral nerves? In normalizing the articular relationship of the dysfunctional vertebral segment and those adjacent to it, are fascial or dorsal strains that compress the vascular and nerve supply being reduced, thereby relieving venous congestion, edema, ischemia, and nerve compression? Are ligaments, muscles, and the posterior facet joint capsule being stretched? Are adhesions being broken?

The posterior facet joints, sacroiliac joints, and muscles are all potential sources of primary low back pain with radiation to the lower extremities. By means not entirely understood, each can produce pseudoradicular pain. The pseudoradicular syndromes differ from true radicular syndromes in that they lack the tension signs and neurologic deficit common to the true radiculopathies. Furthermore, referred pain is characterized as deep, boring, and diffuse, whereas radicular pain is described as sharp and well defined.

Sacroiliac Joint Syndrome

Sacroiliac joint syndrome is due to somatic dysfunction of this joint and must be differentiated from lumbar radiculopathy. Sacral motion is restricted, and changes in tissue texture occur over the sacroiliac joint. The patient's pain may be reproduced during the examination. Associated spasm of one or more muscles attaching to the sacrum is usually present. These muscles include the piriformis, gluteus maximus, coccygeal, iliac, and erector spinae via the thoracolumbar fascia. Muscle spasm and trigger points, if bilateral, are usually worse on the side of the dysfunction.

Symptoms include pain at the sacroiliac area with possible radiation to the lower extremity. Neurologic deficit does not accompany this syndrome. The condition is diagnosed from clinical findings and a favorable response to osteopathic manipulation. Radiography is useful to rule out other pathologic conditions and early ankylosing spondylitis.

Manipulative treatment includes any of the soft tissue techniques: myofascial, muscle energy, counterstrain for tender points, myofascial release, facilitated positional release, and, when indicated, thrusting techniques.

The use of a vapocoolant spray and injection of a local anesthetic into the affected joint may be therapeutic as well as diagnostic. The cause of sacroiliac joint pain is not clear. It has been speculated to originate from the joint itself or to be secondary to prolonged contraction of one of the muscles that attach to it.

Posterior Facet Joint Syndrome

Posterior facet joint syndrome is also not a true radiculopathy; however, its presentation is similar to that of other causes of radiating pain. Posterior facet joint syndrome and sacroiliac syndrome are the most common causes of low back pain referred to the lower extremities. Proposed causes include synovitis and the pinching of folds of synovial tissue (pseudomenisci) within the facet joints, degenerative changes of the facet joint, and spinal segmental instability.

Less clearly understood is the cause of radiating pain associated with posterior facet joint pathology. Innervation of the facet joints by the recurrent sinovertebral nerve and its branches overlaps considerably. Clinically, specific pain patterns corresponding to a specific lumbar level have generally not been shown.

Maigne's syndrome is one Parisian doctor's claim to fame for describing a lesion at the T12-

L1 posterior facet joints. In addition to local pain and tenderness in the region of the facet joints, there is irritation of the superior cluneal nerves, producing tenderness over the iliac crest of the involved side.

The typical history associated with posterior facet joint syndrome is unilateral or bilateral low back pain (usually at the L4–S1 levels), often radiating to the buttock, trochanteric region, and posterior thigh or groin and occasionally extending as far as the calf or ankle. Complaints of muscle weakness or sensory loss do not typically accompany this syndrome. The physical examination generally reveals motion restriction of one or more vertebral segments, local paravertebral muscle spasm, focal paraspinal tenderness, limited spinal range of motion, and exacerbation of pain with lateral side-bending or extension and rotation on the symptomatic side. Straight leg raising is often limited, probably because of accompanying hamstring muscle spasm. Findings on neurologic examination are normal or minimally abnormal. Oblique and lateral radiographs may reveal abnormal posterior facets.

Posterior facet joint syndrome is diagnosed initially from the history and physical examination findings. Without radiography, the diagnosis is often presumptive and is based on the patient's response to manipulative treatment or facet joint injection with a corticosteroid and a local anesthetic agent under fluoroscopy. This type of injection may relieve symptoms in 20% to 50% of suspected cases of posterior facet joint syndrome.

Osteopathic manipulation is effective in the treatment of the facet syndrome. It is directed toward specific palpatory findings. Kirkaldy-Willis and Cassidy conducted a prospective study of high-velocity, low-amplitude thrusting techniques in 283 patients with chronic low back and radicular pain. Results were reported for specific diagnoses—sacroiliac joint and/or posterior facet joint syndrome, lateral stenosis (fixed or dynamic), and central stenosis. Some 79% of 56 patients with posterior facet joint syndrome, 92% of 69 patients with sacroiliac joint syndrome, and 88% of 48 patients with both joint syndromes reported significant improvement in symptoms and ability to resume daily activities. Daily treatment for 2 weeks was most efficacious. Patients who did not respond to this regimen were unlikely to

respond to manipulative treatment. No patient's condition was worsened by the thrusting therapy.

Piriformis Syndrome

Piriformis syndrome is a peripheral neuritis of the sciatic nerve caused by an abnormal condition of the piriformis muscle. The piriformis muscle is an external rotator and abductor of the thigh, located deep to the gluteal muscles. It originates on the anterolateral border of the sacrum, at the sacroiliac joint capsule, and on the anterior portion of the sacrotuberous ligament, and inserts into the superomedial aspect of the greater trochanter of the femur.

After passing through the greater sciatic foramen, the sciatic nerve courses under the piriformis muscle on its way to the posterior thigh. Factors thought to cause sciatic nerve irritation or inflammation include piriformis muscle spasm or contracture, local trauma to the buttocks, repeated mechanical stressors (e.g., running), sacral base unleveling or pelvic instability, excessive local pressure, especially in thin or cachectic patients ("hip pocket neuritis"), anatomic variation, and local perineural inflammation secondary to the endogenous release of vasoactive substances from an inflamed piriformis muscle.

In approximately 10% of the general population the common peroneal and tibial components of the sciatic nerve remain separate. One, usually the common peroneal, passes directly through the piriformis muscle. In another 10%, the piriformis muscle arises from two tendinous origins, with the sciatic nerve passing between them.

The piriformis syndrome produces symptoms easily confused with those of a herniated lumbar disk or facet joint pathology. The patient often complains of hip and buttock pain radiating down the posterior thigh, possibly to the calf or foot. Low back pain is usually not a major component. The piriformis syndrome generally differs from disk herniation by the absence of neurologic deficit. Rarely, severe piriformis compression produces a sciatic nerve palsy and all of the accompanying neurologic sequelae.

On physical examination muscle strength, sensation, and deep tendon reflexes are normal (unless the syndrome is extreme). Most notable is exquisite tenderness with or without trigger points anywhere along the piriformis muscle. When palpated, these trigger points may reproduce the radicular pain. Gluteal tender points may also be present.

Contracture of the piriformis muscle can be grossly assessed with the patient prone. Flex the knees to 90 degrees and, while holding the ankles, internally rotate both hip joints until resistance is met. Compare the relative freedom of motions on each side. Sacral motion is often restricted.

Osteopathic manipulative medicine is espe-cially effective in the treatment of this syndrome. Manipulation is directed toward palpatory findings, not subjective complaints. A combination of soft tissue techniques such as muscle energy treatment, active and passive myofascial techniques to the lumbar and lumbosacral region, counterstrain treatment for tender points, and myofascial release of the sacrum and pelvis, as well as thrusting techniques, when indicated, is especially effective. Trigger points can be treated with a vapocoolant spray and local injection of an anesthetic.

SPONDYLOLISTHESIS AND SPONDYLOLYSIS
Barbara Polstein

The term *spondylolisthesis* is derived from the Greek words *spondyl*, meaning spine, and *olisthesis*, meaning to fall or to slip. Spondylolisthesis refers to forward slippage of one vertebral body over the vertebral body immediately below it. Retrolisthesis, or backward displacement, is much less common but can occur. *Spondylolysis* refers to fracture and separation of the pars interarticularis of the vertebral arch.

Spondylolisthesis occurs in 20% to 70% of patients with spondylolysis. Spondylolisthesis is usually found in the lumbar spine and occasionally in the cervical spine. If found in the thoracic region, it is always secondary to trauma. Approximately 75% of all cases occur with L5 slipping on S1, 20% with L4 slipping on L5, and 5% at higher levels (Figs. 27-5 and 27-6).

Classification
Wiltze, Newman, and McNab have classified spondylolisthesis into five categories, according to etiology. These are described below.

DYSPLASTIC SPONDYLOLISTHESIS
Dysplastic spondylolisthesis is a congenital abnormality of the first sacral or fifth lumbar neural arch. Unable to withstand normal forces exerted on the lumbar spine, this defect permits slippage of the L5-S1 facet joint articulation during childhood or adolescence. Approximately 25% to 35% of symptomatic children have dysplastic spondy-lolisthesis. Standing lateral radiographs show subluxation with forward slipping of the entire neural arch of L5, including the spinous process. Progression of slippage may occur with attenuation of the pedicles. If the posterior elements and lamina are present, spondylolisthesis does not usually exceed 25%. If it does, cauda equina syndrome or frank paralysis can result.

ISTHMIC SPONDYLOLISTHESIS
Isthmic spondylolisthesis is a primary defect of the pars interarticularis (located within the lamina). There are three types:

1. Elongation of the pars interarticularis
2. Fatigue fracture of the pars interarticularis
3. Acute fracture of the pars interarticularis secondary to trauma

Isthmic spondylolisthesis is the most common type of spondylolisthesis in the general population less than 50 years of age. It is thought to be an inherited defect of the cartilaginous model of the vertebral arch. The familial incidence of spondylolysis with or without spondylolisthesis ranges from 27% to 69%. This is in contrast to a 4.4% to 6.0% occurrence in the general population. Some authors report a male-female ratio of 2:1 or 3:1; others have found no sex difference. The most common age of onset of spondylolysis is between 5 and 7 years. Onset is generally painless. The condition is seldom seen in children less than

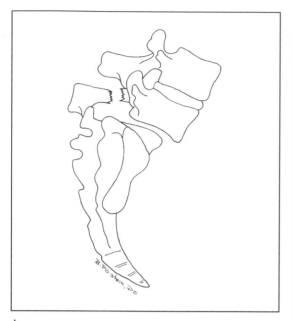

A

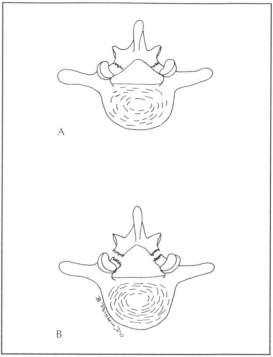

Figure 27-6. Cross-sectional view of bilateral spondylolysis at the pars interarticularis. (Adapted, with permission, from Rosse K. 1980. The Musculoskeletal System in Health and Disease. New York: Harper & Row, p. 132.)

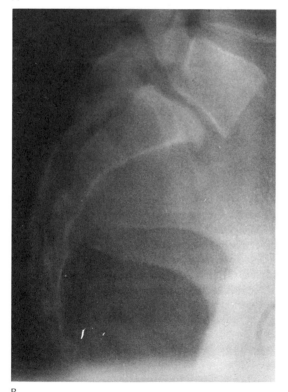

B

Figure 27-5. **(A)** Spondylolysis and spondylolisthesis of L5 on S1. (Adapted from Rothman R, Simeone AF. 1982. The Spine, 2nd ed., Vol. 1. Philadelphia: Saunders, pp. 263–284.) **(B)** Radiograph of same condition.

5 years old. This observation supports the belief that spondylolysis and spondylolisthesis are not anomalies present at birth.

Fredrickson et al. found that approximately 90% to 95% of 500 cases of spondylolysis with or without spondylolisthesis involved L5 on S1. Approximately 75% of the cases were bilateral. No patient with unilateral spondylolysis had concurrent spondylolisthesis.

Analysis of various mechanical loads on the lumbar spine has shown that the L5 vertebra, particularly the pars interarticularis, is subject to the greatest mechanical stress. It is easy to imagine how a defect in the L5 vertebra might predispose it to elongation or to spondylolytic cracks in the pars interarticularis. Farfan et al. identified three mechanisms thought to result in disruption of the neural arch: unbalanced shear force, forced rotation, and flexion overload.

Progression of spondylolisthesis is most rapid at 10 to 15 years of age, during adolescent growth.

Like spondylolysis, it is also generally painless. From 16% to 31% of children with spondylolysis or spondylolisthesis have a significant history of trauma to the low back. Progression of slippage after 20 years of age is rare.

Fredrickson and others have shown that 7% of patients with pars interarticularis defects have concurrent lumbarization or sacralization of the spine. Spina bifida occulta is also 13 times more prevalent in patients with spondylolysis or spondylolisthesis.

DEGENERATIVE SPONDYLOLISTHESIS

This condition is most common in persons aged 50 years and older. Forward displacement of the vertebra is caused by degenerative changes in the posterior facet joints. Commonly, L4 slips on L5. There is a reported female-male ratio of 4:1. Degenerative spondylolisthesis at the L4-L5 level is four times more common in patients with sacralization of the fifth lumbar vertebra. This is because sacralization of L5 subjects the L4 vertebra to greater mechanical forces.

It is believed that degenerative spondylolisthesis the result of spondylosis. Degeneration with erosion of the posterior facet joints and degenerative changes in the disk eventually allow the inferior facets and body of the L4 vertebra to slip forward on the L5 vertebra. Degenerative spondylolisthesis usually does not exceed 30% unless there is a history of previous back surgery, in which case disruption of the lamina or pseudoarthrosis formation exacerbates instability.

TRAUMATIC SPONDYLOLISTHESIS

Traumatic spondylolisthesis involves acute fracture anywhere in the neural arch other than the pars interarticularis, such as the pedicle or the inferior or superior articular facets.

PATHOLOGIC FRACTURE

Pathologic fracture may occur with localized or generalized bone disease anywhere in the neural arch. General causes include metastatic bone disease, Paget's disease, and spinal tuberculosis. A localized cause is fracture of the vertebra one level above a previous spinal fusion.

Findings and Examination

Most cases of spondylolysis and spondylolisthesis in children and adolescents are painless. About a quarter of all cases have low back pain with or without radiation to the lower extremity. Very few seek medical attention before the age of 20. In the majority of cases, symptoms associated with spondylolisthesis begin during the second or third decade of life.

The most common symptom is persistent low back ache with or without radiation to the buttocks, posterior thigh, and occasionally to the leg and foot. These symptoms are aggravated by standing for long periods of time or by increased activity, and are relieved by rest.

The sole complaint of radicular pain or neurologic deficit is less common. In degenerative spondylolisthesis, the pedicles of the forwardly displaced vertebra compress the nerve root at the same level in a guillotinelike manner. A third cause of nerve root compression is intervertebral disk herniation. Spondylolisthesis produces instability, which in turn causes greater stress, with subsequent degenerative changes in the disk and facet joints. Typically, herniation of the L4 disk occurs with spondylolisthesis of L5 on S1.

Hamstring muscle spasm of varying degree is frequently seen with spondylolysis or spondylolisthesis, occurring in 80% of symptomatic children. The hamstring muscles are secondary hip extensors and the major knee flexors. Contracture produces limited forward flexion at the hips, diminished knee extension, and backward tilting of the pelvis. If severe enough, the result is a characteristic stiff-legged, short-strided gait with the hips rotating forward with each step. This gait has been referred to by Wiltze as the pelvic waddle. Some children with hamstring involvement run instead of walk, or walk on their toes with their knees flexed. These children may also sleep with their knees and hips markedly flexed.

The mechanism of hamstring muscle involvement is not clearly understood. Some believe it is due to nerve root irritation. Others suspect it is a mechanical attempt by the body to stabilize the lumbosacral articulation. The postural and gait changes associated with hamstring muscle spasm spontaneously resolve following spinal fusion without the need for nerve root decompression. The straight leg raising test is often positive with minimal degrees of flexion, reflecting the severity of hamstring muscle spasm.

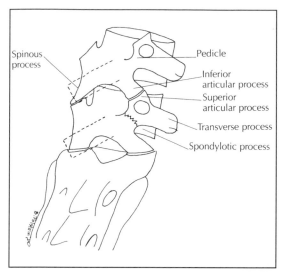

Figure 27-7. Spondylolysis of the L5 pars interarticularis, oblique view. Note the appearance of a collar around the neck of a Scottie dog. (Adapted from McGee, 1987, p. 212.)

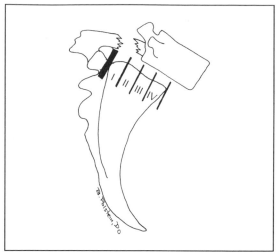

Figure 27-8. Spondylolisthesis, grades I to IV.

Diagnosis

The diagnosis of spondylolysis and spondylolisthesis is made with standing radiography of the lumbar spine, which best demonstrates the degree of spondylolisthesis. Bilateral oblique views allow for the diagnosis of spondylolysis. A spondylolytic defect of the pars interarticularis appears as a collar around the neck of a Scottie dog (Fig. 27-7).

Lowe et al. compared recumbent and standing lateral roentgenograms in 50 patients with spondylolisthesis. Approximately 26% of the patients showed dynamic changes with a 2-mm or greater increase in forward displacement on standing. A comparison of supine and standing radiographs will help evaluate the degree of instability of the defect. Patients with a greater degree of slippage on weight-bearing also tended to have more severe symptoms.

One system of grading spondylolisthesis is on a scale of I to IV. This grading system estimates the degree of forward slip of one vertebra over another on standing lateral radiographs of the lumbar spine. The sacrum or vertebral body below the slipped segment is divided into four equal parts. In grade I spondylolisthesis, vertebral displacement is between 0% and 25% of the anteroposterior (AP) diameter of the vertebra below; in grade

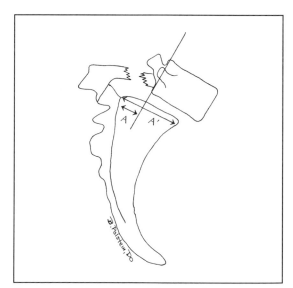

Figure 27-9. The degree of forward slippage is expressed as the percentage $\frac{A}{A'} \times 100$.

II, between 25% and 50%; in grade III, between 50% and 75%; and in grade IV, greater than 75% (Fig. 27-8).

A more accurate measurement expresses spondylolisthesis as a percentage (Fig. 27-9). A is that portion of the AP diameter of the lower segment over which the upper segment has slipped; A' is the total AP diameter of the lower segment. This

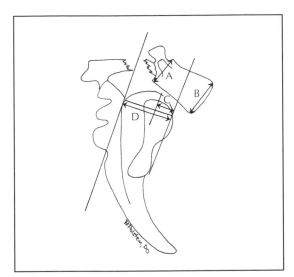

Figure 27-10. Vertebral wedging due to spondylolisthesis is calculated as the percentage $\frac{A}{B} \times 100$. The percent rounding of the sacral base is calculated as $\frac{C}{D} \times 100$. Both measurements have been used as a method of following the progression of slippage of L5 on S1. (Figs. 27-9 and 27-10 adapted from Wiltze LL, Winter RB. 1983. Terminology and measurement of spondylolisthes. J. Bone Joint Surg. 65:6.)

method of measurement is preferred for accurate follow-up of the progression of the spondylolisthesis. It is only possible if roentgenograms are taken the same way each time. Other methods of measuring progression are shown in Figure 27-10).

Patients with grade I or early grade II spondylolisthesis often have relatively normal physical examinations. Limited forward flexion and hamstring muscle tightness might be the only abnormal physical findings. It is usually not until late grade II or grade III slippage occurs that postural deformity becomes apparent. Typically there are marked exaggeration of the lumbar lordosis, backward tilting of the pelvis, and forward thrusting of the lower abdomen. A transverse abdominal crease at the level of the umbilicus is often present.

In isthmic spondylolisthesis, a stepoff or depression directly above the spinous process of the slipped segment (L5) may be palpated. In the degenerative type, the posterior elements are displaced with the rest of the vertebra. Therefore, this stepoff will be palpable just below the spinous process of the slipped segment. In more advanced cases, nerve root irritation causes protective muscle spasm in the lower back, producing a compensatory scoliosis. If not treated, this functional scoliosis can convert into a structural scoliosis.

Treatment

The majority of symptomatic patients respond to conservative treatment without the need for surgical stabilization. Conservative therapy for spondylolisthesis includes the following:

1. A daily exercise program, including the Williams flexion exercises and quarter situps.
2. Weight loss in overweight patients, to help relieve postural stress on the spondylolytic defect.
3. Osteopathic treatment: Manipulative treatment will probably not reduce the lesion. However, it can help to identify the other sources of referred pain that commonly accompany spondylolisthesis or spondylolysis. These include the posterior facet joints (typically one level above the defect), the sacroiliac joints, and myofascial trigger points.

The posterior facet joint and SI joint syndromes are diagnosed clinically, primarily from the presence of motion restriction and lack of neurologic deficit. Myofascial syndromes are recognized from the presence of trigger points. All identified somatic dysfunctions should be treated. Alleviation or significant reduction of the patient's symptoms after one or two treatments confirms the diagnosis.

Surgery is indicated for the following:

1. Symptomatic grade I or II spondylolisthesis unrelieved by an adequate trial of conservative therapy.
2. Progression of forward displacement.
3. Grade III spondylolisthesis.
4. Postural deformity or significant gait abnormality due to hamstring spasm not relieved by physical therapy.

It is important to follow any progression of spondylolisthesis. This is accomplished by serial radiographs with measurement of the percentage of forward slip, as described earlier. Instability of L5 on S1 is responsible for wear and tear of these vertebrae. Gradual erosion of both the anterior and posterior portions of the sacral base produces a rounded or dome shape. The body of L5 becomes wedge-shaped, with the posterior portion narrower than the anterior portion. Both of these changes reflect the degree of slip.

Forward slippage can occur laterally as well as in a purely anterior direction. The *slip angle*, or the angular relationship between L5 and S1, is measured at the intersection of one line drawn along the posterior aspect of S1 and another along the anterior aspect of the body of L5.

Progression is also noted from accentuation of the lumbar lordosis and an increase in the lumbosacral angle. These changes can be followed by measuring the percent of rounding of the sacrum, wedging of the fifth lumbar vertebra, the angle of lumbar lordosis, and the lumbosacral angle.

COCCYGODYNIA
Paula D. Scariati

In 1859, Sir J. V. Simpson coined the term *coccygodynia*, using it to describe persistent pain in the coccyx. He noted that when injury to the coccyx or coccygeal joint occurred, or when the surrounding tissue was inflamed, contraction of the muscles attached to the coccyx would elicit the characteristic pain of coccygodynia. Further observations since that time have confirmed the presence of spasm of the levator ani and coccygeus muscles in a significant percentage of cases of coccygodynia.

Anatomy
THE BONY PELVIS
The word *coccyx* comes from the Greek word *kokkue*, meaning cuckoo, as the coccyx resembles a cuckoo's beak. The coccyx is a result of fusion of four evolutionarily separate vertebrae. It is not unusual to visualize the coccyx as three to five distinct vertebrae in a child, but by adulthood, these bones are united into a single bone. In later life, the coccyx may even fuse with the sacrum. The coccyx is a triangular osseous formation that is concave anteriorly, following the curve of the sacrum.

The bones of the pelvis vary from male to female. The female pelvis is more delicate than the male pelvis. The sacrum is shorter, wider, and less curved. The greater sciatic notch has a greater diameter; the ischial tuberosities are wider apart and everted; and the inferior aperture is larger, and hence the coccyx is more variable in position. The position of the sacrum and coccyx in the female tends to be backward and thus more prone to trauma. The male pelvis has a narrower sciatic notch and the inclination of the sacrum and coccyx is forward into the pelvic cavity tucked between the ischia. This shields the coccyx from external trauma to a great extent in males.

THE MUSCLES
The pelvic diaphragm is a thin sheet of muscle consisting of the coccygeus muscle posteriorly and the more extensive levator ani muscle anterolaterally. Its halves form the sloping floor of the pelvis through which the urethra, vagina, and anal canal pass. The diaphragm closes the inferior pelvic outlet somewhat as a funnel would were it placed in the pelvic cavity.

Levator Ani
This broad, thin muscle unites with its contralateral partner to form the largest portion of the pelvic diaphragm.

Origin: pelvic surface of the body of the pubis to the ischial spine.
Insertion: central perineal tendon, wall of the anal canal, anococcygeal ligament, and coccyx.
Innervation: fibers from the third and fourth sacral nerves which enter its pelvic surface, and the inferior rectal nerve (a branch of the pudendal nerve which originates from S2–S4 nerve roots), which enters its perineal surface.
Functions: The muscular pelvic diaphragm supports the pelvic viscera and resists the inferior

thrust accompanying increases in intraabdominal pressure (e.g., such as occurs during coughing, defecation, and normal thoracolumbar respiration). Parts of the levator ani also support the prostate (males) and the posterior wall of the vagina (females), holds the anorectal junction anteriorly, and supports the fetal head during parturition while the cervix of the uterus is dilating.

Coccygeus
This triangular sheet of muscle lies against and blends with the posterior portion of the levator ani. It forms the smaller, posterior portion of the pelvic diaphragm.

Origin: pelvic surfaces of the ischial spine and the sacrospinal ligament.
Insertion: lateral margins of the fifth sacral vertebra and the coccyx.
Innervation: branches from the ventral rami of the fourth and fifth sacral nerves.
Function: supports the coccyx. In women, it pulls the coccyx forward after it has been pressed posteriorly during childbirth.

Physiology
In *Visceral Manipulation*, Jean-Pierre Barral and Pierre Mercier define the sacrococcygeal articulation as a diarthrosis with an articular motion of up to 30 degrees. This joint is surrounded by anterior, posterior, and lateral sacrococcygeal ligaments that allow good mobility while ensuring appropriate tension on the coccyx and associated structures. The motion of this joint is best exemplified during childbirth, where its posterior flexion allows some vital centimeters to be gained. On a daily basis, the sacrococcygeal joint and pelvic diaphragm play a role in copulation, defecation, and micturition. They also contribute to lumbosacral biomechanics, and thus coccygeal dysfunction can manifest as lumbosacral restriction.

Motion at the sacrococcygeal articulation can be restricted to various degrees following retraction or spasm of the soft tissue structures that attach to or help to maintain the joint. Coccygeal displacement can impede pelvic physiology. For example, when the coccyx moves closer to the pubic symphysis (e.g., anterior flexion), the pelvic diaphragm becomes lax and loses tone. The levator

ani and coccygeal muscles lose power, and thus the structures that pierce the diaphragm are affected. It is not uncommon for patients to complain of incontinence of stool and urine, impotence (males), and painful intercourse (females).

Etiology
The causes of coccygodynia are many. They include infections such as tuberculosis and osteomyelitis, fractures, dislocations, ligamentous tears, postnatal injuries, and other types of trauma.

Signs and Symptoms
The presenting signs and symptoms of coccygodynia are consistent regardless of the etiology.

ACUTE COCCYGODYNIA
A. Symptoms
   1. Pain with sitting
   2. Pain with bowel movements
   3. Proctalgia fugax
   4. Tenesmus (rarer)
   5. Painful intercourse
   6. Occasionally, pain when lying supine, if the sacrococcygeal joint is very convex (the prone position may afford some relief from pain)
B. Signs
   1. Point tenderness at the tip of the coccyx, sacrococcygeal joint, and along the coccygeal ligaments
   2. Muscle pain in the levator ani and coccygeus muscles
   3. Decreased range of motion in the sacrococcygeal joint
   4. Hypermobile distal coccygeal segments secondary to ligamentous tear or fracture
   5. Side-bending and rotation lesions of the sacrococcygeal joint
   6. Sharp pain on distraction and compression of the coccyx
   7. Pain with passive flexion or extension of the coccyx

CHRONIC COCCYGODYNIA
A. Some or all of the signs and symptoms of acute coccygodynia
B. Gastrointestinal
   1. Constipation

2. Hemorrhoids secondary to decreased venous drainage
3. Proctalgia fugax
4. Incontinence

C. Genitourinary
1. Urethral syndromes—nonspecific urinary tract infections secondary to stasis or poor drainage
2. Urethritis secondary to spasm of the periurethral muscles
3. Decreased venous and lymphatic drainage
4. Incontinence
5. Impotence
6. Cystitis
7. Prostatitis

D. Gynecology
1. Painful intercourse
2. Pelvic anhedonia—loss of orgasm secondary to nervous system shock (loss of genital vasomotor response and decrease in uterovaginal mobility)
3. Ligamentous strain causing congestion
4. Uterine retroversion

E. Musculoskeletal
1. Stretched iliolumbar ligaments. If the coccyx is restricted, the sacrotuberous ligament cannot stretch as the ischia spread during the act of sitting. Instead, the iliolumbar ligaments are forced to accommodate.
2. Spasm of associated adjacent muscles (e.g., the piriform muscle, which has its origin on the anterior surface of the sacrum)

F. Psychology
Depression—generalized devitalization secondary to a decrease in the mobility of the entire body or a decrease in the craniosacral respiratory impulse

Evaluation

Evaluation begins as the patient walks in the door. Does he walk stiffly and sit cautiously? A complete history is important. The physician must inquire as to any signs and symptoms relative to the genitourinary and gastrointestinal systems, as well as sexual dysfunctions.

Next the mobility of the coccyx is tested. An external route is employed first. A rectal examination is done only if necessary. The patient sits with his legs hanging slightly apart so that the sacrococcygeal attachments are taut. With his index finger, the physician follows the patient's gluteal crease to a point 1 cm posterior to the anus. At the tip of the coccyx, located at this point, a posterosuperior force is exerted. Sharp pain is an indication of dysfunction and a reason to perform a rectal examination.

To facilitate rectal examination, the patient is placed in the lateral decubitis position with his legs slightly separated. Donning a lubricated glove, the physician enters the rectum with his index finger, leaving the finger in the rectal ampulla with the pad posteriorly against the coccyx and sacrum. The mobility of the sacrococcygeal articulation is checked by placing a thumb, externally, parallel to the index finger. The coccyx is moved anteriorly and then side to side. Anterior restrictions are the most common, but lateral displacements also occur.

Range of motion testing of the coccyx evaluates the integrity of the sacrococcygeal joint and the associated ligaments and muscles. Normally there are asymmetries and minimal tenderness.

Osteopathic Manipulative Techniques

Conservative, noninvasive treatment of coccygodynia seems to produce the best results. Some authors have proposed coccygotomies and injections as first-line therapy. This seems premature and irrational when one considers the combined cure and improvement rate of manipulation in various studies is anywhere from 50% to 100%.

MOBILIZATION OF THE SACROCOCCYGEAL JOINT

1. **Patient position:** lying on the table in the lateral decubitus position.
2. **Physician position:** standing beside the table, facing the back of the patient.
3. **Technique:**
   a. The physician places the palm of his cephalad hand on the patient's sacrum (used for counterpressure).
   b. The physician inserts the index finger of his other hand gently into the patient's rectum.
   c. Thereafter different techniques are used.
      i. For anterior displacement, the tip of the coccyx is pushed posteriorly and up.
      ii. For posterior displacement, the tip of the coccyx is pushed anteriorly.

iii. For lateral displacement, the coccyx is mobilized from side to side.

iv. For pure fixation, the coccyx is moved in an anterior-posterior motion.

d. With each repetition, the force exerted is increased to help facilitate the fullest motion possible at the sacrococcygeal joint.

e. All the techniques are done gently. The goal is to free stiffened tissue, release joint restriction, and restore full mobility.

RELEASE OF THE PELVIC DIAPHRAGM AND ASSOCIATED MUSCLES

1. **Patient position:** lying on the table in the lateral decubitus position.

2. **Physician position:** standing beside the table, facing the back of the patient.

3. **Technique:**

a. The physician inserts the full length of his index finger into the patient's rectum. (The physician should position the palm of his other hand on the patient's sacrum as a stabilizing force.)

b. The physician exerts a lateroposterior pressure with a concomitant horizontal stroking motion to the fibers of the levator ani and coccygeus muscles.

c. The piriformis is immediately beyond the sacrospinous ligament and is touched by fingertip in such a manner that lateral motion of the finger will stroke lengthwise those portions of the muscles in the pelvis.

d. It is wise to begin this technique as lightly as possible, since the muscles involved are tender. Pressure may be increased in the course of several treatments.

MYOFASCIAL RELEASE OF THE PELVIC DIAPHRAGM

This technique may be done from an external approach. The principles were described earlier.

Dysfunctions of the coccyx and the sacrococcygeal joint can cause increased tension on the dural tube, which in turn can affect attachments of the tube (dura) in the spine and cranium. Upledger and Vredevoogd found a cause-and-effect relationship between sacrococcygeal somatic dysfunction and pain of the head and back.

TOTAL TREATMENT PROGRAM

1. Osteopathic manipulative treatment every other day for 7 to 10 days

2. Improved posture, because sitting erect pulls the buttocks together and causes natural cushioning

3. Laxatives for constipation

4. Hot sitz baths daily for 7 to 10 days.

5. Tricyclics for depression

Conclusion

Coccygodynia is a painful symptom complex that can affect major organ systems. It is the job of osteopathic physicians to look at the entire picture and realize the far-reaching interactions. Only by restoring proper structure is the body allowed its fullest potential to heal.

DYSMENORRHEA AND PREMENSTRUAL SYNDROME

Charles J. Smutney III
Mary E. Hitchcock

Two of the most frequent ailments of females of reproductive age are dysmenorrhea and premenstrual syndrome. Dysmenorrhea can be subdivided into two distinctive forms, primary and secondary. These three entities are separate, though they can be found together in the same patient. They can be defined as follows:

1. **Primary dysmenorrhea** (functional dysmenor-

rhea): painful* menses in the absence of discrete organic disease.**

* Pain, a highly subjective part of our history taking, is not sufficient to make a diagnosis. Symptoms must persist and significantly alter the patient's activities of daily living (ADL) for several hours at a minimum. The symptoms often last as long as several days. In the case of secondary dysmenorrhea, weeks to months may pass with major ADL changes prior to the patient seeking attention.

2. **Secondary dysmenorrhea** (acquired dysmenorrhea): painful* menses associated with definable pathology.**
3. **Premenstrual syndrome** (PMS): an interrelated constellation of physical, metabolic, hormonal, and psychological imbalances, variable in nature, and beginning an average of 7–10 days (range 2–14 days) before menses. Symptoms include headache, bloating or abdominal swelling, irritability, tiredness, and food cravings such as sweets and/or salt. Hormonal imbalances may predispose a woman to anxiety, depression, and even open hostility. Symptom complexes often potentiate mood swings. Symptoms and imbalances decrease rapidly with onset and progression of menses.**

An osteopathic thinker must have a clear understanding of the physiology, anatomy, structure, and function involved to better differentiate these entities. This knowledge facilitates a clearer understanding of what a healthy system does. A treatment plan may then assist the patient back to health quickly and efficiently.

Dysmenorrhea tends to be a diagnosis made in women in their teens and twenties. PMS tends to be more frequently found and treated in women in their thirties and forties. However, there is significant overlap in the age criteria and frequent simultaneous occurrences or mixed diagnoses.

In secondary dysmenorrhea, pathologies may include, but are not limited to, endometriosis, intrauterine device, fibroids (especially submucous fibroids, which may cause a ball-valve effect and/or pooling of fluids and breakdown products), anovulatory menorrhagia, pelvic congestion syndrome (associated with a retroverted uterus, venous stasis, and lymphatic stasis), polyps, strictures, hydrosalpinx, ectopic pregnancy (a surgical emergency), and retention of endometrial fragments that act as foreign bodies. An anteflexed uterus, hyperplasia or fibrosis, and estrogen-progesterone imbalances may play significant roles. Poor physical conditioning, multiparous uterus, and/or weakness or damage to the suspensory ligaments must also be considered as contributing factors.

Primary dysmenorrhea may be considered after secondary dysmenorrhea has been effectively ruled out. The physiology of menses and the mechanism of uterine contracture, in particular,

is significant. In addition to some of the physical conditioning problems mentioned above, functional contraction for expulsion of endometrial products is essential. This is largely regulated by the hormonally controlled production of specific prostaglandins (PG).

The PGs are produced as a result of the disintegration of the endometrial lining. The higher the concentration of PG in pooling menstrual fluid, the more severe the subsequent cramping. This trigger of severe contracture and the increased potential for ischemia secondary to the contracture predisposes for pain "that feels like I'm in labor," as many women describe it. This pain may be localized to the abdomen or extend to the back and to the thighs. It may last hours to days, may present as an annoyance or, at its worst, may be totally incapacitating.

Because of these symptoms, the drug of choice has now become a nonsteroidal anti-inflammatory drug (NSAID), which is a PG inhibitor.

The osteopathic physician sees another opportunity here as well. Although NSAIDs break a chain of events leading to pain, they do not treat the whole problem. The machinery is simply not functioning up to its designed potential. The vasculature and the lymphatics that help drain the debris of breakdown products internally, as well as the structures that may be assisted in draining the intrauterine debris to the outside world, must be addressed. Preventing pooling or assisting in maintaining physiologic drainage can help the patient move toward a more healthful state (structure and function).

The etiology of PMS is complex and less well understood. Some theories propose progesterone deficiency, endogenous opiate peptide excess, or pyridoxine deficiency as potential causes. Blood serum studies clearly show that there is some transported element or elements that can trigger symptoms. No specific agents have been identified as yet. Studies of a variety of pharmacologic agents used to treat PMS show as high as 30% to 40% of patients responding to placebo.

These inconclusive studies may lead many practitioners to ascribe a psychological diagnosis without giving consideration to other factors. The placebo side of the equation is less well studied, and much may be gained by a thorough investigation in this area. Part of the placebo effect is related to the psyche and its effects on the limbic system. The final effect of pharmacochemical treatment remains unclear. Certain structural considera-

---

** All three entities may be associated with a vaso-vagal effect and its associated nausea.

tions, however, may play a large role in each individual's response to the onset of menses.

The status of the psycho-neuro-endocrine system is often reflected in the somatic system via the autonomics. A structural examination will show much of this connection. The 10th, 11th, and 12th thoracic vertebrae along with the 1st and 2nd lumbar vertebrae are associated with the sympathetic innervation of the uterus, ovary, salpinx, bladder, large intestine, and sigmoid colon. These same structures share interneurons with musculoskeletal elements of the low back, pelvis, and upper leg. In other words, somatic afferent pain fibers share interneurons with visceral fibers at the same levels. "Any stimulation of the somatic sensory nerves may affect the skeletal muscles, visceral muscles, the blood vessels, and the glands which receive innervation from the same cord level either directly or via the sympathetic ganglia" (Burns).

In those segments of the cord supplying innervation to somatic structures that have shown altered mobility and palpable changes in texture, a lower reflex threshold exists that is called *facilitation*. These areas require less stimulation to sustain neuronal activity. For example, a facilitated segment involving the uterus at T12 and its muscular counterpart, slips of the internal and external oblique and the inferior segments of the rectus abdominus and pyramidalis muscles, can now feed into each other with small amounts of neurologic stimulation. A simple bending and twisting movement can as easily set off a pain cycle as an inflammatory response of the uterine myometrium to retained elements. Either of these alone might not be noticed if the facilitated segment were not present.

One goal of osteopathic manipulative medicine (OMM) is to reduce facilitation, thus allowing for an increased pain signal threshold. This would result in the interneurons sending fewer pain messages into the reflex arc at the cord level; consequently, less input would be sent up the spinothalamic tract to be centrally processed.

The technique chosen as treatment is of less importance than the understanding of the physiologic and anatomic mechanisms involved. Once an understanding of the local phenomenon is gained, a treatment program may be developed.

Integration of the local situation into the patient's whole body function is critical to osteopathic thinking. Environment, diet, stress, support systems within the patient's family, hydration sta-

tus, fitness, and the interaction of other body systems with the local phenomenon must all be considered carefully.

The whole patient must be appraised in examining the musculoskeletal system. Changes cannot occur in one organ or tissue without affecting others through the communication between the visceral and somatic systems. Osteopathic treatment is directed toward normalization of musculoskeletal function and restoration of normal physiology through reflex mechanisms. Bimanual manipulation of the uterus itself, to correct retroversion or anteflexion anomalies, during the process of a proper vaginal examination can begin the osteopathic program. Treating the facilitated segments that are at the levels of innervation of the visceral segments could be the next step.

Consideration of other areas should become evident in the surveillance structural screen. Upper thoracic vertebrae and ribs as well as cervical vertebrae may affect hormonal secretion via their postganglionic fibers, which course upward through the superior cervical ganglion, along the carotid vessels to the adenohypophysis. Similarly, adrenal function can be influenced by vasomotor efferents in the lower thoracic spine, disturbing the balance of this gland with the hypothalamic pituitary axis. This could lead to an imbalance in the systemic sympathetic dynamic equilibrium. Leg length differences can create increased neurologic tone to the facilitated segment. A simple heel lift can reduce that tone. The articulations of the pelvis and muscles of the pelvic diaphragm should be addressed to improve venous and lymphatic drainage and to help the sacral parasympathetic side of the equation function freely.

The sacral counterpart and its parasympathetic role can and should be balanced along with the vagal parasympathetics and its associated bony structural dysfunctions at C2 and the cranial base.

In addressing the treatment plan, a few simple techniques can be used. Inhibitory pressure over the lower thoracic, lumbar, and sacral vertebral structures may be used to quiet uterine contractions at the height of painful menstruation. With the patient prone, the physician maintains deep steady pressure on the sacrum until the contractions are released (Fig. 27-11). Pressure on the symphysis pubis with the patient supine may relieve lower abdominal and lumbar discomfort (Fig. 27-12).

In teaching the patient to self-treat, sacral pressure may be maintained by placing a book under

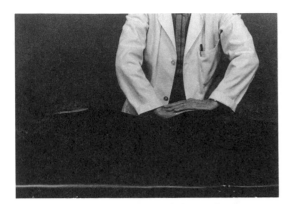

Figure 27-11. Sacral pressure for the relief of dysmenorrhea.

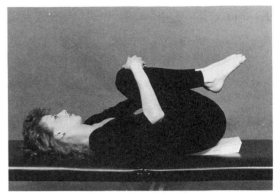

Figure 27-14. Increasing sacral pressure by flexing legs on trunk.

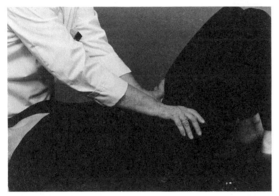

Figure 27-12. Deep inhibiting pressure on tissues overlying the pubic symphysis.

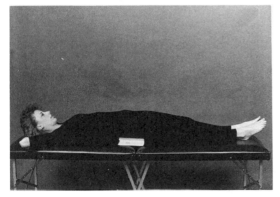

Figure 27-13. Self-treatment by sacral pressure using a book.

the sacral body near the S2-S3 junction, keeping clear of the ilia (Figs. 27-13, 27-14). The position of the book can be shifted toward the sacral base or apex as the patient determines which area is more effective at alleviating the cramping pain.

Patients may also be taught to treat their own anterior tender points.

Appropriate treatment may include one or more of the following; OMM, tailored rest and exercise programs, diet, vitamin replacement, mineral replacement, thyroid treatment, estrogen and/or progesterone hormone therapy, antispasmodics, NSAIDs, muscle relaxants, antidepressants, anxiolytics, hypnotic-sedatives, other psychoactive drugs, diuretics, and analgesics.

Diet and nutrition status can play a major role in effective management of both PMS and dysmenorrhea. Nutrition studies indicate that there can be a major reduction in symptoms in patients with nutritional deficiencies. Patients may need vitamin and electrolyte replacement as a result of the hormone-regulated catabolic and anabolic processes engaged in the monthly restructuring of the uterus. Calcium and magnesium supplements may reduce or relieve cramping. Vitamin B complex may reduce water retention and stress and supply needed nutrients to the adrenal glands. Vitamin E may reduce breast tenderness. It functions in efficient oxygen utilization and scavenges free radicals that may abound in this metabolically, highly active state. Reduction in the intake of processed sugars, processed foods, caffeine, alcohol, red meats, fatty foods, salt, and dairy products can favorably reduce PMS. This complements the well-known improvement in general health that a sensible diet can provide. Complex carbohydrates will alleviate the relative and sometimes frank hypoglycemia that can occur while providing the necessary energy sources to facilitate refurbishing of the uterine home.

Carefully chosen pharmacologic agents with a plan for early reevaluation and tapering of drugs where possible are important in treating the symptom complex.

A well-designed osteopathic treatment program considering all of the above, with scheduled follow-up and attention to the mind, body, and spirit, can help the patient return toward and maintain health.

THE OBSTETRIC PATIENT
Charles J. Smutney III
Mary E. Hitchcock

Osteopathic care throughout pregnancy provides a woman with the special benefit of adjusting the functions of her body to the demands of a progressing pregnancy. Seemingly minor problems, especially those involving the back, may be the beginning of a lifetime of musculoskeletal difficulties. Childbearing women without other clear traumatic or visceral causes of back pain can often trace part of their own history to a difficult labor and/or postpartum onset.

An exercise program begun in the early prenatal period, or, ideally, prior to conception, may strongly reduce the potential for developing low back dysfunctions. If manipulation and an exercise regimen are developed and continued postpartum, the patient may return to normal function much more rapidly.

In a discussion of obstetric back pain, the pelvis may serve as a starting point. It is the foundation upon which the entire spinal column is balanced. Forward tilting of the pelvis occurs during pregnancy, with a resulting increased lumbar lordosis as a counterbalance. Often this increase in spinal curves may extend as far as the cranial base and may induce craniosacral strains. This may lead to acute and, if uncorrected, chronic backache as well as a host of other symptoms. Lordosis is commonly more marked in women than in men. Obesity and/or a growing fetus compound the stresses, exaggerating the curve (Fig. 27-15). Alterations in posture shift the stresses from their normally ligamentous and disk-oriented balance to a strenuous muscle-controlled balance. As the pregnancy continues to develop, distension of the abdomen further reduces the muscular capacity to counterbalance. This is a living example of the physiological

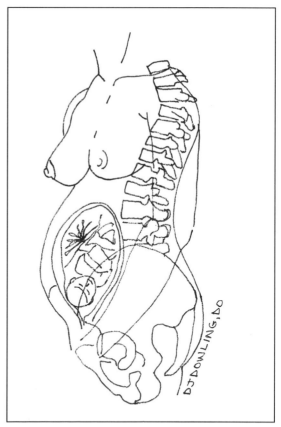

Figure 27-15. Pregnancy increases the curvature of the spine, especially the lumbar lordosis.

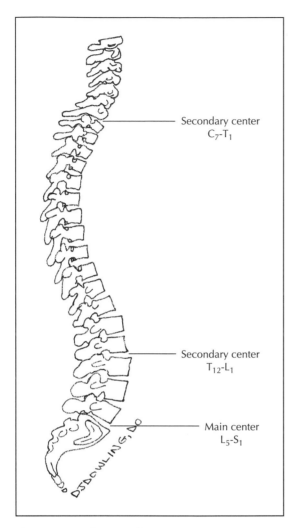

Secondary center
C_7-T_1

Secondary center
T_{12}-L_1

Main center
L_5-S_1

Figure 27-16. Centers of gravity.

principle of the length-tension relationship where muscles can be stretched beyond their capacity to contract efficiently.

Anatomically, the body is designed to resist gravity through one primary and two subsidiary centers of transition (Fig. 27-16). These transition zones at the C7-T1, T12-L1, and L5-S1 junctions serve as fulcrums for the transmission of force upward and downward through the column. They serve as balance points for the anterior-posterior (A-P) curve and may serve as proprioceptive references to the longitudinal center of gravity. The compound functions at these points subject them to higher stresses than at other spinal areas. This adaptation is to human advantage, however, because this arrangement can resist ten times that of a straight column. With an engineer's eye, the spinal column can be viewed as the mast of a ship with a series of muscular and ligamentous stays placed for balance and control through a range of motion. A good example is the trapezius and its wedge-shaped form from spinous process to scapular spine. A-P curve changes in the column result in an increase of the thoracic A-P diameter and transverse diameter and a shortening of the longitudinal axis. This reduces the efficiency of the "stay and mast" system.

The iliopsoas muscle is often considered the "mainstay" in the column support system. It therefore has the potential for a significant role in the back pain of pregnancy and in back pain in general. Crossing the critical area of the L5-S1 junction, it can help distribute forces from the large range of motion above through to the relatively limited movement of the sacrum. Equally important is its capacity to help distribute forces from below upward. Its origins at the inferior borders of the transverse processes of L1-L5, the anterolateral surfaces of the vertebral bodies of T12-L5, and the intervertebral disks between them give this muscle a unique range of functions similar in some respects to the sternocleidomastoid. As a result, its structure and function require complex innervation, great recruitment capacity, and significant power capacity.

The iliopsoas may be involved in respiratory function as an anchoring mechanism for the crura of the diaphragm. It is involved in the stabilization of the lumbar spine in standing, sitting, and locomotion. It supports the viscera and forms a major part of the posterior and lateral bowl of the faux pelvis. It may also support the growing fetus, keeping the body of the uterus in the faux pelvis and the abdomen until descent at term begins.

One key may be understanding the iliopsoas's role in nutation and counternutation (physiologic anterior-posterior rocking of the sacrum). The psoas muscle may act as a prime mover of the lumbosacral junction and may strongly influence sacral mechanics. This becomes focal in studying the mechanics of gait, respiration, and the sequence of engagement, flexion, descent, and internal rotation of the fetus. The muscularly controlled counternutation of delivery is assisted by progesterone and relaxin, which induces ligamentous laxity. This facilitates the opening of the true pelvic inlet, which must occur for engagement to begin.

During delivery, the hip, pelvic, and abdominal musculature undergoes maximum physical strain, with resulting stress on the back and the pelvic

Figure 27-17. Sympathetic and parasympathetic innervation of the female pelvis.

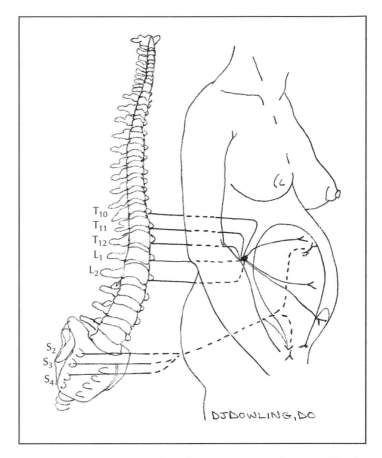

and sacroiliac ligaments. The lithotomy position further exacerbates stress because gravity cannot assist in the process (squatting perhaps being the most natural position).

The sympathetic innervation to the female pelvic structures is derived from nerves at the spinal levels of T10–T12 and L1–L2. Nociceptive fibers also follow these tracts and share interneurons with musculoskeletal nociceptive fibers at the same levels. Parasympathetic innervation arises from S2–S4 through the pelvic splanchnic nerve (Fig. 27-17). Changes in A-P curves can facilitate segments and lower pain thresholds. This information becomes more useful diagnostically when one is attempting to separate out other visceral problems that may occur during pregnancy.

As the curves progress, there may be an increase in the tortuosity of viscera as they traverse the pelvic brim. This may lead to compression of some of the structures that are normally suspended freely. The biomass of the uterus and the fetus may further compound these restrictions. Respiratory and circulatory function may be altered, leading to commonly found constipation, edema, and backache. Urinary frequency, susceptibility to infection, leg cramps, varicosities, acrodyesthesia (tingling and numbness of the hands), breast soreness, and joint pains are also common complaints. Each of these has structural strain as a component to be considered.

Although lumbar and sacral backaches are the most common musculoskeletal complaints of pregnancy, complaints from the apex of the skull to the plantar surface of the foot may frequently be encountered. Secondary to large postural changes, muscle fatigue and discomfort initiate many complaints. Increasing breast mass may exaggerate this. Rib dysfunctions and thoracic and cervical pain may increase in frequency and duration. Muscle tension headache may occur more frequently as these dysfunctions accumulate. Postural changes may alter the weight-bearing distribution of the seated patient toward the coccyx, predisposing to coccygodynia.

These manifestations might be heralding the

oncoming hypertension, edema, altered glucose balance, preeclampsia, and other symptoms that define a pregnancy in difficulty. Allopathic medicine relies on frequent checkups for early intervention, nutritional supplements, and dietary advice as the tools to prevent them. The true battle with these entities only begins once they have arrived. Pharmacology becomes the only avenue for holding the symptoms at bay until delivery or termination.

The osteopathic concept provides a great deal more treatment, quite literally at the practitioner's fingertips. "Traditionally, osteopathic manipulative management of the obstetric patient has been limited to soft tissue relaxation especially to the lumbar region and, occasionally, to making corrections of the isolated somatic dysfunctions" (Zink). This is often effective in improving the comfort of the patient but does not directly address (1) gravitational strains, (2) optimization of external or pulmonary respiration, or (3) facilitation of drainage of the venous and lymphatic systems. It certainly does not address optimization of the primary respiratory mechanism.

To treat the patient as a unit, we must consider the neurologic model, the respiratory-circulatory model, the energy model, the fluid model, and osteopathy in the cranial field in an integrated manner. It may also be important to consider other models of function. The key is to integrate the information into the understanding of the patient as a unique, interrelated unit of function.

We are taught the practice of observation, palpation, motion testing, and special testing as a matter of course. These skills may take on refined meaning here. Alterations in normal respiratory mechanics can often yield signs of other problems beginning. The mechanics of pulmonary respiration is often a good place to begin the diagnostic and therapeutic process of assisting the patient back toward health.

Normal breathing is dependent, both anatomically and physiologically, on a level pelvis and a straight spine (in which the movement of all segments is unhindered). This allows the thoracic cage, which is suspended from the spine, to function properly, thereby ensuring maximum external respiration. When proper external respiration occurs, there is an effective negative pressure in the thorax that guarantees the continuous return of blood from the central nervous system. This, in turn, allows the cerebrospinal fluid to move more freely. At the same time an effective negative pressure in the thorax aspirates the venous blood from the rest of the body as well as promoting terminal lymphatic drainage. (Zink)
Tettambel stated,

A well tuned engine or balanced musculoskeletal system is capable of good performance. It's prepared to accommodate the traveling fetus by regulating its own contractions and assisting the muscles to cooperate with the flexion, extension, and rotations of the fetal skull. . . . By maintaining the body fluid homeostasis and reevaluating the ever changing pregnant posture and gait, the obstetrician helps the kidneys to maintain their efficiency and regulate their filtration system and the heart to maintain a healthy beat, keeping the pumping station running without being on overload. Therefore, edema and late breaking preeclampsia may be kept at bay.

Treatment programs must be designed to address all of the above issues, from prenatal planning and treatment to postpartum follow-up. It must be emphasized that the treatment protocol will evolve from a good medical, surgical, gynecological, social, nutritional, psychological, and trauma history combined with a thorough diagnostic and structural examination. This will elucidate a fair portion of the balances and imbalances as they affect the intricate workings of the patient.

Some additional treatment techniques and exercises included here may add to the battery of tools to assist the patient in seeking and maintaining a healthy pregnancy and delivery. Still stated,

The knee chest position will place the abdomen in the proper form for unloading the pelvis and any impacted condition. Then place the hands low down on the abdomen and draw the contents of the pelvis forward toward the umbilicus and up from the pelvis, to give free passage of blood and other fluids circulating in the lower part of the abdomen.

Sacral rocking may be used to release sacral restrictions, both before delivery and during early delivery (Fig. 27-18). After delivery, the woman's legs are removed from the stirrups and her hips are put through adduction and internal rotation while still flexed, followed by extension (Figs. 27-19, 27-20). This reduces the potential for sacroiliac dysfunction, which may result from the increased elasticity of pelvic ligaments combined with the intense ligamentous strain of delivery.

In breech presentations, an external cephalic version may be attempted, which has a success

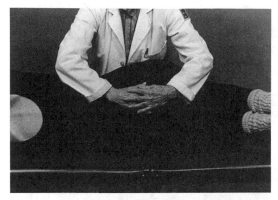

Figure 27-18. Sacral rocking on obstetric patient.

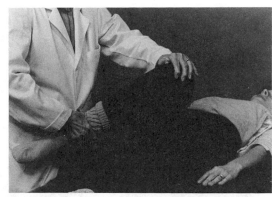

Figure 27-19. Adduction and internal rotation of the hips.

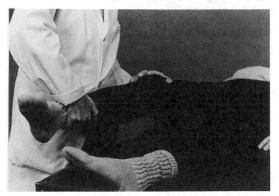

Figure 27-20. Adduction, internal rotation, and extension of the hips.

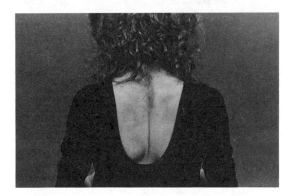

Figure 27-21. Approximation of the scapulae.

rate as high as 75%. Since the major risk is abruptio placentae, it may be prudent to attempt this with delicate hands and gentle forces over a period of time.

Manipulation may also be used postpartum as early as 4 or 5 hours after a cesarean section, and then up to three times a day, to alleviate hyperextension of the lumbar spine.

Within minutes to a few hours after delivery, simple in-bed exercises may begin. The patient may be instructed to approximate the scapulae while sitting (Fig. 27-21). This encourages motion of the chest and shoulder girdle and may reduce some of the muscular stress accumulated during delivery. Within hours to the next day, the woman may lie in bed with her knees bent and raise the buttocks an inch or so, pressing the lumbar area against the bed and thus tilting the pelvis (Fig. 27-22). This may be beginning the abdominal and low

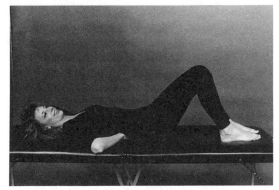

Figure 27-22. Tilting the pelvis posteriorly by flattening the lumbar lordosis.

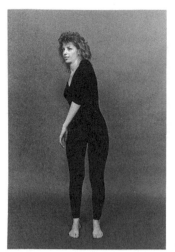

Figure 27-23. Trunk twists.

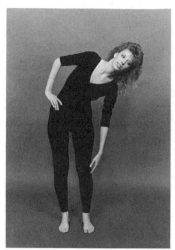

Figure 27-24. Bending the trunk sideways.

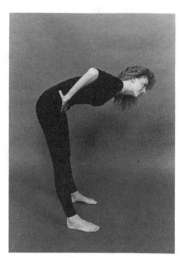

Figure 27-25. Forward bending of the trunk.

back rehabilitation process. As tolerated, she may stand with legs apart about shoulder width and twist the trunk from right to left and back slowly (Fig. 27-23). Emphasis should be placed on slow motion and maximal range of motion without incurring pain. Now is not the time for a "no pain, no gain" mentality. In the same position, she may bend the trunk sideways and forward (Figs. 27-24, 27-25). This may help strengthen and stretch both internal and external obliques, restoring more normal abdominal muscle function. The woman may continue adding exercises as tolerated.

Advancing to lying on the floor with her legs straight and arms out to the sides, she reaches with one knee to the opposite arm, returns, and does the same with the other arm and knee (Fig. 27-26).

When the iliopsoas is severely contracted, an initial stretching exercise is suggested. The unaffected leg is placed at a height of 2 to 2½ feet from the floor, on a chair or stool. The affected leg is stretched about 3 feet behind in neutral rotation attitude. With continuous gentle stretch, the foot of the affected leg is gradually rotated internally. The woman then applies pressure over the buttock on the affected side, adding full body weight to the stretch at the level of the compromised hip (Fig. 27-27).

A passive stretch may be accomplished by lying supine on a rolled-up towel that has been placed at the thoracolumbar junction. This should relieve some of the flexion stress accumulated during the day.

Leg raising with the legs not more than 6 inches from the floor will strengthen abdominal muscles (Fig. 27-28). If the legs are raised higher than this, the psoas muscle becomes involved in flexion, which is not desirable in some low back problems.

All exercises should be repeated 10 times without pain. Mild to moderate discomfort is to be expected. Patients should strive to work up to 10 repetitions and then, as tolerated, work toward exercising two and three times per day. Gentle passive stretching should follow each exercise period. Moving on to more strenuous aerobic and anaerobic exercises gradually may speed the return toward normal with reduced risk of injury. High-impact aerobics may cause more trouble than good because of increased risk of injury.

Gentle encouragement from the physician is in order, and involvement of a supportive family is welcome. In addition to exercise, the physician must pay attention to, and frequently reassess, nutritional and psychological factors throughout patient care. Nutritional research is only recently being added to medical school and residency curricula.

Studies by Myers, Muller-tyl and Wimmer-Puchinger, Ringrose, Copper, and McDonald each point out that psychological stress and emotional turmoil may manifest themselves via the hypothalamic-autonomic axis as the physical phenomena of obstetric complications.

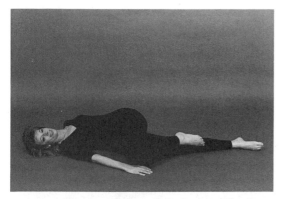

Figure 27-26. Trunk twists while lying on the floor.

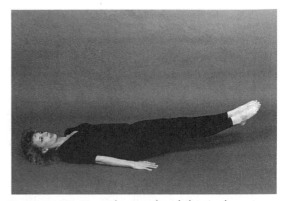

Figure 27-28. Strengthening the abdominal muscles.

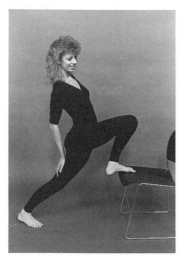

Figure 27-27. Iliopsoas stretch.

Contraindications to manipulation are of great import:

1. Do not use stimulatory treatments during premature labor. Stimulation of spinal nerves may be sufficient to continue a labor that might otherwise have been halted by complete rest.
2. Do not use stimulatory treatment in the presence of abruptio placentae. Abruption is considered a medical urgency or emergency and may require a "crash" cesarean section. Abruptio placentae occurs after the 20th week of gestation and most commonly in the last 10 weeks of pregnancy. Any detachment earlier in pregnancy is regarded as abortion. When symptoms of shock or changes in fetal activity and heart sounds occur, placenta previa should be suspected.
3. Treat with extreme caution if membranes rupture without labor. Without amniotic fluid protection, the fetus is more vulnerable to outside trauma. External cephalic version is more difficult in the absence of amniotic fluid. The use of fetal movements in response to gentle sustained pressure may be effective but may take time.
4. An ectopic pregnancy requires emergent surgery.

The list of contraindications is short, itself giving some hint to the extensive applications of osteopathic philosophy and practice to the obstetric patient. "Osteopathic obstetrics can be a reality. Integration of structure, function, and palpatory skills can expand the diagnostic acumen that can't be appreciated through technology or textbook" (Tettambel).

Today's environment of cost conservation and ever-tightening regulation requires greater clinical ability and less reliance on technology. Now more than ever, it is the job of the student and prudent practitioner of osteopathic philosophy to develop clinical knowledge of the psychological, nutritional, and structural aspects of the patient. A. T. Still wrote about this about 100 years ago. The application of Dr. William Garner Sutherland's concept of developing "thinking fingers" has never been more appropriate. As a physician treating obstetrics patients, this has a twofold application. We are, after all, treating two patients simultaneously.

THE PULMONARY PATIENT
Eileen L. DiGiovanna

Treating the pulmonary patient, particularly one with chronic disease, is a challenge to the physician. The use of osteopathic manipulation adds a dimension to the care of patients with respiratory problems.

Pulmonary conditions may be divided into the acute, infectious type and the chronic, progressive type. Acute pulmonary diseases include the various pneumonias and infectious bronchitis. These are of rather sudden onset and are bacterial or viral in etiology. Chronic pulmonary diseases are frequently gradual in onset and slowly progressive. Although persons with these conditions are susceptible to secondary infections, the primary cause is seldom of an infectious nature. Included are asthma and chronic obstructive pulmonary diseases (COPDs) such as chronic bronchitis and emphysema.

Other pulmonary conditions, such as lung cancer, pulmonary embolus, and tuberculosis, are less likely to respond with manipulation, although it may prove a valuable adjunctive treatment.

Somatic Diagnosis of Pulmonary Diseases

Osteopathic somatic dysfunction diagnosis may be a valuable tool in identifying the presence of pulmonary pathology. Numerous studies have been done over the years to find the best somatic predictors of respiratory disease. Myron Beal reviewed many previous studies and also reported one of his own. The most consistent findings were at T2–T7, with significant representation at C2–C3. Beal found somatic dysfunction of two or more adjacent vertebrae in this region, deep muscle splinting, and resistance to compressive springing of the involved area. These areas represent viscerosomatic reflexes from the lung to the soma.

When evaluating the pulmonary patient, it is also important to evaluate all components involved in respiration, including rib motion, ability of the spine to straighten during inspiration, diaphragmatic motion, and accessory muscles of respiration such as the scalenes, sternocleidomastoids, and abdominal muscles.

The physician should keep in mind that there is more involved in respiration than just thoracic cage motion. For tissues to be healthy, they require the following:

1. Good arterial supply
2. Motor and sensory impulses
3. Trophins
4. Adequate biochemical environment
5. Venous and lymphatic return

Each of these needs to be evaluated and addressed.

Entities
BRONCHITIS AND PNEUMONIA
Although the causes and manifestations may differ, the goals of therapy are relatively the same in any of these conditions:

1. To improve lymphatic and venous flow
2. To improve arterial circulation to carry immune system products to the lungs
3. To ease removal of accumulated bronchial secretions and phlegm
4. To decrease the workload of breathing

Osteopathic manipulation should address these goals to assist the body's fight against infection.

Various forms of lymphatic pump or thoracic pump will aid in improving venous and lymphatic flow as well as favorably affecting arterial circulation. Rib-raising techniques may be used to free bronchial secretions so they may be more easily expectorated and to normalize sympathetic innervation to the lung. The workload of breathing may be decreased by improving the compliance of the thorax—that is, by freeing the ribs, vertebrae, clavicles, and sternum to restore the intrinsic elastic forces in the thorax.

BRONCHIAL ASTHMA
Asthma represents a group of symptoms of various causes. The lungs of asthmatics are highly sensitized and react to such varied stimuli as allergens,

irritants, emotion, and exercise. Whatever the trigger, the allergic attack is manifested through an inflammatory response, including spasm of the bronchioles, edema of the mucous membrane, and increased production of thick, tenacious mucus. These three incidences create difficulty in emptying air out of the alveoli, with resultant dyspnea and a wheezing sound on expiration.

In managing an acute attack of asthma, it is essential to address the patient's immediate needs first. Medications such as epinephrine should be given or nebulized albutenol should be used. Then, as breathing quiets, rib raising is useful in easing the patient's respiratory efforts and in loosening mucous plugs.

Between acute attacks, it is important to treat all components of the respiratory system. In particular, all viscerosomatic reflex areas should be treated to prevent possible abnormal autonomic feedback to the lungs. Possible increased vagal involvement may be treated by freeing the occipitoatlantal area.

Because of the emotional involvement in asthma as an etiologic factor and the fear elicited by the dyspnea, the very act of placing the hands on the patient will have beneficial effects and serve to calm him as you treat. This alone can be a significant therapeutic factor.

CHRONIC OBSTRUCTIVE PULMONARY DISEASE

As a result of cigarette smoking and pollution, COPD has become a major cause of pulmonary illness in the world today. It is of insidious onset and is devastating to its victims. Dyspnea may become quite significant. As dyspnea increases, physical activity is curtailed. Chronic bronchitis produces large amounts of thick mucus; emphysema produces lesser amounts.

Muscoloskeletal changes occur during the course of the disease. The chest assumes a barrel shape in which the AP diameter equals the transverse diameter. The accessory muscles of respiration gradually hypertrophy. Hypertrophied scalene muscles may cause neurovascular compression at the scalene triangle. Rib motion is markedly restricted and eventually contributes to the dyspnea. The thoracic spine becomes kyphotic and immobile. Motion of the diaphragm is restricted.

Osteopathic manipulation contributes to the overall well-being of the patient, even though the basic pathophysiology may not be reversible. The thoracic spine is treated to restore mobility and to address the viscerosomatic reflex changes in the upper thoracic spine. Rib motion may be improved with muscle energy or counterstrain techniques. It may be well to avoid thrusting techniques, since many COPD patients require corticosteroids, which may lead to osteoporosis. Rib-raising techniques are helpful. Fascial release of the diaphragm should be done. Thoracic pumping will improve lymphatic flow and the expectoration of tenacious mucus.

The cervical area should be treated, with attention given to the accessory respiratory muscles. The clavicles should be freed and any sternal restrictions treated.

Upper extremity motion restriction may be found in chronic lung disease. Sternal release and Spencer techniques may be used to improve this condition.

After osteopathic manipulation, COPD patients frequently report a subjective increase in their sense of well-being. They experience less effort breathing and improved physical functioning.

Because of the relationship of the muscoloskeletal system to the respiratory system, the osteopathic physician must evaluate all components of each system when diagnosing and treating the pulmonary patient.

THE CARDIAC PATIENT
Charles J. Smutney III

The demonstration of the fundamentals of osteopathic philosophy is clearly expressed in the understanding and treatment of the cardiac patient.

It is useful to begin with the concept of segmental facilitation, which will affect the patient's response to myocardial infarction or angina. These patients may present themselves in a variety of ways, from being silent and asymptomatic to having the classic acute crushing chest pain, shortness of breath, diaphoresis, and pain radiating to the left shoulder and down the left arm. This nociceptive response may be perceived in the central nervous system (CNS) as pain, discomfort, or weakness in the muscoloskeletal system, when in fact the problem is entirely within the confines of the myocardium, its vasculature, and its electrochemical environment. The CNS receives reports from the soma and acts on somatic information in a highly organized fashion.

Research has demonstrated that the visceral components use the same somatic system for reporting their status. Mechanoreceptors within the myocardium and the vascular structures relay information concerning pressure and stretch characteristics back to the CNS via afferent pathways. Similarly, chemoreceptors report information about the chemical environment along the same pathways, which terminate on interneurons that also process somatic nociceptive information.

Knowledge of the anatomy of those pathways is useful. The heart reports its nociceptive information through the cardiac plexus to fine nerves that synapse in the superior, middle, and inferior cervical ganglia near the levels of C2, C5, and C7, respectively. Information is passed from there to the spinal chain ganglia and then back to the dorsal horn at the levels of T1–T5. The signal is transferred to an interneuron that is shared by a somatic afferent neuron from the same segmental level. It then travels up the spinothalamic tracts to present information to higher centers for interpretation and action.

The heart's central role in survival is demonstrated by the sophistication and redundancy of its sensory gathering systems. Vagal sensory afferents duplicate data transmission of nociception but bypass the gating mechanism of the spinal cord. The vagus also carries its own rate-regulating fibers directly toward the sinoatrial and atrioventricular nodes, where it can override the inherent cardiac rhythm generators.

The great vessels on the superior aspect of the heart are surrounded by a mixed plexus of parasympathetic vagal fibers and sympathetic fibers from the cardiac nerves. Embedded in the plexus are parasympathetic ganglia that receive the vagal preganglionic fibers. The plexus supplies postganglionic fibers to the sinoatrial and atrioventricular nodes, cardiac muscle itself, and to the coronary vasculature of the heart. Stimulation of the sympathetic fibers accelerates cardiac output and can be arrhythmogenic, especially left sided stimulation of the sympathetic pathways. . . . Stimulation of the parasympathetic vagal fibers stabilizes the heart rate. Thus the balance between the sympathetic and parasympathetic pathways is crucial to cardiac function. (Willard and Carreiro, 1994)

Distant pressure and chemoreceptors in the hypothalamus, the carotid bodies, the arch of the aorta, and the kidney further duplicate nociceptive feedback. There is some evidence that cells of the neuro-endocrine-immune system can also directly and indirectly regulate the heart.

Pain (nociception) plays a large role in visceral function and dysfunction. Still said, "Drive a shingle nail through one toe. Would you be surprised if the heart made seventy-five (beats per minute)? Or even 125 beats per minute?" Consider what other systems are affected and how they are affected when epinephrine is released by the adrenals. What are the mechanisms of this release?

A look at a partial list of common painful presentations elucidates the role of pain in the acute patient. This may include left-sided chest pain, left shoulder and arm pain, jaw pain, neck pain, epigastric pain, right-sided chest pain, back pain, and rib pain.

The significance of pain is its effect on the heart and other systems. Pain is a stimulator of the sympathetic nervous system. Exertion is often the initiating event creating increased oxygen demand.

When demand is high enough and supply is insufficient to meet it, chemoreceptors signal pain. This leads to increases in heart rate, stroke volume, cardiac output, coronary blood flow, systolic blood pressure, pulmonary blood pressure, cerebral blood flow, muscle blood flow, oxygen consumption, lactic acid production, respiration, and alertness. This is accompanied by a decrease in total peripheral resistance, cutaneous blood flow, and renal blood flow. These demands on a heart that is less than healthy can precipitate a "feed forward" effect, further increasing demands. This may quickly outstrip the ability of the heart to adapt. Both the chemicals consumed and the ones released can further activate the pain cycle. The endpoint of this cycle is often myocardial infarction (MI).

Treatment of the patient experiencing angina or MI is targeted at breaking this cycle in one or more areas simultaneously. The standard use of oxygen, morphine, nitrates, and one aspirin or other antiplatelet aggregation agent underscores some of the pharmacologic approaches. Addressing the facilitated segments at T1–T4 may down-regulate the sympathetic nervous system enough to alter oxygen demands.

The absence of pain does not diminish the potential for danger. Hypertension and the silent MI of diabetes are examples of this at different ends of the spectrum. Hypertension shows a consistent somatic dysfunction pattern of C6–T2–T6 (Johnson). Frequently this is associated with point tenderness at one or more of these segments.

The peripheral neuropathy of diabetes is responsible, at least in part, for the painless aspect of silent MI. The diabetic patient continues to demonstrate other signs of sympathetic up-regulation, most notably diaphoresis and shortness of breath. In both circumstances, nociceptive function is still facilitating segments even though frank pain is not part of the picture.

The osteopathic physician finds certain avenues to use in the acute situation and also as a preventive means. Decreasing facilitation of the first four thoracic and the cervical segments, particularly at C2, may break a variety of arrhythmias, decrease heart rate, and decrease nociceptive firing. Treatment of the cranial base may aid in balancing the sympathetic and the peripheral nervous systems, further down-regulating demand on the heart. Treatment of the structures involved in pulmonary respiration may increase the efficiency of respiration. This in turn increases the venous and lymphatic return without increasing and often decreasing energy demands. It may also increase oxygen supplies.

By extending these thought processes to preventive medicine, one can do much for the cardiac patient. Manipulation may reduce factors contributing to decompensation. It may also increase time between events and decrease severity.

Patients with congestive heart failure (CHF) and cardiomyopathy may benefit from lymphatic fluid management protocols and improvement in respiratory mechanics. Patients with coronary artery disease, arrhythmias, and hypertension may also benefit from treatments that decrease energy demands. Treatment of postcatheterization patients and post–coronary artery bypass graft patients may include carefully planned and executed manipulation, targeting the dysfunction caused by the procedures themselves. A focus on balancing the autonomics in all situations may be warranted.

Good palpatory skills can raise suspicion about specific cardiac anomalies. Cardone describes the structural findings that are frequently associated with certain conditions:

1. Coarctation of the aorta: greater muscular development of the upper extremities than the lower extremities.
2. Ventricular septal defect—children: bilateral prominence of the anterior part of the chest with bulging of the upper two thirds of the sternum and a drawing in of the lower third.
3. Ventricular septal defect—adult: unilateral bulge at the fourth and fifth intercostal spaces at the left lower sternal border.
4. Atrial septal defect: bulging in the area of the second and third intercostal spaces at the left sternal border.
5. Constrictive pericarditis or isolated tricuspid valve regurgitation: drawing in of the precordium during systole.

The importance of collecting historical, physical, nutritional, social, trauma, familial, and structural data can never be emphasized enough. A structural screen of the entire person followed by a targeted scan will direct the diagnosis and treatment protocols to be developed. An osteopathic screen and scan can help to differentiate cardiac from noncardiac origins. This may provide the intern, resident, and attending physician with more information to diagnose and treat the patient more accurately and efficiently.

GASTROINTESTINAL CONSIDERATIONS
Michael F. Oliverio

A thorough knowledge of segmental and autonomic innervation of the gastrointestinal (GI) tract aids the osteopathic physician in both the diagnosis and treatment of GI disease. The "enteric" nervous system provides a baseline peristaltic rate and sphincter tone. Activity of the viscera is modulated through the autonomic nervous system. In addition to the autonomic nervous system, the lymphatic drainage of the abdomen is an important consideration in the treatment of inflammatory bowel disease and in the resolution of ileus. Decongestion of the lymphatic drainage channels and improvement of lymphatic flow are crucial to success.

Autonomic Nervous System

Parasympathetic innervation increases peristalsis, relaxes sphincter tone, increases enzyme secretion, and increases blood flow to the intestines. Parasympathetic supply begins in the medulla and exits the skull as the vagus nerve through the jugular foramen. The left vagus innervates the esophagus, the greater curvature of the stomach, and the proximal duodenum. The right vagus supplies the lesser curvature, the small intestine, and the large intestine to the area of the mid–transverse colon. The pelvic splanchnic nerves derived from S2–S4 levels complete the supply from the mid–transverse colon to the rectum.

Normal GI function is not dependent on sympathetic stimulation. Strong sympathetic outflow decreases peristalsis and glandular secretion while increasing sphincter tone. Paradoxically, sympathetic stimulation does enhance gallbladder contraction. Sympathetic innervation derives from the plexi located just anterior to the heads of the thoracic ribs. A segmental arrangement exists. Knowledge of this arrangement is invaluable in diagnosis and is essential to efficient and successful treatment. Three additional collateral sympathetic ganglia lie anterior to the aorta. The celiac, superior mesenteric, and inferior mesenteric ganglia serve the areas of the stomach to the duodenum, the duodenum to the mid–transverse colon, and the mid–transverse colon to the rectum, re-

spectively. Early inflammatory processes stimulate these ganglia and initiate tissue texture changes that are palpable in the skin and subcutaneous tissues over the involved ganglia. Prolonged facilitation in the form of increased afferent input to the collateral ganglia leads to reflex segmental changes in the posterior sympathetic ganglia and eventually viscerosomatic dysfunction patterns.

Viscerosomatic reflex dysfunctions may be diagnosed by cool, rough skin, marked contraction of the superficial muscles over a broad area, and pain relieved by heat. There is a boggy feel to the tissues with a rubbery feel at the physiological barrier to joint motion. With an advanced disease process mere correction of the osteopathic dysfunction will not lead to cure, and at best the response to manipulation will be slow until the gross pathology has been removed.

The segmental arrangement of the sympathetic chain is as follows:

Esophagus: T6
Lower esophagus and stomach: T6–T9
Liver and gallbladder: T6–T9 on the right
Spleen and pancreas: T6–T9 on the left
Small intestine: T7–T9
Ascending and transverse colon: T10–L1 on the right
Descending colon and rectum: T12–L2 on the left.

Slow type C pain fibers, in conjunction with the sympathetic fibers, transmit information to the brain regarding damage such as ischemia, chemical irritation, spasm, wall distension, and stretching of ligaments. This information is interpreted by the patient as a cramping sensation. Visceral pain patterns are referred to the surface of the body.

Parietal pain is transmitted via fast delta fibers and are perceived as sharp, prickling pain. It is caused by inflammation or irritation of the peritoneum. These pain patterns are localized directly over the affected areas.

Acute gastritis may exhibit facilitated segments at T6–T9. This allows for differentiation from myocardial infarction, which would have the facilitated segments at T1–T5 on the left. Gallbladder inflammation or infection demonstrates facilitation of segments at T7–T12 on the right. Facilitation of these segments on the left would make one suspicious of peptic ulcer disease.

Gastric ulcer will first manifest as irritation of the gastric mucosa, which is reflected in increased sympathetic activity initially through the celiac plexus. With continued insult, the collateral ganglia will become overwhelmed and the T6–T9 segments will be reflexly recruited. Eventually somatic dysfunction will occur at this level. The hypersympathetic state perpetuated by the somatic dysfunction must be relieved to aid in the healing process.

Treatment
Harold I. Magoun, Sr., states,

A general osteopathic treatment is far less effective in the therapeutic approach to specific body functioning than manipulation confined to establishing normal physiology to the segment most intimately connected neurologically with that one function.

The goal of osteopathic manipulation in the treatment of GI disease is to remove the facilitation and hypersympathetic state as well as normalize the parasympathetic influence to the area. Rib raising and inhibition of both posterior muscle spasm and of midline collateral ganglia are the two main techniques used to target the sympathetic supply. Release of the vagus nerve at the jugular foramen may be accomplished by occipitomastoid suture decompression and treatment of the occip-

ito-atlantal-axial (OAA) complex. Parasympathetic irritation may also be decreased by treatment of the sacroiliac joints and sacral decompression.

Improvement of the lymphatic drainage may be achieved through mesenteric lifts, treatment of the abdominal diaphragm, and thoracic inlet mobilization. Lifting of the ventral mesenteries will assist lymphatic drainage of the intestinal tract.

Osteopathic treatment of postoperative patients will result in a decrease in postoperative ileus. Rib raising is performed with the patient supine. The physician places his fingertips on the rib heads at the site of facilitation. Gentle traction is exerted toward the physician and upward. This is held until a release of tissue tension is perceived.

Inhibition of collateral ganglia is accomplished by using inhibition in conjunction with respiratory cooperation. The physician first diagnoses the area of greatest tissue tension over the ganglia and then inserts fingertips into the patient's anterior abdominal wall. The physician follows the tension down into the abdomen by holding against the patient's inhalation and taking up the slack of exhalation and then awaiting a release, which will be palpated as a softening of the tissues.

The occipito-atlantal-axial area may be treated using any standard technique. Cranially, the occipitomastoid suture should be evaluated and treated if any restriction is found. The temporal bones need to be evaluated for normal motion and the motion improved where necessary. The cranial treatment may conclude with CV4 to assist in relaxing and regulating movement of the thoracic and other diaphragms, both to decrease sympathetic tone and to improve lymphatic return.

GENITOURINARY CONSIDERATIONS
Mary Banihashem

Poor posture and body mechanics can result in altered homeostasis of any organ in the body. The diaphragmatic pump and the pelvic diaphragm have a close link with the healthy functioning of the kidney. Poor posture can cause the diaphragmatic pump to work ineffectively, and as a result the blood, nerve supply, and free drainage of the kidney can be affected. Hence, when evaluating

patients with urinary tract disorders, a full structural examination is required.

Altered Body Mechanics That Affect Diaphragmatic Motion
1. Somatic dysfunctions at the thoracolumbar junction L1–L3 (diaphragm attachment).

2. Lower rib dysfunctions and the quadratus lumborum.
3. The psoas muscle. This will have a direct effect on the lordosis of the lumbar spine. Because of the close approximation to the kidney, any psoas contracture or spasm may cause fascial pulls and hence restriction of motion of the kidney and ureter.

Autonomic Supply of the Urinary Tract

The autonomic supply of the urinary tract is important to the osteopathic physician when considering treatment. The sympathetic innervation to the kidney and ureters is at the level of T10–L1. Sympathetic stimulation will cause the following:

1. **Vasoconstriction of the ureters**, so any increase in sympathetic tone will decrease ureteral peristaltic waves and may cause ureterospasm.
2. **Relaxed bladder wall**, which will result in incomplete emptying of the bladder.
3. **Chronic sympathicotonia to the kidney:** continual sympathetic stimulation to the kidney can cause essential hypertension.

The parasympathetic supply of the kidney arises from the vagus nerve. The proximal portion of the *ureters* is supplied by the *vagus nerve*, and the distal portion is supplied by the pelvic *splanchnic nerve S2–S4*. The *bladder's* parasympathetic supply comes from the pelvic splanchnic nerves S2–S4.

Any increase in parasympathetic tone will cause the following:

1. Relaxation of the internal urinary sphincter
2. Increase in peristalsis of the ureters
3. Increase in bladder wall tone

Any decrease in parasympathetic tone will cause the following:

1. Impotence
2. Tightening of the internal urinary sphincter.
3. Incomplete emptying of the bladder

Osteopathic treatment adds to the functional capacity of the kidneys and prevents further irritation. It does not attempt to force injured tissues to try to do more work, but instead improves the blood supply, nerve supply, and lymphatic drainage.

Treatment

The general approach to renal disease in osteopathic medicine is to eliminate the somatic dysfunction component with its related effect on the neural, lymphatic, and vascular elements so that the diseased kidney will function maximally. This will be completed with medication and dialysis as required.

SYMPATHETIC PATHOPHYSIOLOGY

1. Sympathetic hyperactivity can be reduced by treatment of somatic dysfunction at the level T10–L1.
2. Somatic dysfunction in the upper cervical region interferes with the activity of the renal nerve fibers passing to the kidney by way of the superior cervical ganglion of the sympathetic system.

PARASYMPATHETIC PATHOPHYSIOLOGY

1. Treatment involves removal of any somatic dysfunction at the occipitoatlantal joint. (The vagus nerve will be affected.)
2. Parasympathetic output at the pelvic splanchnic nerves (S2–S4) can be stimulated at the sacrum. The technique that can be used is referred to as *sacral pounding*:
   a. The patient is prone.
   b. A pillow is placed over the sacrum.
   c. The physician locates the sacrum and with a fist beats over the sacrum.
   d. The pounding action on the sacrum will have a stimulatory effect on the parasympathetic system.

Treatment of sacroiliac somatic dysfunctions, the psoas, and the quadratus lumborum will keep the parasympathetic supply to the ureters healthy and keep the area mobile.

LYMPHATICS

The thoracic and pelvic diaphragms are vital to the drainage of the urinary system.

The following areas are examined and treated for somatic dysfunctions:

1. Cervicothoracic junction

2. Scalenes for muscle hypertonia
3. The first rib for restrictions

The techniques that should be used are rib raising and lymphatic pump.

DIRECT TREATMENT TO THE KIDNEY

The kidney can be treated through the abdomen on either side of the umbilicus by lightly working and directing each kidney upward and outward. This treatment relaxes any tissues around the blood vessels, nerves, and lymphatics to and from the kidney that may be contracted and thus aids in establishing the normal activity of the organs. It also helps in relaxing tissues around the ureters. The treatment of the kidney can be further aided by keeping the bowels active and functioning effectively.

References

WHIPLASH INJURIES

Becker RE. 1958. Whiplash injuries. In: Yearbook of Selected Osteopathic Papers. Carmel, Calif: Academy of Applied Osteopathy, pp 65–68.

———. 1961. Whiplash injury. In: Yearbook of Selected Osteopathic Papers. Carmel, Calif: Academy of Applied Osteopathy, pp 90–98.

Cailliet R. 1981. Neck and Arm Pain. Philadelphia: F.A. Davis.

Harakal JH. 1975. An osteopathically integrated approach to the whiplash complex. J Am Osteopath Assoc 74:59–73.

Heilig D. 1963. Whiplash, mechanics of injury: Management of cervical and dorsal involvement. J Am Osteopath Assoc 63:52–59.

Lalli JJ. 1972. Cervical vertebral syndromes. J Am Osteopath Assoc 72:43–50.

Macnab MB. 1971. The whiplash syndrome. Orthop Clin North Am 2:389–403.

McKeever DC. 1960. The so-called whiplash injury. Orthopedics 2:14.

Mealy K, Brennan H, Fenelon GCC. 1986. Early mobilization of whiplash injuries. Br Med J 292:656–657.

HEADACHES

Friedman AP. 1979. Tice's Practice of Medicine. Vol X. Hagerstown, Pa: Harper & Row.

Guyton AC. 1981. Textbook of Medical Physiology. Philadelphia: W.B. Saunders.

Isselbacker KJ, et al. 1980. Harrison's Principles of Internal Medicine, 9th ed. New York: McGraw-Hill.

Jones LH. 1981. Strain and Counterstrain. Colorado Springs: American Academy of Osteopathy.

Magoun HI. 1951. Osteopathy in the Cranial Field. Kirksville, Mo: Journal Printing Co.

———. 1978. Practical Osteopathic Procedures. Kirksville, Mo: Journal Printing Co.

Upledger JE, Vredevoogd JD. 1983. Craniosacral Therapy. Seattle: Eastland Press.

Warwick R. 1973. Gray's Anatomy, 35th British ed. Philadelphia: W.B. Saunders.

Wyngaarden JB, ed. et al. 1982. Cecil's Textbook of Medicine. Philadelphia: W.B. Saunders.

SCOLIOSIS

Arbuckle BE. 1970. Scoliosis capitis. Am Osteopath Assoc 70:131–137.

Ascani E, et al. 1986. Natural history of untreated idiopathic scoliosis after skeletal maturity. Spine 11:784–789.

Brookes HL, Bunnel WD, Mitchell FL. 1981. You can help patients with scoliosis. Patient Care 11:111–127.

Bunnel WD. 1986. The natural history of idiopathic scoliosis before skeletal maturity. Spine 11:773–776.

Fryette HH. 1978. Principles of Osteopathic Technique. Kirksville, Mo: Journal Printing Co.

Kahanovitz N, et al. 1986. Lateral electrical surface stimulation (TENS) compliance in adolescent female scoliosis patients. Spine 11:753–755.

Kein HA. 1972. Scoliosis. Ciba Found Symp 24:2–32.

Magoun HI. 1978. Practical Osteopathic Procedures. Kirksville, Mo: Journal Printing Co.

McCollough NC III. 1986. Nonoperative treatment of idiopathic scoliosis using surface electric stimulation. Spine 11:802–803.

Meranda JT. 1988. Evaluation and management of childhood scoliosis. Female Patient 13:49–60.

Ogilvie JW. 1984. Conservative management of childhood scoliosis. J Musculoskel Med 1:67–77.

Picault C, et al. 1986. Natural history of scolioses in girls and boys. Spine 11:777–778.

Roaf R. 1987. Posture. New York: Academic Press.

Schiowitz S, et al. 1983. Biomechanics of vertebral motion. In: An Osteopathic Approach to Diagnosis and Treatment. Old Westbury, NY: New York College of Osteopathic Medicine.

Stiachano WF. 1953. Scoliosis. In: Yearbook of the American Academy of Osteopathy. Vol 52, pp 377–378.

Sullivan JA, et al. 1986. Further evaluation of the scolition treatment of idiopathic adolescent scoliosis. Spine 8:903–906.

Weinstein SL. 1986. Idiopathic scoliosis: Natural history. Spine 11:780–783.

THORACIC OUTLET SYNDROME

Cailliet R. 1977. Neck and Arm Pain, 2nd ed. Philadelphia: F.A. Davis.

Sheon RP, Moskowitz RW, Goldberg VM. 1982. Soft Tissue Rheumatic Pain: Recognition, Management, Prevention.

Turek SL. 1984. Orthopaedics: Principles and Their Application, 4th ed. Philadelphia: Lippincott.

Tyson RR, Kaplan AF. 1975. Modern concepts of diagnosis and treatment of thoracic outlet syndrome. Orthop Clin North Am 6(2).

LUMBAR RADICULOPATHIES

Arnoldi X, et al. 1976. Lumbar spinal stenosis and nerve root entrapment. Clin Orthop 115:4.

Bernard T, Kirkaldy-Willis WH. 1987. Recognizing specific characteristics of nonspecific back pain. Clin Orthop 217:266.

Cathie AG. 1974. American Academy of Osteopathy 1974 Year Book. Special manipulative procedures for the normalization of the L-S and S-1 areas. AAO Year Book 1974, pp 131–139.

Cathie A. 1950. Anatomical relationships of the sciatic nerve. Academy of Applied Osteopathy Year Book, pp 70–72.

———. Academy of Applied Osteopathy Yearbook 1952, Academy of Applied Osteopathy.

Chrisman D, et al. 1964. A study of the results following rotary manipulation in the lumbar intervertebral disc syndrome. J Bone Joint Surg [Am] 46:524–557.

Davis H. 1950. Technic for the removal of still lesions usually found in the S-1 area and associated low back conditions. Academy of Applied Osteopathy Year Book. Academy of Applied Osteopathy, pp 73–75.

Dooley JF, et al. 1988. Nerve root infiltration in the diagnosis of radicular pain. Spine 13:79–83.

Doran DML, Newell DJ. 1975. Manipulation in the treatment of low back pain: A multicenter study. Br Med J 2:161.

Dvorak J, Gauchat M-H, Valach L. 1988. The outcome of surgery for lumbar disc herniation: I. A 4–17 year follow-up with emphasis on somatic aspects. Spine 13:1418.

Eaton J. 1952. Differential diagnosis of low back syndrome. Academy of Applied Osteopathy Year Book. 1952. Academy of Applied Osteopathy, pp 79–85.

Frymoyer J. 1988. Back pain and sciatica: Medical progress. N Engl J Med 318:291.

Hadler N, et al. 1987. A benefit of spinal manipulation as adjunctive therapy for acute low back pain: A stratified controlled trial. Spine 12:703.

Haldeman S. 1983. Spinal manipulative therapy: Status report, Clin Orthop 179:62.

Helbig T, Lee C. 1988. Lumbar facet syndrome. Spine 13:61–64.

Hockburger R. 1986. The lowdown on low back pain. Emerg Med. 18:123.

Hoeler FK, Tobis JS, Buerger AA. 1981. Spinal manipulation for low back pain. JAMA 245:1835.

Jackson R, Jacobs R, Montesano P. 1988. Facet joint injection: A prospective, statistical study. Spine 13:966.

Johnson J, et al. 1988. Extraspinal pathology and incidental disc herniation in patients with sciatica. Spine 13:393.

Kirkaldy-Willis WH. 1981. Musculoskeletal disorders: A three-article symposium. Postgrad Med 70:166.

———. 1978. Five common back disorders. How to diagnose and treat them. Geriatrics. 33:32–41.

———. Hill RJ. 1987. A more precise diagnosis for low back pain. Spine 4:102.

———. McIvor G. 1976. Editorial: Lumbar spinal stenosis. Clin Orthop 115:2.

———. ed. 1988. Managing Low Back Pain, 2nd ed. Edinburgh: Churchill Livingstone.

Kosteljanetz M, et al. 1988. The clinical significance of straight leg raising (Lasegue's sign) in the diagnosis of prolapsed lumbar discs. Spine 13:393.

Kostiuk JP, et al. 1986. Cauda equina syndrome and lumbar disc herniation. J Bone Joint Surg [Am] 68:386.

Kuo PP-F, Loh Z-C. 1987. Treatment of lumbar intervertebral disc protrusions by manipulation. Clin Orthop 215:47.

Lee CK, Rauschning W, Glenn W. 1988. Lateral lumbar spinal canal stenosis: Classification, pathology, anatomy, and surgical decompression. Spine 13:313.

Levine RL, Schutta HS. 1987. Lumbo-sacral root syndromes. In Camins MB, O'Leary PF, eds. The Lumbar Spine. New York: Raven Press, pp 163–170.

Mensor MC. 1955. Non-operative treatment, including manipulation, for lumbar intervertebral disc syndrome. J Bone Joint Surg 1955;37-A:925.

Mooney V. 1983. Syndromes of low back disease. Orthop Clin North Am 14:505–515.

———. Robertson J. 1976. The facet syndrome. Clin Orthop 11:149.

Nakano K. 1987. Sciatic nerve entrapment: The piriformis syndrome. J Musculoskel Med 33.

Paris S. 1983. Spinal manipulative therapy. Clin Orthop 179:55.

Porter RW, Miller CG. 1988. Neurologic claudication and root claudication treated with calcitonin: A double blind trial. Spine 13:1061.

Selby DK. 1983. When to operate and what to operate on. Orthop Clin North Am 14:577.

Siehl D. 1967. Manipulation of the spine under general anesthesia. American Academy of Osteopathy Yearbook 1967. M. Barnes (ed.). Carmel, CA: American Academy of Osteopathy, 147–151.

Simons P, Traudl J. 1983. Myofascial origins of low back pain: Parts 1–3. Postgrad Med 73:66.

Soliday H. 1978. Review of low back pain and treatment in general practice. Osteopath Med 2.

Spitzer W, LeBlanc F, Dupuis M. 1987. Scientific approach to the assessment and management of activity related spinal disorders: A monograph for clinicians. Spine (suppl), vol 12.

Steiner C. 1977. Ambulatory treatment of disc syndrome. J Am Osteopath Assoc 77:290–299.

———. 1987. Piriformis syndrome: Pathogenesis, diagnosis, and treatment. J Am Osteopath Assoc 87: 318–323.

Weinstein X, et al. 1986. Lumbar disc herniation. J Bone Joint Surg [Am] 68:43.

Yong-Hing K, Kirkaldy-Willis WH. 1983. Pathophysiology of degenerative disease of the lumbar spine. Orthop Clin North Am 14:491.

SPONDYLOLISTHESIS AND SPONDYLOLYSIS

Dietrich M, Kurowski P. 1985. The importance of mechanical factor in the etiology of spondylolysis. Spine 10:532.

Farfan HF, Osteria V, Lamy C. 1976. The mechanical etiology of spondylolysis and spondylolisthesis. Clin Orthop Rel Res 117:40.

Fredrickson B, Mettolick W, Lusicky J. 1984. The natural history of spondylolysis and spondylolisthesis. J Bone Joint Surg [Am] 66(5):699.

Kirkaldy-Willis WH, ed. 1988. Managing Low Back Pain, 2nd ed. Edinburgh: Churchill Livingstone.

Lowe R, et al. 1976. Standing roentgenograms in spondylolisthesis. Clin Orthop Rel Res 117:80.

McGee D. 1987. Orthopedic Physical Assessment. Philadelphia: W.B. Saunders.

Mierau D, et al. 1987. A comparison of the effectiveness of spinal manipulative therapy for low back pain patients with and without spondylolisthesis. J Manip Phys Ther 10(2):49.

Russe K. 1980. The Musculoskeletal System in Health and Disease. New York: Harper & Row, p. 132.

Rothman R, Simeone AF. 1982. The Spine, 2nd ed. Vol. 1. Philadelphia: W.B. Saunders, pp 263–284.

Soren A, Waugh T. 1985. Spondylolisthesis and related disorders: A correlative study of 105 patients. Clin Orthop Rel Res 193:171.

Turners R, Bianco A. 1971. Spondylolysis and spondylolisthesis in children and teen-agers. J Bone Joint Surg [Am] 53:1298.

Wiltze L, Newman P, McNab I. 1976. Classification of spondylolysis and spondylolisthesis. Clin Orthop Rel Res 117:23.

———. Winter R. 1983. Terminology and measurement of spondylolisthesis. J Bone Joint Surg [Am] 65(6):768.

COCCYGODYNIA

Barral JP, Mercier P. 1988. Visceral Manipulation. Seattle: Eastland Press.

Borgia CA. 1964. Coccygodynia: Its diagnosis and treatment. Milit Med 335–338.

Dubrovsky B, et al. 1985. Spinal control of pelvic floor muscles. Exp Neurol 88:277–287.

Duncan GA. Painful coccyx. Arch Surg 1088–1104.

Edwards M. Trauma of the coccyx and coccygodynia. Am J Surg 42:591–594.

Karpinski MRK, Piggott H. 1985. Greater trochanteric pain syndrome. J Bone Joint Surg [Br] 67.

Llourie J, et al. 1985. Avascular necrosis of the coccyx: A cause of coccygodynia. Br J Clin Pract 247–248.

Nicosia JF, Abcarian H. 1985. Levator syndrome: A treatment that works. Dis Colon Rectum 28:406–408.

Postacchin F, Massobrio M, Marco. 1983. Idiopathic coccygodynia. J Bone Joint Surg [Am].

Sinaki M, et al. 1977. Tension myalgia of the pelvic floor. Mayo Clin Proc 52:717–722.

Stern FH. 1967. Coccygodynia among the geriatric population. J Am Geriatr Soc 15:100–102.

Thiele GH. 1937. Coccygodynia and pain in the superior gluteal region. JAMA 1271–1275.

Upledger JE, Vredevoogd JD. 1983. Craniosacral therapy. Seattle: Eastland.

Wilensky T. The levator ani, coccygeus and piriformis muscles. Am J Surg 59:44–49.

DYSMENORRHEA AND PREMENSTRUAL SYNDROME

Burns L. 1911. Studies in Osteopathic Sciences. Vol. 2. The Nerve Centers. Cincinnati: Monfort & Co.

Buster JE. 1986. Dysmenorrhea and premenstrual syndrome. In: N Hacker and JG Moore. Essentials of Obstetrics and Gynecology. Philadelphia: W.B. Saunders.

Dalton K. 1977. Premenstrual Syndrome and Progesterone Therapy. London: Heinemann.

Day ML, Snell BJ. 1993. Use of prostaglandins for the induction of labor. J Nurse Midwifery 38 (suppl 2): 42S–48S.

DiGiovanna EL, Schiowitz S. 1991. An Osteopathic Approach to Diagnosis and Treatment. Philadelphia: J.B. Lippincott.

Guyton AC. 1986. Textbook of Medical Physiology, 7th ed. Philadelphia: W.B. Saunders.

Irwin J, Morse E, Riddick D. 1981. Dysmenorrhea induced by autologous transfusion. Obstet Gynecol 58: 286–290.

Korr IM. 1979. The Collected Papers of Irvin M. Korr. Indianapolis, IN: American Academy of Osteopathy.

Koor IM. 1974. Research and practice a century later. Andrew Taylor Still Memorial Lecture. J Am Osteopath Assoc 73:362–369.

Nies AS. 1990. Principles of therapeutics. In: LS Goodman and A Gilman, eds., Pharmacological Basis of Therapeutics, 8th ed. New York: Pergamon Press, pp 62–84.

Northrup C. 1994. Women's Bodies, Women's Wisdom. New York: Bantam.

Pickles VR, Hall WJ, Best FA, et al. 1965. Prostaglandins in endometrium and menstrual fluid from normal and dysmenorrheic subjects. J Obstet Gynecol Br Commonw 72:185.

Reid SL, Yen SSC. 1983. The premenstrual syndrome. Clin Obstet Gynecol 26:710.

Still AT. 1902. Philosophy and Mechanical Principles of Osteopathy. Kansas City: Hudson-Kimberly.

West JB. 1986. Best and Taylor's Physiological Basis of Medical Practice, 11th ed. Baltimore: Williams & Wilkins.

Willard F. 1993. Medical Neuroanatomy. Philadelphia: J.B. Lippincott.

Willard F, Carreiro J. 1994. Neurological and anatomical considerations in low back pain. Colorado Springs, CO: American Academy of Osteopathy Conclave of Fellows Lecture.

THE OBSTETRIC PATIENT

Copper AJ. 1958. Psychosomatic aspects of pre-eclamptic toxemia. J Psychosom Res 2.

DiGiovanna EL, Schiowitz S. 1991. An Osteopathic Approach to Diagnosis and Treatment. Philadelphia: J.B. Lippincott.

Golay J, Vedam S, Sorgen L. 1993. The squatting position for the second stage of labor: Effect on labor and on maternal and fetal well being. Birth 20(2):73–78.

Gray's Anatomy. 1995. London: Churchill Livingstone.

Guyton AC. 1986. Textbook of Medical Physiology. Philadelphia: W.B. Saunders, pp 125–126.

Hacker NF, Moore JG. 1986. Essentials of Obstetrics and Gynecology. Philadelphia: W.B. Saunders.

Kapandji IA. 1974. The Physiology of the Joints. Vol. 3. The Vertebral Column Taken as a Whole. London: Churchill Livingstone.

Kimberly, 1902; Somatic Dysfunction. Reprints via Osteopathic Enterprise, Kirksville, Mo., 1986.

Korr IM. 1979. The Collected Papers of Irvin M. Korr. Indianapolis: American Academy of Osteopathy.

McDonald RL. 1965. Personality characteristics in patients with three obstetric complications. Psychosom Med 27(4):

Moore KL. 1985. Clinically oriented anatomy. In: The Abdomen, pp. 275–276. Baltimore: Williams & Wilkins.

Muller-tyl E, and Wimmer-Puchinger B. Psychosomatic aspects of toxemia of pregnancy. J Psychosom Obstet Gynecol 1(3–4):

Myers R. 1979. Maternal anxiety and fetal death. In: Zichella and Pancheri, Psychoneuroendocrinology and Reproduction. New York: Elsevier.

Northrup C. 1994. Women's Bodies, Women's Minds. New York: Bantam.

Periti E, Nannini R. 1995. Il rivolgimento per manoure esterne nella presentazione pudalica. Minerva Ginecol 47(1–2):9–15.

Ringrose C. 1961. Psychosomatic influence in the genesis of toxemia of pregnancy. Can Med Assoc J 84:

Still AT. 1902. The Philosophy and Mechanical Principles of Osteopathy. Kirksville, Mo: Hudson.

Sutherland WG. 1939. The Cranial Bowl. Mankato, Mn: Free Press.

———. 1990. Teachings in the Science of Osteopathy. Cambridge, MA: Rudra Press.

———. 1962. With Thinking Fingers. Kansas City, Mo: The Cranial Academy. Limited reprint 1994.

Tettambel MA. 1994. An Interview: Structural focus: Key to osteopathic obstetrics concept. ICI Pharma, 1994.

West JB. 1985. Best and Taylor's Physiological Basis of Medical Practice. Baltimore: Williams & Wilkins, pp 58–101.

Willard F, Patterson MM. 1993. Nociception and the Neuro Endocrine Immune Connection. Proceedings of the 1992 American Academy of Osteopathy International Symposium. Indianapolis: American Academy of Osteopathy.

Zink G, Lawson WB. 1970. Pressure gradients in the osteopathic manipulative management of the obstetric patient. Osteopath Ann

THE PULMONARY PATIENT

Beal M, Morlock J. 1984. Somatic dysfunction associated with pulmonary disease. J Am Osteopath Assoc 84: 179–183.

Greenman P. 1977. Manipulative therapy for the thoracic cage. Osteopath Ann 3:140–149.

Howell RK, Allen TW, Kappler RE. 1975. The influence of osteopathic manipulative therapy in the management of patients with chronic obstructive lung disease. J Am Osteopath Assoc 74:757–760.

Kline JA. 1959. An examination of the management of bronchial asthma. American Academy of Osteopathy Yearbook 1959. M. Barnes (Ed.). Carmel, CA: American Academy of Osteopathy, pp 127–132.

Magoun HI. 1978. Practical Osteopathic Procedures. Kirksville, Mo: Journal Printing Co.

Stiles E. 1981. Manipulative management of chronic lung disease. Osteopath Ann 9:300–304.

Zink J. 1977. Respiratory and circulatory care: The conceptual model. Osteopath Ann 3:108–112.

THE CARDIAC PATIENT

Burns L. 1911. Studies in Osteopathic Sciences: Vol. 2. The Nerve Centers. Cincinnati: Monfort.

DiGiovanna EL, Schiowitz S. 1991. An Osteopathic Approach to Diagnosis and Treatment. Philadelphia: J.B. Lippincott.

Goodman LS, Gilman A. Principles of Therapeutics: Pharmacological Basis of Therapeutics, 8th ed. New York: Pergamon Press.

Gray's Anatomy. 1995. London: Churchill Livingstone.

Guyton AC. 1986. Textbook of Medical Physiology, 7th ed. Philadelphia: W.B. Saunders.

Kandel E, Schwartz J. 1994. Principles of Neural Science, 3rd ed. New York: Elsevier.

Kimberly, 1902; Somatic Dysfunction. Reprints via Osteopathic Enterprise, Kirksville, Mo, 1986.

Korr IM. 1979. The Collected Papers of Irvin M. Koor. Indianapolis: American Academy of Osteopathy.

———. 1974. Research and practice a century later. Andrew Taylor Still Memorial Lecture. J Am Osteopath Assoc 73:362–369.

Still AT. 1902. The Philosophy and Mechanical Principles of Osteopathy. Kirksville, Mo: Hudson.

Sutherland WG. 1939. The Cranial Bowl. Mankato, Mn: Free Press.

———. 1990. Teachings in the Science of Osteopathy. Cambridge, MA: Rudra Press.

———. 1962. With Thinking Fingers. Kansas City, Mo: The Cranial Academy. Limited reprint 1994.

Talman WT. 1993. The central nervous system and cardiovascular control in health and disease. In: PA Low, eds, Clinical Autonomic Disorders. Boston: Little, Brown, pp 39–53.

West JB. 1986. Best and Taylor's Physiological Basis of Medical Practice, 11th ed. Baltimore: Williams & Wilkins.

Willard F. 1993. Medical Neuroanatomy. Philadelphia: J.B. Lippincott.

Willard F, Carreiro J. 1994. Neurological and anatomical considerations in low back pain. American Academy of Osteopathy Conclave of Fellows Lecture.

Willard F, Patterson MM. 1993. Nociception and the Neuro Endocrine Immune Connection. Proceedings of the 1992 American Academy of Osteopathy International Symposium. Indianapolis: American Academy of Osteopathy.

GASTROINTESTINAL CONSIDERATIONS

Andreoli et al. eds. 1993. Cecil Essentials of Medicine, 3rd ed. Philadelphia: W.B. Saunders.

Guyton C. 1981. Textbook of Medical Physiology VI. Philadelphia: W.B. Saunders.

Kuchera M. 1994. Osteopathic Considerations in Systemic Disease, 2nd ed. Ohio: Greyden Press.

Magoon HI, Sr. 1978. Practical Osteopathic Procedures. Kirksville, Mo: Journal Printing Co.

Magoun, HI. 1976. Osteopathy in the Cranial Field, 3rd ed. Kirksville, Mo.: Journal Printing Co.

Pick T, Pickering, et al., eds. 1977. Gray's Anatomy. Revised American, from the 15th English Ed. New York: Bounty Books.

28 Alternative Modes of Treatment

TRIGGER POINT THERAPY
Joseph A. DiGiovanna

Trigger point therapy gained prominence as an important modality in treating myofascial pain in the 1960s. Although it had been a recognized type of therapy for many years, it was brought to the forefront by Janet Travell, who treated John F. Kennedy, the president of the United States. For years, Travell worked to document the existence of the myofascial trigger point. Although trigger points could be palpated and treated successfully, no scientific data were available. Eventually David Simons, clinical professor of physical medicine and rehabilitation at the University of California, supplied much of the needed neurophysiologic information, and trigger point therapy became an accepted therapeutic modality. Travell and Simons cooperated in writing a book on the diagnosis, treatment, and aftercare of patients with trigger points. *Myofascial Pain and Dysfunction: The Trigger Point Manual* was published in 1983.

What Is a Trigger Point?

A trigger point is best described as an area of hypersensitivity in a muscle from which impulses travel to the central nervous system, giving rise to referred pain. The area from which the pain arises is the *trigger point*. The area at which pain is noticed is the *reference point*. The reference point

and the trigger point may be in the same area; however, in most instances the reference point is distant.

A trigger point may be latent or clinically active. A latent trigger point may exist for a long time without producing symptoms. It may become clinically active—symptomatic—if disturbed by any one of many factors, which will be described later. A clinically active trigger point has the capacity to refer pain.

In the examination of a clinically active trigger point, one or several of the following may be noted:

1. On palpation, a hard, usually rounded (although it may form various shapes) mass is felt. This area is sensitive or painful to the patient.
2. The clinician may feel a tremor or fasciculation under the palpating finger.
3. When pressure is applied to the trigger point, the patient may complain of pain not only under the palpating finger but at a distant area (reference area). Pain felt only at the reference area is an indication that a specific pathway exists. Therefore, before trigger point therapy is started on any patient, the clinician should review the various pathways. If a patient complains of pain at a distant or reference area, the

An Osteopathic Approach to Diagnosis and Treatment, second edition
Eileen L. DiGiovanna and Stanley Schiowitz
Lippincott–Raven Publishers, Philadelphia © 1997.

clinician will then be able to locate the trigger point.

Causes of Trigger Points

Causes of trigger points include the following:

1. Acute injury to tissue from a fall, an automobile accident, a strain, and so forth.
2. Excessive repetitive movements.
3. Another primary point, causing a secondary trigger point.
4. Nervous tension or stress.
5. A previously latent, asymptomatic trigger point that is activated by any of the above.
6. A preexisting Jones tender point. There is some question as to whether the Jones tender point is an early untreated trigger point. I feel that an untreated, long-standing tender point may undergo certain chronic changes, at which time it may be classified as a trigger point requiring intensive treatment. Studies done by Miehlke and reported by Travell and Simons indicate that the myofascial trigger point process begins as a neuromuscular dysfunction, but can evolve into a histologically demonstrable dystrophic phase. Miehlke's study related the clinical symptoms to the biopsy findings. It supported the fact that the initial dysfunctional phase, after a period of time, develops into the dystrophic phase.

Trigger points are not dependent on muscular activity to exist, as demonstrated by autopsy studies of trigger point tissue. Trigger points are true pathologic entities. Some of the changes noted in such tissues at autopsy were fatty infiltration, an increased number of nuclei, fibrosis, and serous exudates and mucopolysaccharide deposits.

Treatment

Several methods of therapy are presently being used by physicians. The specific method depends on several factors, including the duration of the trigger point, its location, the expertise of the physician, and the cooperation of the patient.

Travell used the spray-and-stretch technique initially, first with ethyl chloride and subsequently with fluorimethane, which causes less freezing to the skin and is not flammable. Later she used injection therapy. At present, Travell often uses a combination of techniques. Hans Kraus, initially an advocate of injection therapy, often uses both modalities. Other types of modalities are transcutaneous electrical nerve stimulation, ultrasound, and electrical muscle stimulation. The use of fluorimethane and injection therapy is discussed in more detail.

FLUORIMETHANE

Fluorimethane is a vapocoolant spray that is applied in the following manner:

1. First the nozzle function is checked. When depressed, the nozzle should produce a direct stream that travels approximately 3 feet.
2. The skin is sprayed from the trigger point to the reference point, at a 45-degree angle, at a rate of 4 inches per second, in one direction only.
3. Three or four sweeps are made while the area being treated is simultaneously stretched gently. This process should be repeated three to four times. An effective method is to use passive stretching after the first series of sweeps, isometric resistant contractions after the second series of sweeps, and isokinetic resistant contractions after the third series of sweeps.
4. The treatment should not be rushed.
5. Myofascial treatment, muscle energy techniques, counterstrain treatment, high-velocity techniques, fascial release, or facilitated positional release may be used as indicated.
6. The patient should be sent home with instructions for a series of gentle, progressive stretching exercises.
7. Follow-up treatment should be within a week or less.
8. The patient should be warned of a possible exacerbation of pain in the first 24 to 48 hours. If pain occurs, ice should be applied intermittently to the trigger point for the first 24 hours, followed by wet warm compresses for the next 24 hours. Analgesics may be given.

INJECTION THERAPY

Trigger points may be treated by direct injection of lidocaine. The size and length of the needle are determined by the site being injected. For a large muscle mass, such as in the hip, a $1\frac{1}{2}$-inch, 22- or 23-gauge needle may be used. If the upper border of the trapezius or an intercostal muscle is to be injected, a $\frac{5}{8}$-inch, 25-gauge needle is usually used. Care must be taken to avoid injecting into the lung.

Technique

Approximately 1½ to 3 ml of 1% lidocaine is injected into the trigger point and the four quadrants surrounding it in equal amounts. Always aspirate before injecting. Most patients will respond to the lidocaine; however, a short-acting steroid may be added. I usually use lidocaine alone for the first or second treatment. If the response is poor, a steroid may be added.

The patient should be warned of possible increased pain the following day, although in most cases there is improvement. If there is increased pain, ice should be applied intermittently for 24 hours, followed by moist heat for 24 hours. If the trigger point does not completely resolve, it may be reinjected in approximately one week.

The combination of fluorimethane spray and lidocaine injection may be used, although either may be used alone.

MECHANISM OF ACTION

Although the exact mechanism of action of trigger point therapy is not known, several theories have been proposed. At present, the theory of greatest acceptance hypothesizes interruption of the reflex arc by the action of the modality used. Afferent sensory nerve fibers travel from the muscle to the spinal cord. The fibers are classified as A fibers and C fibers. Stimulation of the A fibers, the large myelinated fibers, decreases pain. (These fibers respond to phasic stimulation.) Stimulation of the C fibers, the small unmyelinated fibers, results in increased pain, such as occurs when one burns one's fingers. Efferent fibers return to the muscle from the cord. Interruption of the cycle either toward or away from the cord, that is, either the afferent or the efferent fibers, breaks the pain cycle, and the pain is relieved. If the cause of the pain is not addressed, the pain cycle will most likely return, or a new pain cycle will be established.

A second theory suggests that trigger point treatment releases endorphins, which decrease the pain. Clinical experience indicates that one or more mechanisms of action are operative, because symptoms and pain are relieved when trigger points are appropriately treated.

CHAPMAN'S REFLEXES
Eileen L. DiGiovanna

Frank Chapman graduated from the American School of Osteopathy in 1897. In his practice he became aware of areas in the soft tissues of the body that were palpably different from the surrounding tissue. As various investigators have proposed reflex linkage of somatic structures with visceral structures, so Chapman believed his gangliaform contractures were neurolymphatic reflexes. Each reflex area seemed to be consistently related to a specific viscera. Particularly significant to Chapman was the interrelatedness with the endocrine system.

The reflex area can be palpated in the deep fascia at specific points on the anterior and posterior parts of the body. The areas feel tense and are about the size of a small bean. The patient describes tenderness as pressure is applied to the area.

Many osteopathic physicians find Chapman's reflexes of particular use in the differential diagnosis of visceral disease. By knowing the patterns of distribution of reflex areas, they are able to relate the reflex area to a specific viscera. For example, reflex areas along the lateral thigh are related to colon problems. The gallbladder produces a reflex in the forearm just below the elbow.

Chapman and his successor, Charles Owens, believed these reflex areas lay in lymphoid tissues. A student, H. R. Small, who worked with Owens reported, "In the intercostal space between the anterior and posterior fascia is located some lymphoid tissue. It is within this tissue that a Chapman's Reflex will be found."

Fred Mitchell describes the method of treatment in his foreword to Owens' book, *An Endocrine Interpretation of Chapman's Reflexes.* The pad of the finger is placed over the area to be treated, and "firm gentle contact is maintained and a rotary motion imparted to the finger through the arm and hand so as to express the fluid content of the locus into the surrounding tissues (i.e., dissipate the swelling)." Each reflex area involved with a particular viscus must be treated.

Today many physicians believe there is a relationship among trigger points, acupuncture points, Jones tender points, and Chapman's reflexes. Precisely what the relationship may be is unknown. George Northup states in an editorial, "One cannot escape the feeling that all of these seemingly diverse observations are but views of the same iceberg, the tip of which we are beginning to see without understanding either its magnitude or its depth of importance."

References

Gunn CC, Milbrandt WE. 1977. Tenderness at motor points: An aid in the diagnosis of pain in the shoulder referred from the cervical spine. J Am Osteopath Assoc 77:196–212.

Johnson DM. 1979. Time, gravity, and the motion barrier. Osteopath Ann 7(1):31–44.

Kraus H. 1970. Clinical Treatment of Back and Neck Pain. New York: McGraw-Hill.

Northup GW. 1977. Same subject—different views (editorial). J Am Osteopath Assoc 77:288–289.

Northup TL. 1941. Role of the reflexes in manipulative therapy. J Am Osteopath Assoc 40:521–524.

Owens C. 1980. An Endocrine Interpretation of Chapman's Reflexes. Indianapolis, IN: American Academy of Osteopathy.

Reeves JL, Jaeger B, Poletti CE. 1984. Trigger points in headache. Aches Pains 5:22–25.

Travell JG, Simons DG. 1983. Myofascial Pain and Dysfunction: The Trigger Point Manual. Baltimore: Williams & Wilkins.

Index